IMPLANT TREATMENT PLANNING FOR THE EDENTULOUS PATIENT

A Graftless Approach to Immediate Loading

IMPLANT TREATMENT PLANNING FOR THE EDENTULOUS PATIENT

A Graftless Approach to Immediate Loading

Edmond Bedrossian, DDS, FACD, FACOMS

Diplomate, American Board of Oral and Maxillofacial Surgery
Associate Professor, Department of Oral and Maxillofacial Surgery
University of the Pacific, Arthur A. Dugoni School of Dentistry
Director, Implant Training
University of the Pacific, Oral and Maxillofacial Residency Training Program
Private Practice
San Francisco, California

MOSBY
ELSEVIER

MOSBY
ELSEVIER

3251 Riverport Lane
St. Louis, Missouri 63043

IMPLANT TREATMENT PLANNING FOR THE EDENTULOUS PATIENT: A GRAFTLESS APPROACH TO IMMEDIATE LOADING

ISBN 978-0-323-07368-4

Library of Congress Control Number 2010920810

This publication was sponsored in part by a special sale to Nobel Biocare USA.

This book is not intended to be used as a surgical manual. For detailed instruction on using specific NobelBiocare product systems portrayed in this book, please consult the appropriate clinical manual available at www.nobelbiocare.com or +1 800 322 5001.

Vice President and Publishing Director: Linda Duncan
Executive Editor: John Dolan
Developmental Editor: Brian S. Loehr
Publishing Services Manager: Catherine Jackson
Senior Project Manager: Karen M. Rehwinkel
Design Direction: Paula Catalano

Printed in China

Last digit is the print number: 9 8 7 6 5 4 3 2

To my parents, who lived by example and instilled dedication, loyalty, integrity, and passion into the lives of everyone they met. To my lovely wife Jasmine, and my wonderful sons Armand and Aram, I will forever be grateful to all of you for always being there for me. This book is dedicated to you.

FOREWORD

In *Implant Treatment Planning for the Edentulous Patient: A Graftless Approach to Immediate Loading,* Edmond Bedrossian emphasizes the importance of safe, reliable, and affordable osseointegration therapies in reconstruction of anatomical and functional defects in the oral, maxillofacial, and cranial regions.

A decisive factor in patient care is simplification of treatment, which should be based on identifying and utilizing the enormous capacity of existing original anchoring tissues. When possible, one should avoid unnecessary advanced and complicated major grafting procedures.

It is important to inform each patient about alternatives, referring to long-term clinical experiences and emphasizing the prognostic consequence of the close interaction between surgery, prosthetics function, and the quality of life.

P-I Brånemark
Professor, MD, PhD, ODhc

PREFACE

The science of osseointegration has given dentistry an understanding of the physiologic rehabilitation of edentulous patients in a simplified, safe, and predictable manner. Collaberation between multicenter international groups has lent credibility to the concept of graftless surgery and immediate loading. Expansion of the original protocol of the two-stage approach by Professor P-I Brånemark to the current concept of immediate loading of endosseous implants is the result of an appreciation of distance, contact osteogenesis, and load control.

The purpose of this publication is to present the current philosophy, as well as surgical and prosthetic techniques for the treatment of edentulous patients with dental implants to support a fixed prosthesis. The various chapters review the biology, biomechanics, and surgical and prosthetic technical steps for delivering simplified and predictable treatment plans for patients.

ACKNOWLEDGMENTS

Many thanks to Professor Per-Ingvar Brånemark, a scientist, visionary, mentor, and friend. Without his guidance, inspiration, education, and unselfish dedication to patient care, completion of this book would not be possible. His subtle encouragements to expand the limits of biology and osseointegration in a predictable and simplified manner have been the road map for the cautious approach in developing the concept of graftless techniques and immediate loading of dental implants.

The team approach, as advocated by Professor Brånemark, involves the contribution of several dedicated experts to this project. To all my restorative colleagues, I extend my deepest gratitude. To the University of the Pacific's Dugoni School of Dentistry and my colleagues at the Department of Oral and Maxillofacial Surgery Residency Training Program, many thanks for believing in our long-term vision and providing the environment for developing our surgical and prosthetic protocols.

The completion of each patient's treatment would not be possible without the cooperation of skilled laboratory technicians. We have been fortunate to have the dedication and support of Todd Brusco, Anezka G. Felton, and Vatche Makasdjian. We are very grateful for all their hard work in helping us realize our goal in rehabilitating edentulous patients with fixed prostheses.

We also recognize the support of Nobel Biocare, Kevin Mosher, Robert Gottlander, and Dominico Scala in providing the latest technical support, including their continued interest in developing the concept of computer-guided treatment planning.

CONTENTS

. . . and the second section presents cases from the author's actual archives.

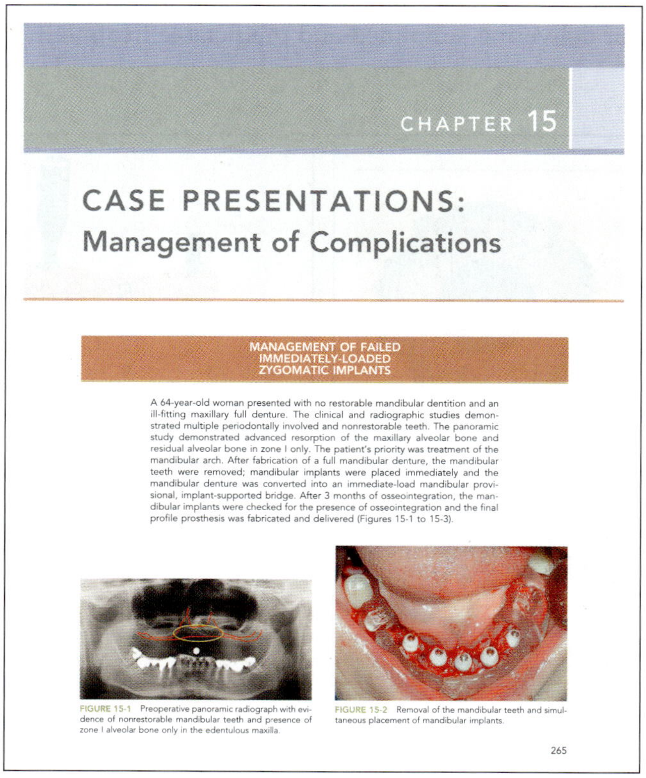

CHAPTER 15

CASE PRESENTATIONS: Management of Complications

MANAGEMENT OF FAILED IMMEDIATELY-LOADED ZYGOMATIC IMPLANTS

A 64-year-old woman presented with no restorable mandibular dentition and an ill-fitting maxillary full denture. The clinical and radiographic studies demonstrated multiple periodontally involved and nonrestorable teeth. The panoramic study demonstrated advanced resorption of the maxillary alveolar bone and residual alveolar bone in zone I only. The patient's priority was treatment of the mandibular arch. After fabrication of a full mandibular denture, the mandibular teeth were removed; mandibular implants were placed immediately and the mandibular denture was converted into an immediate-load mandibular provisional, implant-supported bridge. After 3 months of osseointegration, the mandibular implants were checked for the presence of osseointegration and the final profile prosthesis was fabricated and delivered (Figures 15-1 to 15-3).

FIGURE 15-1 Preoperative panoramic radiograph with evidence of nonrestorable mandibular teeth and presence of zone I alveolar bone only in the edentulous maxilla.

FIGURE 15-2 Removal of the mandibular teeth and simultaneous placement of mandibular implants.

265

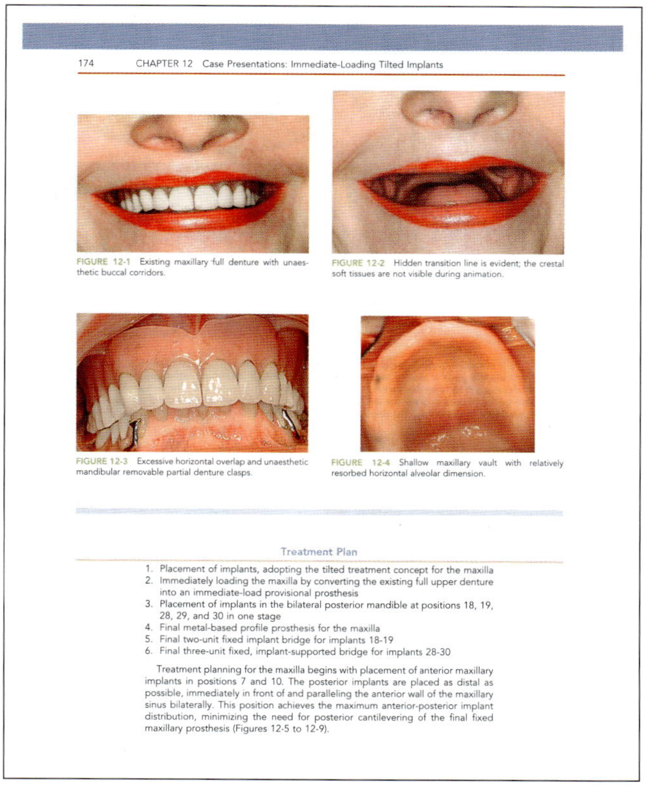

174 CHAPTER 12 Case Presentations: Immediate-Loading Tilted Implants

FIGURE 12-1 Existing maxillary full denture with unaesthetic buccal corridors.

FIGURE 12-2 Hidden transition line is evident; the crestal soft tissues are not visible during animation.

FIGURE 12-3 Excessive horizontal overlap and unaesthetic mandibular removable partial denture clasps.

FIGURE 12-4 Shallow maxillary vault with relatively resorbed horizontal alveolar dimension.

Treatment Plan

1. Placement of implants, adopting the tilted treatment concept for the maxilla
2. Immediately loading the maxilla by converting the existing full upper denture into an immediate-load provisional prosthesis
3. Placement of implants in the bilateral posterior mandible at positions 18, 19, 28, 29, and 30 in one stage
4. Final metal-based profile prosthesis for the maxilla
5. Final two-unit fixed implant bridge for implants 18-19
6. Final three-unit fixed, implant-supported bridge for implants 28-30

Treatment planning for the maxilla begins with placement of anterior maxillary implants in positions 7 and 10. The posterior implants are placed as distal as possible, immediately in front of and paralleling the anterior wall of the maxillary sinus bilaterally. This position achieves the maximum anterior-posterior implant distribution, minimizing the need for posterior cantilevering of the final fixed maxillary prosthesis (Figures 12-5 to 12-9).

Outstanding photos and illustrations!

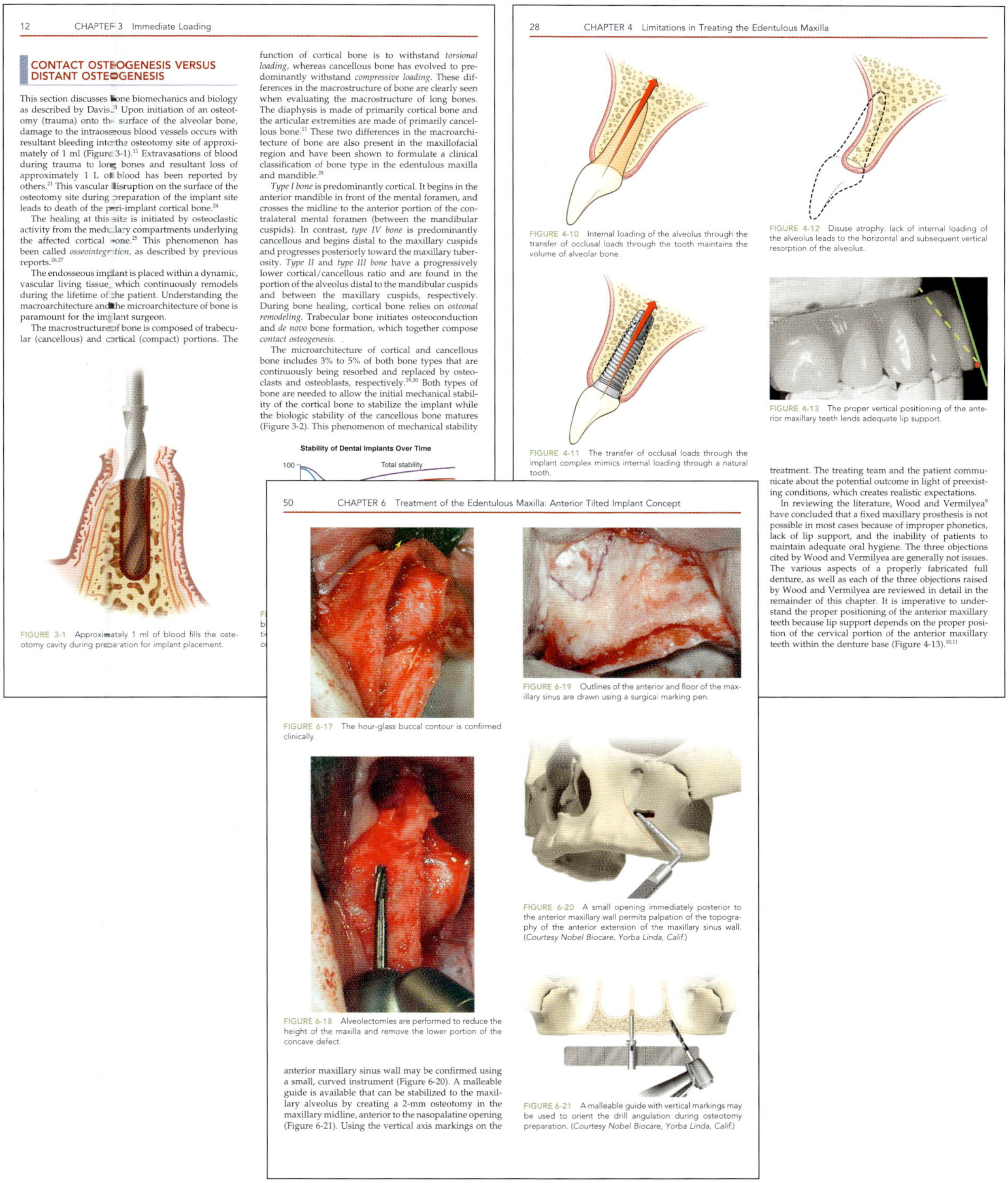

12 CHAPTER 3 Immediate Loading

CONTACT OSTEOGENESIS VERSUS DISTANT OSTEOGENESIS

This section discusses bone biomechanics and biology as described by Davis.[3] Upon initiation of an osteotomy (trauma) onto the surface of the alveolar bone, damage to the intraosseous blood vessels occurs with resultant bleeding into the osteotomy site of approximately of 1 ml (Figure 3-1).[11] Extravasations of blood during trauma to long bones and resultant loss of approximately 1 L of blood has been reported by others.[21] This vascular disruption on the surface of the osteotomy site during preparation of the implant site leads to death of the peri-implant cortical bone.[24]

The healing at this site is initiated by osteoclastic activity from the medullary compartments underlying the affected cortical bone.[25] This phenomenon has been called *osseointegration*, as described by previous reports.[26,27]

The endosseous implant is placed within a dynamic, vascular living tissue, which continuously remodels during the lifetime of the patient. Understanding the macroarchitecture and the microarchitecture of bone is paramount for the implant surgeon.

The macrostructure of bone is composed of trabecular (cancellous) and cortical (compact) portions. The function of cortical bone is to withstand *torsional loading*, whereas cancellous bone has evolved to predominantly withstand *compressive loading*. These differences in the macrostructure of bone are clearly seen when evaluating the macrostructure of long bones. The diaphysis is made of primarily cortical bone and the articular extremities are made of primarily cancellous bone.[11] These two differences in the macroarchitecture of bone are also present in the maxillofacial region and have been shown to formulate a clinical classification of bone type in the edentulous maxilla and mandible.[28]

Type I bone is predominantly cortical. It begins in the anterior mandible in front of the mental foramen, and crosses the midline to the anterior portion of the contralateral mental foramen (between the mandibular cuspids). In contrast, *type IV bone* is predominantly cancellous and begins distal to the maxillary cuspids and progresses posteriorly toward the maxillary tuberosity. *Type II* and *type III bone* have a progressively lower cortical/cancellous ratio and are found in the portion of the alveolus distal to the mandibular cuspids and between the maxillary cuspids, respectively. During bone healing, cortical bone relies on *osteonal remodeling*. Trabecular bone initiates osteoconduction and *de novo* bone formation, which together compose *contact osteogenesis*.

The microarchitecture of cortical and cancellous bone includes 3% to 5% of both bone types that are continuously being resorbed and replaced by osteoclasts and osteoblasts, respectively.[29,30] Both types of bone are needed to allow the initial mechanical stability of the cortical bone to stabilize the implant while the biologic stability of the cancellous bone matures (Figure 3-2). This phenomenon of mechanical stability

Stability of Dental Implants Over Time

100

Total stability

FIGURE 3-1 Approximately 1 ml of blood fills the osteotomy cavity during preparation for implant placement.

28 CHAPTER 4 Limitations in Treating the Edentulous Maxilla

FIGURE 4-10 Internal loading of the alveolus through the transfer of occlusal loads through the tooth maintains the volume of alveolar bone.

FIGURE 4-12 Disuse atrophy: lack of internal loading of the alveolus leads to the horizontal and subsequent vertical resorption of the alveolus.

FIGURE 4-11 The transfer of occlusal loads through the implant complex mimics internal loading through a natural tooth.

FIGURE 4-13 The proper vertical positioning of the anterior maxillary teeth lends adequate lip support.

treatment. The treating team and the patient communicate about the potential outcome in light of preexisting conditions, which creates realistic expectations.

In reviewing the literature, Wood and Vermilyea[9] have concluded that a fixed maxillary prosthesis is not possible in most cases because of improper phonetics, lack of lip support, and the inability of patients to maintain adequate oral hygiene. The three objections cited by Wood and Vermilyea are generally not issues. The various aspects of a properly fabricated full denture, as well as each of the three objections raised by Wood and Vermilyea are reviewed in detail in the remainder of this chapter. It is imperative to understand the proper positioning of the anterior maxillary teeth because lip support depends on the proper position of the cervical portion of the anterior maxillary teeth within the denture base (Figure 4-13).[10,11]

50 CHAPTER 6 Treatment of the Edentulous Maxilla: Anterior Tilted Implant Concept

FIGURE 6-17 The hour-glass buccal contour is confirmed clinically.

FIGURE 6-19 Outlines of the anterior and floor of the maxillary sinus are drawn using a surgical marking pen.

FIGURE 6-18 Alveolectomies are performed to reduce the height of the maxilla and remove the lower portion of the concave defect.

FIGURE 6-20 A small opening immediately posterior to the anterior maxillary wall permits palpation of the topography of the anterior extension of the maxillary sinus wall. (*Courtesy Nobel Biocare, Yorba Linda, Calif.*)

anterior maxillary sinus wall may be confirmed using a small, curved instrument (Figure 6-20). A malleable guide is available that can be stabilized to the maxillary alveolus by creating a 2-mm osteotomy in the maxillary midline, anterior to the nasopalatine opening (Figure 6-21). Using the vertical axis markings on the

FIGURE 6-21 A malleable guide with vertical markings may be used to orient the drill angulation during osteotomy preparation. (*Courtesy Nobel Biocare, Yorba Linda, Calif.*)

CHAPTER 1

Demographics of Edentulous Patients

As dentists, we devote our lives to helping our patients maintain their oral structures in the highest possible state of health. But some patients still become fully edentulous, despite our efforts.

This book is devoted to presenting the physiologic treatment option for fully edentulous patients. Placement of dental implants followed by immediate loading with a fixed, implant-supported prosthesis mimics the biomechanics of teeth within alveolar bone.[1] Biologic benefits for this group of patients are internal loading on the alveolus and preventing continued resorption of the patient's jaw. The psychologic benefits are the ability of the patients to feel confident during speech and mastication without the constant reminder of having a mobile full denture. An understanding of the biomechanics and the strategic placement of implants throughout the edentulous arch permits use of a physiologic treatment protocol in even the most severely atrophic mandibles and maxillae. It is important to remember that this treatment option can typically be accomplished in a 4-hour, surgical-prosthetic appointment and results in only minimal postoperative discomfort for most patients.

Despite universal concurrence within the academic and scientific dental communities that this approach best serves patients, it continues to be grossly underused. Only a limited fraction of Americans missing all their teeth in one or both arches have been treated with implant-supported, fixed prostheses.[2] A major reason for the underuse of this treatment option, especially in the maxilla, is the misconception that a flangeless, fixed maxillary prosthesis cannot be fabricated because of lack of lip support and difficulties with phonetics. Similarly, the position of the mental foramen in the mandibular arch limits the anterior-posterior distribution of the implants, once again eliminating this option for most practitioners. Hence, a tissue-supported, implant-retained overdenture is fabricated for these patients.

Financial considerations also affect the treatment options. Although insurers increasingly are covering some of the costs, patients still bear—and for the foreseeable future will continue to bear—the biggest share of the financial responsibility. But economic constraints only partially explain the relatively low percentage of edentulous patients who are living with implant-supported fixed prostheses. Several studies have looked at the socioeconomic concerns of edentulous patients. It is helpful to summarize the findings of some of these studies.

A 2008 quantitative survey of more than 54,000 U.S. consumers[3] found that almost 90% ranked their smile as their most important attribute, followed by the appearance of their teeth (87%) (Figure 1-1). Both were considered to be more important than hair, clothing, eyes, facial features, and physique. Respondents revealed that they not only understood the aesthetic deficit created by edentulism, but furthermore associated it with lower social status, lower income, and a lack of concern for one's health. Individuals who were missing teeth reported covering their mouths when they smiled or laughed or avoiding smiling altogether, particularly when being photographed. The financial costs of implant treatment often did not surprise respondents familiar with the cost of dental work. However, respondents also frequently assumed that dental implants could only be delivered via a lengthy and complex procedure involving significant pain. Furthermore, some felt that implant treatment could not be justified because they thought the main benefits of implants were restored appearance and masticatory function—benefits that

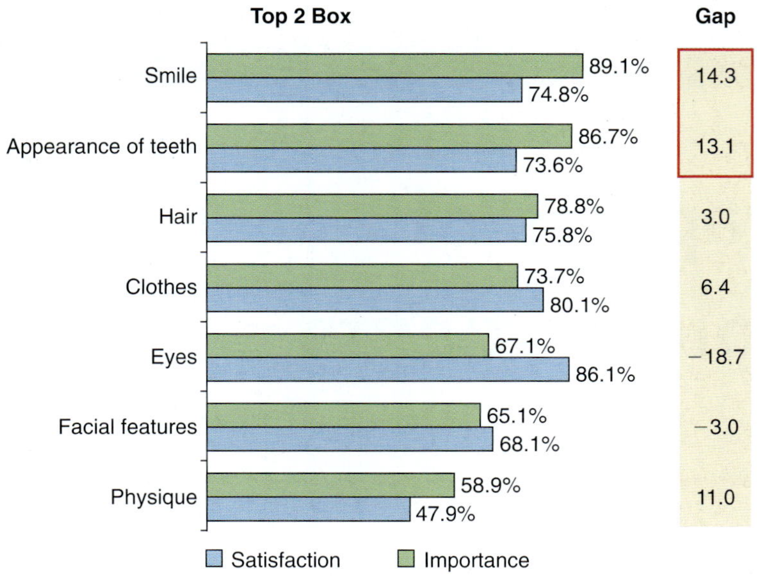

FIGURE 1-1 U.S. consumers ranked their smile as well as the appearance of their teeth as their top two most important attributes. *(Data from Nobel Biocare survey, August 2008.)*

could be delivered by (less expensive) removable dentures with equal effectiveness.

As the various chapters of this book explain, the psychosocial and the physiologic consequences of edentulism are profound. Inevitable alveolar bone resorption occurs in the absence of sustained loading, with dramatic consequences for the overall facial contours. As the resorption progresses, dentures cease to fit, a challenge that cannot be overcome by the best of practitioners.[4,5]

Looking into the patient profiles in most urban practices, it is evident that the retention rates for natural teeth have steadily increased[6] and percentage rates for edentulism have declined.[7] The suggestion has even surfaced that in the future dentists may not need to treat edentulism. That is a significant misconception (Figure 1-2). Many fully edentulous patients tolerate essentially nonfunctional full dentures because they have been told that they are not candidates for implants. The reason for this statement could be anatomic; patients with large maxillary sinuses or resorbed posterior mandibular alveolus are not candidates. However, an even higher percentage of patients today *would* be edentulous were it not for the attempts to maintain otherwise nonrestorable teeth as long as possible, avoiding the need to have a removable appliance. Patients do understand that further destruction of the alveolus occurs with the progression of their periodontal or peri-implant disease, but the fear of edentulism and the use of a full denture lead these patients to ignore their failing oral conditions.

The time to discuss with patients the risks as well as the benefits of the graftless approach to immediate

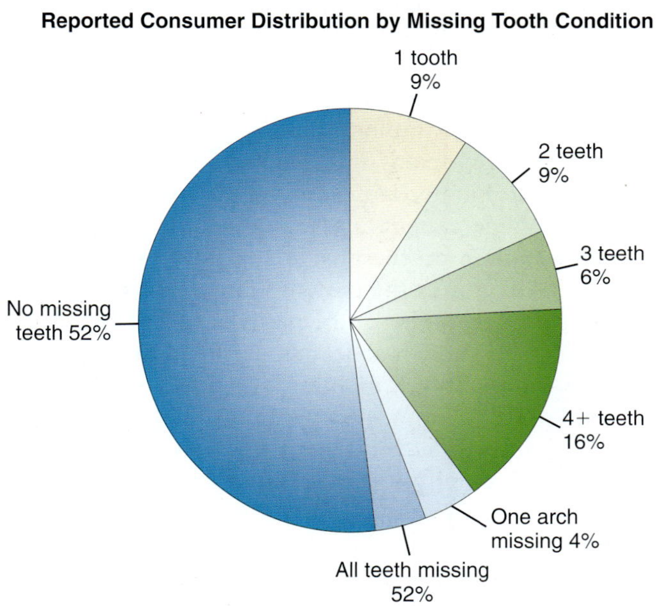

FIGURE 1-2 Demographics of population surveyed missing one to all of their teeth. *(Data from Nobel Biocare survey, August 2008.)*

loading with an implant-supported prosthesis is now. It is essential for our profession to have an appreciation for the concept of immediate loading, as well as an updated understanding of the biomechanical sciences of bone and bone-implant interface as presented by Davis, Rangert, and Brunski.[8-10] The graftless approach to treatment of the edentulous patients and immediate loading has been evolving for the last 15 years,[11-16] and communicating this predictable treatment concept within our profession is timely.

As an analysis by Douglass et al.[17] has demonstrated, the future is on the horizon. The researchers estimate that by 2020, the decrease in the percentage of the overall U.S. population that is edentulous will be more than offset by a 79% growth in the population aged 55 years and older. The result will be an increase in the overall need for some form of full-mouth restoration—from 53.8 million in 1991 to 61 million in 2020; the researchers warn that their estimates may be *"significantly conservative."* Other sources confirm that the loss of multiple teeth continues to be a common condition, particularly among older individuals. Data gathered in 2004 by the Centers for Disease Control and Prevention, Division of Oral Health,[18] indicate that 45.9% of Americans aged 65 or older have lost six or more teeth because of tooth decay or gum disease. Although tooth loss correlates strongly with decreased income, it is significant to note that more than 30% of individuals earning more than $150,000 per year nonetheless report having lost four or more teeth.[18]

The following chapters summarize and synthesize 30 years of research into dental implants for the edentulous patient. Every aspect of the delivery of implant-supported, fixed prostheses—from review of contact and distant osteogenesis to discussion of two-stage versus one-stage protocols and the scientific bases for immediate loading of implants (see Chapter 3)—is reviewed. The systematic pretreatment evaluation protocols establishing the correct diagnosis and restorative planning for the implant-supported, fixed prosthesis are reviewed in Chapter 4. Additional chapters present alternative surgical protocols for delivery of the graftless approach for immediate loading of the edentulous maxilla and the mandible.

Recent literature compares the results of immediate loading with early loading (generally accepted as the connection of the prosthesis between 4 to 6 weeks after implant placement). Fischer et al.[19] report no significant differences between the outcomes of immediate versus early loading of the edentulous maxilla. Fischer reports a 94.7% success rate in immediate-load cases and 95.7% rate in early-load cases. This study is consistent with the findings of Degidi et al.[20] (2005), in which they report a success rate of 96.30% to 99.37% for immediate-load maxillary implants. Ioannidou and Doufexi in 2005[21] performed a meta-analysis of loading time of implants in the maxilla and the mandible and found no difference between patients with edentulous maxillary or mandibular arches, as well as no difference between implants that were immediately or conventionally loaded.

Many patients understand the compelling benefits of an implant-supported prosthesis and want to do whatever it takes to preserve their appearance, function, and health. Demographics dictate that baby boomers who are just beginning to turn 65 constitute the affluent sector of the American public. Yet they also include the individuals who will have the largest number of teeth missing and the most severe periodontal problems. Dentists who understand and are able to provide these individuals with implant-supported prostheses will be better able to serve their patients' needs. If patients are clearly informed of the benefits of the graftless approach for the placement

Awareness of Consequences of Missing Teeth

		Awareness by missing teeth concern	
	Total	Not concerned	Concerned
Sample size–have missing teeth	26,422	11,582	9,130
Difficulty chewing food	59.0%	52.1%	66.5%
Shifting of surrounding teeth to fill gap	52.4%	52.8%	54.9%
Impact to appearance of smile	50.0%	41.2%	61.4%
Impact to overall facial contour (sunken face)	37.2%	31.6%	44.4%
Loss of jaw bone	24.2%	20.2%	28.3%
Increased risk of heart disease	10.7%	7.6%	14.9%
I have not heard of any of the above	20.2%	24.3%	15.4%

FIGURE 1-3 Awareness level of the consequence of missing teeth in the population surveyed. *(Data from Nobel Biocare survey, August 2008.)*

and immediate loading of implants to support a fixed prosthesis, it is my opinion that most patients would opt for this treatment approach. However, there are patients who will choose an alternative option. Figure 1-3 summarizes the results from 26,422 respondents on their awareness of the consequences of missing teeth. As long as patients truly understand the future consequences and need for continued treatment of their condition, dentists can present the alternatives, including conventional full denture, overdenture, or no treatment at all, in good conscience.

This book is intended for general dentists as well as dental specialists. The content of the following chapters will help in the planning and the execution of the various treatment approaches available to provide our patients with the most physiologically sound and functional rehabilitation for practical, aesthetic, and predictable long-term care.

REFERENCES

1. Brånemark PI, Zarb G, Albrektsson T, editors: *Tissue-integrated prostheses.* Hanover Park, Ill, 1985, Quintessence.
2. Wood M, Vermilyea SG: A review of selected dental literature on evidence-based treatment planning for dental implants: Report of the Committee on Research in Fixed Prosthodontics of the Academy of Fixed Prosthodontics. *J Prosthet Dent* 92:447-462, 2004.
3. The survey was conducted by Nobel Biocare in August of 2008 and included 54,680 participants.
4. Sutton DN, Lewis BRK, Patel M, et al: Changes in facial form relative to progressive atrophy of the edentulous jaws. *Int J Oral Maxillofac Surg* 2004:33:676-682.
5. Henry PJ: A review of guidelines for implant rehabilitation of the edentulous maxilla. *J Prosthet Dent* 87:281-288, 2002.
6. Marcys SE, Drury TF, Brown LJ, et al: Tooth retention and tooth loss in the permanent dentition of adults: United States, 1988-1991. *J Dent Res* 75(Spec No):684-695, 1996.
7. Weintraub JA, Burt BA: Oral health status in the United States: Tooth loss and edentulism. *J Dent Educ* 49, 368-376, 1985.
8. Davis JE: Understanding peri-implant endosseous healing. *J Dent Educ* 67(8), 2003.
9. Brunski JE: Biomechanical factors affecting the bone-dental implant interface. *Clin Mater* 3:153-201, 1992.
10. Brunski JE: In vivo bone response to biomechanical loading at the bone/dental implant interface. *Adv Dent Res* 13:99-119, 1999.
11. Schnitman PA: Ten-year result for Brånemark implants immediately loaded with fixed prostheses at implant placement. *Int J Oral Maxillofac Implants* 12:495-503, 1997.
12. Chow J, Hui E, Lee P, et al: Zygomatic implants—Protocol for immediate loading: A preliminary report. *J Oral Maxillofac Surg* 64:804-811, 2006.
13. Zhao Y, Skalak R, Brånemark PI: *Analysis of a dental prosthesis supported by zygomatic fixtures.* The Institute for Applied Biotechnology, Gothenberg, Sweden, unpublished.
14. Bedrossian E: Immediate function with the zygomatic implant: A graftless solution for the patient with mild to advanced atrophy of the maxilla. *Int J Oral Maxillofac Implants* 21(6):937-942, 2006.
15. Brånemark PI: Introduction to Brånemark Novum concept. In Brånemark P-I, editor: *The Brånemark Novum protocol for same-day teeth.* A global perspective, Berlin, 2001, Quintessenz.
16. Maló P, Rangert B, Nobre M: All-on-4 immediate-function concept with Brånemark system implants for completely edentulous maxillae: A 1-year retrospective clinical study. *Clin Implant Dent Relat Res* 7(Suppl 1):S88-S94, 2005.
17. Douglass CW, Shih A, Ostry L: Will there be a need for complete dentures in the United States in 2020? *J Prosthet Dent* 87:5-8, 2002.
18. Centers for Disease Control and Prevention, Division of Oral Health: *Lost 6 or more teeth (website)*: http://apps.nccd.cdc.gov/nohss/ListV.asp?qkey=7&DataSet=2. Accessed September 17, 2009.
19. Fischer K, Bäckström M, Sennerby L: Immediate and early loading of oxidized tapered implants in the partially edentulous maxilla: A 1-year prospective clinical, radiographic, and resonance frequency analysis study. *Clin Implant Dent Relat Res* 7(suppl 1), 2008.
20. Degidi M, Piattelli A, Felice P, et al: Immediate functional loading of edentulous maxilla: A 5-year retrospective study of 388 titanium implants, *J Periodontol* 76:1016-1024, 2005.
21. Ioannidou E, Doufexi A: Does loading time affect implant survival? A meta-analysis of 1,266 implants. *J Periodontol* 76:1252-1258, 2005.

CHAPTER 2

Osseointegration: Rationale for Two-Stage versus One-Stage Protocols

The word *osseointegration* consists of *os,* the Latin word for bone, and *integration,* derived from the Latin words meaning *the state of being combined into a complete whole.* Osseointegration is defined as direct bone anchorage to an implant body that can provide a foundation to support a freestanding fixed prosthesis; it has the ability to transmit occlusal forces directly to bone.[1-3] To achieve osseointegration between the implant and the bone, the implant surface must be made of an inert material with affinity to establish a direct contact with the bony tissue, without a soft tissue interface. As Brånemark explains, "*the bases for osseointegration, leading to permanent, functional and interactive coexistence between titanium and bone, is established when a topographically harmonious and precise recipient site—geometrically adjacent to the anatomy of the fixture—is gently prepared in bone.*"[4]

The concept of osseointegration was initially discovered by accident as Brånemark was studying microcirculation in bone using titanium chambers inserted in the tibia of rabbits.[5] Upon completion of the study, removal of the titanium chambers proved to be difficult. Further studies led to the understanding that titanium is the most favorable material for replacement of lost roots in the human alveolar bone.[2,6,7] Once osseointegration was established, the junction of the implant and the bone—*direct* anchorage—was so strong that a 100-kg force did not separate and dislodge the implant,[8] and further application of force would have led to fracture of the bone itself and not the osseointegrated junction between the bone and the implant. Therefore, a direct implant-to-bone contact without a soft tissue interface is paramount.

Considering a different point of view, Linkow and Chercheve[9] and Weiss[10] believed that a peri-implant membrane established between the implant surface and the bony osteotomy site acted like the periodontal membrane of teeth, cushioning the occlusal forces placed onto the prosthesis and transmitted to the alveolar bone. In later studies[11] this fibrointegration could not withstand the forces applied under functional load and became larger, with an inflammatory reaction, gradual bone resorption, and loss of the fixtures. Brånemark further demonstrated that use of peri-implant membranes is consistent with failure of implants under load. In his studies, Brånemark[12] described the biologic and the biomechanical differences between natural teeth, fibrointegrated implants, and osseointegrated implants. Three separate models were described as follows:

1. Teeth supported by periodontium
2. Implants anchored in nonmineralized connective tissue
3. Implants anchored by osseointegration

Teeth supported by differentiated, functionally oriented periodontal ligaments have a high threshold for tissue injury and demonstrate height mechanical resistance to applied occlusal loads. On the other hand, implants anchored in nonmineralized connective tissue demonstrate low resistance to injury with low mechanical resistance as the implants are surrounded by tissues that have low differentiation and functional fibers that are not generally functionally oriented. Osseointegrated implants, however, are surrounded by continuously remodeling differentiated and functionally oriented bone tissues with a high threshold for injury under functional load. From this observation, it was clear that implant-to-bone contact without a fibrous interface was needed for functional support under occlusal loading. To achieve predictable bone anchorage, a consistent composition and finish of the implant's surface is essential,[13] as is an intimate contact between the implant and the osteotomy site—the bone—which is achieved by threading the implant into the prepared site.[14] The objective of a threaded endosteal implant is to establish stabilization of the fixture immediately after preparation of the osteotomy and during the initial healing period to achieve osseointegration. The dynamics of osseointegration and the relationship of an endosteal implant with its surrounding alveolar bone can be distinguished over time as three distinct and partially overlapping intervals or periods: healing, remodeling, and dynamic equilibrium (Figure 2-1).

During the first 18 months, referred to as the *healing phase,* primary and secondary bone healing occurs. The *remodeling phase,* which begins at 3 months and overlaps with the healing phase, ends at 18 months. After this period, the *dynamic equilibrium phase* begins, in which a balance is established between the forces acting on the fixture and the remodeling capacity of the anchorage bone.[15]

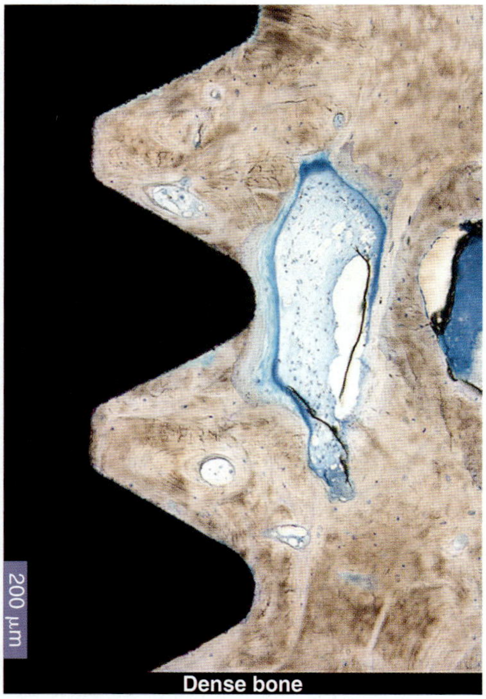

FIGURE 2-1 Osseointegration: the intimate contact of titanium oxide with bone without an interpositional soft tissue interface.

KEY FACTORS INFLUENCING OSSEOINTEGRATION

Four main criteria influence the predictability of achieving osseointegration after insertion of the implant in the bony osteotomy.

1. Composition and characteristics of the material (commercially pure titanium)[1,6,16,17]
2. A threaded fixture design, allowing placement into the osteotomy with initial stability and increased surface area for force distribution[11,18,19]; lack of an intimate fit of the threads against the bony wall of the osteotomy site, which results in soft tissue proliferation instead of direct bone fill[11]; and a precise fit of the endosteal implant within the vital bony osteotomy, which is essential for the success of the procedure
3. Preventing excessive heat generation and avoiding temperatures higher than 39° C by maintaining a maximum speed control of 2000 rpm during creation of the osteotomy and 15 to 20 rpm during implant insertion[5,20-22]
4. Maintaining a stress-free healing period: 6 months for the maxilla and 3 months for the mandible are the standard for osseointegration after the two-stage protocol[1,23]

Bone healing begins within the first week after placement of the implant and reaches its peak around the fourth week. The interface between the implant and the osteotomy matures and gradually becomes bone tissue around 8 weeks.[1] The dynamic condition of the bone continues after insertion of the prosthesis. Bony remodeling occurs for up to 18 months after insertion of the definitive prosthesis, with the resultant woven bone maturing into the denser laminar bone.[5] Understanding the occlusal forces generated under functional loads, it was possible to develop a set of criteria for the evaluation of the continued maintenance of osseointegration over time. The occlusal forces generated by the dentate patient are approximately 100 psi. The occlusal forces generated by conventional complete denture patients are 15 to 20 psi.[24-26] Patients with fully bone-anchored prostheses generate the same occlusal forces as dentate patients.[27] In 1986, Albrektsson et al. proposed a standard for clinically defining osseointegrated implants under function as successful.[28] The following criteria define successful implants:

1. The individual implant remains immobile clinically.
2. Peri-implant radiolucency is not seen on periapical radiographs.
3. One year after loading of the implant, vertical bone loss should not exceed 0.2 mm annually.

4. Individual implants should be free of pain, infection, neuropathies, or violation of the mandibular canal.
5. At the end of the 5-year and 10-year observation periods, a success rate of 85% and 80% is appreciated, respectively.

Since 1965, Brånemark and others have conducted clinical research to establish better appreciation of osseointegration. They recommend the following three criteria for ongoing clinical studies:

1. Controlled behavior of titanium in vitro
2. Continued development of a host-preparation technique that elicits a favorable and predictable healing process
3. Implant and prosthetic design and performance that withstands long-term functional and parafunctional forces.[8,29,30]

THE BIOLOGIC BASES FOR THE EVOLUTION OF THE IMMEDIATE-LOAD CONCEPT

The original protocol for the placement of implants as described by Brånemark[8] adopted the two-stage protocol. After preparation of the osteotomy and atraumatic installation of implants within the osteotomy, cover screws were placed and the soft tissues over the implant were primarily closed. Soft tissues over submerged implants were not loaded by any type of removable, tissue-supported prosthesis. This protocol was adopted to minimize the chance of infection and the migration of epithelial tissues between the osteotomy and the implant during the healing period. The submerged, two-stage implants were allowed to heal for 3 months in the denser mandibular bone and 6 months in the less-dense maxillary bone. At the end of the waiting period, the soft tissues over the implants were entered and the cover screws were replaced by temporary healing abutments, with adaptation of the surgical flap around these abutments forming a soft tissue collar. By exposing the implants into the oral cavity, the restorative dentist would have access for fabrication of the definitive prosthesis.

OSSEOINTEGRATION ACCORDING TO SKALAK AND BRÅNEMARK

Osseointegration at the *light microscope level* is defined as the close apposition of new and remodeled bone immediately next to the implant without interpositioned connective or fibrous tissues. This relationship must be biologically responsive and remain vital under normal physiologic load without excessive deformation or initiation of rejection mechanisms.

The lack of relative motion between the osseointegrated implant and the bone supports osseointegration from the biomechanical point of view. Deformation of the implant–bone interface should mimic the same deformation as within bone itself under functional loads throughout the patient's lifetime.

From a biophysical point of view, the components of tissues within a thin zone around the fixture (as seen under light and electron microscope) are considered. The mineralized tissues in this zone are in contact with the implant within nanometers over most of its surface, which does not allow formation of any other intervening material (Figure 2-2).

To understand osseointegration, the clinician must be aware of the healing, repairing, and remodeling capacity of bone under functional load. Adaptation of

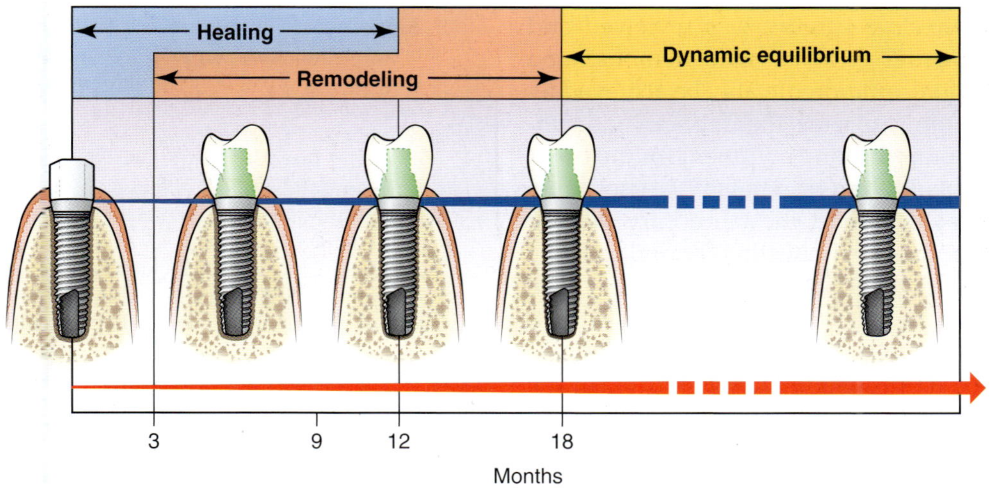

FIGURE 2-2 "Dynamics of osseointegration": the dynamic relationship of the implant with bone can be distinguished over time as three distinct periods: (1) healing phase, (2) remodeling phase, and (3) dynamic equilibrium phase reached at 18 months.

the human alveolus to the nonbiologic component placed within it and exposed to unlimited and cyclic functional loads is paramount to maintenance of osseointegration. The original design of the osseointegrated implant was intended to support a fixed prosthesis for the fully edentulous patient.[29] Four to six machine-surfaced implants were placed within the alveolus of the edentulous arch and allowed to heal without loading for 3 to 6 months.[1,23] The final prosthesis was a fixed, implant-supported bridge. The presence of the maxillary sinus in the upper jaw and the mental foramen in the lower jaw limited the distribution of the implants within the edentulous arch; thus the finished fixed prosthesis had cantilevers that extended distally from the most distal fixtures. The length of the cantilever was limited to 10 mm in the maxilla and 20 mm in the mandible; the length of the cantelevers is determined by the anterior-posterior distribution of implants.

In 1982 the landmark Toronto implant meeting allowed critical analysis of the treatment provided to the original group of patients using osseointegration principles developed in the previous two decades.[15] The biomechanical analysis by Skalak[32,33] decisively influenced simplification of the instrumentation and protocols for the ongoing treatment of edentulous patients with osseointegrated implants. Skalak predicted that the dimension and number of implants used to treat edentulous patients could be minimized and the total rehabilitation of patients could be performed in 1 day. The diagrammatic illustrations for the factors controlling the capacity to transfer functional load in one- or two-stage procedures are also well documented.[33-35] Skalak's prediction has been supported by controlled clinical studies that proved the immediate loading of edentulous patients to be safe and predictable.[36-39]

As we move toward immediate loading of implants, a review of the "conventional techniques" is prudent. The concept of *two-stage* surgery was reviewed and modified by Schroeder et al.[40-42] who demonstrated that osseointegration could predictably be achieved by creating the osteotomy, placing the implant, and substituting the temporary healing abutment for the cover screw during implant surgery. The soft tissues were immediately adapted around the temporary healing abutment and the 3-month healing period for the mandible and 6-month period for the maxilla were observed.

The *one-stage* implant protocol exposes the implants to an uncertain level of unavoidable load during the healing phase. The potential for micromotion and non-osseointegration of implants has been reviewed in the literature.[43-46] The adopted one-stage protocol demonstrated favorable outcome in early studies.[47,48] It was observed that the stability of the bone around the implant platform remained the same regardless of whether the surgeon followed the two-stage or one-stage surgical protocol.[49] During the healing phase, the involved tissues seem to tolerate micromotion in the range of 50 to 150 microns. Using machined implant surfaces, it has been reported that the threshold for achieving osseointegration is 100 microns.[45] Understanding micromotion led to the development and evolution of the concept of immediate loading.[38,50-52] Immediate loading of fully edentulous patients is also facilitated by the appreciation for the simultaneous occurrence of *contact osteogenesis* in concert with *distant osteogenesis,* with new bone growth occupying the space between the implant surface and the osteotomy walls. This establishes a clinically immobile union of the implant with the host bone, which is discussed in Chapter 3.

SUMMARY

Osseointegration is defined as the apposition of bone adjacent to an implant surface without interpositional soft tissue. Osseointegration can be achieved by two-stage as well as one-stage surgical protocols. Later chapters discuss the scientific bases for modification of protocols, with the concept of immediate loading fulfilling the prediction made by Skalak and Brånemark that simplification and early loading of implants could be possible.[32,33] Analogue and computer-guided approaches are presented, as is a discussion of techniques for placement of the most distal implant as posterior as possible within the edentulous maxilla and mandible to avoid or limit the cantilevered portion of fixed, implant-supported bridges.[37,38,53]

REFERENCES

1. Albrektsson T, Brånemark PI, Hansson HA, et al: Osseointegrated titanium implants. Requirements for ensuring a long-lasting direct bone-to-implant anchorage in man. *Acta Orthop Scand* 52:155-170, 1981.
2. Brånemark PI: Osseointegration and its experimental background. *J Prosthet Dent* 50:399-410, 1983.
3. Carlsson L, Rostlund T, Albrektsson B, et al: Osseointegration of titanium implants. *Acta Orthop Scand* 57:285-289, 1986.
4. Brånemark PI: *The osseointegration book: From calvarium to calcaneus,* Chicago, 2005, Quintessence, pp 22-25.
5. Brånemark PI, Breine U, Adell R, et al: Intraosseous anchorage of dental prostheses. 1. Experimental studies. *Scand J Plast Reconstr Surg* 3:81-93, 1969.
6. Albrektsson T, Brånemark PI, Hansson HA, et al: The interface zone of inorganic implants in vivo: Titanium implants in bone. *Ann Biomed Eng* 11:1-27, 1983.
7. Zarb GA, Symington JM: Osseointegrated dental implants: Preliminary report on a replication study. *J Prosthet Dent* 50:271-276, 1983.

8. Brånemark PI, et al: Intraosseous anchorage of dental prosthesis. I. Experimental studies. *Scand J Plastic Reconstr Surg* 3:81-93, 1969.
9. Linkow LI, Chercheve R: *Theories and techniques of oral implantology*, St. Louis, 1970, Mosby.
10. Weiss CM: Tissue integration of dental endosseous implant: Description and comparative analysis of the fibro-osseous integration and osseous integration systems. *J Oral Implantol* 12:169-214, 1986.
11. Brunski JB, Moccia AF, Pollack SR, et al: The influence of functional use of endosseous dental implants on the tissue implant interface. II. Clinical aspects. *J Dent Res* 58:1053-1969, 1979.
12. Brånemark PI: *The osseointegration book: From calvarium to calcaneus*, Chicago, 2005, Quintessence.
13. Henry PJ: Comparative surface analysis of two osseo integrated implant systems. *Int J Oral Maxillofac Implants* 2:23-27, 1987.
14. Carlsson L, Rostlund T, Albrektsson B, et al: Removal torques for polished and rough titanium implants. *Int J Oral Maxilfofac Implants* 3:21-24, 1988.
15. Brånemark PI Introduction to osseointegration. In Brånemark P-I, Zarb G, Albrektsson T, editors: *Tissue-integrated prosthesis-osseointegration in clinical dentistry*, Chicago, 1985, Quintessence.
16. Albrektsson T: Direct bone anchorage of dental implants. *J Prosthet Dent* 50:255-261, 1983.
17. Kasemo B: Biocompatibility of titanium implants: Surface science aspects. *J Prosthet Dent* 49:832-837, 1983.
18. Carlsson L, Rostlund T, Albrektsson T, et al: Osseointegration of titanium implants. *Acta Orthop Scand* 57:285-289, 1986.
19. Haraldson T: A photoelastic study of some biomechanical factors affecting the anchorages of osseointegrated implants in the jaw. *Scand J Plast Reconstr Surg* 14:209-214, 1980.
20. Lavelle C, Wedgwood D, Love WB: Some advances in endosseous implants. *J Ora Rehabil* 8:319-331, 1981.
21. Eriksson RA: *Heat-induced bone tissue injury.* An in vivo investigation of heat tolerance of bone tissue and temperature rise in the drilling of cortical bone. Unpublished thesis. Sweden, 1984, University of Gothenburg.
22. Eriksson RA: The effect of heat on bone regeneration. *J Oral Maxillofac Surg* 42:705-711, 1984.
23. Lekholm U: Clinical procedures for treatment with osseointegrated dental implants. *J Prosthet Dent* 50:116-120, 1983.
24. Carr AB, Laney WR: Maximum occlusal force levels in patients with osseointegrated oral implant prostheses and patients with complete dentures. *Int J Oral Maxillofac Implants* 2:101-108, 1987
25. Laney WR, Tolman DE, Keller EE, et al: Dental implants: Tissue integrated prosthesis utilizing the osseointegration concept. *Mayo Clin Proc* 61:91-97, 1986.
26. Haraldson T, Karlsson U, Carlsson GE: Bite force and oral function in complete denture wearers. *J Oral Rehabil* 6:41-48, 1979.
27. Haraldson T: Masticatory muscle function in patients rehabilitated with OIB. *Swed Dent J* 28(Suppl):137-142, 1985.
28. Albrektsson T, Zarb G, Worthington P, et al: The long-term efficacy of currently used dental implants. A review and proposed criteria for success. *Int J Oral Maxillofac Implants* 1:11-25, 1986.
29. Brånemark PI, Hansson BO, Adell R, et al: *Osseointegrated implants in the treatment of the edentulous jaw. Experience from a 10-year period.* Stockholm, 1977, Almgrist Wiksell.
30. Zarb GA, Schmitt A, Baker B: Tissue-integrated prosthesis: Osseointegration research in Toronto. *Int J Periodontics Restorative Dent* 1:26-51, 1987.
31. Meredith N, Shagaldi F, Alleyne D, et al: The application of resonance frequency measurements to study the stability of titanium implants during healing in the rabbit tibia. *Clin Oral Implants Res* 8:234-243, 1997.
32. Brunski JB, Skalak R: Biomechanical considerations. In Worthington PH, Brånemark P-I, editors: *Osseointegration surgery. Application in the maxillofacial region*, Chicago, 1992, Quintessence, pp 15-39.
33. Skalak R: Biomechanics of osseointegration. In Brånemark PI, Rydevik BL, Skalak R, editors: *Osseointegration in skeletal reconstruction and joint replacement*, Chicago, 1997, Quintessence, pp 45-56.
34. Brånemark PI: Introduction to Brånemark Novum concept. In Brånemark PI, editor: *The Brånemark Novum protocol for same-day teeth. A global perspective*, Berlin, 2001, Quintessenz.
35. Engrstrand P, Grondahl K, Ohrnell LO, et al: Prospective followup study of 95 patients with Brånemark Novum concept. *Clin Implant Dent Relat Res* 5:3-11, 2003.
36. Chow J, Hui E, Lee P, et al: Zygomatic implants—Protocol for immediate loading: A preliminary report. *J Oral Maxillofac Surg* 64:804-811, 2006.
37. Bedrossian E, Rangert B, Stumpel L, et al: Immediate function with the zygomatic implant—A graftless solution for the patient with mild to advanced atrophy of the maxilla. *Int J Oral Maxillofac Surg* 21:1-6, 2006.
38. Maló P, Rangert B, Nobre M: All-on-4 immediate-function concept with Brånemark system implants for completely edentulous maxillae: A 1-year retrospective clinical study. *Clin Implant Dent Relat Res* 7(Suppl 1):S88-S94, 2005.
39. Calandriello R, Tomatis M: Simplified treatment of the atrophic posterior maxilla via immediate/early function and tilted implants: A prospective 1-year clinical study. *Clinic Implant Dent Relat Res* 7(Suppl 1):S1-S12, 2005.
40. Schroeder A, Pohler O, Sutter F: Geweb reaktion auf ein Titan–Hohlzylinder Implantat mit Titan-S ritzschichtoberfache. *SSO Schweiz Monatsschr Zahnheilkd* 86:713-727, 1976.
41. Schroder A, Stich H, Straumann F, et al: Uber die Anlagerung Osteocement an eine belasteten Implantat-kbrper. *SSO Schweiz Monatsschr Zahnheikd* 88:1051-1058, 1978.
42. Schroder A, Mffiglin B, Sutter F: Das ITI Hohlzylinderimplantat Typ F zur Prothesenretention b im zahnlosen Kiefer. *SSO Schweiz Monatsschr Zahnheilkd* 93:720-733, 1983.
43. Cameron H, Pilliar RM, Macnab I: The effect of movement on the bonding of porous metal to bone. *J Biomed Mater Res* 7:301-311, 1973.
44. Brunski JE: Biomechanical factors affecting the bone-dental implant interface. *Clin Mater* 3:153-201, 1992.
45. Brunski JE: In vivo bone response to biomechanical loading at the bone/dental implant interface. *Adv Dent Res* 13:99-119, 1999.
46. Pilliar RM: Quantitative evaluation of the effect of movement at a porous coated implant-bone interface. In Davies EJ, editor: *The bone-biomaterial interface*, Toronto, 1995, University of Toronto Press.
47. Abrahamsson I, Berglundh T, Wennström J, et al: The peri-implant hard and soft tissues at different implant systems. A comparative study in the dog. *Clin Oral Implants Res* 7:212-219, 1996.
48. Ericsson I, Nilner K, Klinge B, et al: Radiographical and histological characteristics of submerged and non-

submerged titanium implants. An experiential study in the Labrador dog. *Clin Oral Implants Res* 6:20-26, 1996.

49. Ericsson I, Randow K, Nilner K, et al: Some clinical and radiographical features of submerged and non-submerged titanium implants. A 5-year follow-up study. *Clin Oral Implants Res* 8:422-426, 1997.
50. Schnitman PA, Wöhrle PS, Rubenstein E, et al: Ten-year results for Brånemark implants immediately loaded with fixed prostheses at implant placement. *Int J Oral Maxillofac Implants* 12:495-503, 1997.
51. Ericsson I, Randow K, Nilner K, et al: Early functional loading of Brånemark dental implants. A 5-year follow-up study. *Clin Implant Dent Relat Res* 70-77, 2000.
52. Chow J, Hui E, Li O, et al: Immediate loading of Brånemark system fixtures in the mandible with a fixed provisional prosthesis. *Appl Osseointegration Res* 2:30-35, 2001.
53. Aparicio C: Tilted implants as an alternative to maxillary sinus grafting: A clinical, radiological, and Periotest study. *Clin Implant Dent Relat Res* 1:39-49, 2001.

CHAPTER 3

Immediate Loading

Immediate loading of implants has been reported in the literature by several authors. In 1997, Schnitman[1] and Balshi,[2] in two separate studies of immediate-loading implants, reported surgical success rates of 85% and 80%, respectively. Following the development of the Brånemark Novum protocol, Brånemark and co-workers[3] reported a 98% success rate in 1999; in 2004, van Steenberg and co-workers[4] reported a 93% success rate. The changes in both the surgical and prosthetic protocols are impressive and are a significant departure from the original two-stage protocol. To better understand the significant changes in the immediate-load protocol, it is prudent to understand the biologic bases for this approach.

The two-stage protocol used a machined-surface implant made from commercially pure titanium. The texture and the condition of the implant surface[5]—specifically the outermost atomic layer—is a key factor in osseointegration. Implant surfaces vary based on the handling and preparation methods used.[6] The composition of commercially pure titanium is 99.7% titanium, 0.05% iron, 0.10% oxygen, 0.03% nitrogen, 0.01% carbon, and 0.06% of other elements.[7-9] It is milled in an argon-gas environment. After completion of the milling process, its exposure to air forms a 50- to 100-Å-thick oxide layer.[7-10] The oxide layer of osseointegrated implants is surrounded by glycoprotein with an adjacent calcified layer approximately 100 Å in width. For the machined implant to establish an intimate contact between the titanium oxide, the glycoprotein, and the calcified matrix, the process of osseointegration or distant osteogenesis requires several weeks of undisturbed healing time. The concept of distant osteogenesis[11] is discussed in more detail in the following section.

Immediate loading of implants has been facilitated in part by the modification of the implant surface, generally referred to as *rough* or *microtextured* surfaces. This modification has led to higher predictability when adopting the immediate-load concept. Reports of 98% surgical success have been published using the TiUnite surface.[12-14] These findings are consistent with compositional changes of the implant surface influencing biocompatibility and healing.[15] Rough surfaces influence osseointegration by (1) increasing the implant surface area within the bony osteotomy,[16] (2) enhancing initial stability by fibrin matrix retention,[17] and (3) "accelerating" osseointegration by their osseoconductive properties.[18,19]

The methods for enhancing machined implant surfaces are the application of titanium plasma spray or performing anodic oxidation.[19] Recent literature indicates that the anodic oxidation process, such as is used with the TiUnite implant surface, seems to have higher success rates.[20,21] Such success is in part due to the osseoconductive properties of the roughened surface, which results in better fibrin clot retention on the implant surface and initiates contact osteogenesis over the implant surface.[11] Better primary stability of roughened surfaces versus machined surfaces has been demonstrated in dog models.[22] In 2001, Glauser[23] also demonstrated the superior stability of textured implant surfaces over machined implant surfaces using resonance frequency analysis. The stability of implants was measured during bone healing as well as at the end of the osseointegration period. Throughout the study, the textured implant had higher implant stability quotient (ISQ) values compared with the machined implants.[23]

It is apparent that the biologic bases of immediate loading are correlated with the topography of the implant as well as with its surface morphology. The composition of the implant, limiting micromotion as described by professors Brunski and Skalak,[60] and using a rigid framework during the healing period are all compatible with the biologic healing cascade of bone.

CONTACT OSTEOGENESIS VERSUS DISTANT OSTEOGENESIS

This section discusses bone biomechanics and biology as described by Davis.[11] Upon initiation of an osteotomy (trauma) onto the surface of the alveolar bone, damage to the intraosseous blood vessels occurs with resultant bleeding into the osteotomy site of approximately of 1 ml (Figure 3-1).[11] Extravasations of blood during trauma to long bones and resultant loss of approximately 1 L of blood has been reported by others.[21] This vascular disruption on the surface of the osteotomy site during preparation of the implant site leads to death of the peri-implant cortical bone.[24]

The healing at this site is initiated by osteoclastic activity from the medullary compartments underlying the affected cortical bone.[25] This phenomenon has been called *osseointegration,* as described by previous reports.[26,27]

The endosseous implant is placed within a dynamic, vascular living tissue, which continuously remodels during the lifetime of the patient. Understanding the macroarchitecture and the microarchitecture of bone is paramount for the implant surgeon.

The macrostructure of bone is composed of trabecular (cancellous) and cortical (compact) portions. The function of cortical bone is to withstand *torsional loading,* whereas cancellous bone has evolved to predominantly withstand *compressive loading.* These differences in the macrostructure of bone are clearly seen when evaluating the macrostructure of long bones. The diaphysis is made of primarily cortical bone and the articular extremities are made of primarily cancellous bone.[11] These two differences in the macroarchitecture of bone are also present in the maxillofacial region and have been shown to formulate a clinical classification of bone type in the edentulous maxilla and mandible.[28]

Type I bone is predominantly cortical. It begins in the anterior mandible in front of the mental foramen, and crosses the midline to the anterior portion of the contralateral mental foramen (between the mandibular cuspids). In contrast, *type IV bone* is predominantly cancellous and begins distal to the maxillary cuspids and progresses posteriorly toward the maxillary tuberosity. *Type II* and *type III bone* have a progressively lower cortical/cancellous ratio and are found in the portion of the alveolus distal to the mandibular cuspids and between the maxillary cuspids, respectively. During bone healing, cortical bone relies on *osteonal remodeling.* Trabecular bone initiates osteoconduction and *de novo* bone formation, which together compose *contact osteogenesis.*

The microarchitecture of cortical and cancellous bone includes 3% to 5% of both bone types that are continuously being resorbed and replaced by osteoclasts and osteoblasts, respectively.[29,30] Both types of bone are needed to allow the initial mechanical stability of the cortical bone to stabilize the implant while the biologic stability of the cancellous bone matures (Figure 3-2). This phenomenon of mechanical stability

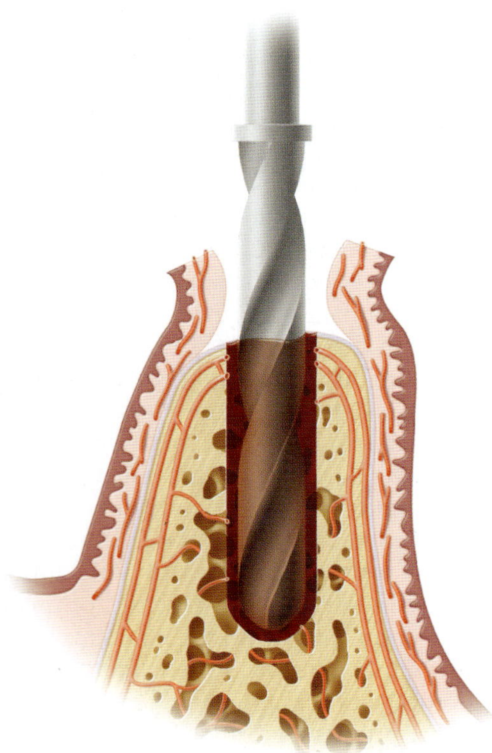

FIGURE 3-1 Approximately 1 ml of blood fills the osteotomy cavity during preparation for implant placement.

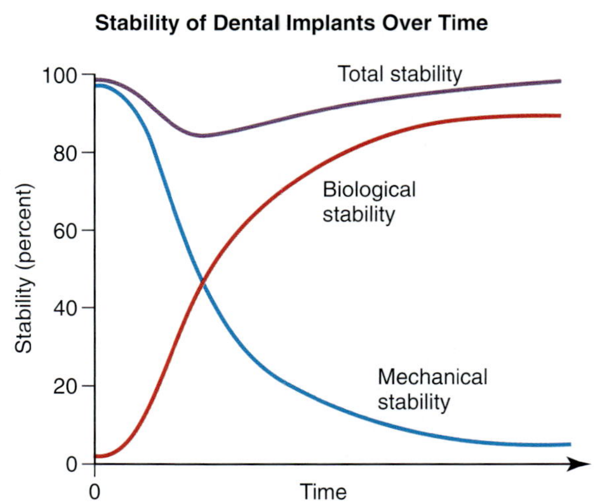

FIGURE 3-2 Mechanical stability declines as biologic stability increases with osseointegration of an implant. Maturation of biologic stability can be described as *osseointegration* or *total stability.*

giving way to biologic stability has been studied by Glauser and others[31-35] using resonance frequency analysis.

Laying down new bone on the walls of the osteotomy site and the implant surface itself are termed *distant* and *contact osteogenesis*, respectively.[11,36] Distant osteogenesis occurs on cortical bone surfaces when new bone forms on the surface of old bone lining the walls of the implant osteotomy site. In contact osteogenesis, new bone is formed for the first time directly on the implant surface.

Contact osteogenesis—new bone formation on the surface of the newly placed implant within the osteotomy by differentiating osteogenic cells—is referred to as *de novo* bone formation.[37,38] The presence of a *cement line matrix*, as described by von Ebner[39] and Davis,[11] is the hallmark for the histologic appreciation of this concept.

Both distant and contact osteogenesis occurs at every endosseous implant osteotomy healing site. The initial stability[31,40] attained by the cortical aspect of the bone is crucial to allow recruitment of osteogenic cells onto the implant surface, initiating contact osteogenesis. Recruitment of the osteogenic cells to the implant surface is related to implant surface design and surface texture.

Contact Osteogenesis

Extravasated blood within the osteotomy site has a composition as outlined in Figure 3-3. Red blood cells are obviously important in oxygen transportation, but do not have a major influence in early bone healing. Platelets, however, play a major role in the mechanism of early bone healing through their degranulation and release of platelet-derived growth factor (PDGF) and transforming growth factor-beta (TGF-β), as well as through vasoactive factors such as serotonin and histamine, which play a major role in regulation of wound healing cascade.[41,42] Stimulation and proliferation of human osteoblasts by PDGF is extensively reported in the literature.[43,44] PDGF and TGF-β are mitogenic and chemotactic factors for fibroblasts, neutrophil, and osteogenic cells.[45-47] Platelet degranulation also results in the release of platelet releasate, which also plays a role in the stimulation, recruitment, migration, and proliferation of bone marrow–derived cells.[48]

Contact osteogenesis begins with activation of platelets and their contact with the implant surface. Glycoprotein (GP) IIb/III integrin binds to the implant surface fibrinogen[21] and mediates the adhesion of platelets. Greater platelet adhesion is seen on implants

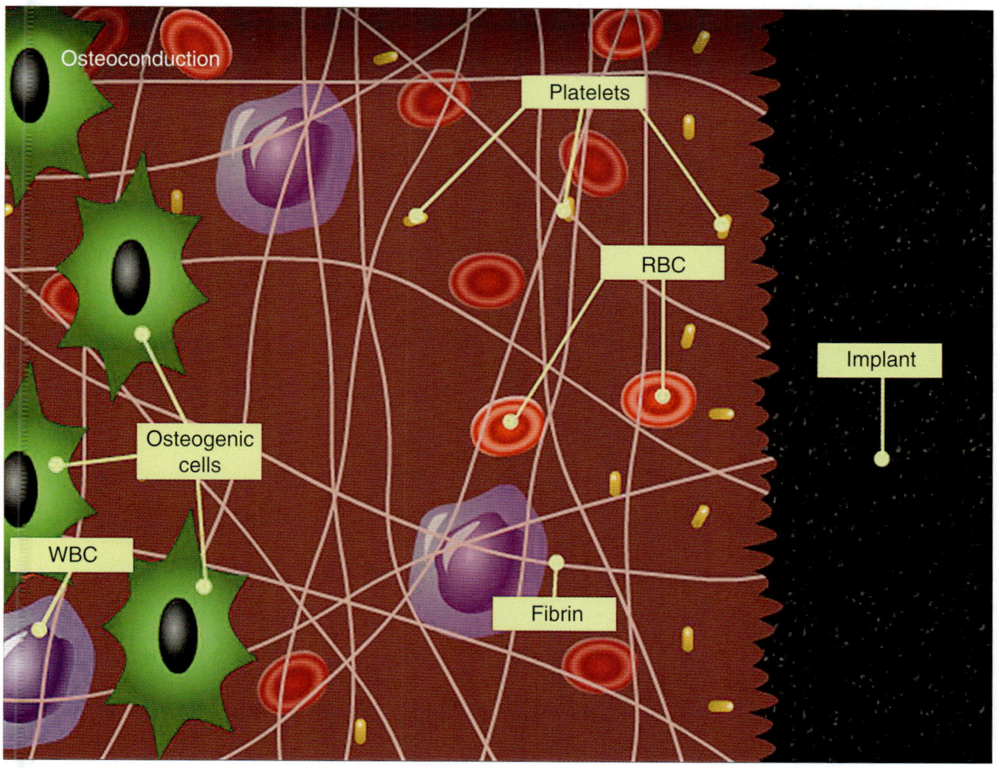

FIGURE 3-3 Composition of various cells found in extravasated blood within the osteotomy site. *(Courtesy Dr. John E. Davies, University of Toronto.)*

that have surfaces of greater porosity.[49] Platelets activated by contacting the implant surface release cytokines, growth factors, and microparticles, which, in conjunction with the three-dimensional matrix formed by the fibrin in the coagulation cascade, results in the migration of osteogenic cells to the implant surface.[50]

The implant surface design plays two important roles in the osteoconduction ability of an implant. It first influences the anchorage of the temporary fibrin matrix and modulates the level of platelet activation. Therefore, microtopographically complex surfaces promote osteoconduction by increasing the surface area for fibrin attachment as well as by potentiating the activation of platelets that produce a cytokines and growth factor gradient, attracting leukocyte and osteogenic cells in the healing compartment.[11]

Platelet degranulation also releases arachidonic acid metabolites that cause vasoconstriction. The osseoconductive influence of the implant depends on the quality of fibrin adhesion to the implant surface. The extravasated blood in the osteotomy site contains factor VII and factor III, which in turn cause the activation of factor X. The activation of factor X together with factor V converts prothrombin to thrombin, which causes the conversion of fibrinogen to fibrin of the clot.[51-53] This transient, fibrin-based matrix of the blood clot creates the scaffold on which osteogenic cells migrate to the implant surface. Fibrin adhesion onto the implant surface is strongly influenced by the texture of the implant surface (Figure 3-4). The migration of the osteogenic cells produces a contractile force on the fibrin matrix. This contractile force has the potential of detaching this transitory fibrin matrix from the implant surface. The unpredictable adherence of fibrin matrix onto a smooth-surfaced implant is demonstrated in Figure 3-5, in which the migration of the osteogenic cells place undo contractile stress on the weakly adhered fibrin matrix, detaching it from the implant surface. On the other hand, the microtextured implant surface demonstrates resistance to forces applied to the organic fibrin matrix, allowing the migration of osteogenic cells onto the implant surface. The direct deposition of organic matrix onto the textured implant surface is contrasted with the formation of bone away from the smooth implant surface in Figure 3-6.

The series of events that lead to the initiation of de novo bone formation on the surface of the implant is summarized as follows. Osteoconduction is initiated by contact between platelets and the implant surface, causing the release of cytokines and growth factors (Figure 3-7). The continued contact with platelets and their degranulation establishes a dense gradient across the organic collagen matrix (Figure 3-8), attracting osteogenic cells onto the implant surface (Figure 3-9). Once the osteogenic cells have reached the implant surface, they polarize and become osteoblasts

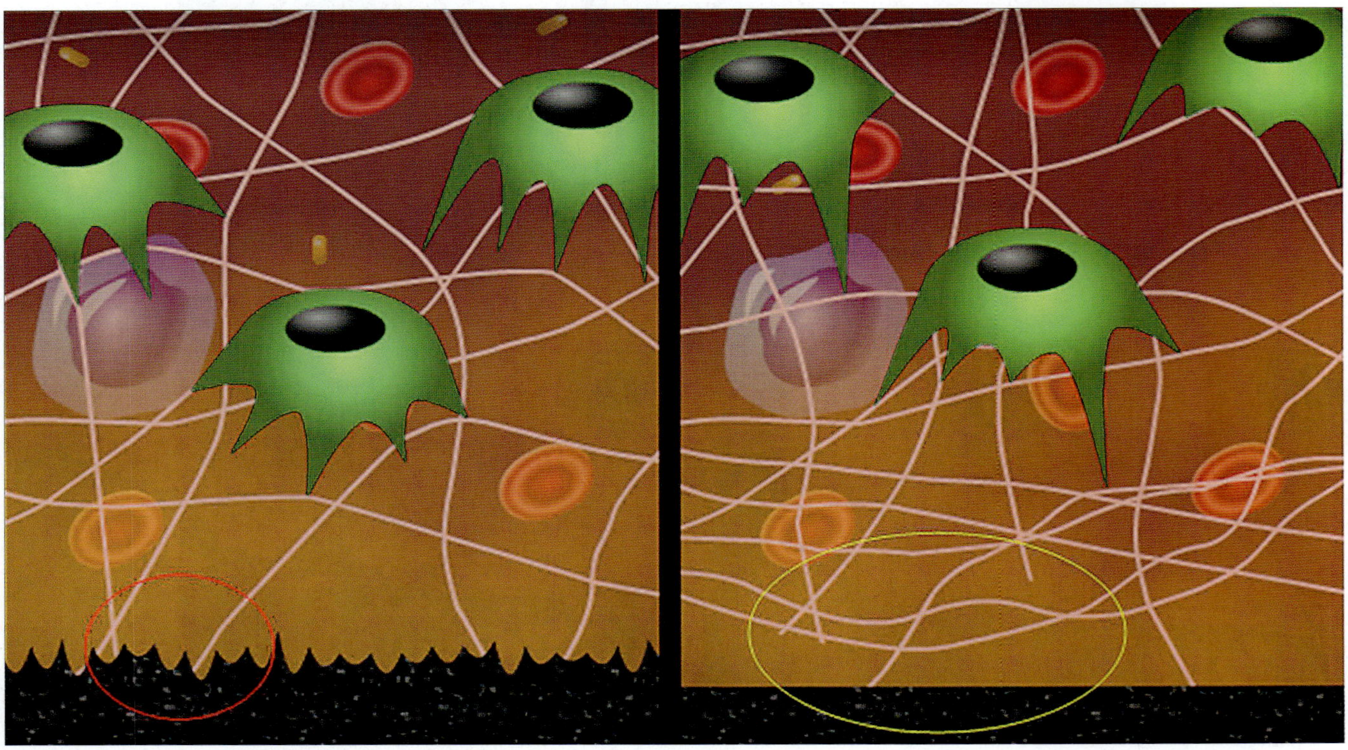

FIGURE 3-4 Textured implant surfaces allow for stronger fibrin adhesion than do smooth implant surfaces. *(Courtesy Dr. John E. Davies, University of Toronto.)*

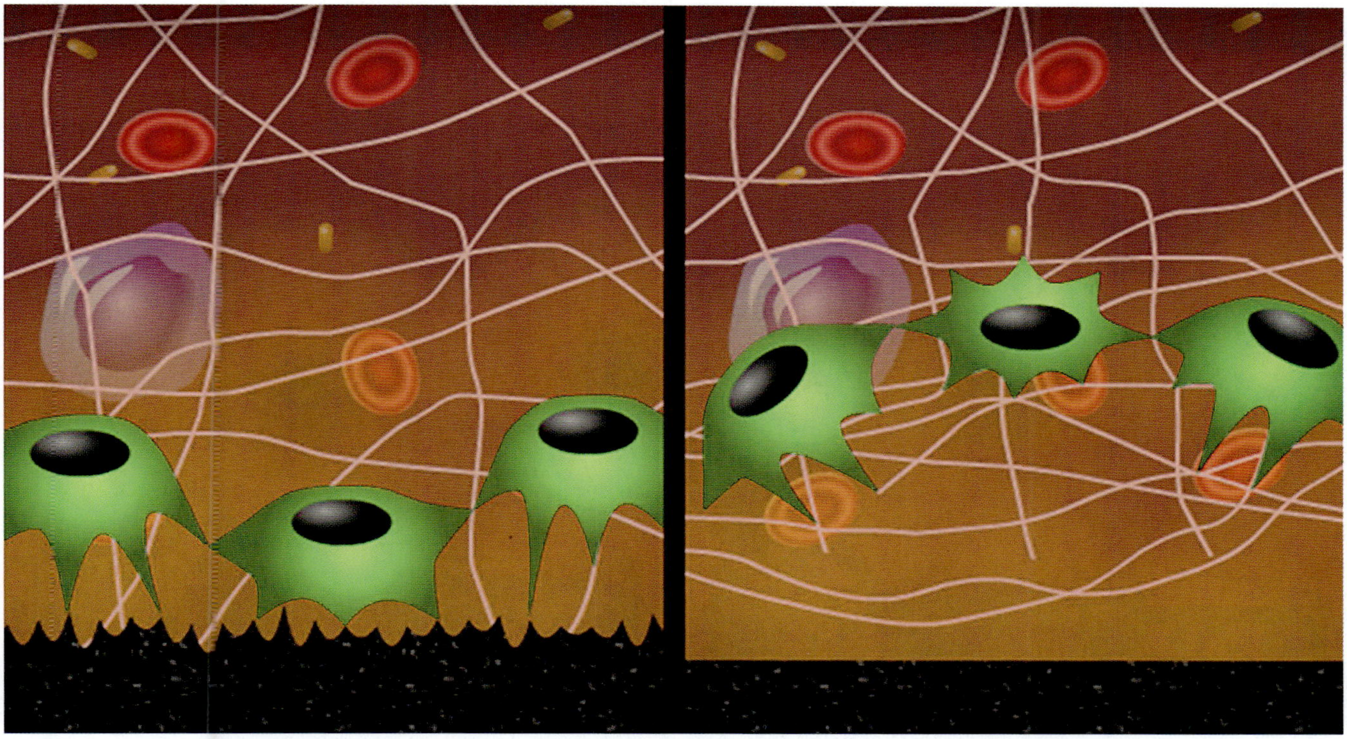

FIGURE 3-5 Contractile forces applied by osteogenic cells to the fibrin matrix result in unpredictable adherence of the fibrin to the smooth implant surface. *(Courtesy Dr. John E. Davies, University of Toronto.)*

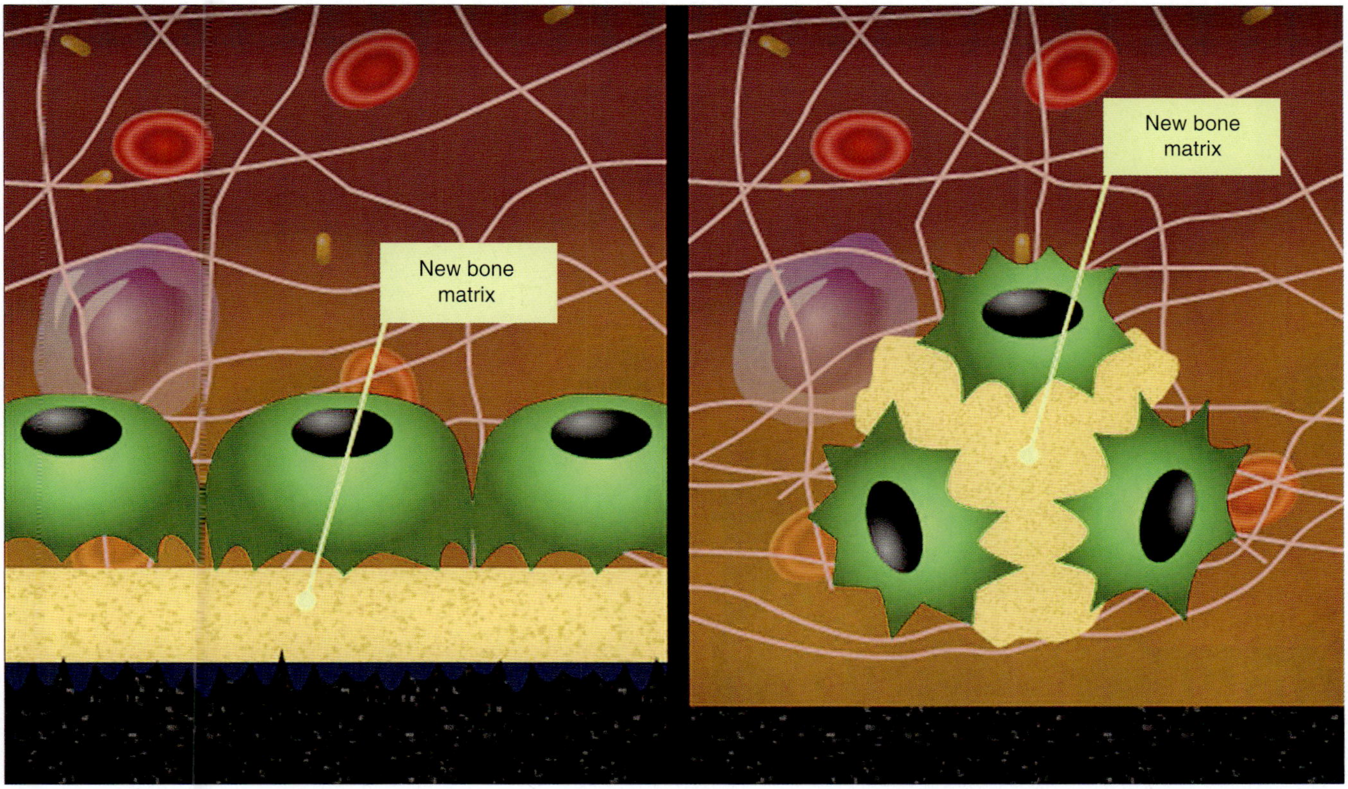

FIGURE 3-6 Implant surface design influences the direct deposition of organic matrix onto the implant surface. *(Courtesy Dr. John E. Davies, University of Toronto.)*

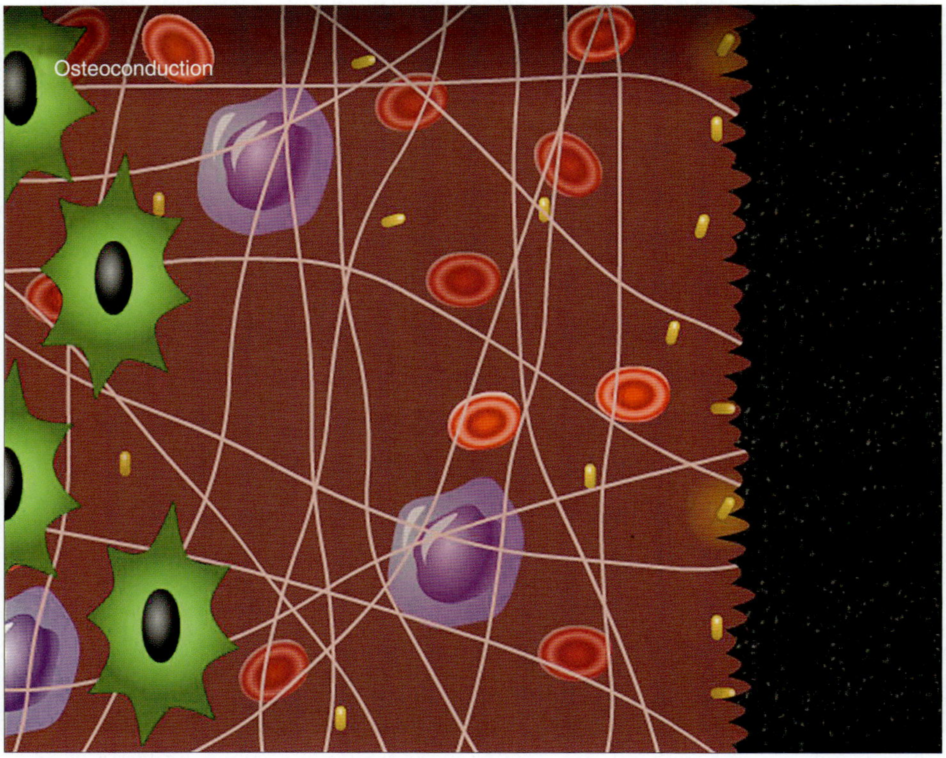

FIGURE 3-7 Platelet contacting the implant surface results in the release of cytokines and multiple growth factors in the osteotomy site. *(Courtesy Dr. John E. Davies, University of Toronto.)*

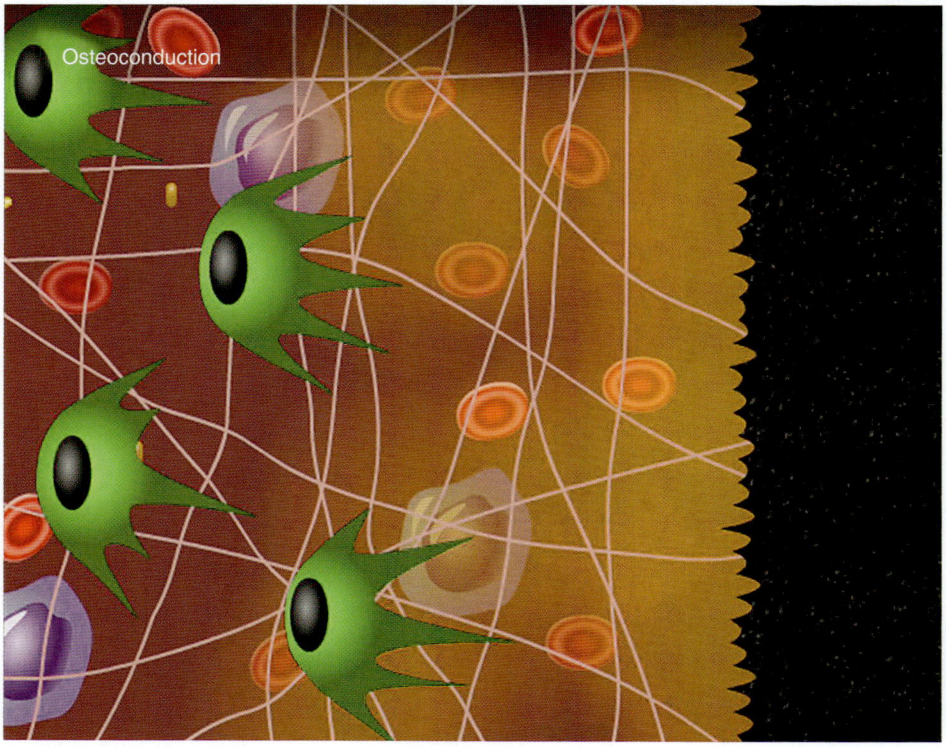

FIGURE 3-8 A cytokine gradient is established as more platelets contact the implant surface. *(Courtesy Dr. John E. Davies, University of Toronto.)*

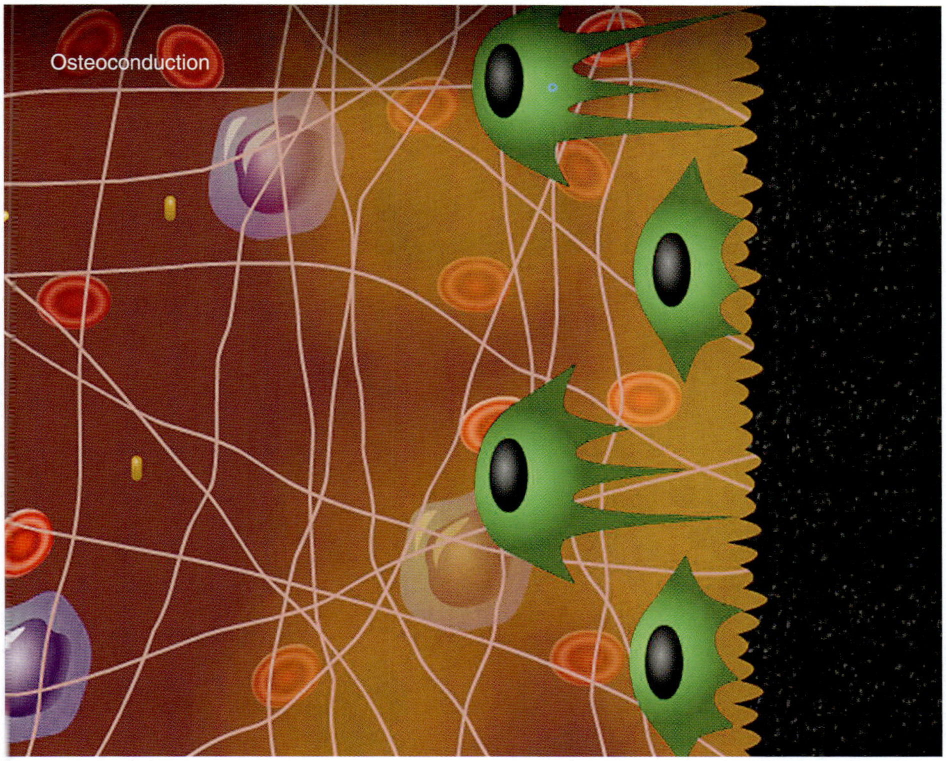

FIGURE 3-9 The cytokine gradient attracts the osteogenic cells toward the implant surface. *(Courtesy Dr. John E. Davies, University of Toronto.)*

(Figure 3-10), initiating new bone formation by secretion of the collagen-free "cement line" (Figure 3-11).[38,54] The formation of new bone, the de novo bone formation cascade, has been confirmed through in vitro and in vivo studies.[55,56] Bone formation has four stages. In *stage one* the differentiating osteogenic cells secrete a collagen-free organic bone matrix composed of bone proteins, osteopontin, and bone sialoprotein, as well as two proteoglycans.[57] This collagen-free matrix provides for *stage two:* nucleation sites for calcium phosphate mineralization. *Stage three* involves growth of calcium phosphate crystals and initiation of collagen fiber assemblies. *Stage four* is the calcification of the collagen compartments. Thus, in contact osteogenesis, bonding of new bone to the implant surface is achieved by micromechanical interdigitation of the cement line with the implant surface.[58]

Initiation of calcium phosphate nuclei and their growth and mineralization allow for the direct growth of new bone onto the implant surface.[59] The entrapment of osteoblasts within the calcifying matrix forms osteocytes. The osteocytes communicate and receive their nutrients from the newly recruited osteoblasts on the leading edge of the new bone, through canaliculi, as seen in Figure 3-12.

Distant Osteogenesis

In distant osteogenesis new bone is formed on the surface of the old bone of the implant osteotomy site. The interruption of the vasculature on the walls of the implant site after preparation of the osteotomy leads to bone death.[24] Subsequent slow remodeling and healing is initiated by the orthoclastic cells derived form underlying medullary compartments of the osteotomy wall.[46] Under the light microscope, distant osteogenesis has been described as the *process of osseointegration* (Figure 3-13). The process of distant osteogenesis is illustrated by recruitment of osteoblasts onto the walls of the osteotomy with new bone formation occurring toward the implant surface (Figures 3-14, 3-15, 3-16, and 3-17).

In contrast, histologically (Figure 3-18), contact osteogenesis depends on the de novo bone formation directly on the surface of the implant growing outward toward the walls of the osteotomy, preceded by a secure anchorage of a three-dimensional fibrin matrix onto the implant surface and osteoconduction (Figures 3-19, 3-20, 3-21, and 3-22).

Osseointegration is generally defined as the apposition of bone adjacent to an implant surface without

Text continued on p. 22.

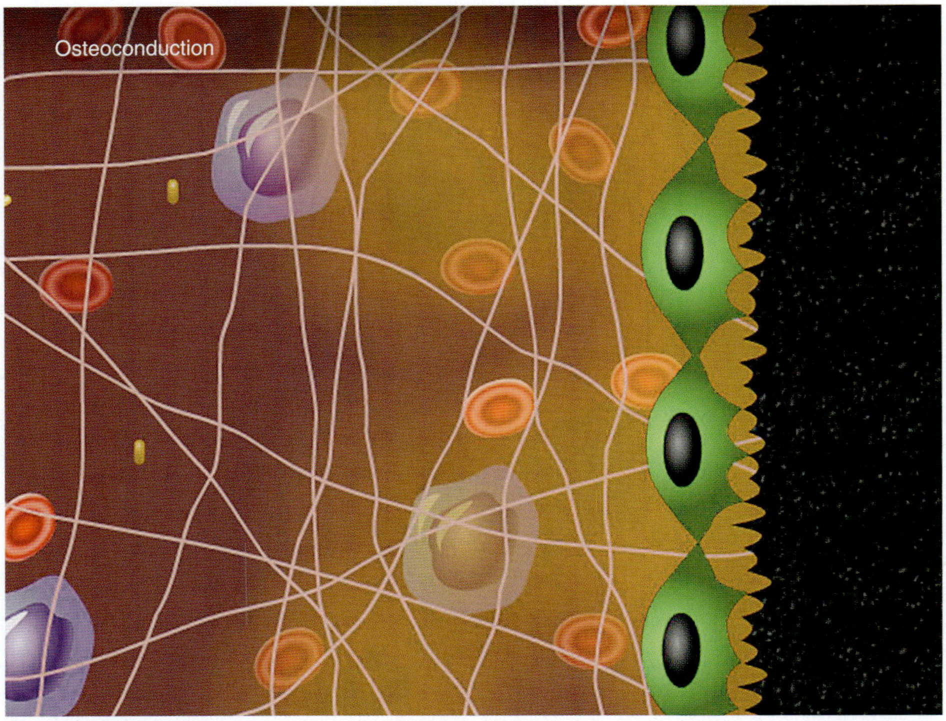

FIGURE 3-10 Polarization of the osteogenic cells to osteoblast on the implant surface. *(Courtesy Dr. John E. Davies, University of Toronto.)*

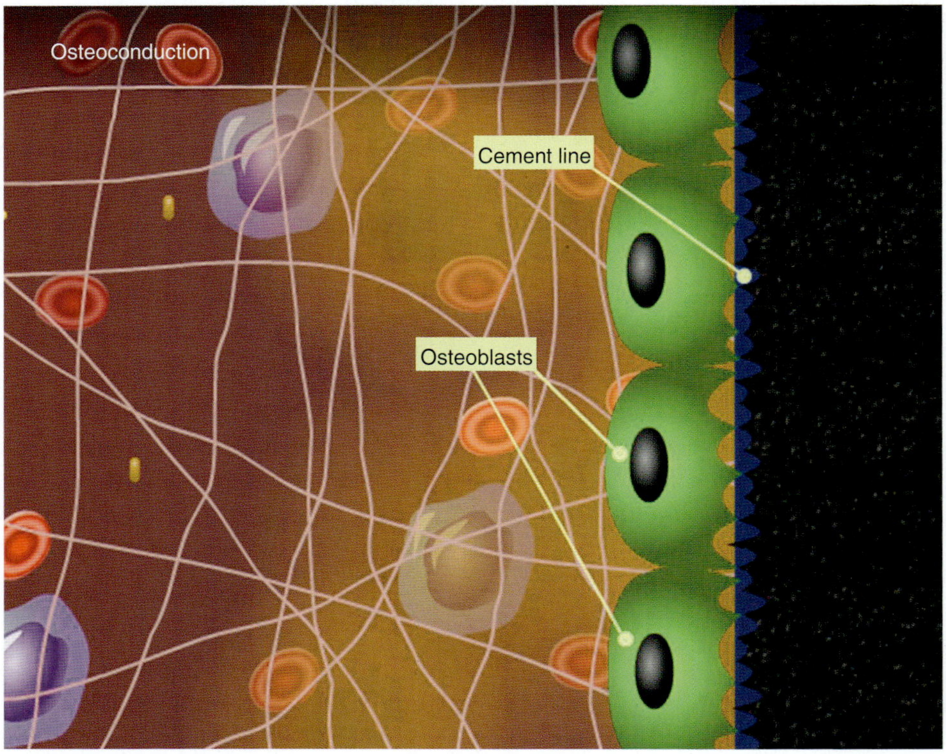

FIGURE 3-11 De novo bone formation: new bone formation on the implant surface. *(Courtesy Dr. John E. Davies, University of Toronto.)*

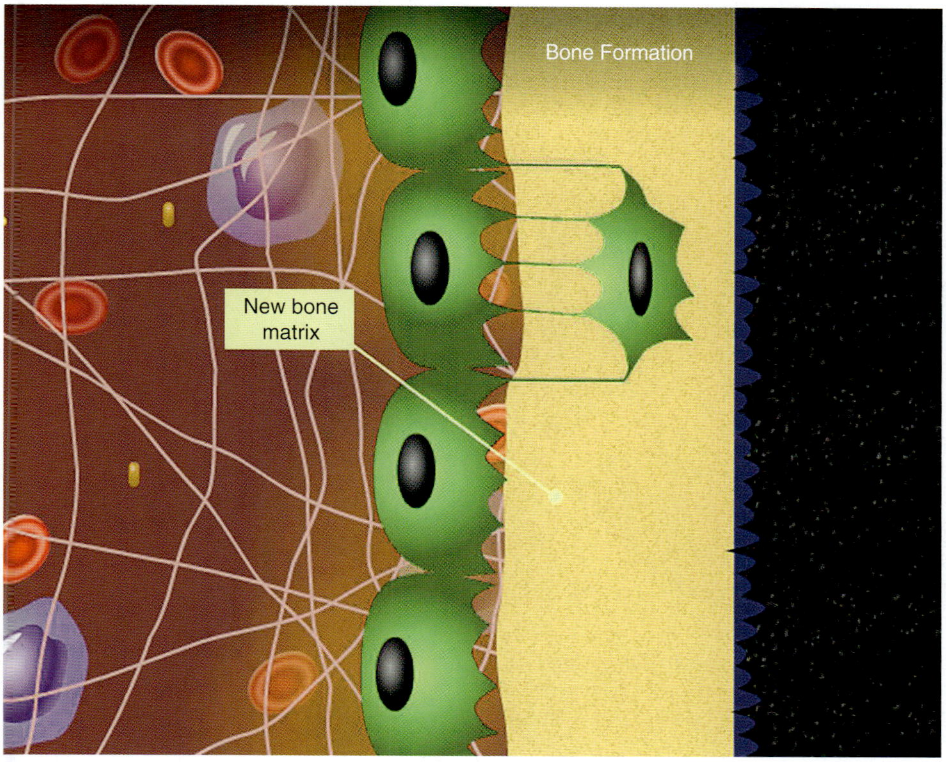

FIGURE 3-12 Canaliculi connect the osteocytes to the nutrient-rich surface of the forming new bone. *(Courtesy Dr. John E. Davies, University of Toronto.)*

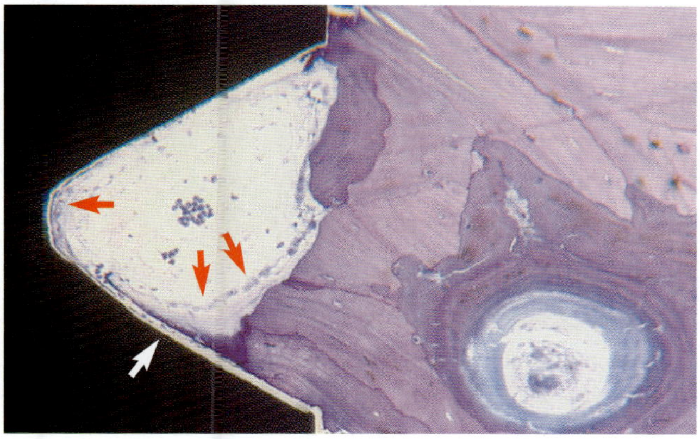

FIGURE 3-13 Light microscopic presentation of distant osteogenesis: osseointegration.

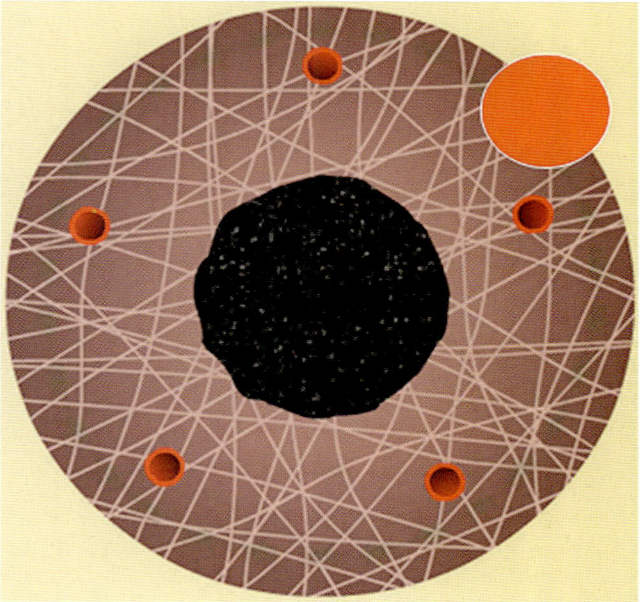

FIGURE 3-14 Distant osteogenesis begins on the surface of the osteotomy wall. *(Courtesy Dr. John E. Davies, University of Toronto.)*

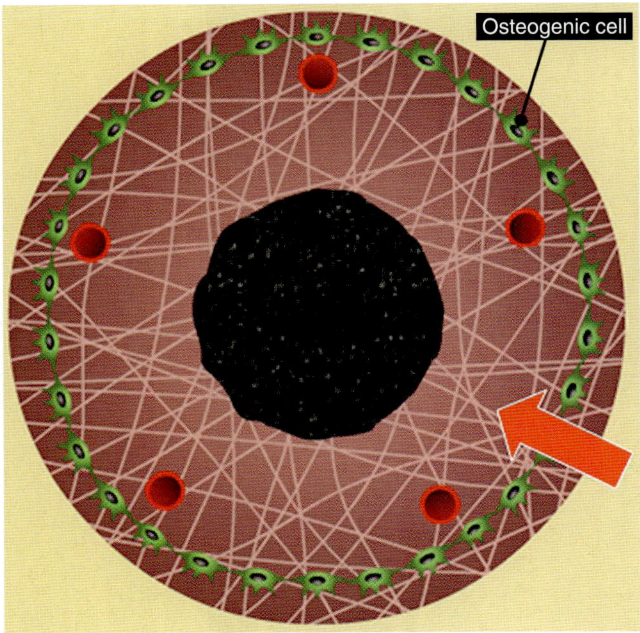

FIGURE 3-15 Osteogenic cells polarize on the surface of the osteotomy, become osteoblasts, and grow toward the implant surface. *(Courtesy Dr. John E. Davies, University of Toronto.)*

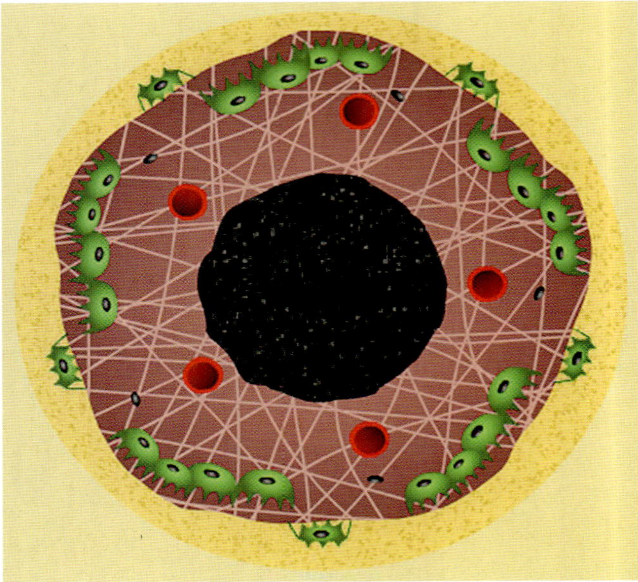

FIGURE 3-16 Osteoblasts are trapped within the new matrix. *(Courtesy Dr. John E. Davies, University of Toronto.)*

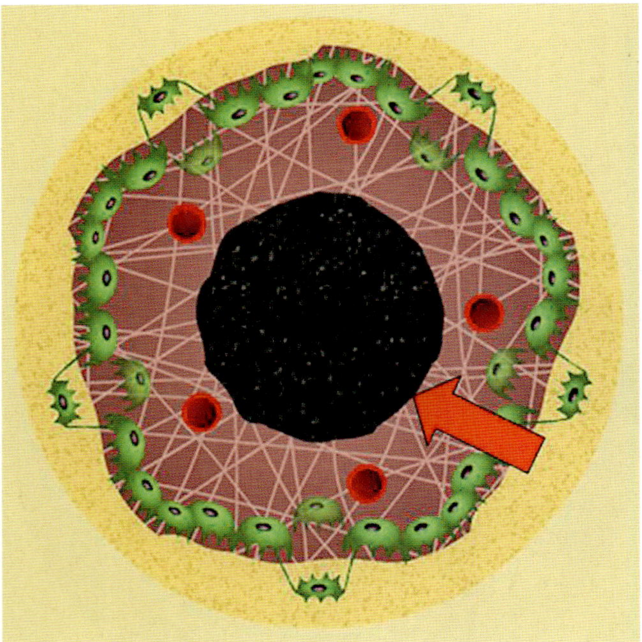

FIGURE 3-17 Osteocytes establishing canaliculi with the leading surface of the new forming bone. *(Courtesy Dr. John E. Davies, University of Toronto.)*

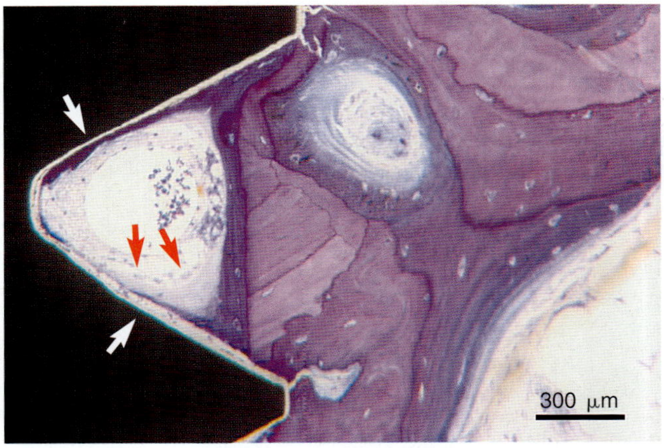

FIGURE 3-18 Light microscope presentation of contact osteogenesis: osseointegration.

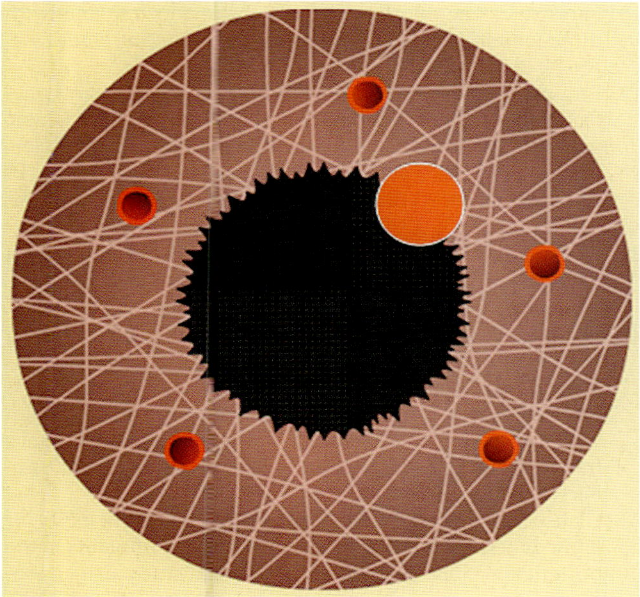

FIGURE 3-19 Contact osteogenesis begins on the surface of the implant. *(Courtesy Dr. John E. Davies, University of Toronto.)*

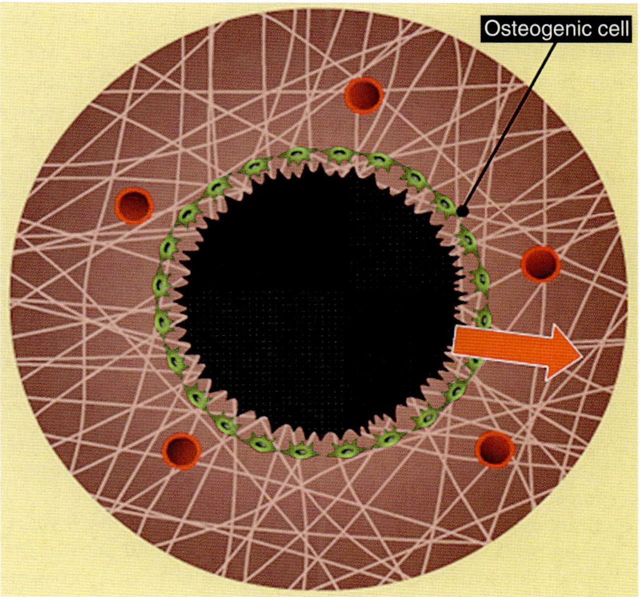

FIGURE 3-20 Osteogenic cells polarize on the surface of the implant, become osteoblasts, and begin growing away from the implant surface. *(Courtesy Dr. John E. Davies, University of Toronto.)*

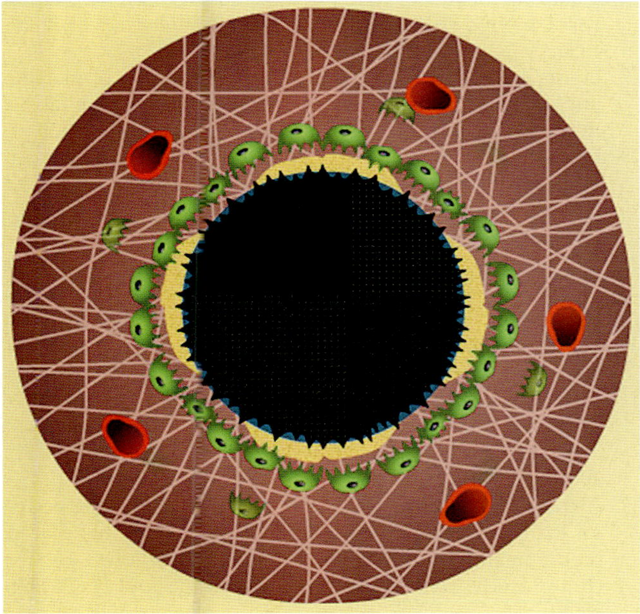

FIGURE 3-21 De novo bone formation represented by the *blue line* of new bone formation directly onto the implant surface. *(Courtesy Dr. John E. Davies, University of Toronto.)*

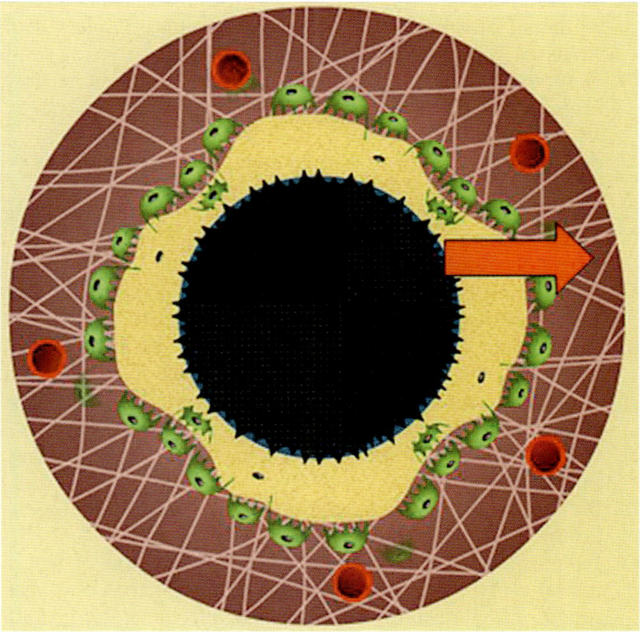

FIGURE 3-22 Formation of osteocytes and growth of bone from the implant surface toward the osteotomy wall. *(Courtesy Dr. John E. Davies, University of Toronto.)*

interpositional soft tissue through the simultaneous occurrence of contact osteogenesis in concert with distant osteogenesis. This phenomenon establishes a clinically stable implant and, in conjunction with a rigid, cross arch–stabilized prosthesis, allows for immediate loading of the implant within the host bone.

REFERENCES

1. Schnitman PA, Wbhrle PS, Rubenstein E, et al: Ten year results for Brånemark implants immediately loaded with fixed prostheses at implant placement. *Int J Oral Maxillofac Implants* 12:495-503, 1997.
2. Balshi TJ, Wolfinger GJ: Immediate loading of Brånemark implants in edentulous mandibles: *A preliminary report. Implant Dent* 6:83-88, 1997.
3. Brånemark P-I, Engstrand P, Ohrnell L-O, et al: Brånemark Novum: A new treatment concept for rehabilitation of the edentulous mandible. Preliminary results from a prospective clinical follow-up study. *Clin Implant Dent Relat Res* 1:2-16, 1999.
4. van Steenberghe D, Molly L, Jacobs R, et al: The immediate rehabilitation by means of a ready-made final fixed prosthesis in the edentulous mandible: A 1-year follow-up study of 50 consecutive patients. *Clin Oral Implant Res* 15:360-365, 2004.
5. Brånemark P-I, Breine U, Adell R: Intraosseous anchorage of dental prosthesis. I. Experimental studies. *Scand J Plast Reconstr Surg* 3:81-93, 1969.
6. Kasemo B, Lausmaa J: Biomaterial and implant surface science: A surface science approach. *Int J Oral Maxillofac Implants* 4:247-259, 1988.
7. Albrektsson T: Direct bone anchorage of dental implants. *J Prosthet Dent* 50:255-261, 1983.
8. Kasemo B: Biocompatibility of titanium implants: Surface science aspects. *J Prosthet Dent* 49:832-837, 1983.
9. Parr GR, Gardner LK, Toth RW: Titanium: The mystery metal of implant dentistry. Dental materials aspect. *J Prosthet Dent* 54:410-413, 1985.
10. Albrektsson T, Brånemark P-I, Hansson H-A, et al: Osseointegrated titanium implants. Requirements for ensuring a long-lasting direct bone-to-implant anchorage in man. *Acta Orthop Scand* 52:155-170, 1981.
11. Davis JE: Understanding peri-implant endosseous healing. *J Dent Educ* 67(8):932-949, 2003.
12. Brånemark P-I: Osseointegration and its experimental background. *J Prosthet Dent* 50:399-410, 1983.
13. Calandriello R, Tomatis M: Immediate function of single implants using Brånemark system: Prospective one year report of final restorations. *Appl Osseointegration Res* 4:32-40, 2004.
14. Malo P, Friberg B, Polozzi G, et al: Immediate and early function of Brånemark implants placed in the esthetic zone: A 1-year prospective clinical multicenter study. *Clin Implant Dent Relat Res* 5(Supple 1):37-46, 2003.
15. Kasemo B, Lausmaa J: Aspects of surface physics on titanium implants. *Swed Dent J* 28(Suppl):19-36, 1985.
16. Wennerberg A: *On surface roughness and implant incorporation.* Unpublished PhD thesis, Department of Biomaterials Handicap Research, Sweden, 1996, Goteborg University.
17. Park JY, Davis JE: Red blood cells and platelet interaction with titanium implant surfaces. *Clin Oral Implants Res* 11:530-539, 2000.
18. Larsson C: The interface between bone and implants with different surface oxide properties. *Appl Osseointegration Res* 1:9-14, 2000.
19. Schupbach P, Glauser R, Rocel A, et al: The human bone-oxidized titanium implant interface: A light microscopic scanning electron microscopic, black-scatter scanning electron microscopic, and energy-dispersive X-ray study of clinically retrieved dental implants. *Clin Implant Dent Relat Res* 7(Suppl 1):36-43, 2005.
20. Henry P, Tan A, Allen B, et al: Removal torque comparison of TiUnite and turned implants in the greyhound dog mandible. *Appl Osseointegration Res* 1:15-17, 2000.
21. Cormack DH: Bone. In: *Ham's histology,* ed 9, Philadelphia, 1987, Lippincott.
22. Rompen E, DaSilva D, Lundgren AK, et al: Stability measurements of a double-threaded titanium implant design with turned or oxidized surface. An experimental resonance frequency analysis study in the dog mandible. *Appl Osseointegration Res* 1:18-20, 2000.
23. Glauser R, Portmann M, Ruhstaller P, et al: Stability of immediately loaded machined and oxidized implants in the posterior maxilla. A comparative clinical study using resonance frequency analysis. *Appl Osseointegration Res* 2:27-29, 2001.
24. Roberts WE: Bone tissue interface. *J Dent Educ* 52:804-809, 1988.
25. Brunski JE: Biomechanical factors affecting the bone-dental implant interface. *Clin Mater* 3:153-201, 1992.
26. Masuda T, Yliheikkila PK, Felton DA, et al: Generalizations regarding the process and phenomenon of osseointegration. Part I. In vivo Studies. *Int J Oral Maxillofac Implants* 13:17-29, 1998.
27. Linder L, Obrant K, Boivin G: Osseointegration of metallic implants. II. Transmission electron microscopy in the rabbit. *Acta Orthop Scand* 60:135-139, 1989.
28. Leckholm U, Zarb GA: Patient selection and preparation. In: Brånemark P-I, Zarb GA, Albrektsson T: *Tissue integrated prostheses: Osseointegration in clinical dentistry,* Chicago, 1985, Quintessence, pp 199-210.
29. Brighton CT: Principles of fracture healing. In Murry JA, editor: *Instructional course lectures.* St. Louis, 1984, Mosby.
30. Walter M, Talbot IC: Wound healing. *In: General pathology,* ed 7, New York, 1996, Churchill Livingstone.
31. Becker W, Sennerby L, Bedrossian E, et al: Implant stability measurements for implants placed at the time of extraction: A cohort, prospective clinical trial. *J Periodontol* 76:391-397, 2005.
32. Glauser R, Ruhstaller P, Windisch S, et al: Immediate occlusal loading of Brånemark system TiUnite implants placed predominantly in soft bone: 4-year results of a prospective clinical study. *Clin Implant Dent Relat Res* 7(Suppl 1):S52-S59, 2005.
33. Sennerby L, Meredith N: Resonance frequency analysis: Measuring implant stability and osseointegration. *Compend Contin Educ Dent* 19:493-498, 500, 502; quiz 504, 1998.
34. Rasmusson L, Kahnberg KE, Tan A: Effects of implant design and surface on bone regeneration and implant stability: An experimental study in the dog mandible. *Clin Implant Dent Relat Res* 3:2-8, 2001.
35. Östman PO, Hellman M, Wendelhag I, et al: Resonance frequency analysis measurements of implants at placement surgery. *Int J Prosthodont* 19:77-83; discussion 84, 2006.
36. Osborn JF, Newesely H: Dynamic aspects of the implant-bone interface. In Heirnke G, editor: *Dental implants: Materials and systems,* Munchen, 1980, Carl Hanser Verlag.

37. Davies JE, Hosseini MM: Histodynamics of end osseous wound healing. In Davies JE, editor: *Bone engineering,* Toronto, 2000, Em Squared.
38. Davies JE, Chernecky R, Lowenberg B, et al: Deposition and resorption of calcified matrix in vitro by rat bone marrow cells. *Cells Mater* 1:3-15, 1991.
39. von Ebner V (Ritter von Rosenheim): Ober den feineren Bau der Knochensubstanz [On the fine structure of bone]. *SB Akad Wiss Math Nat Kl Abt III* 72:49-138, 1875.
40. Lazzara RJ: Bone response to dual acid-etched and machined titanium implant surfaces. In Davies JE, editor: *Bone engineering,* Toronto, 2000, Em Squared.
41. Park JY, Gemmell CH, Davies JE: Platelet interactions with titanium: Modulation of platelet activity by surface topography. *Biomaterials* 22:2671-2682, 2001.
42. Marx RE: Platelet concentrate: A strategy for accelerating and improving bone regeneration. In Davies JE, editor: *Bone engineering,* Toronto, 2000, Em Squared, pp 447-453.
43. Graves DT, Valentin-Opran A, Delgado R, et al: The potential role of platelet-derived growth factor as an autocrine or paracrine factor for human bone cells. *Connect Tissue Res* 23:209-218, 1989.
44. Tsukamoto T, Matsui T, Fukase M, et al: Platelet-derived growth factor β chain homodimer enhances chemotaxis and DNA synthesis in normal osteoblast-like cells (MC3T3-El). *Biochem Biophys Res Commun* 175(3):745-751, 1991.
45. Seppa H, Grotendorst G, Seppa S, et al: Platelet-derived growth factor is chemotactic for fibroblasts. *J Cell Biol* 92(2):584-588, 1982.
46. Postlethwaite AE, Keski-Oja J, Moses HL, et al: Stimulation of the chemotactic migration of human fibroblasts by transforming growth factor beta. *J Exp Med* 165(1):251-256, 1987.
47. Lucas PA, Caplan AI: Chemotactic response of embryonic limb bud mesenchymal cells and muscle-derived fibroblasts to transforming growth factor-beta. *Connect Tissue Res* 18(1):1-7, 1988.
48. Oprea WE, Karp JM, Hosseini MM, et al: Effect of platelet releasate on bone cell migration and recruitment in vitro. *J Craniofac Surg* (in press).
49. Carr AB, Laney WR: Maximum occlusal force levels in patients with osseointegrated oral implant prostheses and patients with complete dentures. *Int J Oral Maxillofac Implant* 2:101-108, 1987.
50. Park JY, Davies JE: Red blood cell and platelet interactions with titanium implant surfaces. *Clin Oral Implant Res* 11:530-539, 2000.
51. Bromberek BA, Enever PA, Shreiber DR, et al: Macrophages influence a competition of contact guidance and chemotaxis for fibroblast alignment in a fibrin gel coculture assay. *Exp Cell Res* 275:230-242, 2002.
52. Colman RW, Marder VJ, Salzman EW, et al: Overview of hemostasis. In Colman RW, Hirsh J, Marder VJ, et al, *editors: Hemostasis and thrombosis: Basic principles and clinical practice,* ed 2, Philadelphia, 1987, Lippincott, 3-17.
53. Halkier T: Blood coagulation. *In: Mechanisms in blood coagulation, fibrinolysis and the complement system,* Cambridge, 1991, Cambridge University Press, pp 1-127.
54. Gemmell CH, Park JY: Initial blood interactions with endosseous implant materials. In Davies JE, editor: *Bone engineering,* Toronto, 2000, Em Squared, pp 108-117.
55. Von Ebner V (Ritter von Rosenheim): Ober den feineren Bau der Knochensubstanz [On the fine structure of bone]. *SB Akad Wiss Math Nat Kl Abt III* 72:49-138, 1875.
56. Davies JE: In vitro modeling of the bone/implant interface. *Anat Rec* 245:426-445, 1996.
57. Bromberek BA, Enever PA, Shreiber DR, et al: Macrophages influence a competition of contact guidance and chemotaxis for fibroblast alignment in a fibrin gel coculture assay. *Exp Cell Res* 275:230-242, 2002.
58. Hosseini MM, Sodek J, Franke R-P, et al: The structure and composition of the bone-implant interface. In Davies JE, editor: *Bone engineering,* Toronto, 2000, Em Squared.
59. Dziedzic DM, Savva IH, Wilkinson DS, et al: Osteoconduction on, and bonding to, calcium phosphate ceramic implants. *Mat Res Soc Symp Proc* 414:147-156, 1996.
60. Brunski JB, Skalak R: Biomechanical considerations. In Worthington PH, Brånemark P-I, editors: *Osseointegration surgery: Application in the maxillofacial region,* Chicago, 1992, Quintessence, pp 15-39.

CHAPTER 4

Limitations in Treating the Edentulous Maxilla

As health care professionals and the general public increasingly understand the benefits of dental implants and accept their use, developing guidelines will allow for predictable treatment outcome for the edentulous patients using fixed, implant-supported prostheses. The use of fixed, implant-supported prostheses in the edentulous mandible has been well studied.[1,2] However, the edentulous maxilla warrants special consideration and is the focus of this chapter.

Treatment of the resorbed edentulous maxilla with a fixed profile prosthesis (Figure 4-1), presents with a set of unique problems. Bilateral maxillary sinuses (Figure 4-2) limit the practitioner's ability to place implants in the posterior portion of the maxilla, which is necessary to establish adequate anterior-posterior distribution (Figure 4-3) of the implants to support the occlusal loads generated and transferred to the alveolus by the fixed prosthesis. Therefore, two to four implants are placed in the premaxilla between edentulous areas 6 through 11 to support the retentive components of an implant-retained, tissue-supported overdenture (Figure 4-4).

Achieving adequate phonetics and stable masticatory function with a fixed prosthesis are the principle concerns in this group of patients. For the surgeon, the limited residual alveolar bone as well as the existence of the maxillary sinuses pose a number of challenges in treating this group of patients with a fixed prosthesis (Figure 4-5). The comprehensive evaluation of the edentulous maxilla is further complicated by the fact that both bone and soft tissue loss can begin before tooth removal as a result of generalized periodontitis, creating the appearance of long teeth (Figure 4-6). However, some edentulous patients may be missing clinical crowns only, without any accompanying soft or hard tissue loss, which is evident in evaluating the relationship of the cervical portion of the teeth in the clear acrylic copy of their existing full denture against the soft tissues of their edentulous ridge (Figure 4-7). Other patients may be missing a combination of teeth, soft tissue, and bone with associated changes in facial form; in this group, the patients' denture may be replacing not only their missing teeth, but in many cases the associated soft and hard tissues (Figure 4-8, *A* and 4-8, *B*). The dental practitioner must be aware of the extent of tissue loss in the edentulous patient to fabricate an aesthetic and functional fixed prosthesis.

Because of the aforementioned concerns, many patients who are missing their maxillary teeth are often treated with a tissue-supported, implant-retained prostheses (i.e., the maxillary overdenture), or, in many cases, patients are informed that they may not be candidates for implant treatment at all. The further use of a tissue-supported prosthesis, whether a full maxillary denture or a tissue-supported maxillary overdenture, leads to further atrophy of the alveolar bone,[3-5] creating a pool of unsatisfied patients who seek alternative treatment options other than the conventional full maxillary denture or the maxillary overdenture.

It is the practice of the author to use physiologic treatment for edentulous patients. The term *physiologic treatment* refers to the execution of a surgical and prosthetic treatment protocol that biomechanically mimics the same physiologic conditions prior to the removal of the patient's teeth. The edentulous alveolus undergoes both horizontal and vertical resorption in the absence of internal loading (Figure 4-9). Maintenance of the edentulous alveolar bone is the goal. The existence of the alveolar bone depends largely on the internal loading such as that provided by the tooth roots (Figure 4-10) or dental implants (Figure 4-11).[6] Lack of internal loading of the alveolus or presence of external pressure placed on the residual alveolar bone by the denture-baring areas during occlusal loading increase the rate of alveolar atrophy and diminish the volume of bone needed for placement of an endosseous implant (Figure 4-12). Fixed-implant restorations are totally implant-supported, without transference of load to denture-bearing areas, avoiding or minimizing the possibility of further resorption associated with tissue-borne prostheses.

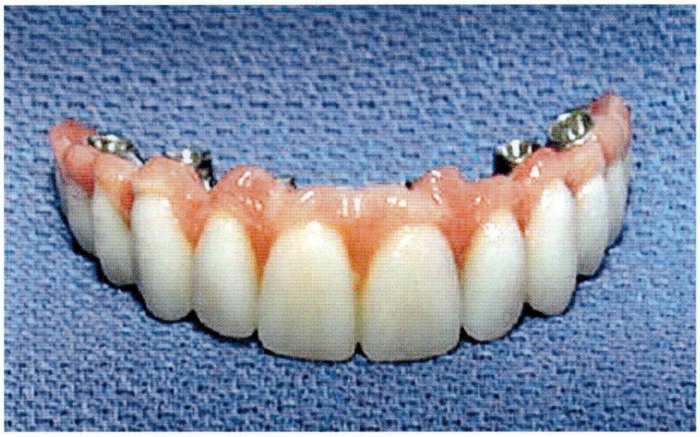

FIGURE 4-1 A fixed profile prosthesis replaces lost teeth and hard and soft tissues.

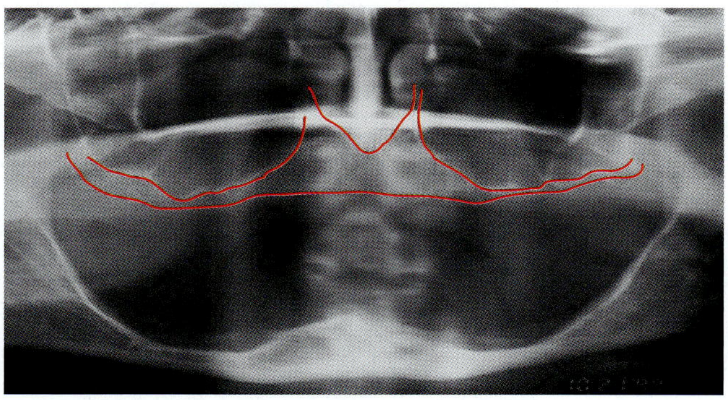

FIGURE 4-2 The posterior placement of implants is limited by the anterior extension of the pneumatized maxillary sinuses.

To predictably plan treatment for this group of patients with a fixed, implant-supported prosthesis, a systematic pretreatment approach to evaluating edentulous patients is essential.[7] This approach to treatment planning allows for better communication between the implant team as well as the patient, leading to predictable aesthetic and phonetic outcomes, as well as a satisfactory functional outcome. Systematic pretreatment planning criteria exist for

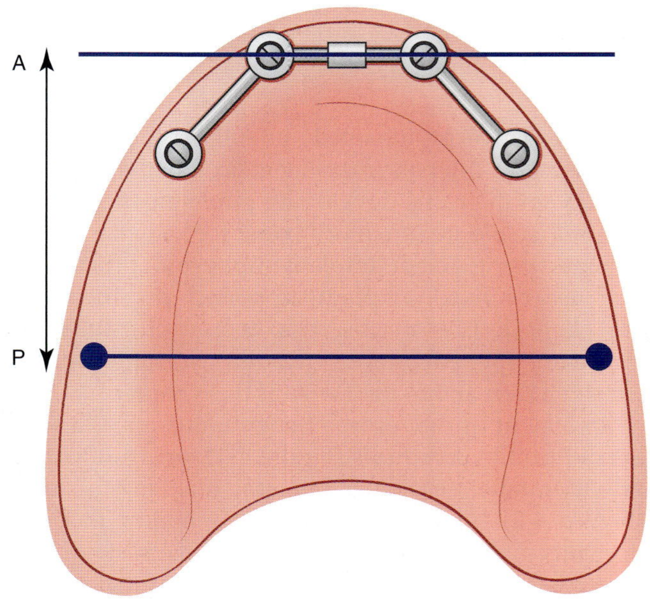

FIGURE 4-3 Appropriate anterior-posterior distribution of implants is necessary to support occlusal forces generated by a fixed prosthesis.

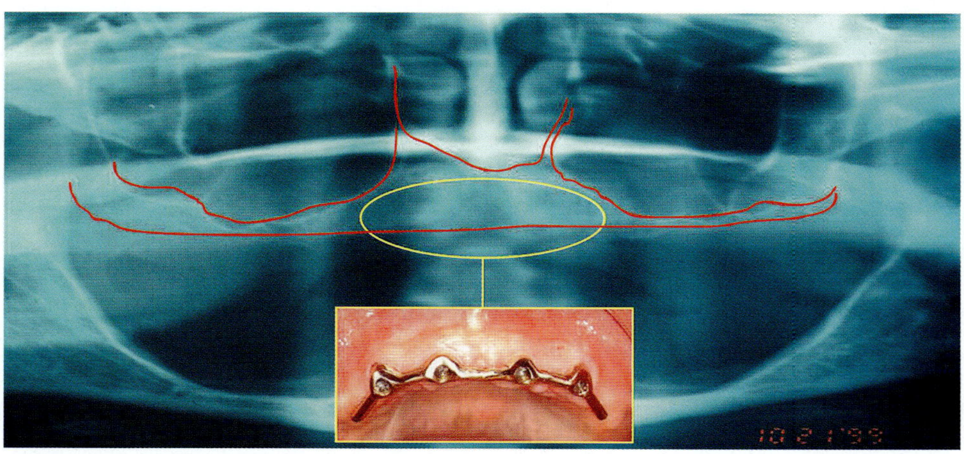

FIGURE 4-4 Placement of an implant in the premaxilla allows for the fabrication of a tissue-supported overdenture prosthesis.

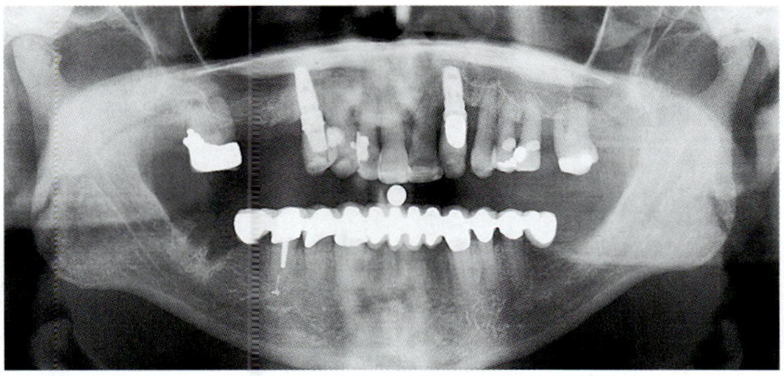

FIGURE 4-5 Lack of adequate bone volume in the premolar-molar region limits placement of implants without grafting.

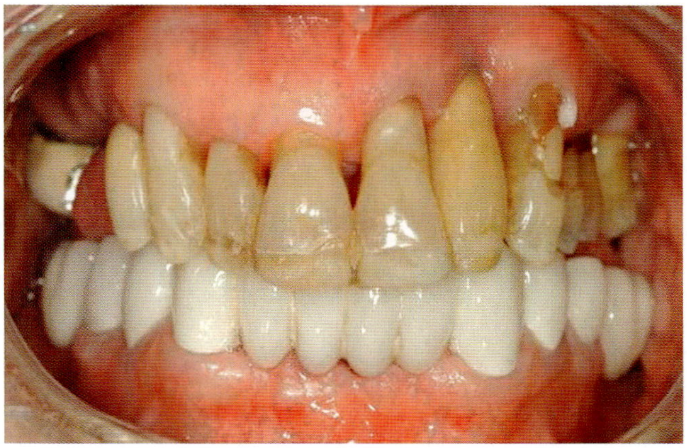

FIGURE 4-6 Secondary to loss of hard and soft tissue volume, unaesthetic appearance of "long teeth" is apparent.

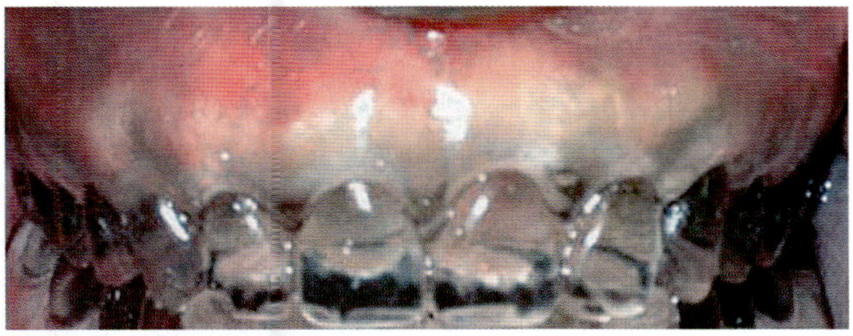

FIGURE 4-7 Intimate contact of the cervical portion of clear denture teeth against soft tissues suggests the loss of tooth structure only.

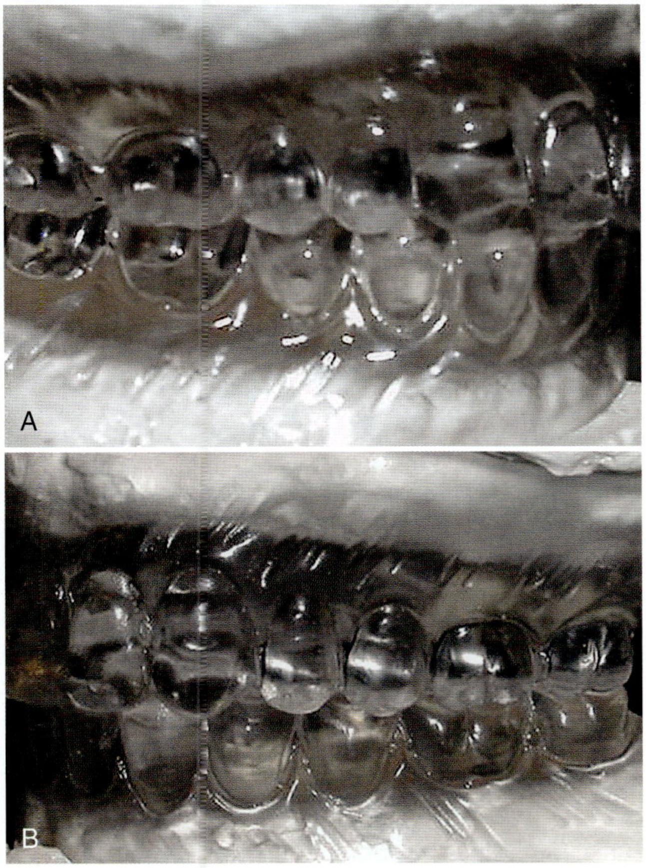

FIGURE 4-8 Space between the cervical portion of clear denture teeth and the edentulous ridge suggests the loss of teeth and hard as well as soft tissues.

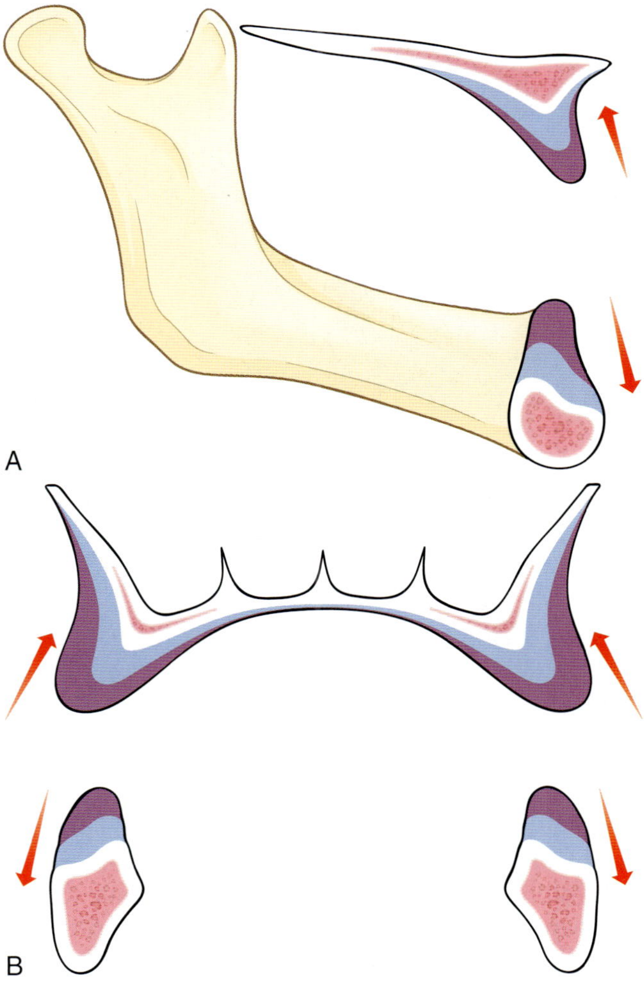

FIGURE 4-9 A, The lack of internal loading of the edentulous mandibular alveolus results in its resorption inferiorly as well as lingually. B, The lack of internal loading of the edentulous maxillary alveolus results in its resorption superiorly as well as palatally.

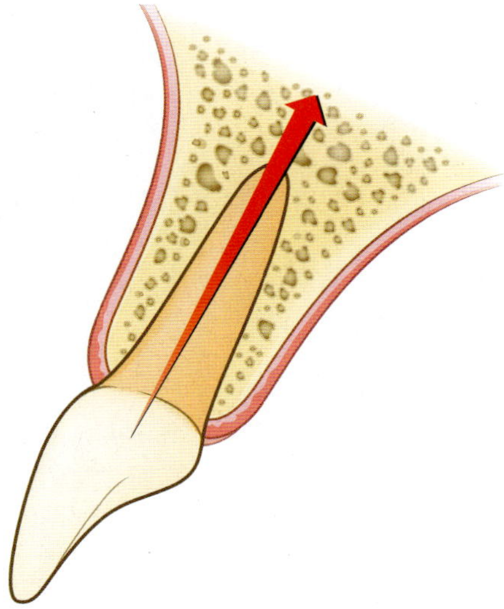

FIGURE 4-10 Internal loading of the alveolus through the transfer of occlusal loads through the tooth maintains the volume of alveolar bone.

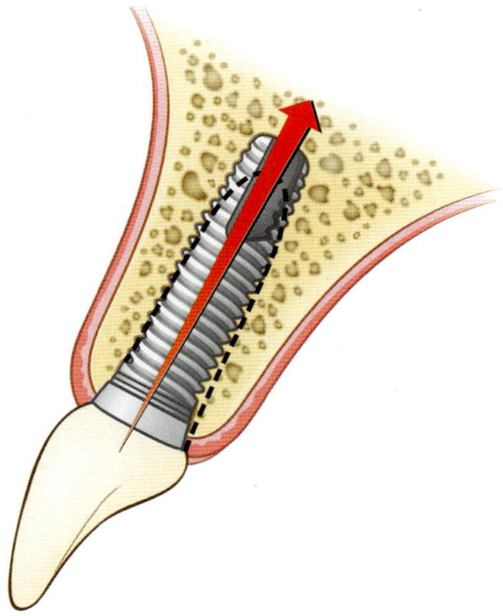

FIGURE 4-11 The transfer of occlusal loads through the implant complex mimics internal loading through a natural tooth.

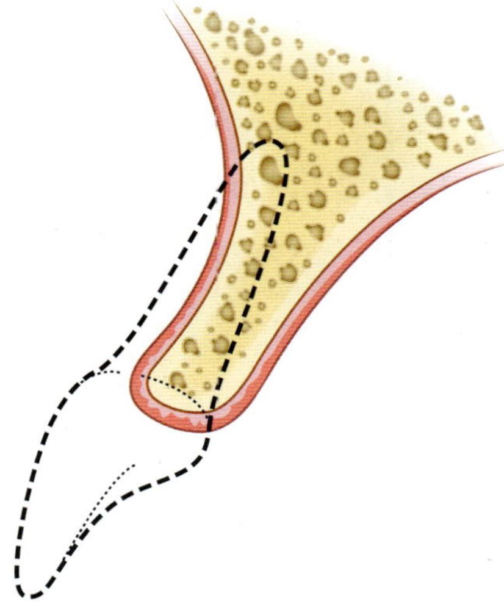

FIGURE 4-12 Disuse atrophy: lack of internal loading of the alveolus leads to the horizontal and subsequent vertical resorption of the alveolus.

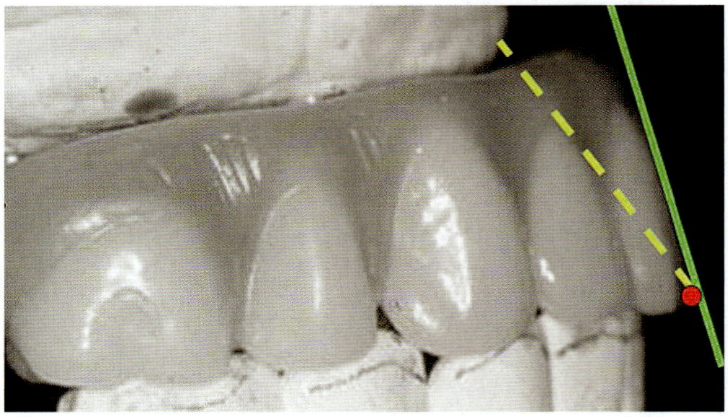

FIGURE 4-13 The proper vertical positioning of the anterior maxillary teeth lends adequate lip support.

evaluation of edentulous patients for fabrication of conventional removable full dentures. McGarry et al.[8] developed a classification of complete edentulism using conventional removable dentures as the final treatment. The classification considers the quantity of the residual edentulous ridge, its morphology or topography, and the relationship of the maxilla to the mandible. Interarch space, tongue anatomy, and attachment of the musculature to the edentulous ridge are considered. The possible need for preprosthetic surgical procedures is also evaluated. These evaluation criteria initially allow the treating team to comprehensively consider all existing conditions and to forecast potential problems prior to the initiation of the treatment. The treating team and the patient communicate about the potential outcome in light of preexisting conditions, which creates realistic expectations.

In reviewing the literature, Wood and Vermilyea[9] have concluded that a fixed maxillary prosthesis is not possible in most cases because of improper phonetics, lack of lip support, and the inability of patients to maintain adequate oral hygiene. The three objections cited by Wood and Vermilyea are generally not issues. The various aspects of a properly fabricated full denture, as well as each of the three objections raised by Wood and Vermilyea are reviewed in detail in the remainder of this chapter. It is imperative to understand the proper positioning of the anterior maxillary teeth because lip support depends on the proper position of the cervical portion of the anterior maxillary teeth within the denture base (Figure 4-13).[10,11]

PHONETICS

The incisal positions of the anterior maxillary teeth are involved with the labiodental sounds "F" and "V" (Figure 4-14). The proper anterior-posterior positioning of the incisal tip is largely determined by the apposing dentition, which plays a vital role in the amount of overjet and overbite needed. Dental technicians and restorative dentists generally are very well aware of the proper positioning of the incisal portion of anterior maxillary teeth. The dentoalveolar sounds "T," "D," and "S" are properly produced by the seal or the lack of space between the necks of the anterior maxillary teeth and the palatal and buccal soft tissues (Figure 4-15). This is predictably achieved by the proper design and processing of the profile prosthesis by a restorative dentist and laboratory technician. Therefore, with the proper tooth positioning and fabrication of the contour of the soft tissue surface of the profile prosthesis, phonetics using a fixed, implant-supported prosthesis should be well controlled for patients with edentulous maxilla.

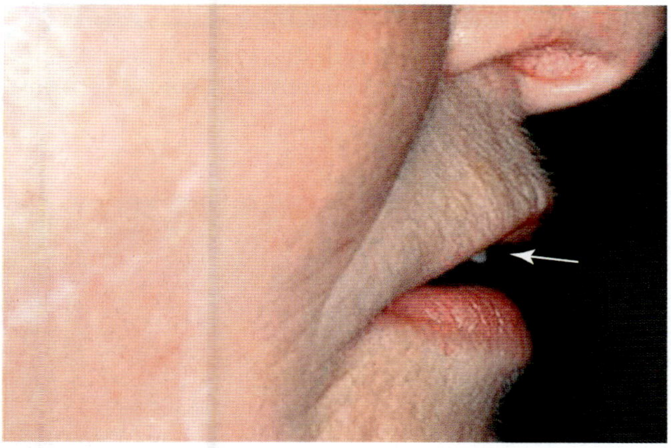

FIGURE 4-14 Labiodental sounds are produced by the incisal portion of the anterior maxillary tooth position.

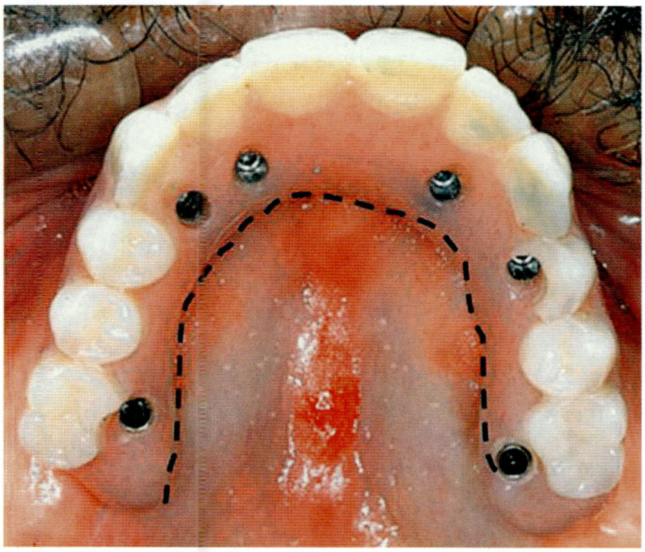

FIGURE 4-15 Dentoalveolar sounds are produced by the palatal seal between the cervical position of the anterior maxillary teeth and the palatal soft tissues.

LIP SUPPORT

It is generally accepted that the flange of the full denture is the primary criterion needed for proper upper lip support. It is the experience of the author that this is not the case in the majority of patients (Figure 4-16, *A*, 16, *B*, and 16, *C*). In cases in which inadequate lip support is identified, the anterior maxillary teeth are generally not positioned properly, leading to the mistaken conclusion that a flange is needed in the final prosthesis to establish lip support. This inaccurate conclusion leads to the fabrication of an overdenture or a new conventional full denture, automatically eliminating this group of patients as candidates for a prosthesis and depriving them of the benefits of a fixed, implant-supported prosthesis.

Lip support is established in part by the proper positioning of the incisal two-thirds of the anterior maxillary teeth.[10] In addition, the cervical one-third of the anterior maxillary teeth are also responsible for upper lip support (Figure 4-17).[11] A common mistake is to set the cervical portion of the anterior maxillary teeth over the edentulous ridge as in a class I edentulous, nonresorbed ridge. A class I edentulous ridge lacks vertical and horizontal alveolar atrophy. The cervical region of the denture teeth are positioned directly over the ridge. However, in most edentulous maxillae, there is vertical and horizontal resorption of the maxilla. The horizontal resorption places the edentulous ridge posterior to the cervical portion of the denture tooth. If the necks of the denture teeth are placed directly over the ridge, a significant lack of upper lip support will be evident clinically. It is essential for the laboratory technician to communicate with the implant team and be aware of the patient's clinical appearance to position the anterior maxillary teeth in the proper axis and avoid the misdiagnosis of inadequate lip support using a fixed prosthesis in this group of patients (see Figure 4-13).

Although the flange of a removable prosthesis may contribute to lip support, the proper positioning of the cervical two-thirds of the anterior maxillary teeth in the anterior-posterior position, independent of the position of the maxillary edentulous ridge and in line with the incisal portion of the tooth, is more effective for proper lip support.

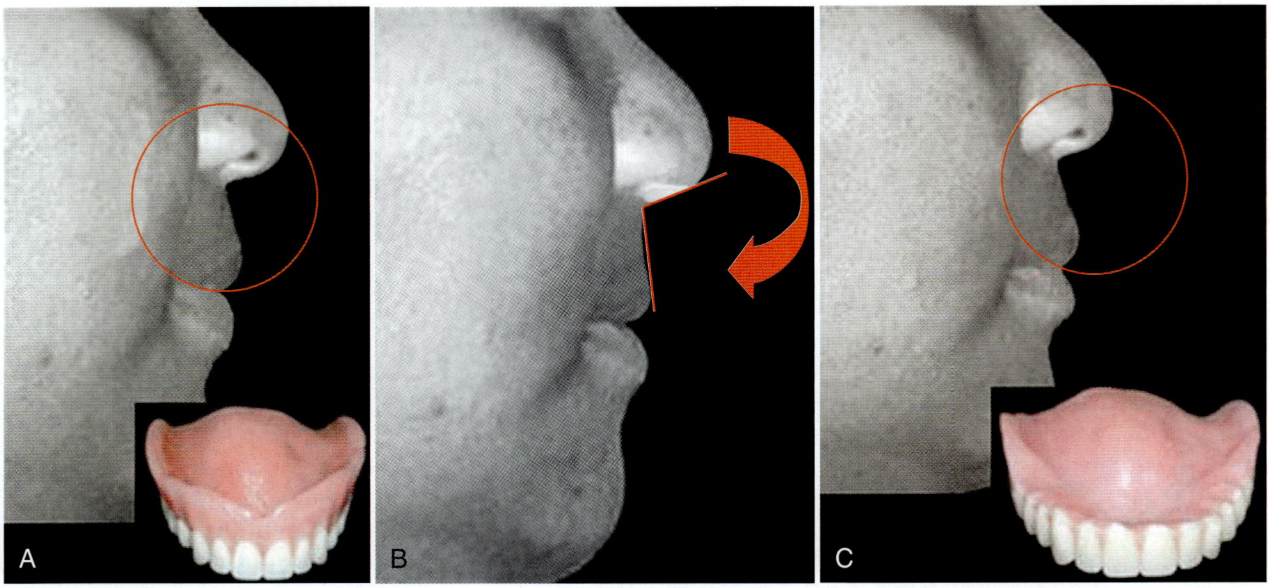

FIGURE 4-16 A, An acute nasolabial angle results from the flange of the full upper denture in the patient's mouth. B, An obtuse nasolabial angle resulting from collapse of the upper lip with the full upper denture removed. C, A natural nasolabial angle with the flange removed between the first bicuspids of the full upper denture in place.

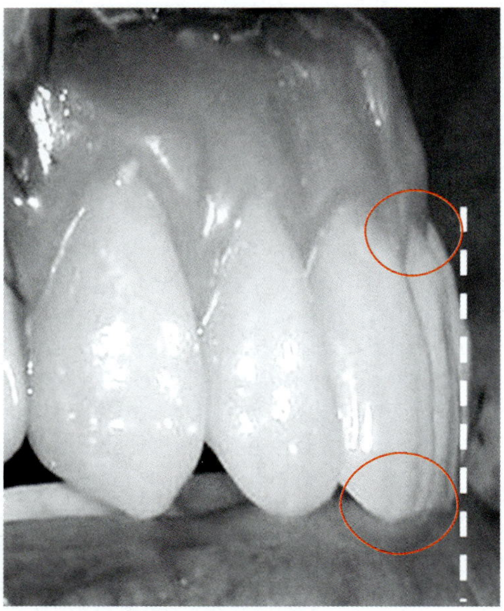

FIGURE 4-17 Proper positioning of the anterior maxillary teeth of the profile prosthesis results in proper lip support.

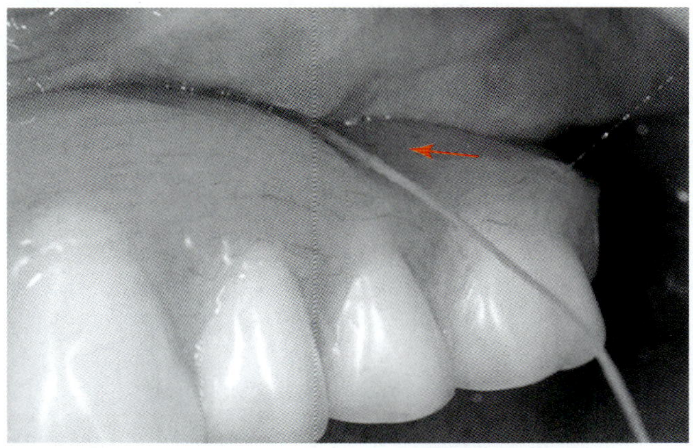

FIGURE 4-18 Channels created within the profile prosthesis to assist in floss threading for oral hygiene purposes.

ORAL HYGIENE

The relationship of the base of the profile prosthesis to the crest of the ridge is identical in contour to the pontic contours in fixed bridges. Patients may easily thread dental floss between implant abutments and clean the undersurface of the profile prosthesis if needed (Figure 4-18). In older patients or for patients with limited dexterity, channels can be created in the bulk of the acrylic to guide the dental floss in between the implants.

It should be clear that a properly fabricated, implant-supported, fixed maxillary prosthesis is a well-tolerated and functional appliance for this group of patients.

The fundamental principles of bone physiology allow for internal loading of the edentulous maxilla, with an implant-supported prosthesis halting further resorption of the residual alveolus. Proper tooth positioning within the prosthesis also allows for a predictable treatment outcome addressing proper facial support and normal phonetics, as well as prosthetic design allowing proper home care for patients with edentulous maxilla treated with a fixed-profile prosthesis.

REFERENCES

1. Schnitman PA: Ten-year result for Brånemark implants immediately loaded with fixed prostheses at implant placement. *Int J Oral Maxillofac Implants* 12:495-503, 1997.
2. Schnitman PA: Immediate fixed interim prostheses supported by two-stage threaded implants: methodology and results. *J Oral Implant* 16:96-105, 1990.
3. Adell R: A long term follow-up study of osseointegrated implants in the treatment of totally edentulous jaws. *J Oral Maxillofac Implants* 5:347-359, 1990.
4. Jemt T: A 5 year prospective multicenter follow-up report on overdentures supported by osseointegrated implants. *J Oral Maxillofac Implants* 11:291-298, 1996.
5. Gilson BS: The sickness impact profile. Development of an outcome measure of health care. *Am J Public Health* 65:1304-1310, 1975.
6. Brånemark P-I, Zarb G, Albrektsson T, editors: *Tissue-integrated prostheses,* Chicago, 1980, Quintessence.
7. Bedrossian E: Fixed-prosthetic implant restoration of the edentulous maxilla: A systematic pretreatment evaluation method. *J Oral Maxillofac Surg* 66:112-122, 2008.
8. McGarry TJ, Nimmo A, Skiba JF, et al: Classification system for complete edentulism. *J Prosthodont* 8:27-39, 1999.
9. Wood M, Vermilyea SG: A review of selected dental literature on evidence-based treatment planning for dental implants: Report of the Committee on Research in Fixed Prosthodontics of the Academy of Fixed Prosthodontics. *J Prosthet Dent* 92:447-462, 2004.
10. Salinas T: Implant treatment and the edentulous maxilla. *Pract Periodontics Aesthet Dent* 6(3):247-248, 2004.
11. Zitzmann NU, et al: Treatment plan for restoring the edentulous maxilla with implant-supported restorations. Removable overdenture verses fixed partial denture design. *J Prosthetic Dent* 82:188-196, 1999.

CHAPTER 5

Systematic Pretreatment Evaluation of the Edentulous Maxilla

Three factors are key determinants for the successful treatment of the completely edentulous maxilla with a fixed restoration. These factors, which can be determined early in the examination process, are (1) the presence or absence of a composite defect; (2) the visibility or lack thereof of the residual ridge crest without the denture in place, with normal smile and without use of retractors; and (3) the amount of bone available in three separate zones of the maxilla, as revealed in a panoramic survey. Prior to discussing each of the three factors for the systematic evaluation of the edentulous maxilla, it may be prudent to establish several baseline criteria. The implant-support requirements of all three fixed restorative options discussed in this chapter are the same as the requirements for a fully implant-supported, nonresilient maxillary restoration. A minimum of four implants should be used, although the option to place more than four may be considered, depending on the available bone volume and other functional considerations.[1,2] The most important factor is the arch-form distribution of those implants with both posterior and anterior support. Evaluation of the three radiographic zones allows for a preoperative determination of whether adequate arch-form support for a fixed restoration is achievable to support the planned occlusal plane. As a general principle, cantilevers in fixed maxillary restorations should be avoided or minimized to one tooth to achieve an adequate functional occlusion.[3-7] Several descriptions of fixed prostheses used to restore completely edentulous maxilla have been published.[8-11] This discussion focuses on the application of three principal designs for implant-supported dental prostheses. These three variations have been chosen based on their ability to restore a broad range of soft tissue deficits. They are (1) metal-ceramic restoration, (2) fixed-hybrid restoration, and (3) fixed-removable restoration.

FIXED-MAXILLARY PROSTHESES

Metal-ceramic restorations may be either screw- or cement-retained.[12-14] Recognizing that ceramic restorations can include teeth that are longer than normal and gingival replacement, emphasis is on metal-ceramic restorations used to replace the clinical crowns of missing teeth only (Figure 5-1).

The hybrid prosthesis is a denture tooth and acrylic design with either a milled titanium or cast-gold framework (Figure 5-2). Practitioners using early designs of implant-supported denture tooth and acrylic fixed prostheses reported phonetic changes as a routine complication, caused by air escaping during speech.[15] A later design known as *profile prosthesis*[16] uses a framework design with subgingival abutment emergence that allows an acrylic resin wrap; the wrap butts up against the tissue as an ovate pontic so that air does not escape and cause phonetic problems. Because a ridge lap is avoided with the convex emergence from the ridge crest, oral hygiene access can be maintained in a manner similar to natural-tooth, fixed, partial-denture pontics.[16] A variation of this design uses gingival porcelains or composite with all-ceramic

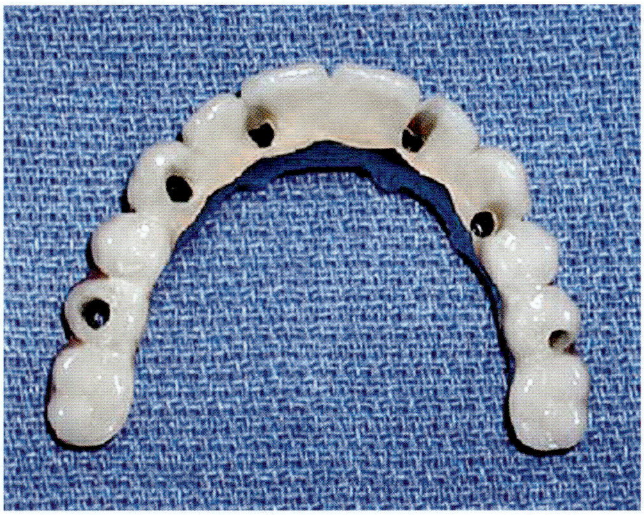

FIGURE 5-1 Ceramo-metal prosthesis may be fabricated for full-arch replacement.

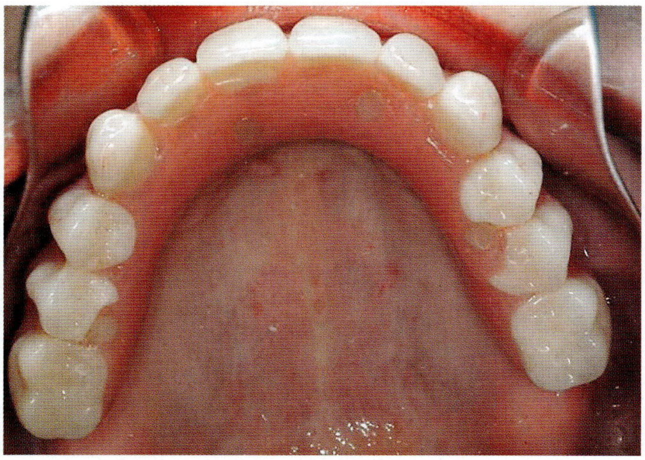

FIGURE 5-2 Profile prosthesis may be fabricated for full-arch replacement.

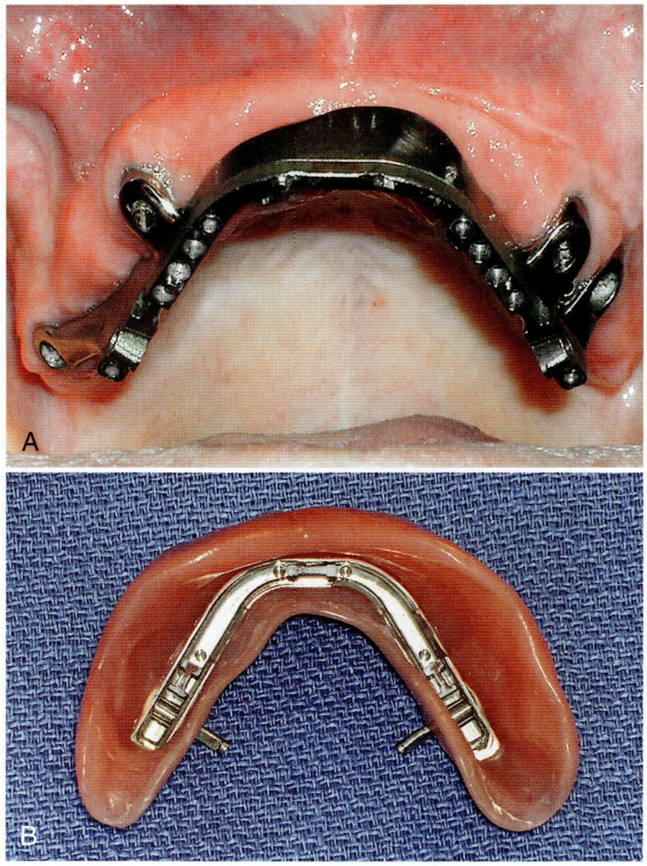

FIGURE 5-3 The Marius bridge, a fixed, detachable prosthesis, may be fabricated for full-arch replacement.

crowns cemented to the framework, which can be used if a porcelain restoration is desired.

For situations in which a labial flange is desirable, a fixed-removable prosthesis can be made with any number of attachments. Figure 5-3 demonstrates a fixed-removable design known as a *Marius bridge* that is nonresilient and fully implant-supported.[17] Fixed-removable designs use a milled titanium or cast meso bar supporting a patient-removable superstructure held in place with a locking mechanism. This allows a ridge lap or flange design, with a suprastructure removable for oral hygiene access. Because a fixed-detachable restoration does not depend on soft tissue support, no unnatural palatal extensions are required.

To determine which of these prostheses is most appropriate, identification of the presence or the lack of a composite defect and the relationship of the transition line to the patient's smile line needs to be made. Evaluation of these factors is not intended to be a substitute for thorough diagnosis and development of a treatment plan. However, such evaluation can provide differential diagnosis information specific to the aesthetic, prosthetic, and biomechanical requirements of fixed, implant-supported maxillary restorations.[18]

PRESENCE OR ABSENCE OF A COMPOSITE DEFECT

The first criterion to consider is the presence or absence of a composite defect. Edentulous patients may present with intact alveolar bone volume and be missing only the clinical crowns, or they may present with missing

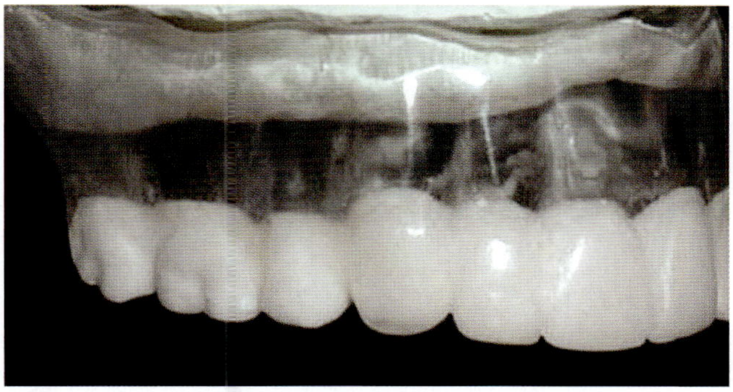

FIGURE 5-4 Composite defect: Patients missing teeth, soft tissues, and hard tissue mass.

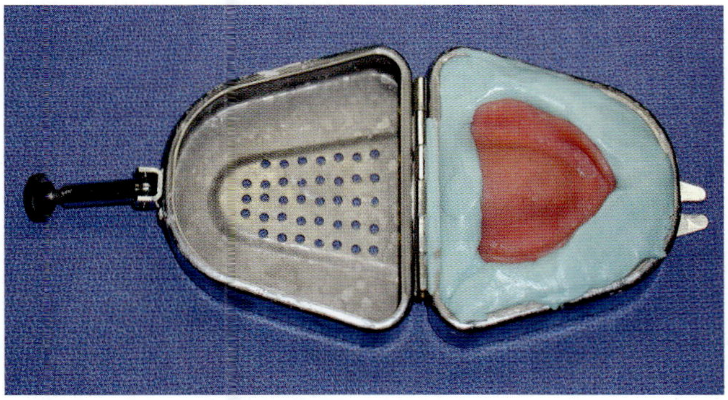

FIGURE 5-5 The Lang duplicator is used to copy the patient's existing full denture.

teeth as well as resorption of their alveolar bone and loss of soft tissues. Differentiating between these two types of patients is essential to creating an aesthetic, definitive fixed prosthesis. Patients missing soft tissue and underlying supporting bone in addition to teeth have a *composite defect* (Figure 5-4). To evaluate the relative soft and hard tissue deficiencies, it is advisable to use a denture or denture set up in wax in which proper tooth position and interarch relationship (proper vertical dimension of occlusion) has been confirmed.

With a satisfactory denture, thickness of the maxillary denture base and flange can be used to assess the presence or absence of composite defect. A thick denture base and flange indicate moderate to advanced resorption of the maxilla. In situations in which minimal soft and hard tissue resorption has occurred, a "tooth-only defect" is present. For this group of patients, a thin denture base and a very thin or absent flange, especially in the anterior sextant, indicate an intact alveolus[19] and therefore the absence of composite defect.

It should be noted that defects resulting from resorption of bone and missing soft tissue occur in both the horizontal and vertical planes, and may not be immediately obvious. To fully assess the presence or absence of a composite defect, duplication of the confirmed denture or tooth set-up by the dental technician or dentist using a denture duplicator can be useful (Figure 5-5). A transparent acrylic resin duplicate of the patient's denture is then placed intraorally, and the position of the cervical portion of the teeth and their relationship to the crest of the edentulous ridge is noted. For patients who present with no space between the cervical portion of the duplicated denture teeth and the edentulous ridge in either horizontal or vertical planes, a tooth-only defect is diagnosed (Figure 5-6). In this situation, interarch space minimum requirements for the implant system and desired restoration still need to be observed. For patients who present with moderate to significant space between the cervical portion of the duplicated denture teeth and the edentulous ridge, a composite defect is identified (Figure 5-7). Table 5-1 illustrates these considerations.

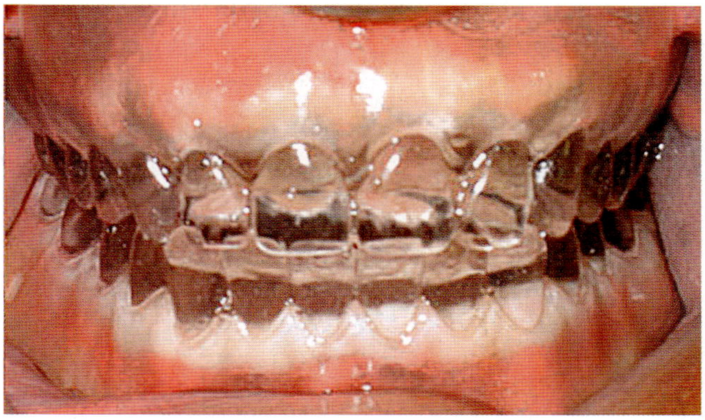

FIGURE 5-6 Clear dentures allow visualization of a tooth-only defect without any soft or hard tissue resorption.

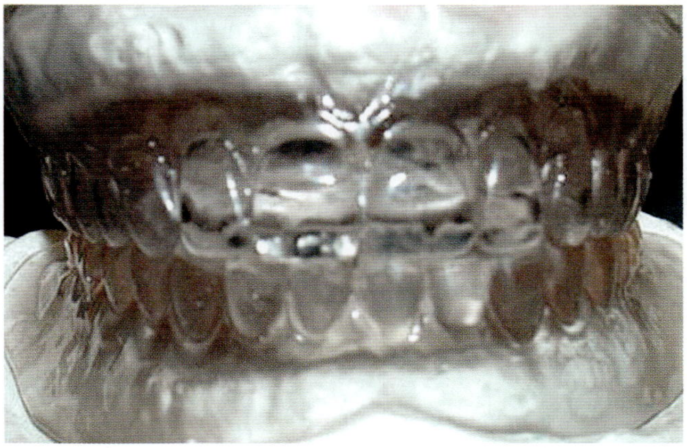

FIGURE 5-7 Moderate composite defect is evident by the space between the cervical portion of the teeth and the edentulous crest.

Preoperative determination of the presence or absence of a composite defect allows the clinician to

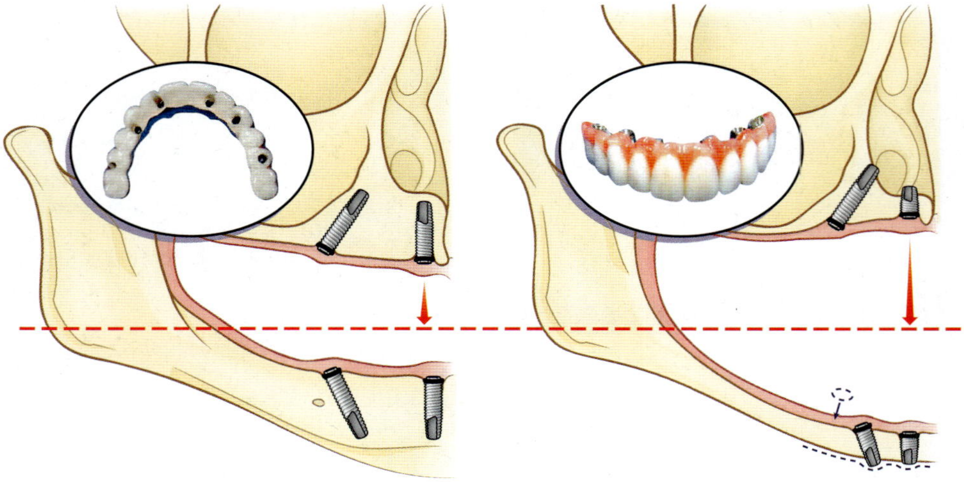

FIGURE 5-8 In the presence of a tooth-only defect, a ceramo-metal prosthesis is fabricated. In the presence of composite defects, a profile prosthesis or a fixed detachable prosthesis is fabricated.

TABLE 5-1

Presence or Absence of a Composite Defect

Intraoral Status	Diagnosis	Definitive Prosthesis
No space between the cervical portion of the duplicate denture teeth and the edentulous ridge	Tooth-only defect	Metal-ceramic
Moderate to significant space between the cervical portion of the duplicate denture teeth and the edentulous ridge	Composite defect	Marius bridge (fixed-detachable) or profile prosthesis (hybrid)

determine the restorative space available for abutments and framework design. In the absence of a composite defect, a metal-ceramic restoration without extensive gingival porcelains can be used. A composite defect requires a fixed dental prosthesis. Either a profile prosthesis or Marius bridge may be used (Figure 5-8).

VISIBILITY OF THE RESIDUAL RIDGE CREST

The second factor to consider in selecting an appropriate prosthesis is the visibility of the edentulous ridge crest at rest and during animation. This section describes evaluation of the *transition line.* To maximize the aesthetic result of a prosthetic, the clinician must evaluate the potential for visibility of the transition between the prosthesis and the soft tissue of the edentulous maxillary ridge without the maxillary denture in place, both in the anterior maxilla and the buccal corridor.

With the patient's maxillary denture removed, the patient should be asked to smile (Figure 5-9). If the soft tissue of the edentulous ridge cannot be seen, the transition between an implant-supported prosthesis and the residual soft tissue crest will not be visible, allowing a degree of flexibility for issues such as color match, shadows, and contour change in the junction of the restoration against soft tissue. A transition line that is hidden during animation results in an aesthetically pleasing outcome (Figure 5-10 and Table 5-2).

If the patient does display the residual ridge soft tissue crest while smiling, the transition between an implant restoration and the soft tissue will be visible, and the aesthetic consequences of this depend on whether the patient also has a composite defect. If the patient is missing teeth but has an intact soft tissue volume, a metal-ceramic restoration can be used, and the visible gingiva will improve the aesthetics rather

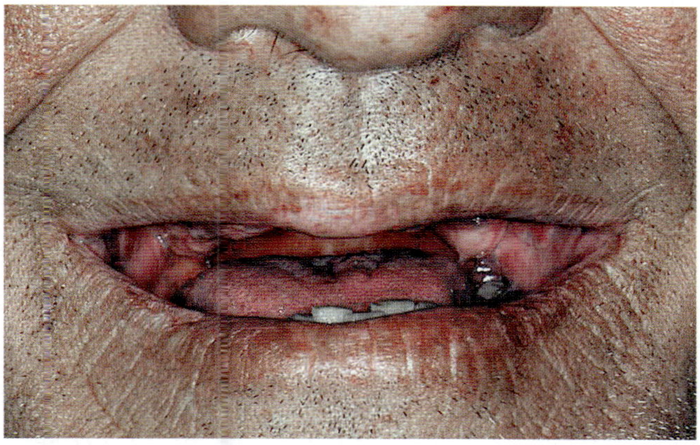

FIGURE 5-9 A hidden transition line: The edentulous ridge of the patient is not visualized during animation.

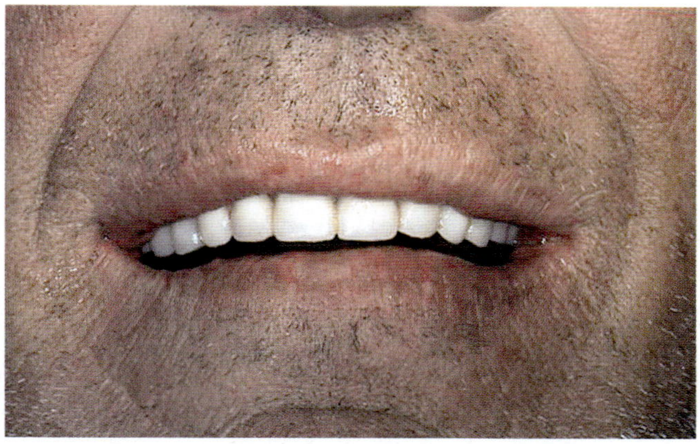

FIGURE 5-10 With the profile prosthesis in place, the transition line of the prosthesis and the patient's soft tissues are not visible during animation.

than detract from them. This assumes that the implants are placed in planned tooth positions. However, when a composite defect is present, a metal-ceramic, tooth-only restoration will result in an aesthetic compromise because the teeth will appear longer than normal. If a profile prosthesis is used with a visible residual ridge crest, the junction of the artificial gingiva and the natural soft tissue will be visible, and the differences in texture and contour between the two may be obvious and unaesthetic (Figure 5-11).

One method for avoiding a visible transition line is to initially reduce the residual ridge height through an alveolectomy and or alveoloplasty to a point at which the crest is no longer visible. Implants can then be placed and restored with provisional as well as final *profile prostheses.* If the ridge is not reduced, the use of a fixed-detachable prosthesis such as the Marius bridge, with a flange that overlaps the gingival junction, is indicated to hide the transition line during animation. This prosthesis can be removed by the patient, so oral hygiene is not compromised; yet it provides the stability and function of a fixed restoration.

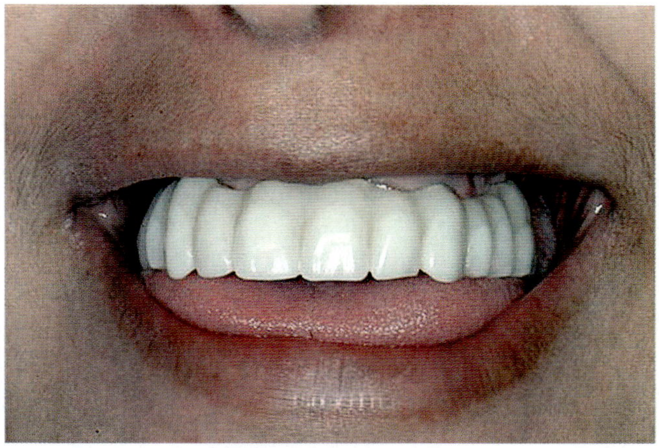

FIGURE 5-11 A visible transition line during animation results in an unaesthetic exposure of the prosthesis and the edentulous ridge.

RADIOGRAPHIC EVALUATION TO ASSESS MAXILLARY ZONES

The third criterion for adoption of a surgical protocol for treatment of the edentulous maxilla with a fixed

TABLE 5-2

Guidelines for Optimal Fixed Dental Prosthetic Choice

	Composite Defect	Tooth-Only Defect
Ridge visible	Marius bridge (Fixed-removable)	Metal-ceramic restoration
Ridge invisible	Profile prosthesis (Fixed hybrid) or Marius bridge (Fixed-removable)	Metal-ceramic restoration

prosthesis is identification of the presence or absence of the *zones of the maxilla.* This is accomplished by reviewing the patient's radiographs. When immediate loading of the maxilla is considered, I recommend a graftless approach. Division of the edentulous maxilla into three radiographic zones allows for a systematic assessment of the residual alveolar bone available for implant placement, which helps determine an appropriate surgical approach. The relationship between the residual maxillary alveolus and the nasal cavity and the position and size of the maxillary sinuses are evaluated radiographically. The alveolar bone of the anterior maxilla from cuspid to cuspid is designated as zone 1, the premolar region is zone II, and the molar region is designated as zone III (Figure 5-12). Analysis of radiographic results according to this schema can enable the surgical and restorative teams to devise a preliminary treatment plan. In complex or borderline situations, three-dimensional radiographic evaluation may still be necessary to confirm preliminary conclusions.

The presence or absence of maxillary zones strongly influences surgical technique (Figure 5-13). If zones I, II, and III are present, axial implants may be placed (Figure 5-14). If zones I and II are present, the tilted-implant prosthesis (Figure 5-15) may be considered. If zone I is the only zone present, zygomatic treatment (Figure 5-16) is considered. A severely atrophied maxilla presents with complete resorption of the maxillary alveolus. Therefore, zones I, II, and III are absent. For these rare cases, quad-zygomatic treatment may be considered (Figure 5-17 and Table 5-3). Because the surgical protocol for these treatments does not involve bone grafting, immediate loading of the implants is considered if the surgical criteria are met.

SPECIAL CONSIDERATIONS

It is paramount to consider the topography of the edentulous ridge and its relationship to the patient's smile line (Figure 5-18). On occasion, the degree of

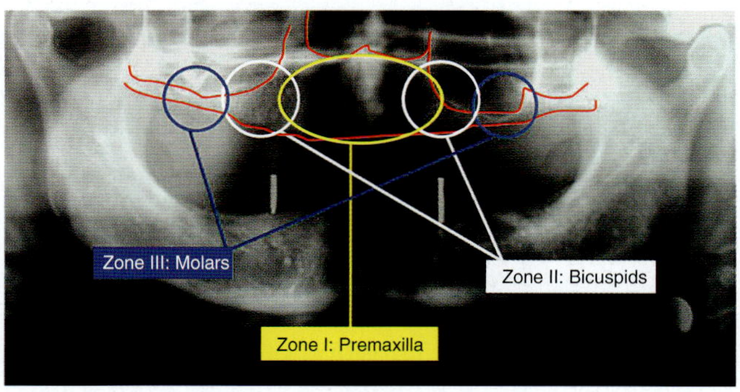

FIGURE 5-12 Zones of the maxilla. The cuspid-cuspid region is zone I. The bicuspid region is zone II. The molar region is zone III.

Presence of Bone	Surgical Approach
Zone I, II, III	Traditional (axial)
Zone I, II	All-on-4
Zone I only	Zygomatic implants
Insufficient bone	Quad zygoma

FIGURE 5-13 The lack of various zones of the maxilla influences the selection of a surgical concept.

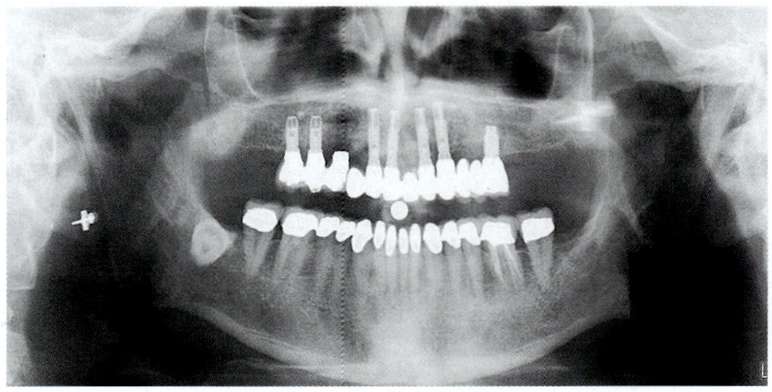

FIGURE 5-14 Axial implants may be considered in the presence of zones I, II, and III.

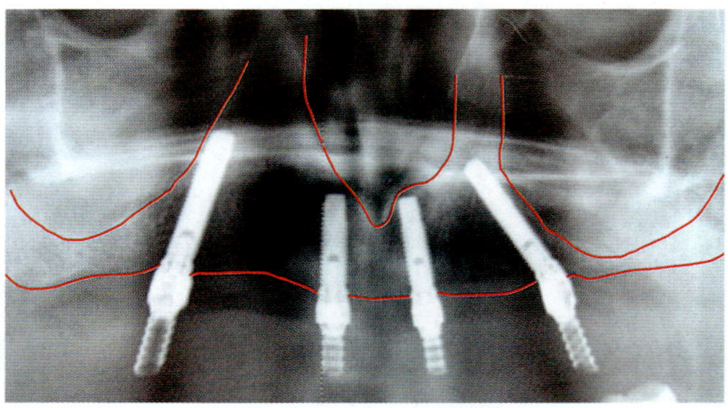

FIGURE 5-15 The tilted concept may be considered in patients with zones I and II only.

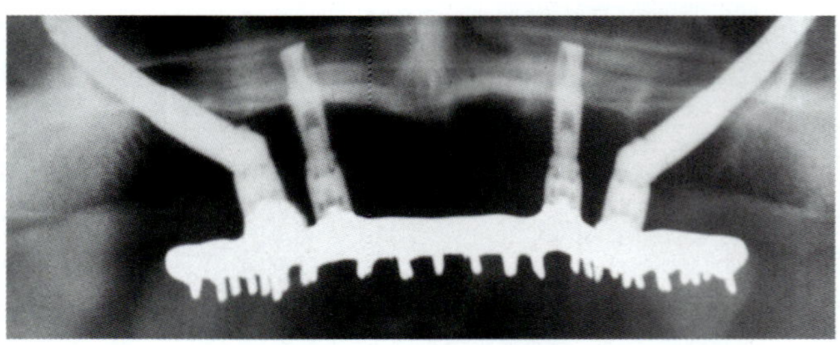

FIGURE 5-16 The zygoma concept may be considered in patients with zone I only.

TABLE 5-3

Guidelines for Optimal Implant Surgical Approach

Bone Present for Implants	Posterior Surgical Approach
Zones I, II, III	Traditional implants
Zones I, II	Inclined implants, posterior implants Traditional anterior implants
Zone I only	Zygomatic implants or Sinus-inlay grafting followed by implants Traditional anterior implants
Insufficient bone in any zone	4 Zygomatic implants or Brånemark horseshoe graft followed by traditional implants

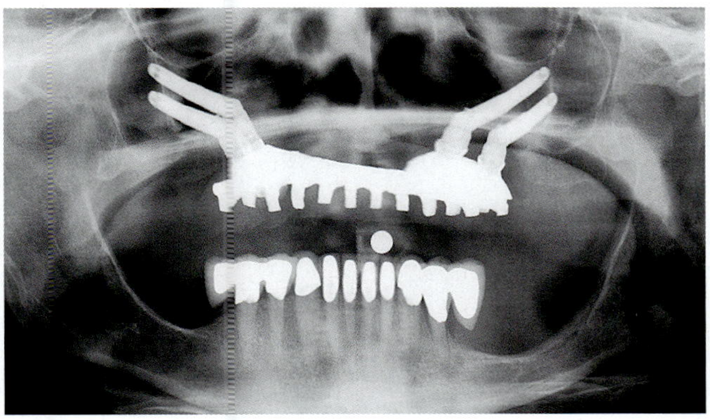

FIGURE 5-17 The quad zygoma concept may be considered in patients lacking zones I, II, and III.

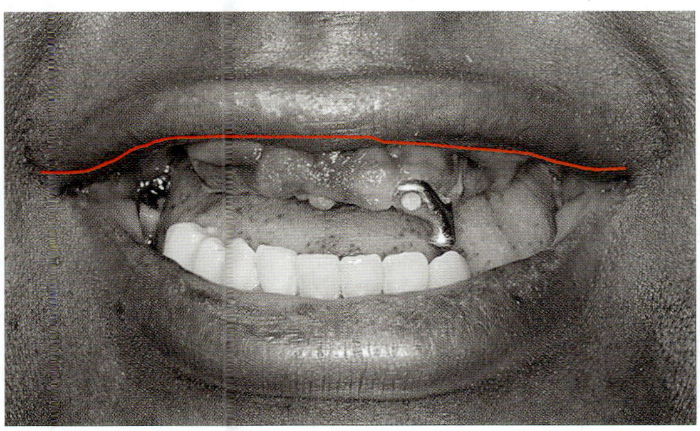

FIGURE 5-18 Transition line evaluation reveals a visible anterior sextant and hidden bilateral buccal corridor transition lines.

anterior maxillary ridge resorption does not correspond to posterior maxillary ridge resorption. Figure 5-19 demonstrates maxillary zones I and II with minimal zone III. Zone I is prominent. The patient demonstrates minimal premaxillary resorption (Figure 5-20). However, a significant resorption of the bilateral buccal corridors is evident (Figure 5-21). To hide the transition line in this group of patients, alveoloplasty of the anterior maxilla may be performed, positioning the transition line more apical to the smile line and equal to that of the posterior maxilla (Figure 5-22). By performing an alveoloplasty, the transition line is positioned in a more apical level as it relates to the patient's smile line. The presence of zones I and II in this patient indicates that the tilted-implant prosthesis (Figure 5-23) should be used for the immediate loading of the maxilla with a provisional profile prosthesis.

In other circumstances, the reverse topography of the edentulous maxilla may be evident in situations in

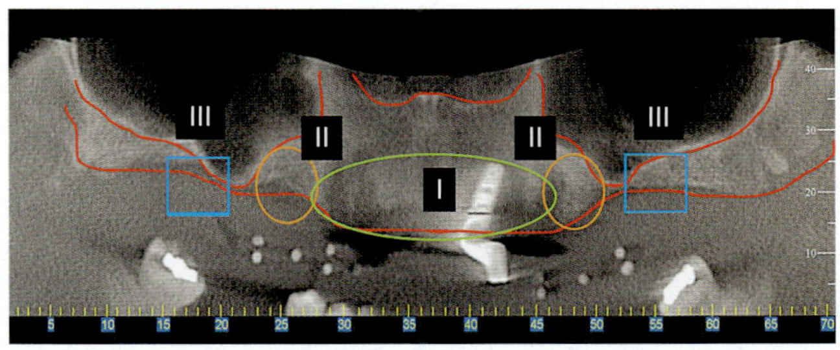

FIGURE 5-19 Evaluation of the zones of the maxilla reveals the presence of zones I and II only.

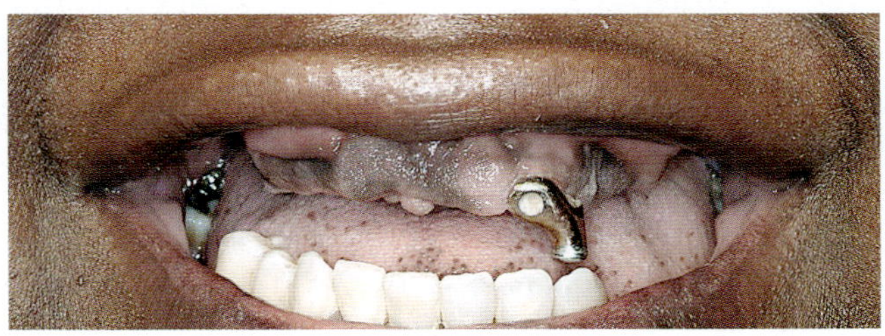

FIGURE 5-20 The discrepancy between a minimal resorbed premaxillary and the significantly resorbed posterior maxillary will have significant aesthetic compromise.

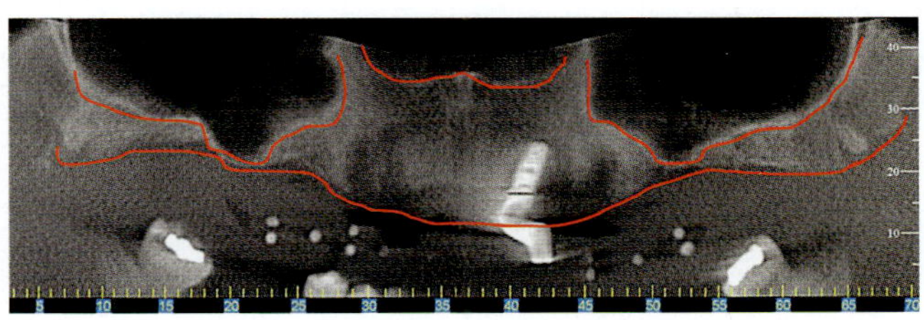

FIGURE 5-21 Total resorption of the posterior maxilla is evident on the reformatted three-dimensional panoramic radiograph.

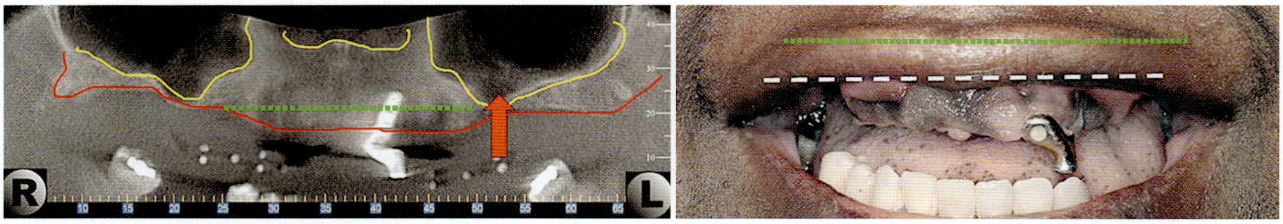

FIGURE 5-22 To hide the anterior transition line, an intraoperative alveolectomy is appropriate.

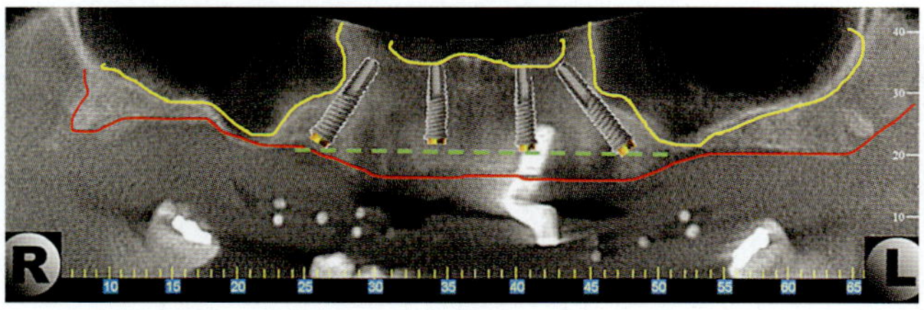

FIGURE 5-23 The presence of zones I and II allows for the adaptation of the "tilted concept" for the treatment of this patient.

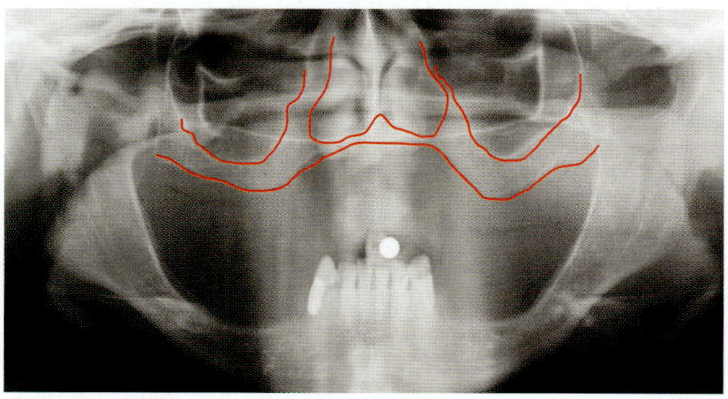

FIGURE 5-24 A reformatted three-dimensional panoramic radiograph demonstrates the complete resorption of the anterior maxilla.

which the complete absence of zone I is further complicated by prominence of edentulous alveolar topography in the buccal corridors (Figure 5-24). In this group of patients, the transition line is apical to the smile line in the anterior maxilla, but in the posterior maxilla, the transition line is visible (Figure 5-25). If this discrepancy is not addressed preoperatively, an unaesthetic outcome for the bilateral buccal corridors will be evident. Bilateral posterior alveolectomies place the posterior maxillary transition line apical to the smile line (Figure 5-26). The presence of zone I bone only suggests that this patient should be treated with the zygoma technique (Figure 5-27). Completion of posterior maxillary alveolectomies allows for the apical positioning of the transition lines in the buccal corridors, which permits an aesthetic outcome of the

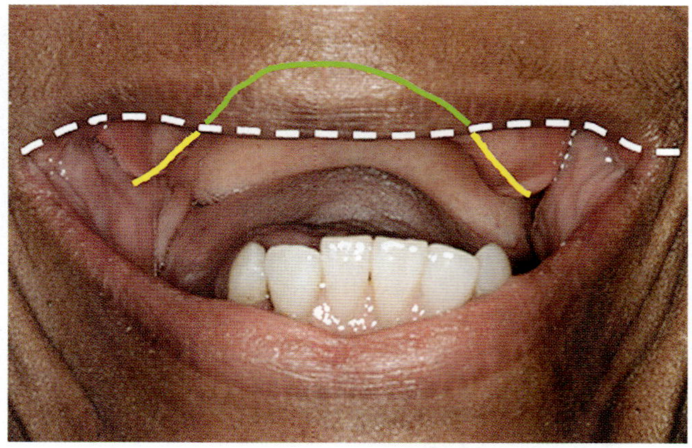

FIGURE 5-25 Bilateral buccal corridor transition lines are visible in this patient.

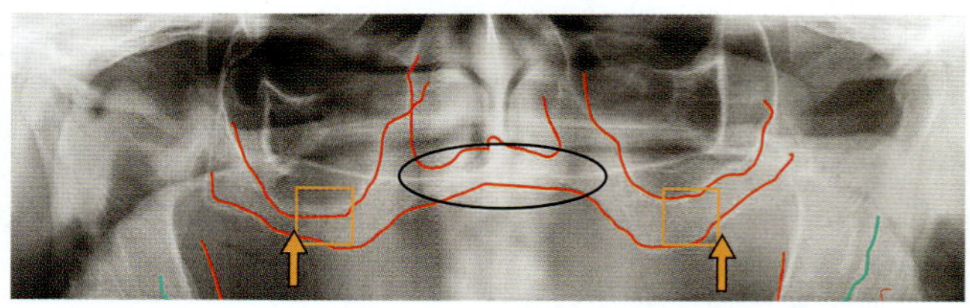

FIGURE 5-26 Intraoperative bilateral posterior alveolectomies will allow for a hidden transition line.

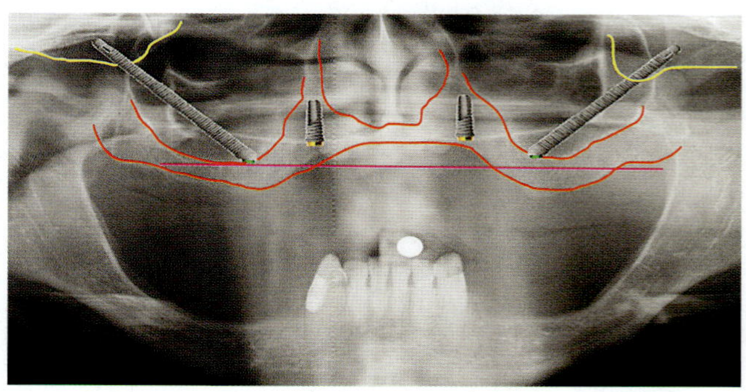

FIGURE 5-27 The presence of zone I only suggests the adaptation of the "zygoma concept" for the treatment of this patient.

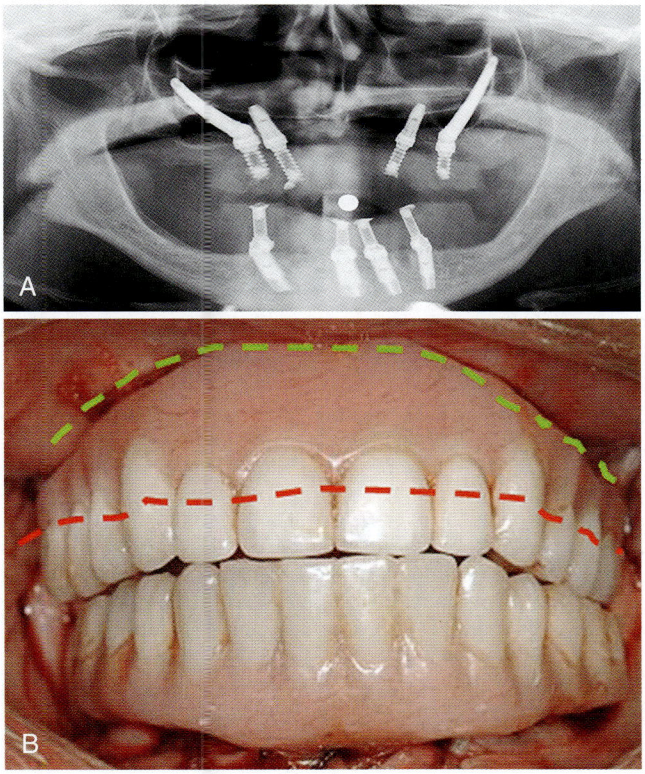

FIGURE 5-28 A, Bilateral posterior maxillary alveolectomies allowed all implant platforms to be on the same alveolar plane. B, Bilateral posterior maxillary alveolectomies allowed for the posterior transition line to be hidden with a resultant aesthetic outcome.

immediate-load profile prosthesis supported by the zygoma surgical technique (Figure 5-28).

If the transition line is not evaluated preoperatively, the unaesthetic outcome of the final transition line may be addressed by removing existing implants and reevaluating and replanning treatment, or by continuing the existing clinical presentation and substituting a fixed-detachable prosthesis such as a Marius bridge for a profile prosthesis. The presence of "flanges" on the Marius bridge will apically move the transition line to the depth of the patient's vestibule, resulting in an aesthetic outcome during animation (Figure 5-29). At the same time, the rigid framework of the Marius bridge (Figure 5-30) allows for cross-arch stabilization of existing implants. The tolerance of the secondary framework within the prosthesis of the Marius bridge is less than 10 microns and the rigid framework cross-arch splints the implants (Figure 5-31), which allows for transfer of occlusal forces to the edentulous ridge, reintroducing internal loading of the alveolus and stopping further resorption of the alveolus for the long term.

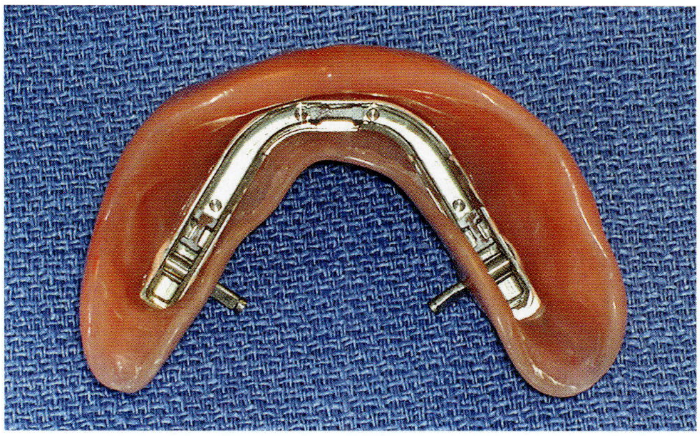

FIGURE 5-29 The flange of the fixed-detachable prosthesis will hide the transition line during animation.

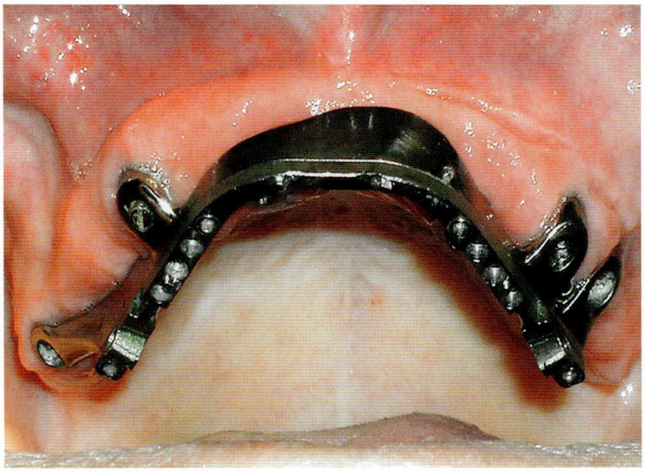

FIGURE 5-30 The rigid cross-arch splinting of the primary bar allows for the transfer of occlusal loads to the implants.

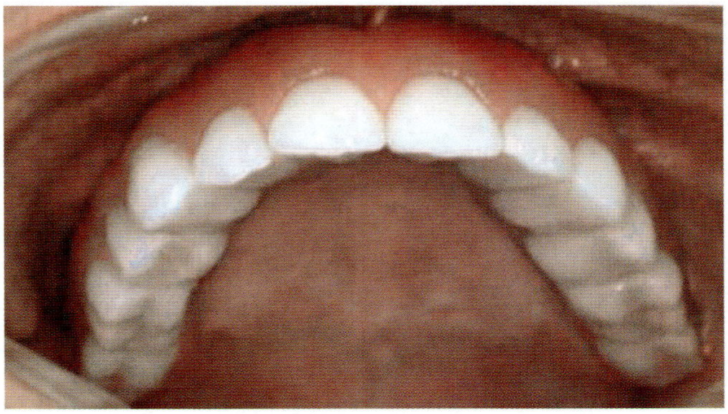

FIGURE 5-31 The "locking" of the superstructure to the framework of the fixed detachable prosthesis allows for the biomechanical transfer of occlusal forces to this implant-supported prosthesis.

REFERENCES

1. Brånemark P-I, Svensson B, van Steenberghe D: Ten-year survival rates of fixed prostheses on four or six implants ad modem Brånemark in full edentulism. *Clin Oral Implant Res* 6:227-231, 1995.
2. Maló P, Rangert B, Nobre M: All-on-4 immediate-function concept with Brånemark system implants for completely edentulous maxillae: A 1-year retrospective clinical study. *Clin Implant Dent Relat Res* 7(Suppl 1):S88-S94, 2005.
3. Taylor T: Fixed implant rehabilitation for the edentulous maxilla. *Int J Oral Maxillofac Implants* 6:332-334, 1991.
4. White G: *Osseointegrated dental technology,* 1993, Quintessence.
5. Sadowsky SJ: The implant-supported prosthesis for the edentulous arch: Design considerations. *J Prosthet Dent* 78:29, 1997.
6. Zitzmann NU, Marinello CP: Fixed or removable implant-supported restorations in the edentulous maxilla: Literature review. *Pract Periodont Aesthet Dent* 12:602, 2000.
7. Henry PJ: A review of guidelines for implant rehabilitation of the edentulous maxilla. *J Prosthet Dent* 87:281-287, 2002.
8. Desjardins R: Prosthesis design for osseointegrated implants in the edentulous maxilla. *Int J Oral Maxillofac Implants* 7:311-320, 1992.
9. Jemt T: Fixed implant-supported prostheses in the edentulous maxilla. *Clin Oral Implant Res* 5:142-147, 1994.
10. Lewis S, Sharma A, Nishimura R: Treatment of edentulous maxillae with osseointegrated implants. *J Prosthet Dent* 68:503-508, 1992.
11. Taylor T: Fixed implant rehabilitation for the edentulous maxilla. *Int J Oral Maxillofac Implants* 6:329-337, 1991.
12. Parel SM, Sullivan DY: *Esthetics and osseointegration,* Dallas, 1989, Taylor Publications, pp 127–153.
13. Zitzman N, Schärer P: Clinical compendium: Oral rehabilitation with dental implants. *Zurich: KBM (Department Fixed and Removable Prostheses and Materials Sciences)* 3:81-89, 1997.
14. Sadowsky SJ: The implant-supported prosthesis for the edentulous arch: Design considerations. *J Prosthet Dent* 78:28, 1997.
15. Jemt T: Failures and complications in 391 consecutively inserted fixed prostheses supported by Brånemark implants in edentulous jaws: A study of treatment from the time of prosthesis placement to the first annual checkup. *Int J Oral Maxillofac Implants* 6:270-276, 1991.
16. Schnitman P: The profile prosthesis: An aesthetic fixed implant-supported restoration for the resorbed maxilla. *Pract Periodont Aesthet Dent* 11:143-151, 1999.
17. Fortin Y, Sullivan RM, Rangert B: The Marius implant bridge: Surgical and prosthetic rehabilitation for the completely edentulous upper jaw with moderate to severe resorption: A 5-year retrospective clinical study. *Clin Implant Dent Relat Res* 4:69-77, 2002.
18. Bedrossian E: Immediate function with the zygomatic implant: A graftless solution for the patient with mild to advanced atrophy of the maxilla. *Int J Oral Maxillofac Implants* 21(6):937-942, 2006.
19. Brånemark P-I, Zarb G, Albrektsson T, editors: *Tissue-integrated prostheses,* 1985, Quintessence.

CHAPTER 6

Treatment of the Edentulous Maxilla: Anterior Tilted Implant Concept

In 1969 Brånemark first suggested topographically positioning four implants in the edentulous maxilla and four implants in the edentulous mandible[1] Four osseointegrated implants distributed along the edentulous arch to support a fixed, implant-supported prosthesis lend structural support and restores edentulous alveolus functionality to a state similar to the dentate alveolus, hence preventing further resorption. This biomechanical reconstruction not only restores form and function, but also has significant psychosocial effects for these patients.[2-5] The use of four implants to support a fixed maxillary prosthesis has also been recently reported with favorable outcomes by this author,[6] Maló,[7] Aparicio,[8] and Krekmanov.[9]

Duyck et al.[10] studied the magnitude and distribution of occlusal forces in vivo using four implants. Their study confirmed the appropriateness of using four implants as long as distribution of the implants is similar to "cornerstones." It has been customary to arbitrarily place six to eight implants in the maxilla for reconstruction with a fixed bridge. Rangert[11] demonstrates, however, that intermediate implants do not support occlusal load, which, in a fixed, implant-supported prosthesis, is biomechanically borne largely by the anterior-most and posterior implants.

Placing four implants to support a fixed prosthesis in the maxilla is useful because the bilateral maxillary sinuses limit available bone for surgical placement of implants without bone grafting.

On occasion, patients with edentulous maxilla may demonstrate on panoramic radiographic examination adequate vertical bone in zone I and limited zone II alveolar bone. Limited available bone in zone II is a function of the anterior extension of the patient's anterior maxillary sinus wall. The thinner the bony septum between the anterior border of the maxillary sinus and the lateral nasal cavity wall, the more limited the available zone II bone. This finding was initially presented by Brånemark in 1978.[12] Brånemark classified the anterior extension of the maxillary sinus from A through E (Figure 6-1). To better appreciate the bone volume available for implant placement, computed tomography or in-office cone beam computed tomography can be used (Figure 6-2). If adequate bone volume is present in zone II, placement of two anterior maxillary implants within zone I and anterior tilting of the posterior implant within zone II allows adequate anterior-posterior (AP) distribution for occlusal force support (Figure 6-3).

RADIOGRAPHIC EVALUATION

The patient's panoramic radiographic examination to establish the presence or absence of zones I and II is the primary radiographic study used (Figure 6-4). To establish adequate width of the residual alveolus, intraoral clinical evaluation, cone beam computed tomography, and, on occasion, "sounding" of the residual alveolus may be considered.

Three-dimensional radiographic evaluation of the residual alveolus is a helpful tool in planning implant sites. As is evidenced by scout films of the cone beam study in Figure 6-5, *A*, adequate bone volume in the vertical dimension is noted; the cross-sectional studies, however, clearly show the limited bone volume present in Figure 6-5, *B*. These studies help the surgeon determine whether to continue the graftless approach or consider alternative treatment options.

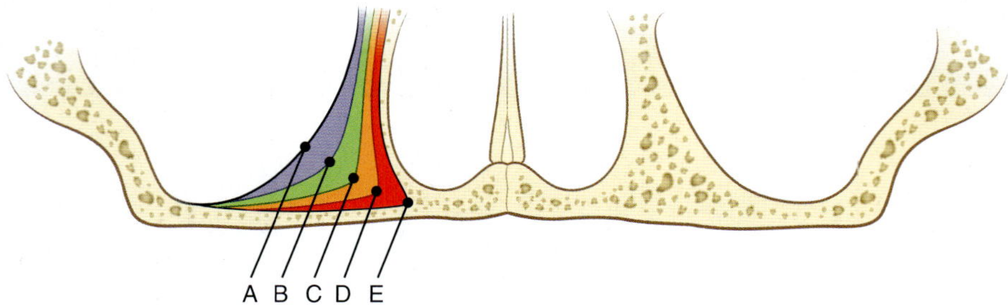

FIGURE 6-1 Brånemark classification for the anterior extension of the maxillary sinus.

TREATMENT PLANNING

Three factors are evaluated in the initial treatment planning phase.[13] Presence or absence of a composite defect is noted. If there is a composite defect, a profile prosthesis is considered (Figure 6-6). The transition line is also evaluated clinically with the patient's existing denture removed to determine whether the edentulous ridge is visible. A favorable outcome is expected if the transition line is not visible in a patient with a composite defect (Figure 6-7). To determine the position and length of the implants to be used in zones I and II, implant templates are superimposed onto the preoperative panoramic radiograph. Using this simple approach, the practitioner can determine the length of the posterior implant in zone II. To avoid collision of the two implants, however, caution must be taken to relate the apex of the tilted implant in zone II with the body of the axially placed implant in zone I (Figure 6-8).

To achieve the most biomechanically stable prosthesis, the largest AP distribution of the implants is preferred. To begin this process, the anterior implants in zone I are planned (Figure 6-9), followed by the two tilted posterior implants in zone II (Figure 6-10). Once the abutment and pontic teeth are selected, the treatment plan is complete (Figure 6-11).

PREOPERATIVE PROTOCOL

The surgical procedure is usually performed in the office setting with intravenous sedation, although the procedure can be performed with local anesthesia or in a hospital operating room with general anesthesia. The patient is premedicated with 2 g of amoxicillin or 600 mg of clindamycin (Cleocin) 1 hour prior to the procedure. If the patient will be edentulated, the immediate denture should be present during the surgical appointment to permit immediate conversion of the patient's "immediate denture" into an immediate-load profile prosthesis (ILPP). If the patient is already edentulous and wears a full maxillary denture, earlier preoperative and treatment planning appointments should have determined whether the existing denture has the proper vertical dimension of occlusion (VDO) and the proper AP tooth position (Figure 6-12) for conversion into an ILPP. If the patient's existing denture does not have the proper VDO and AP tooth position, a restorative dentist should be asked to fabricate a new denture prior to surgery.

SURGICAL PROTOCOL

The preoperative radiographic examination determines the presence or absence of zone I and zone II bone (Figure 6-13). Clinical evaluation of the buccal plate of the edentulous maxilla generally demonstrates either an "hour glass" depression or a straight line between the maxillary alveolus and the maxilla proper. The preoperative models in Figure 6-14 are consistent with "hour glass" topography of the maxillary alveolus; to allow placemat of the implants without perforation of the buccal plate, alveoloplasty is planned prior to implant placement.

Before beginning treatment, the patient is sedated. Local anesthetic administration, including circumvestibular infiltration of the maxilla and greater palatine, and nasopalatine nerve block are completed. A "hockey stick" releasing incision over the tuberosity of the maxilla is initiated and carried full thickness over the edentulous maxillary alveolar ridge to the opposite tuberosity (Figure 6-15). Elevation of a full-thickness flap exposes the maxilla (Figure 6-16). A lateral view of the exposed maxilla confirms the hour glass deformity (Figure 6-17). Alveoloplasty to reduce the depth of the buccal concavity is performed (Figure 6-18). A surgical marking pen may be used to identify the outline of the anterior maxillary wall (Figure 6-19). Transilluminating the lateral maxilla usually makes the anterior wall of the maxillary sinus visible. If the practitioner chooses, prior to initiating the 2-mm osteotomy, a small opening into the maxillary sinus may be made with a round bur. The topography of the

Text continued on p. 50.

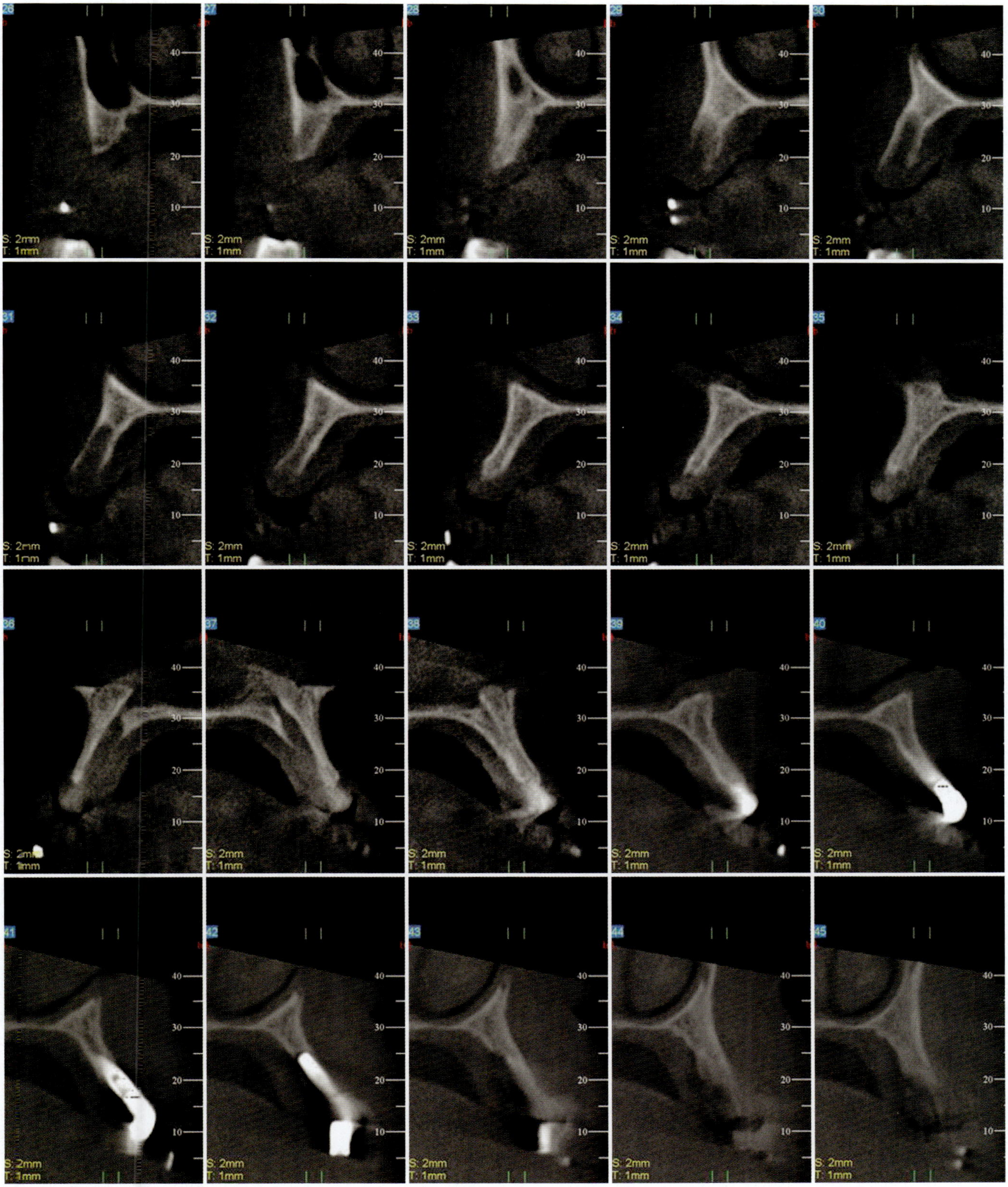

FIGURE 5-2 Preoperative evaluation of a three-dimensional radiographic study of the residual bony volume.

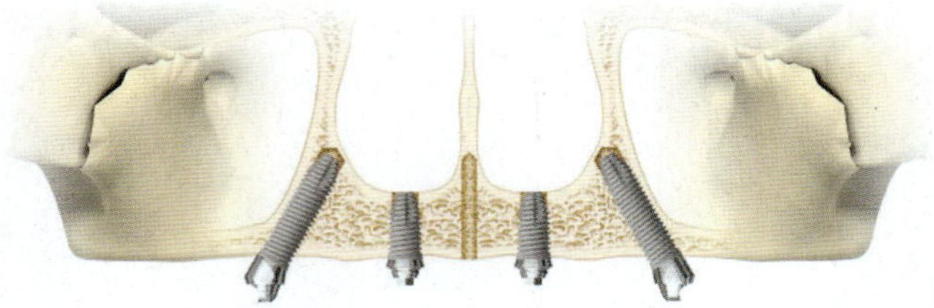

FIGURE 6-3 A "tilted concept" is considered for patients with available bone in zones I and II. (*Courtesy Nobel Biocare, Yorba Linda, Calif.*)

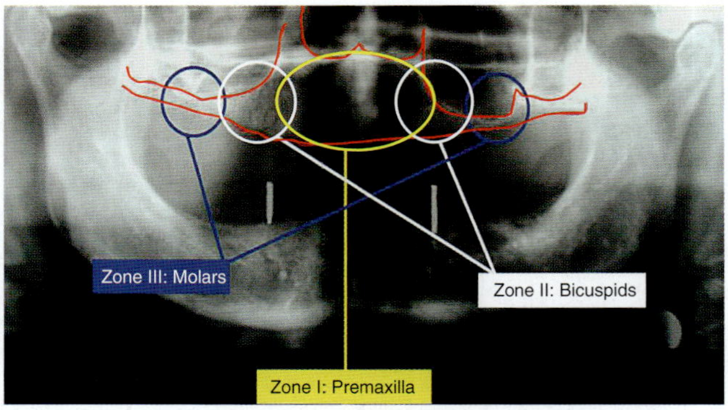

FIGURE 6-4 Available bone in zones I and II observed on a panoramic radiograph.

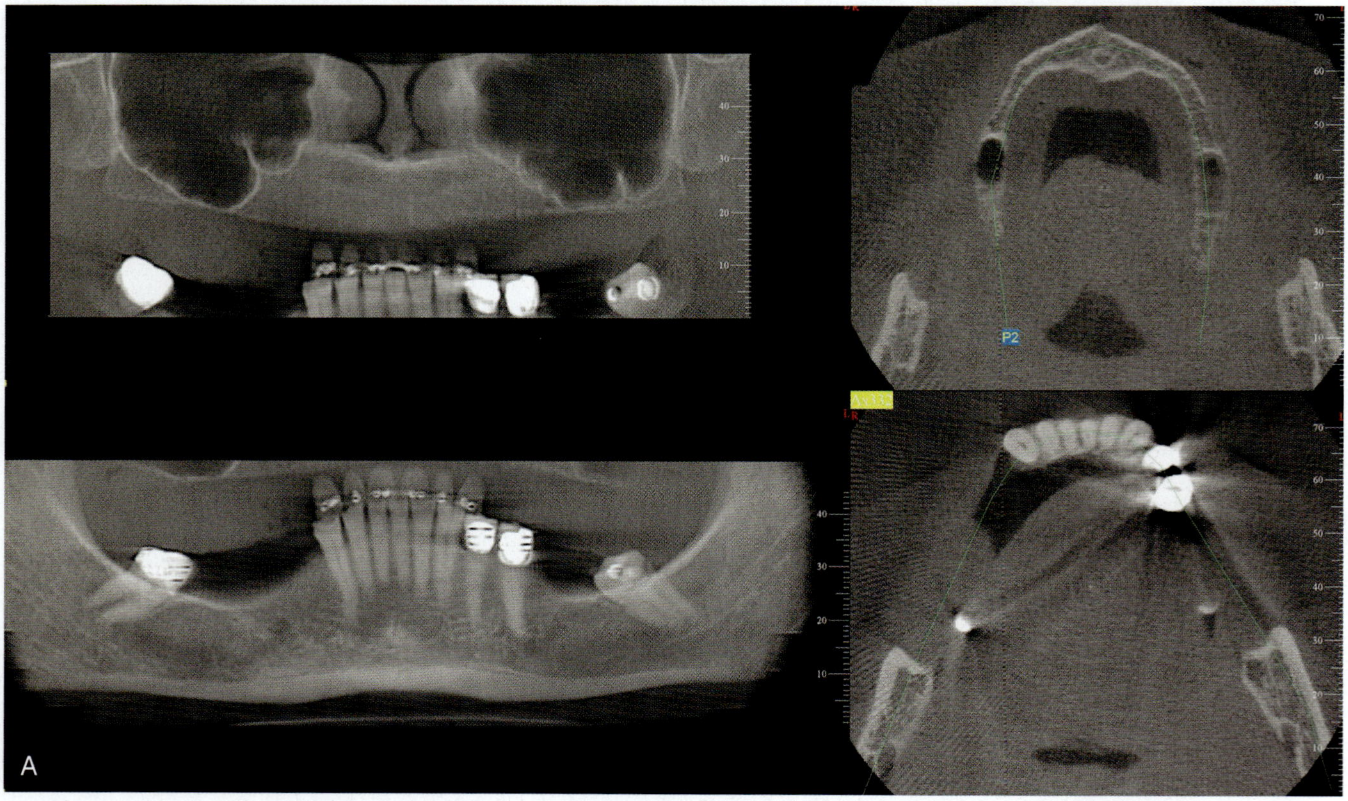

FIGURE 6-5 A, Adequate vertical bony volume seen in the preoperative two-dimensional view.

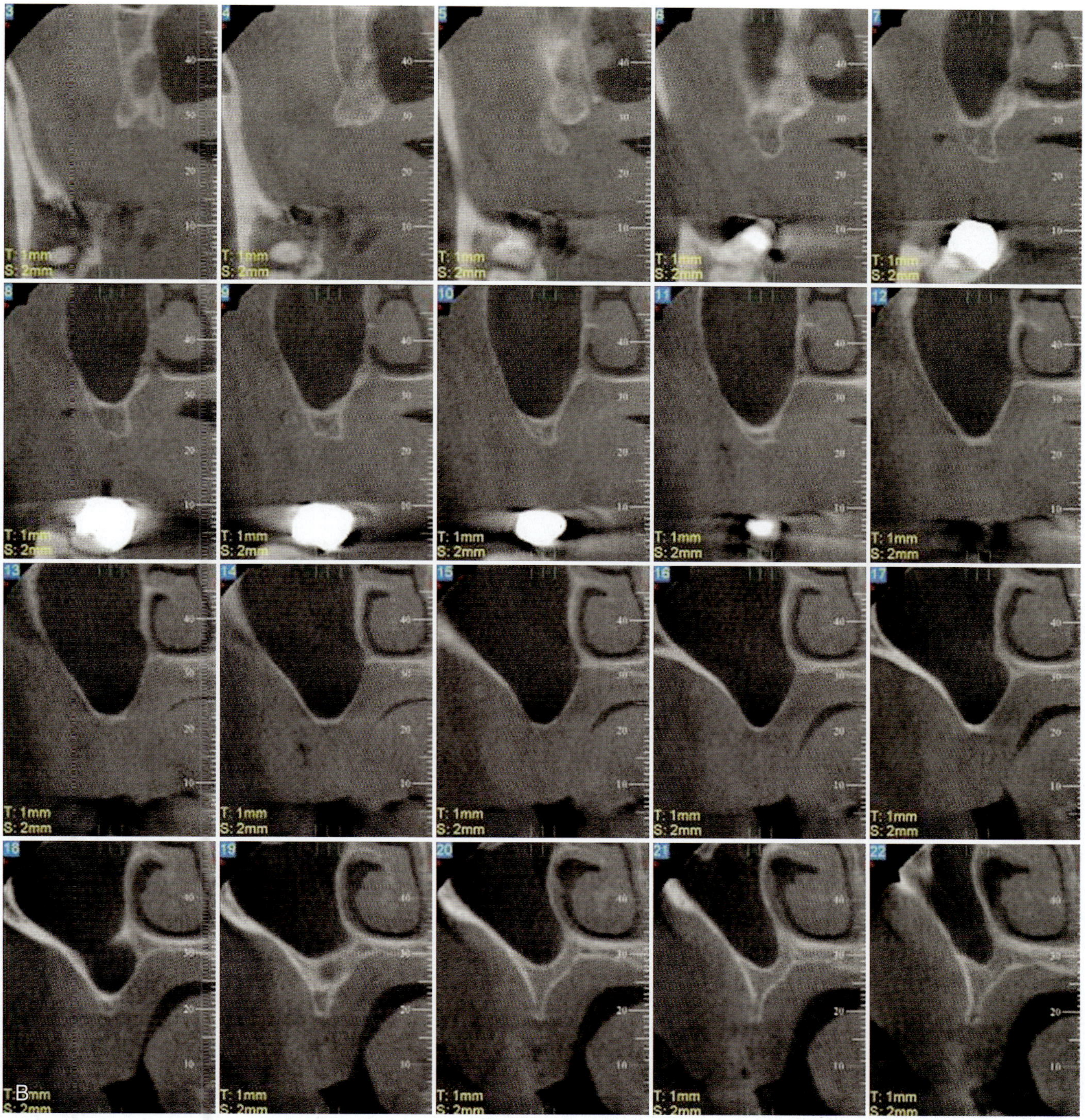

FIGURE 6-5, cont'd B, Resorbed horizontal bone volume seen in the preoperative three-dimensional view.

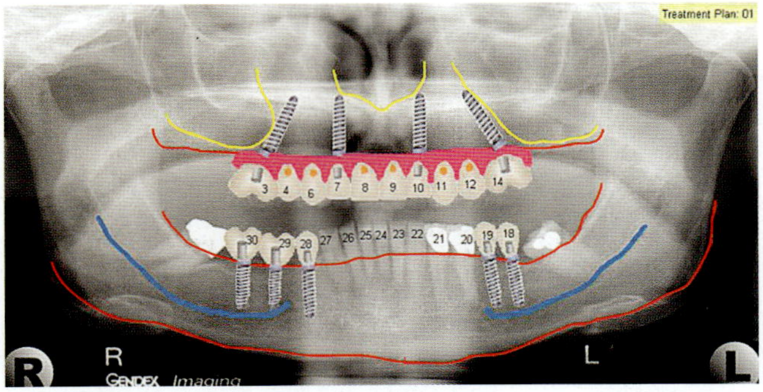

FIGURE 6-6 Preoperative illustration of a profile prosthesis for a patient demonstrating a composite defect of the maxilla.

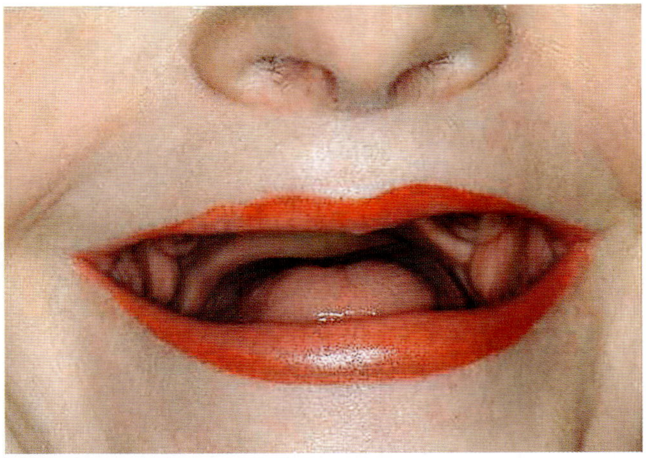

FIGURE 6-7 The hidden transition line allows for an aesthetic outcome with a profile prosthesis.

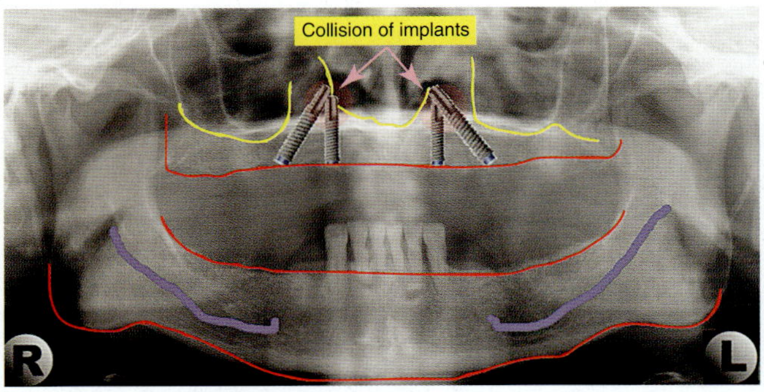

FIGURE 6-8 The length of the axial anterior and tilted posterior implants should be considered to avoid collision of the implant apices.

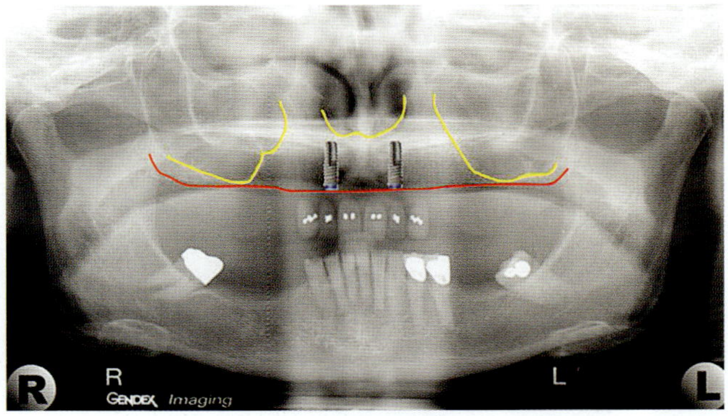

FIGURE 6-9 Anterior 10-mm maxillary implants planned on the preoperative radiograph in zone I.

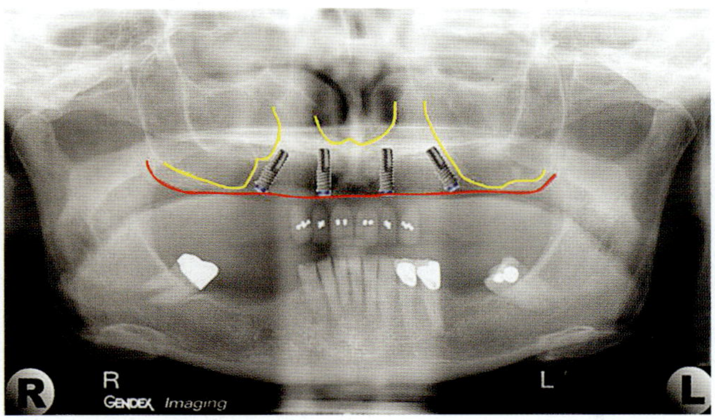

FIGURE 6-10 Tilted 10-mm implants planned in zone II avoid apex collision with the implant apices in zone I.

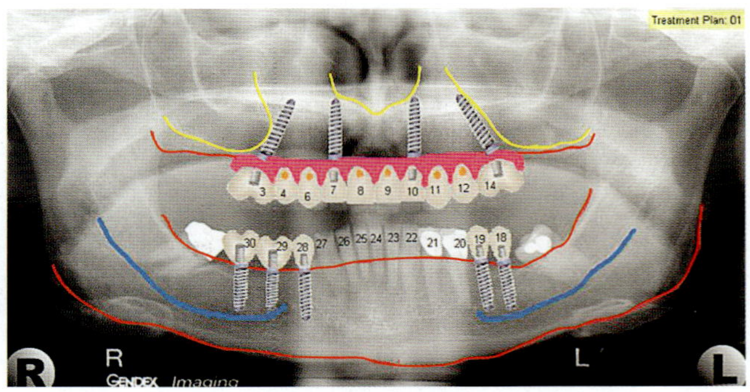

FIGURE 6-11 Four tilted implants provide support for the proposed postoperative profile prosthesis.

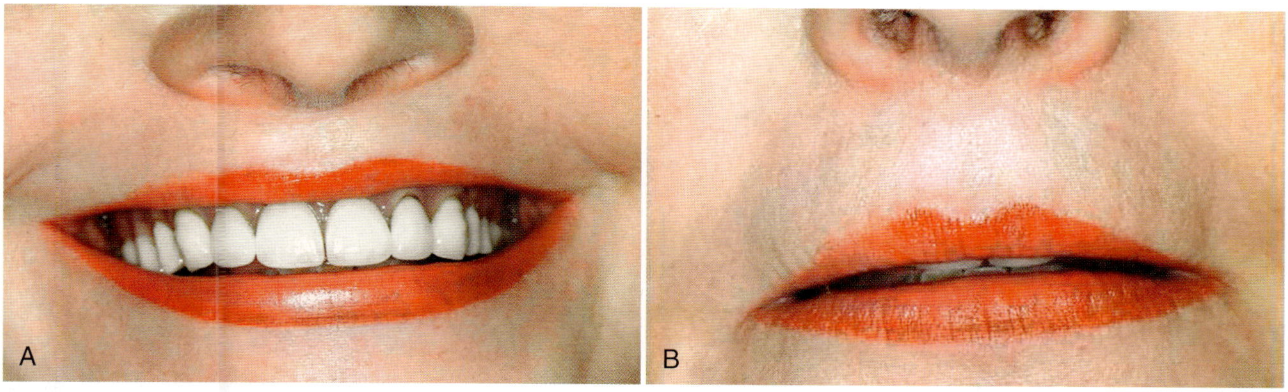

FIGURE 6-12 The preoperative vertical dimension and anterior posterior position of denture teeth are clinically evaluated.

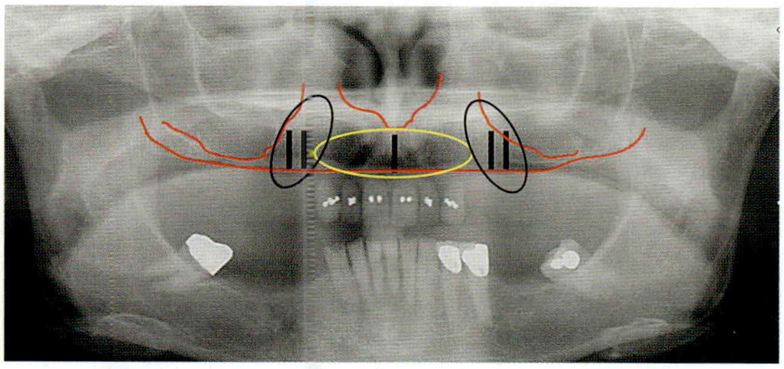

FIGURE 6-13 Preoperative panoramic radiographic examination demonstrates the presence of zone I and zone II of the edentulous maxilla.

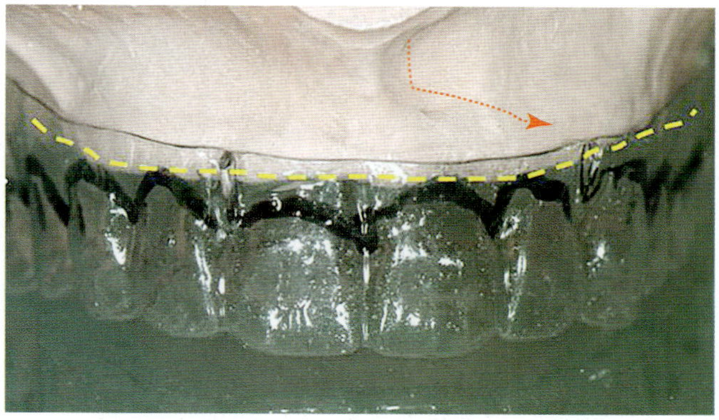

FIGURE 6-14 Hour-glass buccal contour of the maxillary buccal plate is evident on the preoperative cast.

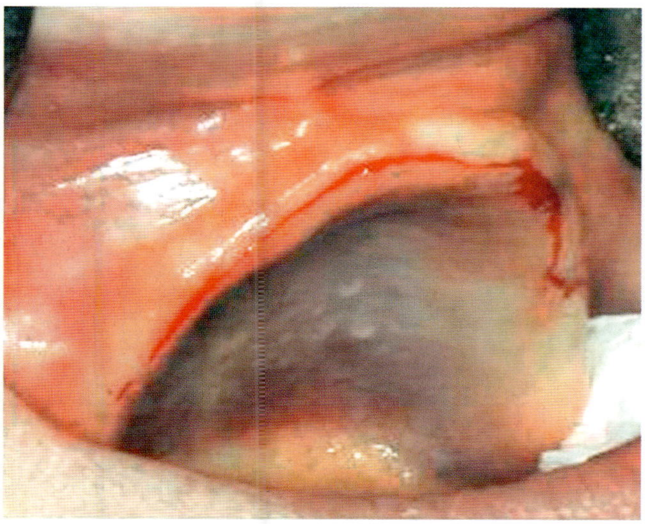

FIGURE 6-15 A midcrestal incision is made to initiate the reflection of a full-thickness flap.

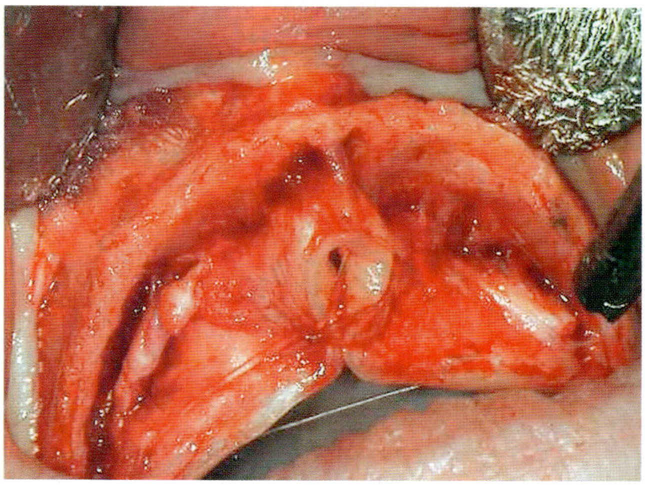

FIGURE 6-16 Reflection of a full-thickness mucoperiosteal flap is extended to directly visualize the buccal and palatal topography of the edentulous maxilla.

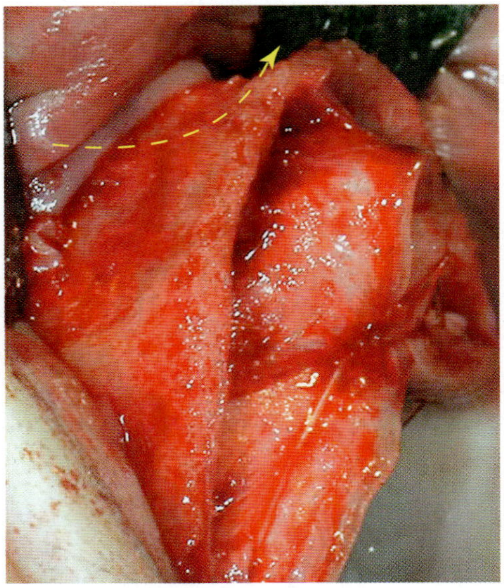

FIGURE 6-17 The hour-glass buccal contour is confirmed clinically.

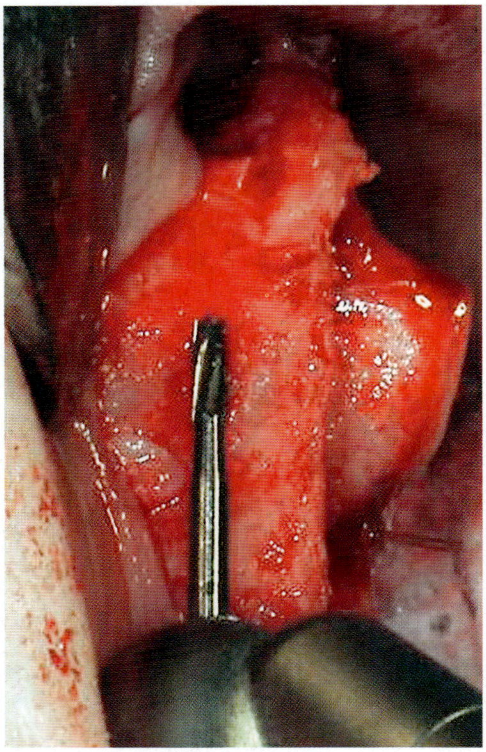

FIGURE 6-18 Alveolectomies are performed to reduce the height of the maxilla and remove the lower portion of the concave defect.

anterior maxillary sinus wall may be confirmed using a small, curved instrument (Figure 6-20). A malleable guide is available that can be stabilized to the maxillary alveolus by creating a 2-mm osteotomy in the maxillary midline, anterior to the nasopalatine opening (Figure 6-21). Using the vertical axis markings on the

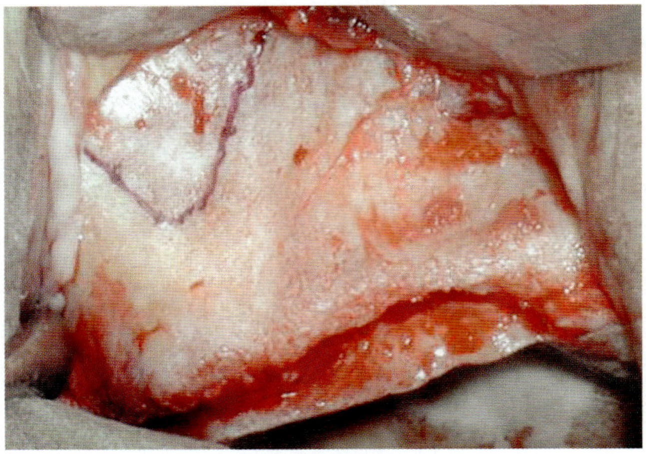

FIGURE 6-19 Outlines of the anterior and floor of the maxillary sinus are drawn using a surgical marking pen.

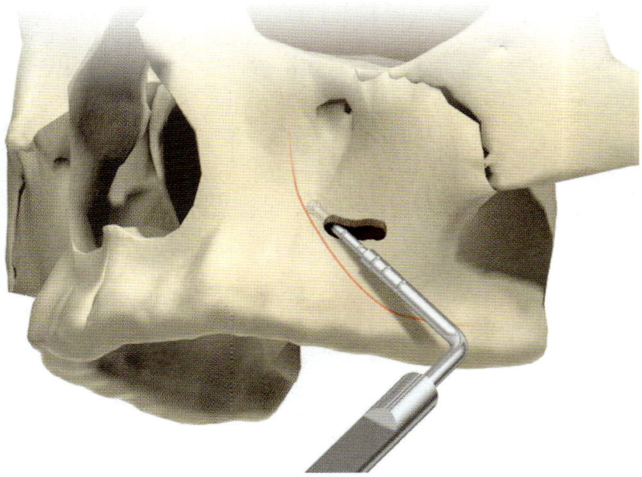

FIGURE 6-20 A small opening immediately posterior to the anterior maxillary wall permits palpation of the topography of the anterior extension of the maxillary sinus wall. (*Courtesy Nobel Biocare, Yorba Linda, Calif.*)

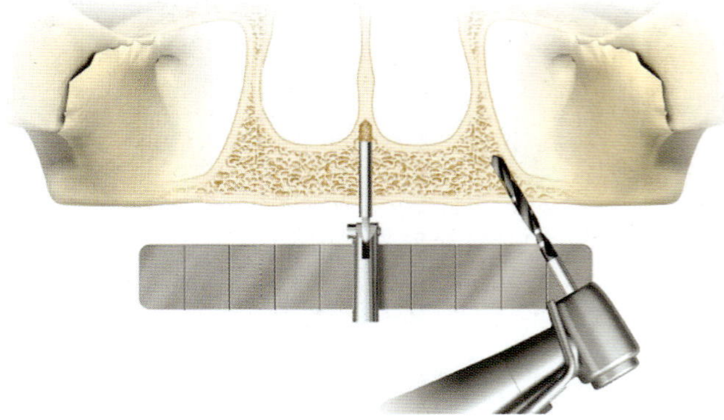

FIGURE 6-21 A malleable guide with vertical markings may be used to orient the drill angulation during osteotomy preparation. (*Courtesy Nobel Biocare, Yorba Linda, Calif.*)

guide, the 2-mm drill can be oriented not to exceed a 45°-tilt from the vertical axis markings while the operator attempts to parallel the anterior maxillary sinus wall (Figure 6-22). The 2-mm drill can be placed over the lateral maxillary wall to simulate the intended angulation for the osteotomy (Figure 6-23). The osteotomy of the tilted implant is now initiated with a 2-mm drill, and the proximity of the drill to the anterior maxillary wall may be viewed by an intraoperative periapical radiograph (Figure 6-24). Once the position of the initial osteotomy 4 mm anterior to the anterior maxillary sinus wall is confirmed, the 2.4-mm drill is used to complete the osteotomy. Regular 4-mm thread diameter platform implants are used. The recommended final osteotomy diameter in type I and II bone is 3 mm. Because the posterior maxilla is primarily cancellous and therefore type III bone, to achieve 40 Ncm of insertion torque, the double-threaded implants are generally inserted in an undersized 2.4-mm osteotomy. The final seating of the implant is confirmed again by an intraoperative periapical radiograph (Figure 6-25).

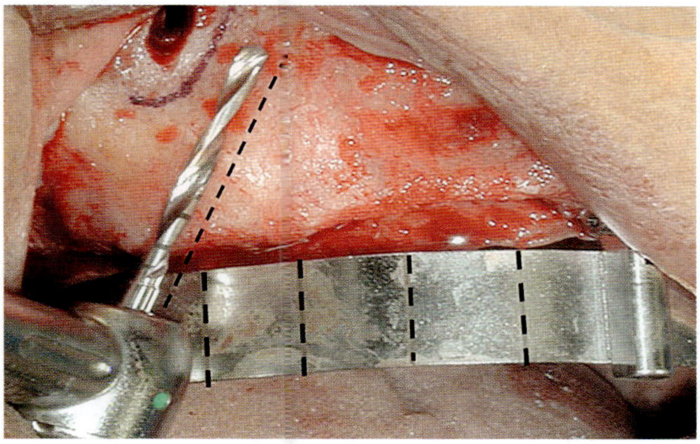

FIGURE 6-22 The angulation of the drill before preparation of the osteotomy for the tilted implant is aided using the malleable guide.

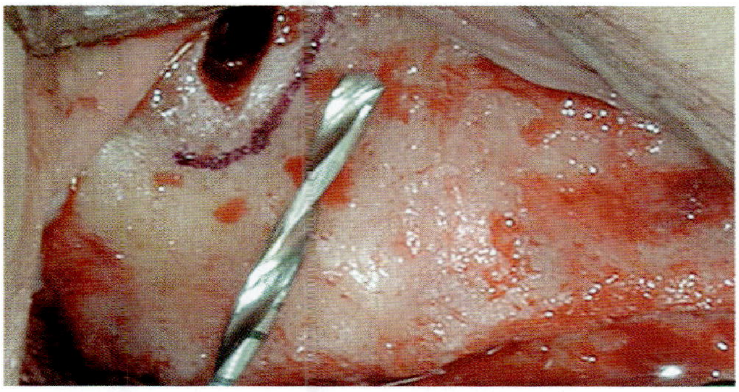

FIGURE 6-23 Simulating the direction of the osteotomy by placing the drill over the intended trajectory helps orient the surgeon prior to initiation of the osteotomy.

The two anterior axial implants are placed per protocol (Figure 6-26). The contralateral tilted implant is placed after the aforementioned surgical procedure. Once all implants are seated (Figure 6-27), the conversion technique for the fabrication of an implant-supported profile prosthesis (ISPP) is followed. It is important to index the position of the anterior implants prior to committing to the final abutments. To index their position, temporary healing abutments are fixated

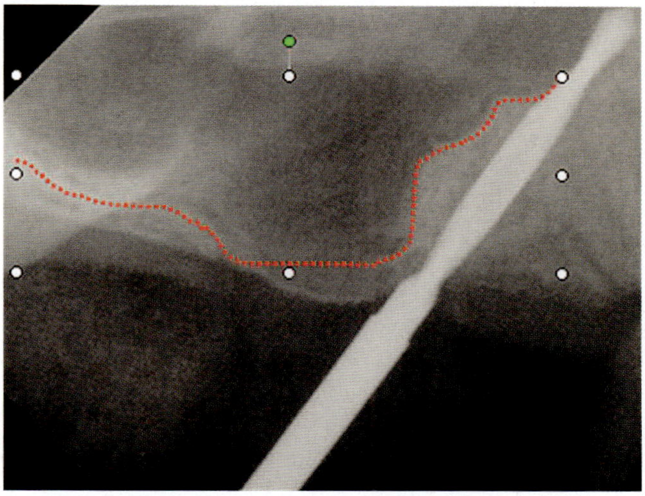

FIGURE 6-24 An intraoperative radiographic examination of the 2-mm drill allows evaluation of the osteotomy site to the anterior maxillary wall. In this case, a decision to move the drill forward may be appropriate.

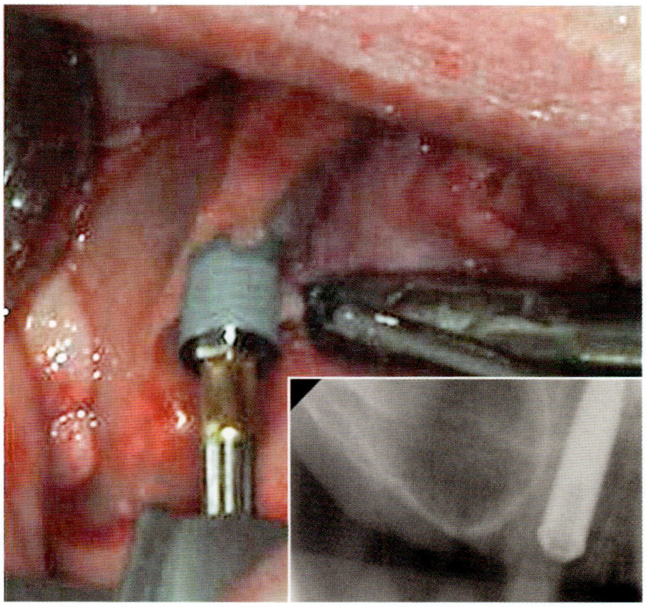

FIGURE 6-25 Final seating of the tilted implant is confirmed using postoperative radiographic examination, which shows the position of the anterior maxillary wall as it relates with the posterior portion of the implant.

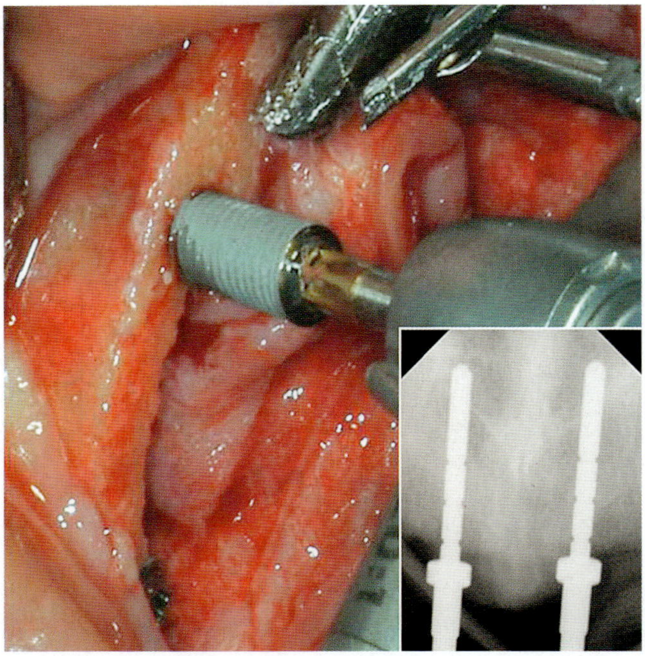

FIGURE 6-26 The angulation of the anterior implants is confirmed with intraoperative radiographs prior to seating the implants.

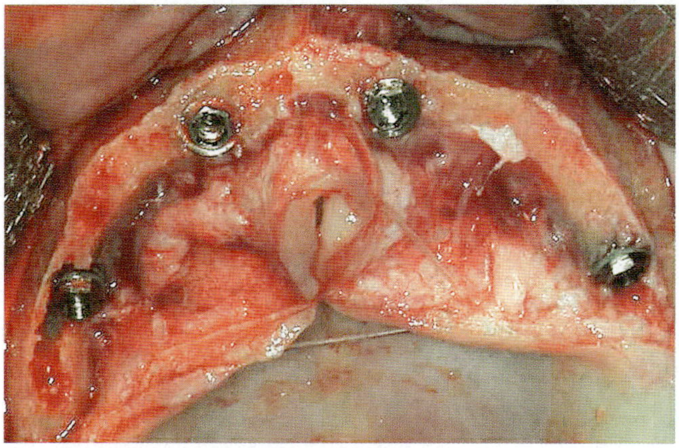

FIGURE 6-27 Complete seating of all implants.

to the two anterior implants (Figure 6-28). To allow prosthetic reconstruction of the two posterior tilted implants, 17° or 30° abutments are used to bring the "working platform" to the proper occlusal orientation (Figure 6-29). The complete seating of the angulated abutment onto the platform of the implant is confirmed by intraoperative radiographs (Figure 6-30). Upon confirmation of complete seating of the angulated abutments, the abutment screw is torqued to the appropriate Ncm as determined by the manufacturer. Prior to suturing the surgical site, plastic temporary healing caps are attached to the posterior abutments

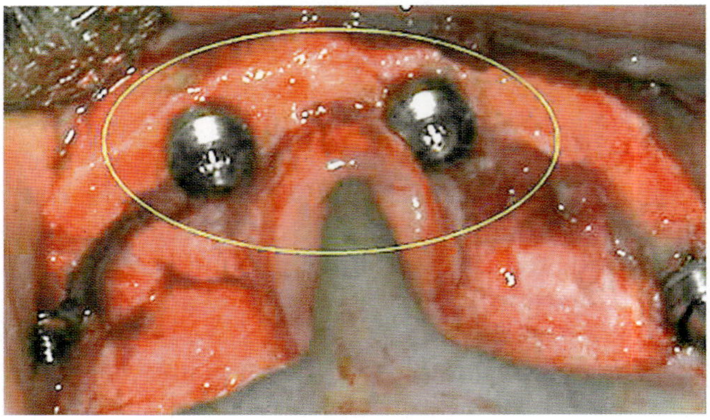

FIGURE 6-28 Temporary healing abutments are placed onto the anterior implants.

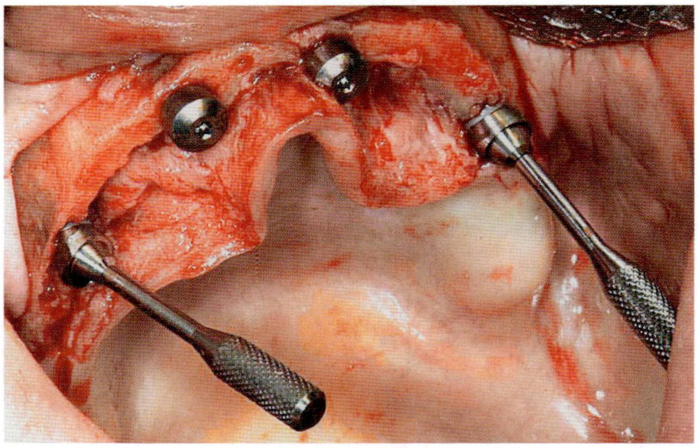

FIGURE 6-29 Depending of the degree of titling of the posterior implants, 17° or 30° multiunit abutments may be used.

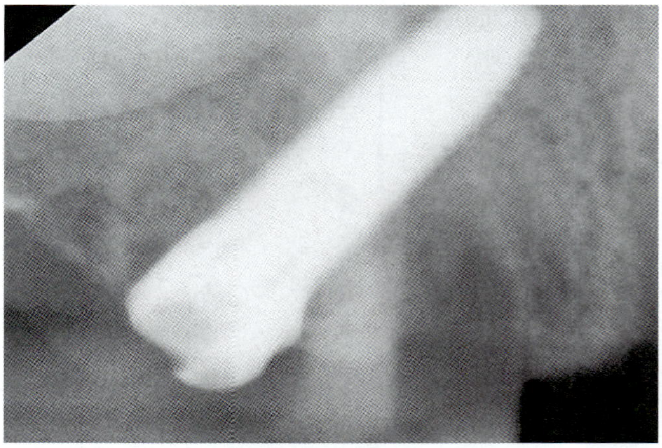

FIGURE 6-30 Periapical radiographic examination confirms complete engagement of the angulated abutment with the implant platform prior to torquing the abutment screw to 20 Ncm.

to allow proper adaptation of the soft tissue flap to the abutments (Figure 6-31).

Indexing material is used (Figure 6-32) to index the position of the implants to the intaglio surface of the patient's denture (Figure 6-33). To begin the process of converting of the immediate denture into an ILPP, the indexed positions of the abutments are perforated through the denture base using a laboratory acrylic bur. Although it is possible to make all four perforations at one time, in this example the decision was made to begin treatment with the two posterior implants only (Figure 6-34). Temporary cylinders were attached to the posterior abutments (Figure 6-35) and the prosthesis was positioned over the temporary cylinders, ensuring circumferential clearance of the cylinder with the denture base (Figure 6-36). Fast-setting acrylic was used to attach the cylinder to the denture using the "salt and pepper" technique (Figure 6-37). The contralateral cylinder is attached using the same fast-setting acrylic (Figure 6-38). The denture is now unscrewed from the patient's mouth and the intaglio side of the cylinder is filled (Figure 6-39).

The prosthetic teeth of the profile prosthesis are mechanically attached to the framework using pink acrylic or pink porcelain. Therefore, the bulk of the acrylic or porcelain between the cingulum of the anterior maxillary teeth and the prosthetic screw axis holes play a significant role in retaining the anterior teeth and preventing them from "popping off" (Figure 6-40). Indexing material is once again placed into the denture

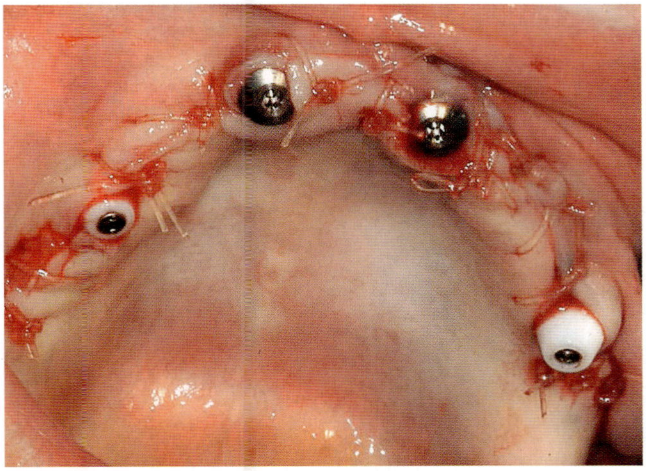

FIGURE 6-31 Angulated abutments correct the prosthetic platform of the posterior implants in line with the anterior axial implant platforms.

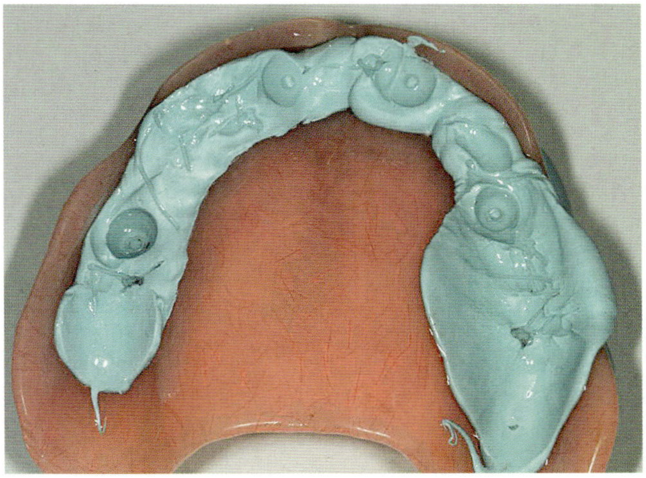

FIGURE 6-33 Transfer of the implant positions to the intaglio surface of the denture.

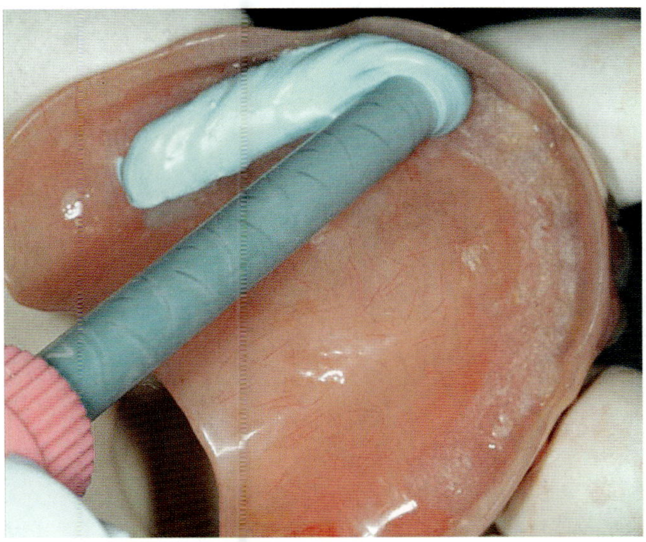

FIGURE 6-32 An indexing material of the dentist's choice is used to transfer the position of the implants to the intaglio surface of the full denture.

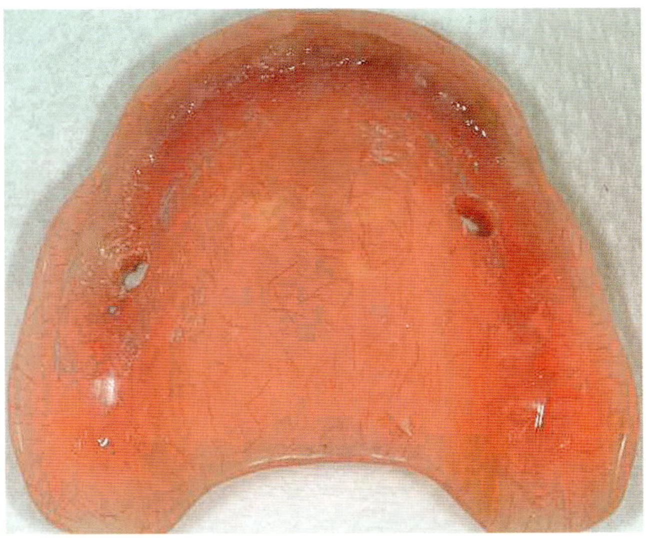

FIGURE 6-34 Positions of the implants are transferred to the acrylic base by drilling through the indexing material and the underlying denture material.

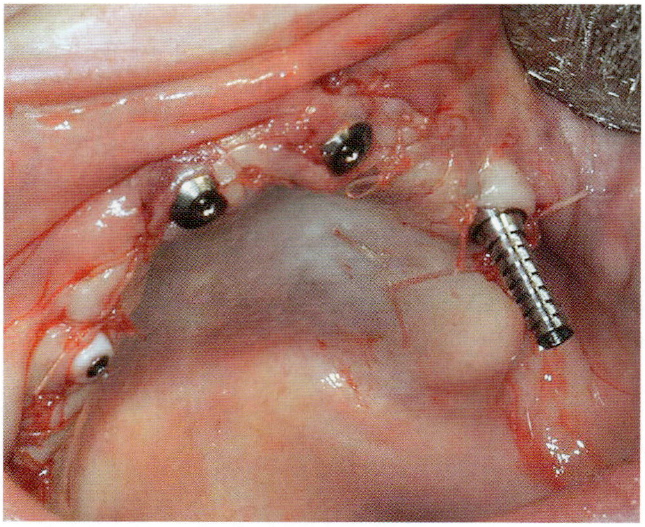

FIGURE 6-35 Temporary titanium cylinders are used to begin conversion of the denture to the provisional fixed prosthesis.

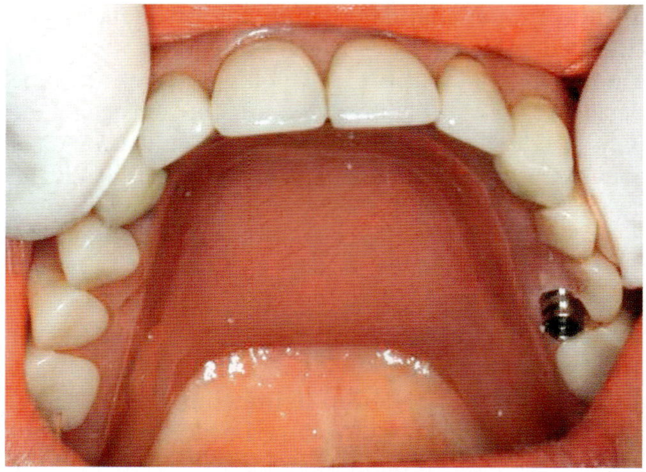

FIGURE 6-36 Prior to luting the cylinder, circumferential space around the cylinder is observed to maintain the proper seating of the denture on the edentulous ridge.

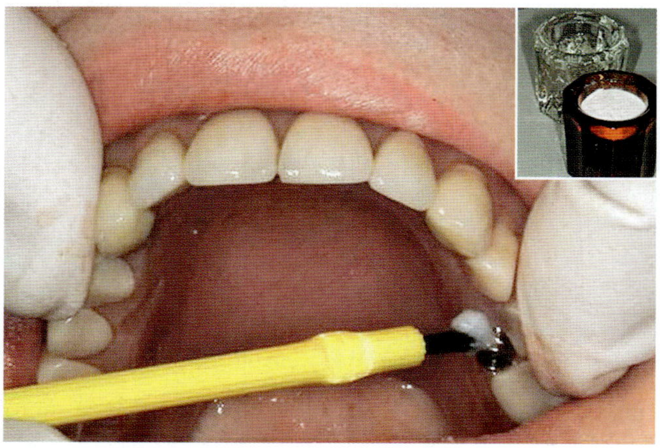

FIGURE 6-37 Fast-setting acrylic material is used in the salt and pepper technique to connect the temporary cylinder to the denture base.

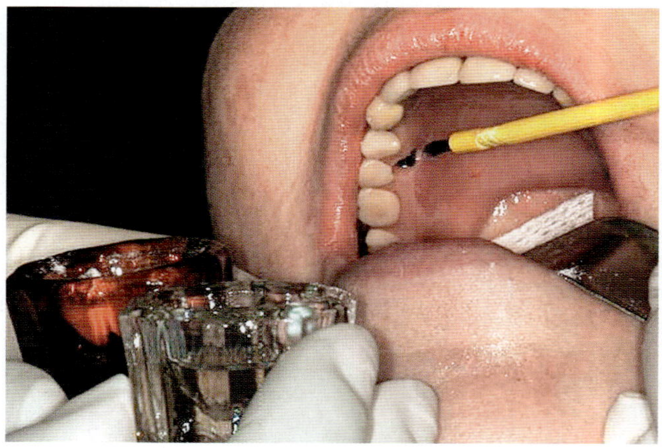

FIGURE 6-38 The contralateral side is luted at the same time as the ipsilateral side, or after acrylic on the ipsilateral side has set.

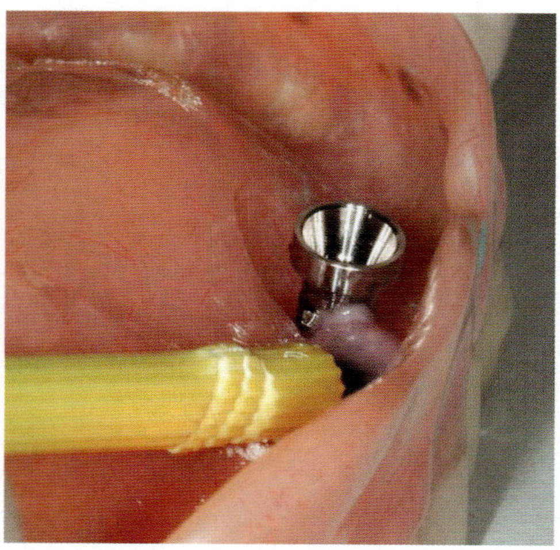

FIGURE 6-39 After the acrylic sets, the temporary titanium screws are carefully removed to allow removal of the prosthesis from the mouth and the addition of acrylic to the intaglio portion of the temporary cylinder.

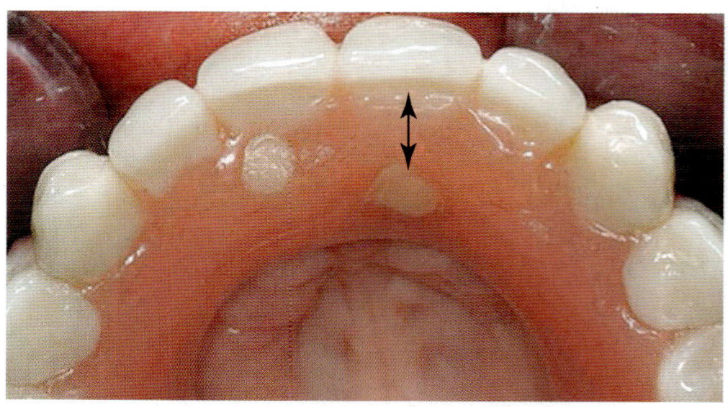

FIGURE 6-40 Adequate thickness of pink acrylic is necessary between the anterior teeth and the position of the titanium cylinder as it protrudes through the denture base. This prevents denture teeth from "popping off" during function.

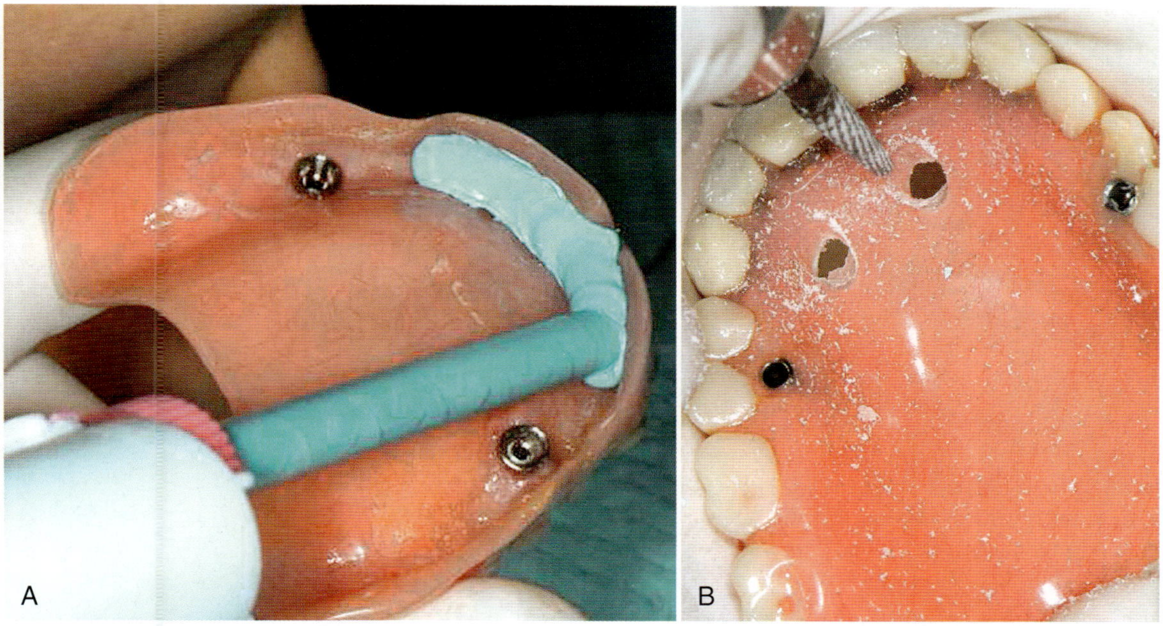

FIGURE 6-41 A, After connection of the posterior implants, the position of the anterior implant is re-indexed. B, A careful opening is made through the denture base, noting the thickness of the pink acrylic remaining palatal to the cingulum of the anterior denture teeth.

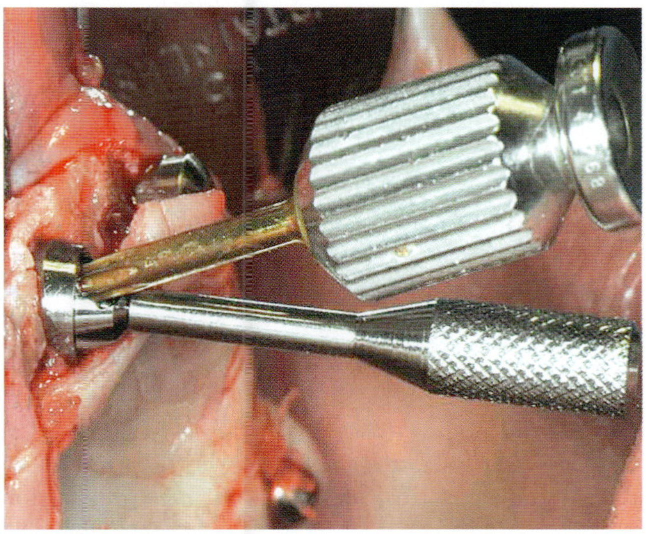

FIGURE 6-42 To place the screw access hole farther palatal from the cingulum of the anterior denture teeth, 17° multi-unit abutments were used.

base to locate the position of the anterior temporary abutments (Figure 6-41). In this example, it was determined that 17° abutments allow the axis of the prosthetic screw hole to be farther away from the cingulum of the anterior teeth, therefore ensuring the greatest bulk of acrylic (Figure 6-42).

The abutments are oriented and secured to the implants. Radiographs confirm complete seating of the abutments (Figure 6-43); the abutment screws are

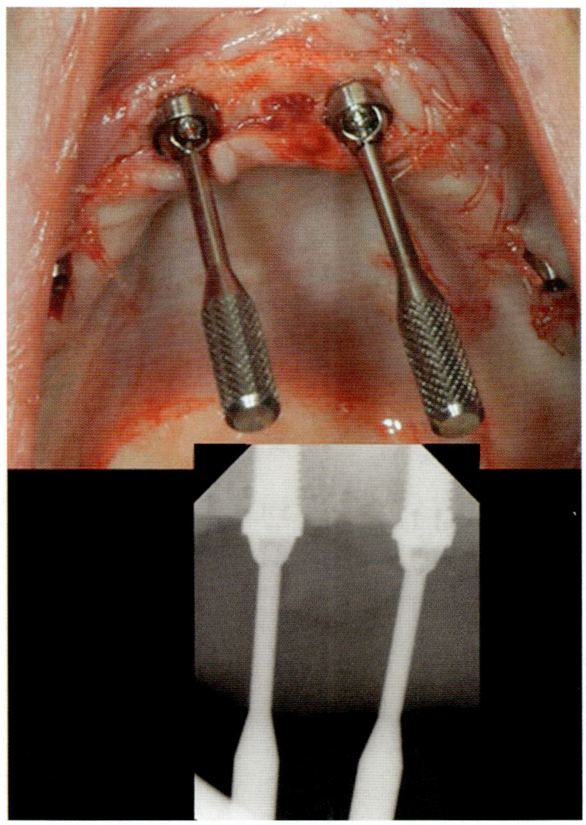

FIGURE 6-43 Periapical radiographic examination is used to confirm complete seating of the abutment to the implant platform prior to torquing the abutment screw to 20 Ncm.

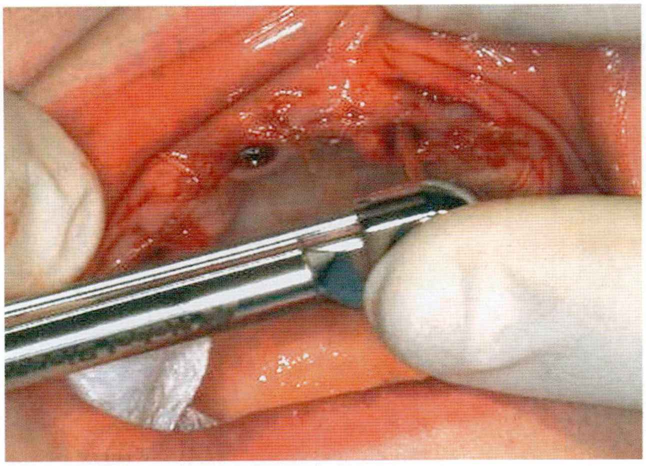

FIGURE 6-44 For angulated multiunit abutments, 20 Ncm of torque is placed, plastically deforming the screw to avoid loosening during function.

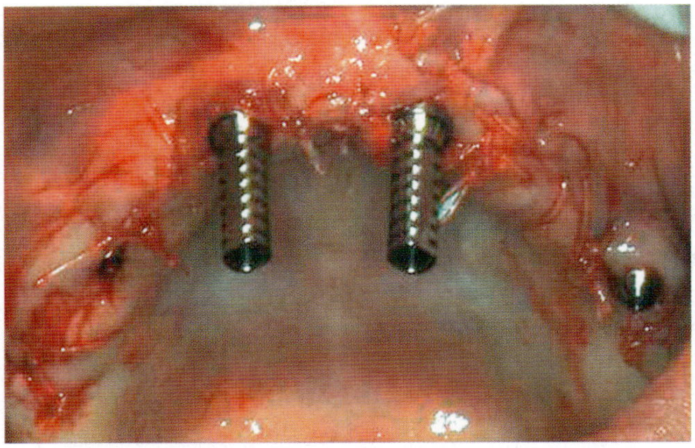

FIGURE 6-45 Temporary titanium cylinders are placed on the anterior 17° abutments, ready for luting to the denture base.

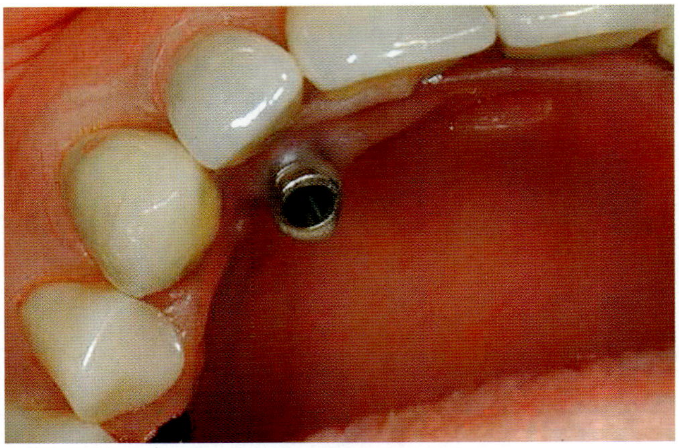

FIGURE 6-46 Circumferential clearing of the acrylic opening around the temporary cylinder is checked prior to luting the cylinder.

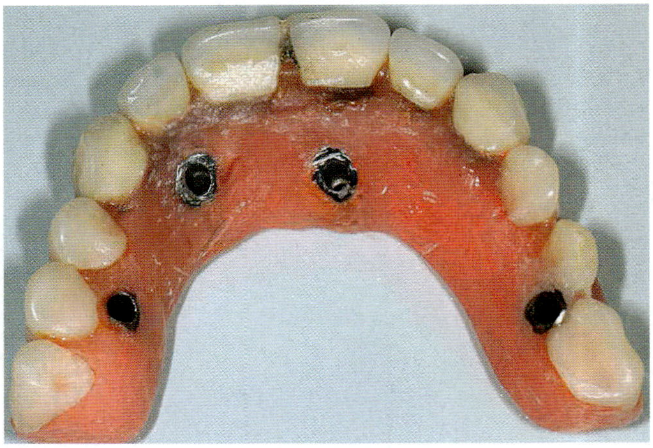

FIGURE 6-47 The denture base and the flange have been removed and recontoured after completion of the luting of all four implant positions to the completed provisional prosthesis.

torqued to 20 Ncm (Figure 6-44). Temporary cylinders are secured to the angulated anterior abutments (Figure 6-45) and the prosthesis is attached using fast-setting acrylic (Figure 6-46). Once the profile prosthesis is completed and polished (Figure 6-47), with the prosthesis fully seated and all four prosthetic screws hand-tightened, the screw access holes are sealed using a cotton pellet and a temporary material of the practitioner's choice, such as cavit. The occlusion is checked (Figure 6-48, *A*) and a final postoperative panoramic radiograph is taken (Figure 6-48, *B*).

POSTOPERATIVE CARE

Postoperative medications are amoxicillin 500 mg four times daily or clindamycin 150 mg three times daily for 1 week, as well as an analgesic as needed. A chlorhexidine rinse in a 0.12% solution is used every day at bedtime during the 6-month osseointegration period. Patients are advised to maintain a soft diet, with foods of a consistency no harder than well-cooked chicken or fish.

The patient's occlusion is checked at the 1-week postoperative appointment (Figure 6-49). Group function with bilateral, equal centric occlusion is the goal for the next 6 months during the osseointegration period. Patients are advised to call immediately if they feel that they are biting more heavily on one side than the other. They are also advised to report any swelling, pain, or mobility of the prosthesis encountered at any time after surgery. Intraoral examination of the prosthesis in 1 week should show normal soft tissue contours and sealed prosthetic screw axis holes (Figure 6-50).

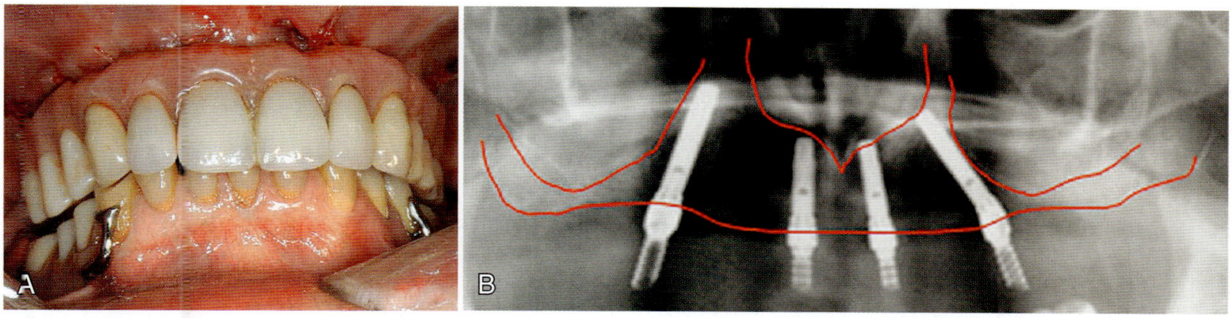

FIGURE 6-48 A, The reproducible centric occlusion and the correct position of the midline confirm proper occlusion of the converted denture into the provisional prosthesis. B, Postoperative panoramic radiographic examination demonstrates the position of the implants, complete seating of the abutments onto the implant platforms, and complete seating of the temporary titanium cylinders to the abutments.

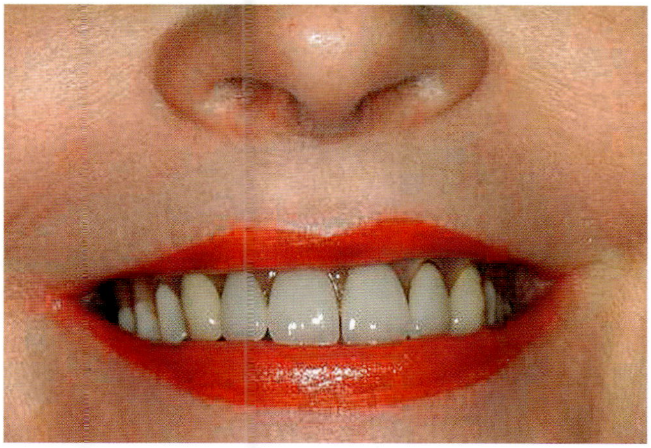

FIGURE 6-49 Postoperative examination at 1 week demonstrates proper function and aesthetics of the provisional prosthesis.

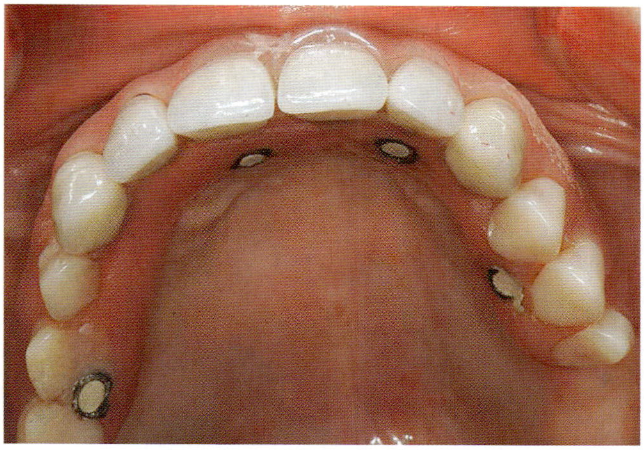

FIGURE 6-50 Intraoral examination 1 week postoperatively is consistent with favorable tissue-to-prosthesis contours, which can be easily maintained by the patient during osseointegration.

PHASE II APPOINTMENT

At the phase II appointment in 6 months, the prosthesis is removed and all abutments are checked by applying the torque driver at 20 Ncm for angulated abutments and 35 Ncm for straight abutments. Lack of screw loosening, implant immobility, and pain-free application of the torque driver confirms osseointegration (Figure 6-51). At this point, the prosthesis is reconnected to the abutments using the prosthetic retaining screws. Cotton pellet and cavit is applied to seal the screw access holes and the patient is referred to a restorative dentist for fabrication of a definitive profile prosthesis.

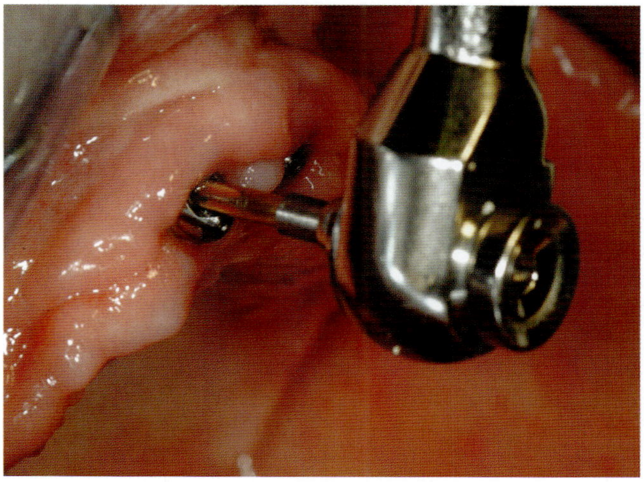

FIGURE 6-51 After 6 months of osseointegration, the provisional implant is removed; the abutment screw torque is confirmed prior to final prosthesis fabrication.

FINAL PROSTHESIS

A final profile prosthesis is fabricated using a metal framework of gold or titanium in conjunction with

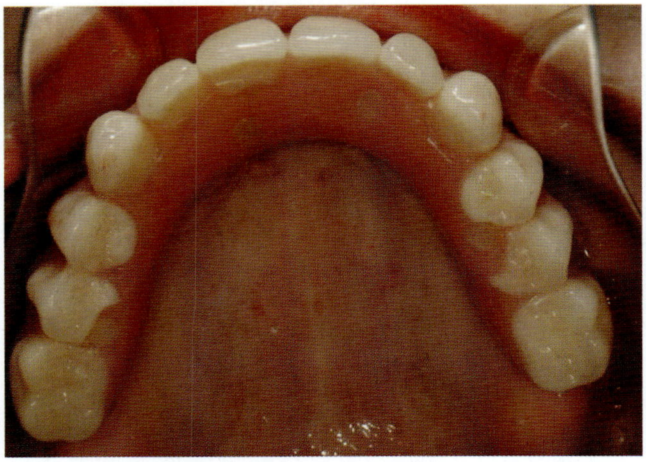

FIGURE 6-52 The final profile prosthesis replaces the patient's composite defect.

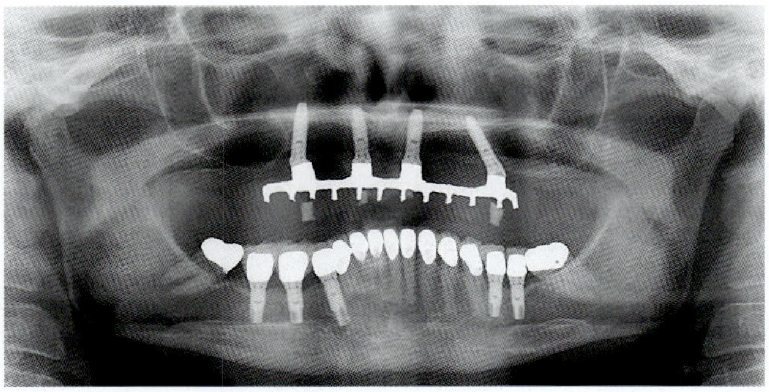

FIGURE 6-53 Final radiographic examination confirms complete seating of all implant components.

pink acrylic and plastic teeth or pink porcelain and porcelain teeth (Figure 6-52). The final radiograph demonstrates complete seating of all components (Figure 6-53). The patient's transition line is hidden during animation, allowing for a natural and aesthetic clinical presentation of the profile prosthesis (Figure 6-54).

DISCUSSION

For many patients, the graftless approach allows implant placement and immediate loading of the edentulous maxilla without bone grafting in one surgical appointment. The single surgery and elimination of additional grafting procedures are factors that make this treatment plan more appealing to patients. Some patients, however, demonstrate adequate vertical bone in zones I and II, but have severe atrophy of the horizontal bony volume. In this group of patients, placement of tilted implants and immediate loading may need to follow an initial bone grafting procedure to increase horizontal bony volume.

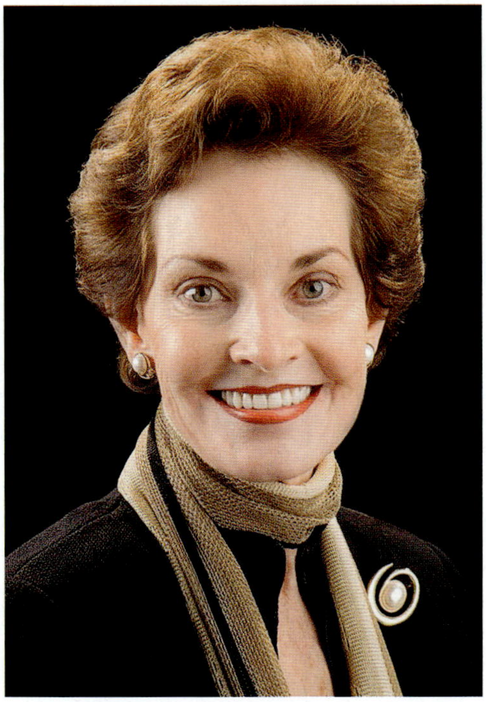

FIGURE 6-54 A well-hidden transition line during animation allows an aesthetic outcome using a profile prosthesis.

REFERENCES

1. Brånemark PI, Hansson BO, Adell R, et al: Osseointegrated implants in treatment of the edentulous jaw. Experience from a 10-year period. *Scand J Plast Reconstr Surg Suppl* 16:1-32, 1977.
2. Adell R, Hansson BO, Brånemark PI, et al: Intraosseous anchorage of dental prosthesis. II. Review of clinical approaches. *Scand J Plast Reconstr Surg* 19-34, 1970.
3. Brånemark PI, Lindstrom J, Hallen O, et al: Reconstruction of the defective mandible. *Scand J Plast Reconstr Surg* 9:116-128, 1975.
4. Breine U, Brånemark PI: Reconstruction of alveolar jaw bone. An experimental and clinical study of immediate and performed autologous bone grafts in combination with osseointegrated implants. *Scand J Plast Reconstr Surg* 14:23-48, 1980.
5. Brånemark PI: Introduction to osseointegration. In Brånemark PI, Zarb G, Albrektsson T, editors. *Tissue-integrated prosthesis—Osseointegration in clinical dentistry,* Chicago, 1985, Quintessence.
6. Bedrossian E: Immediate function with the zygomatic implant: A graftless solution for the patient with mild to advanced atrophy of the maxilla. *Int J Oral Maxillofac Implants* 21(6):937-942, 2006.
7. Maló P, Rangert B, Nobre M: All-on-4 immediate-function concept with Brånemark system implants for completely edentulous maxillae: A 1-year retrospective clinical study. *Clin Implant Dent Relat Res* 7(Suppl 1):S88-S94, 2005.

8. Aparicio C, Ouazzani W, Garcia R, et al: A prospective clinical study on titanium implants in the zygomatic arch for prosthetic rehabilitation of the atrophic maxilla: A follow-up of 6 months to 5 years. *Clin Implant Dent Res* 8:114-122, 2006.
9. Krekmanov L, Kahn M, Rangert B, et al: Tilting of posterior mandibular and maxillary implants for improved prosthesis support. *Int J Oral Maxillofac Implants* 15:405-414, 2000.
10. Duyck J, et al: Magnitude and distribution of occlusal forces on oral implants supporting fixed prosthesis: An in vivo study. *Clin Oral Implants Res* 11:465-475, 2000.
11. Rangert B, Jempt T, Jorneus L: Forces and moments on Brånemark implants. *Int J Oral Maxillofac Implants* 4:241-247, 1989.
12. Brånemark PI, Grondahl K, Worthington P: *Osseointegration and autogenous onlay bone grafts: Reconstruction of the edentulous maxilla,* 2001, Quintessence.
13. Bedrossian E: Fixed-prosthetic implant restoration of the edentulous maxilla: A systematic pretreatment evaluation method. *J Oral Maxillofac Surg* 66:112-122, 2008.

CHAPTER 7

Treatment of the Edentulous Maxilla: Zygoma Implant Concept

Presence of alveolar bone in the premaxilla (zone I) and lack of bone in the bicuspid and molar regions (zones II and III, respectively) is an indication for considering a zygomatic implant. The zygomatic implant establishes posterior maxillary support by using the limited crestal alveolar bone in the bicuspid region and the os zygomaticus for establishing initial implant stability.

RADIOGRAPHIC EVALUATION

Although computed tomography (CT) or conventional tomography can be used, the panoramic radiograph is critical in initial patient evaluation.[1-3] Axial CT scans and cone beam technology can be used to further evaluate the maxillary sinus. The width of the residual alveolar bone and the width and height of the zygomatic body can be visualized in frontal (Figure 7-1) or axial (Figure 7-2) reformatted sections.

Further evaluation of the zygomatic bone has also been described.[4] Although not absolutely necessary, the reformatted frontal images in 0.5- to 1-mm cuts afford the less experienced operator more information for surgery planning (Figure 7-3). Pathologic conditions in the sinus, including but not limited to thickening of the Schneiderian membrane as well as air-fluid levels, may be ruled out in both the panoramic radiographic examination as well as the tomographic studies (Figure 7-4).

Cone beam CT scan can also be used effectively to manipulate postoperative radiographs (Figure 7-5, *A*). The ability to manipulate the cone beam images to demonstrate apex positioning of the zygoma implant within the zygoma body (Figure 7-5, *B*), as well as the relationship of the zygoma implant platform to the crestal portion of the alveolus, leads to a better understanding of surgical technique (Figure 7-5, *C*).

PREOPERATIVE CONSIDERATIONS

The surgical procedure is usually performed in the office setting under intravenous (IV) sedation,[1,5] although the procedure can be performed under local anesthesia or in the operating room under general anesthesia. All patients are premedicated with 2 g of penicillin or 600 mg of clindamycin 1 hour prior to the procedure. Proper administration of sufficient local anesthesia is critical to manage patients under IV sedation. The various infiltrations and nerve blocks include circumvestibular infiltration of the maxilla and greater palatine nerve blocks, as well as bilateral transcutaneous infiltration of the temporal areas over the zygomatic body. Bilateral inferior alveolar nerve blocks are considered to allow retraction of the lower jaw during surgery without undo stimulation of the sedated patient. It is recommended that the path of the implant from the premolar area to the base of the zygoma be directly visualized whenever possible.[1,6] Direct visualization of the base of the zygoma body has also been advocated by clinicians who have used computer-assisted treatment planning and surgical templates for placement of zygomatic implants.[6] Having a clear view of the instruments' path while establishing the osteotomy, as well as visualizing the path of the implant during its insertion, avoids disorientation and potential complications. Generally, three potential axes for implant insertion are possible. The proper axis is a path extending from the bicuspid region through the maxillary sinus, entering the mid portion of the zygomatic body. If the entry point in the zygomatic

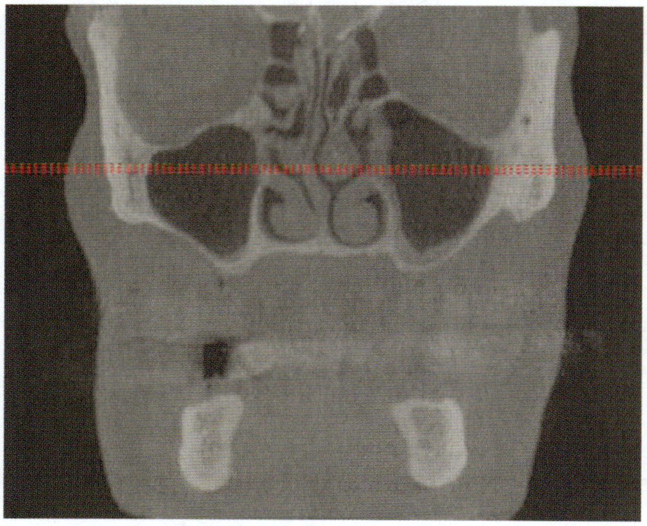

FIGURE 7-1 Coronal cone beam computed tomographic scan of the bilateral maxillary sinuses and the body of the zygomatic bone.

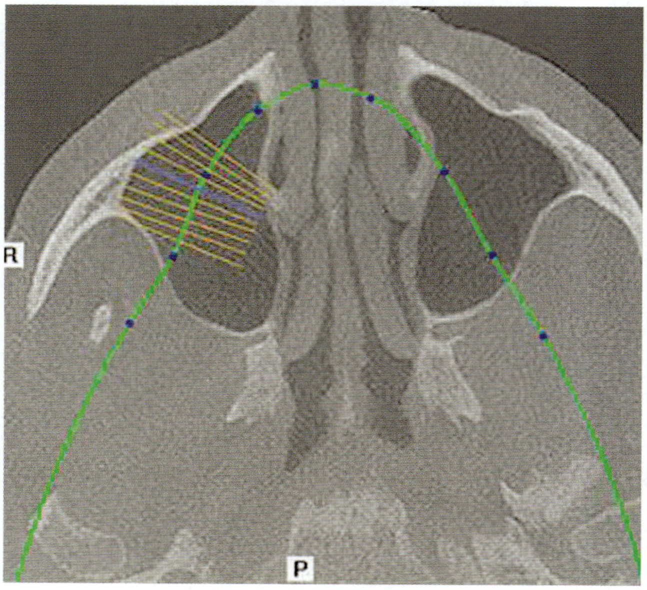

FIGURE 7-2 Axial cone beam computed tomographic scan showing the body and arch of the zygoma.

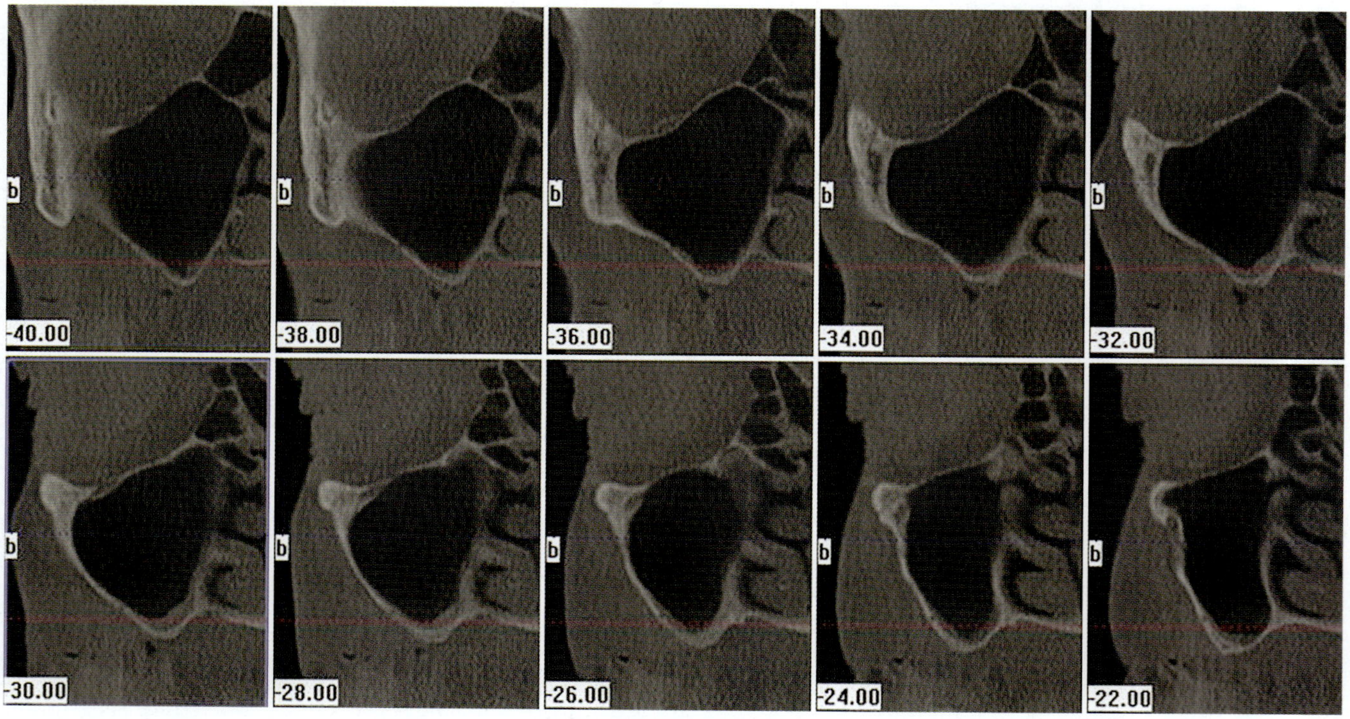

FIGURE 7-3 Coronal series of the zygoma body.

body is anterior to this line axis, potential exists for penetration into the orbit. If the line axis is posterior to this line, potential exists for entering the pterygomaxillary space, which leads to soft tissue envelopment and subsequent lack of osseointegration of the implant, causing unexpected hemorrhage (Figure 7-6).

The zygomatic implant has a unique design. The diameter of the apical two-thirds of the implant is 4 mm and the alveolar one-third widens to a diameter of 5 mm. Zygomatic implants are available in lengths ranging from 30 to 52.5 mm. A specialized series of long zygoma drills are used to prepare the osteotomy (Figure 7-7).

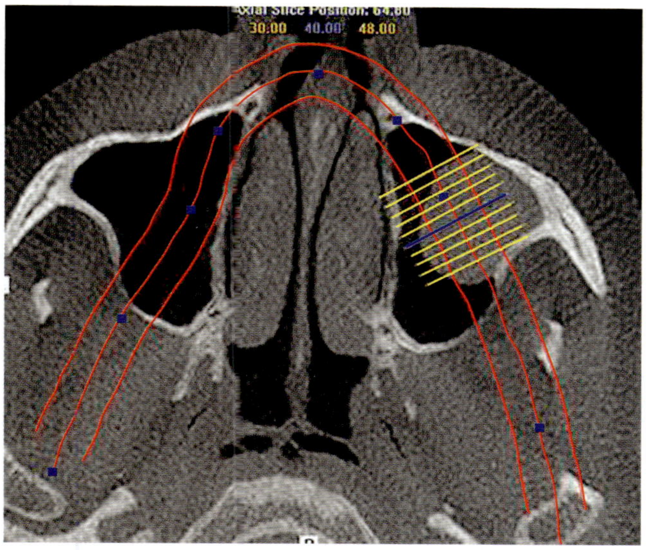

FIGURE 7-4 Axial cone beam computed tomographic scan showing the presence of a maxillary polyp.

SURGICAL OPTIONS

To reconstruct an edentulous maxilla with a zygomatic implant, the traditional two-stage protocol[1,7,8] or the immediate-load protocol[1,6] may be considered. The two-stage protocol requires immediate cross-arch splinting of the zygoma implant at the time of the uncovering procedure. This can be accomplished efficiently using the CAL technique for fabrication of a passive bar prior to the uncovering procedure.[9] Uncovered zygoma implants that have temporary abutment should not be placed under occlusal loads without having been cross-arch stabilized. To expedite the stage II surgery and deliver a passive bar in the two-stage approach, fixture-level impressions of the implants are taken prior to closure of the soft tissues at stage I (Figure 7-8). During the 6-month

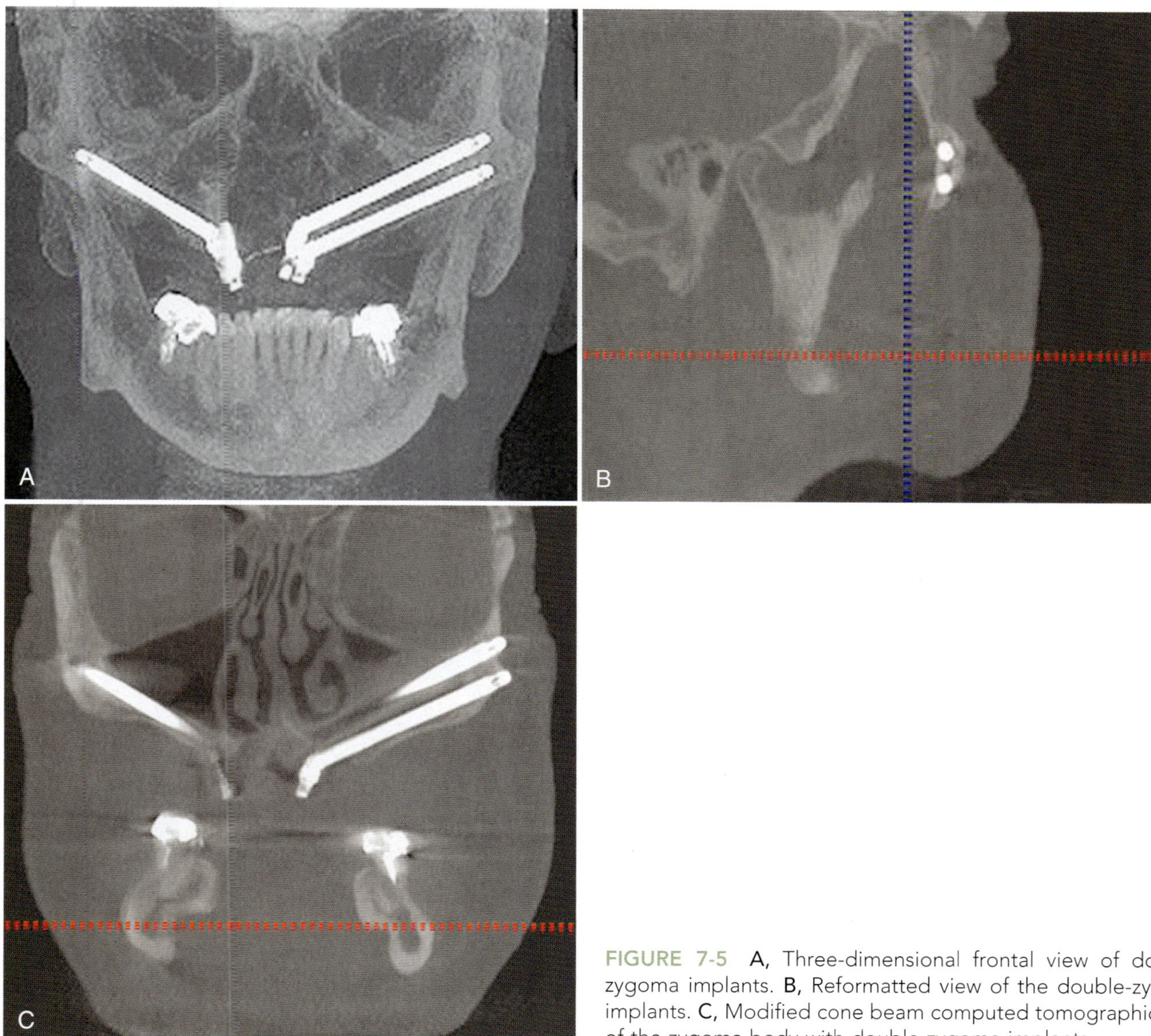

FIGURE 7-5 A, Three-dimensional frontal view of double-zygoma implants. B, Reformatted view of the double-zygoma implants. C, Modified cone beam computed tomographic scan of the zygoma body with double-zygoma implants.

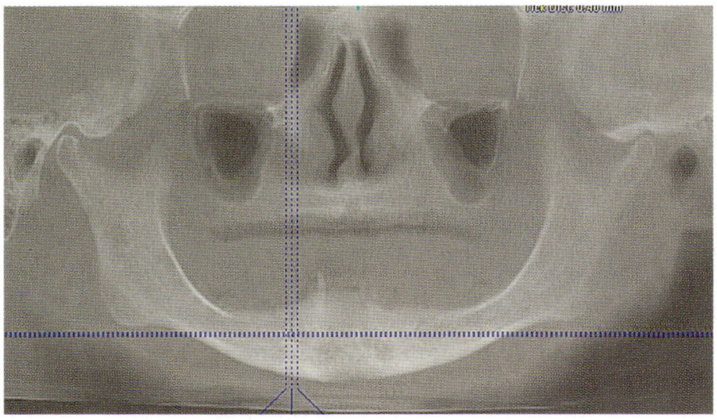

FIGURE 8-15 The panoramic radiograph only allows for evaluation of the vertical edentulous ridge and its length.

existing denture has the proper vertical dimension of occlusion (VDO) and the proper AP tooth position for conversion to an immediate-load provisional profile prosthesis (Figure 8-18).

For edentulous patients who wear an existing full mandibular denture, a restorative dentist should be asked to fabricate a new denture prior to surgery if the patient's existing denture does not have the proper VDO and AP tooth position. For patients with nonrestorable teeth who are to be edentulated (Figure 8-19), the mandibular immediate denture should also be fabricate at the proper VDO (Figure 8-20) because immediate conversion of the patient's "immediate denture" into the mandibular immediate-load profile prosthesis is intended (Figure 8-21).

The systematic preoperative treatment planning protocol for the edentulous mandible permits consideration of:

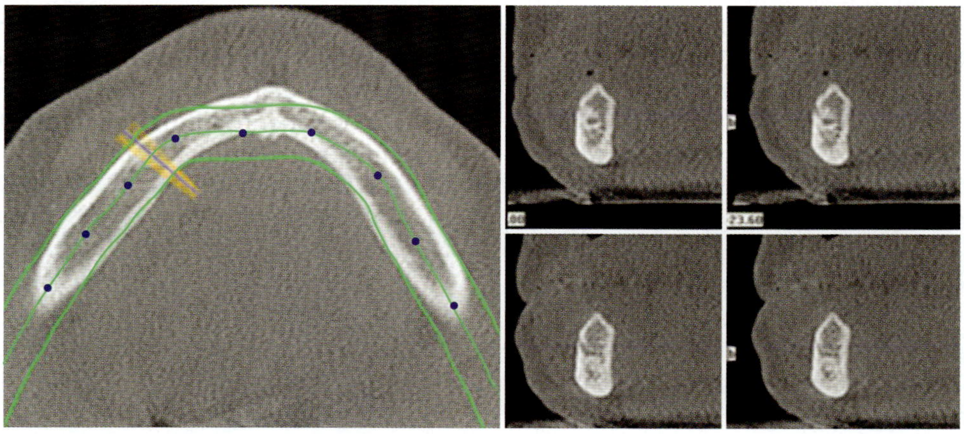

FIGURE 8-16 The width of the residual edentulous mandible is easily studied using a cone beam radiograph.

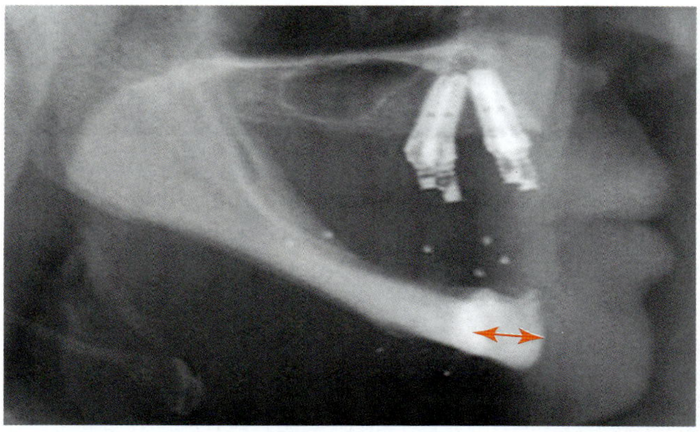

FIGURE 8-17 A conventional lateral cephalometric study demonstrates the width of the anterior mandible, as well as the position of the genial tubercle and its relationship to the residual crest of the edentulous anterior mandibular alveolus.

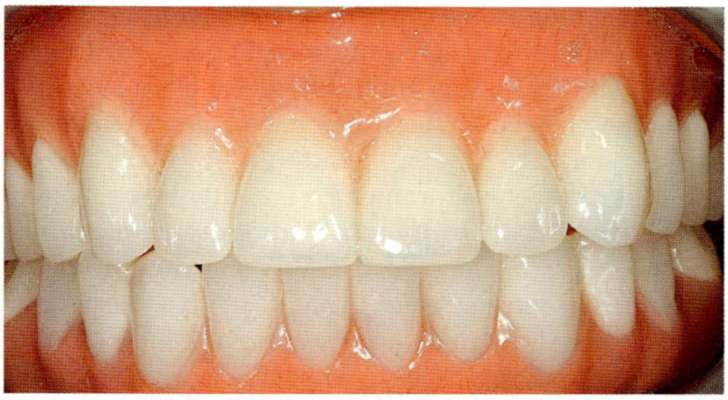

FIGURE 8-18 Determination of the proper vertical dimension occlusion and anterior-posterior tooth position of the existing prosthesis is recommended prior to initiation of the immediate-load protocol.

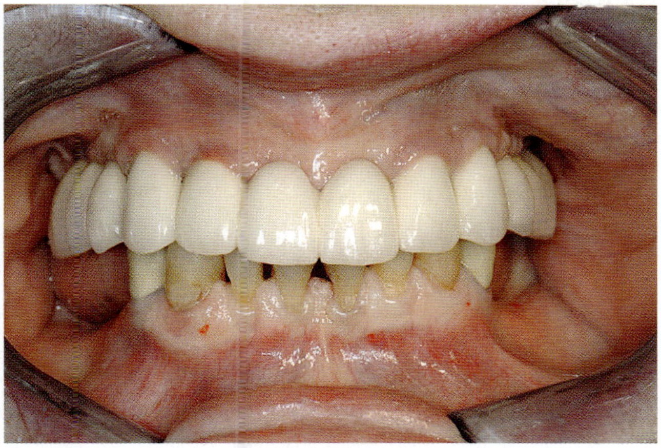

FIGURE 8-19 For patients with collapsed vertical dimension of occlusion (VDO), fabrication of the immediate denture should take into consideration the desired increase in VDO.

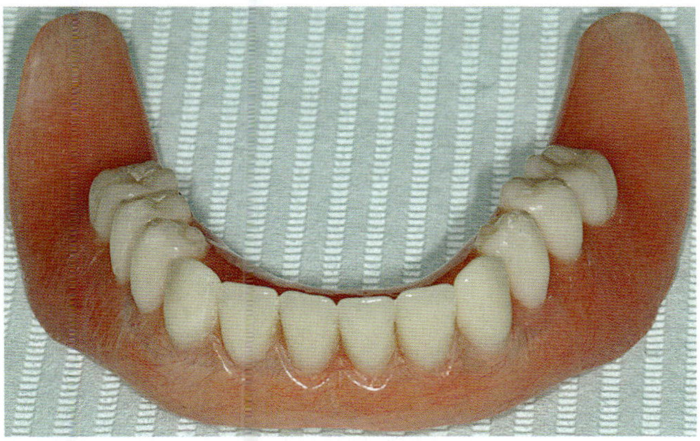

FIGURE 8-20 An immediate denture, which will be used for conversion to immediate-load prosthesis, is fabricated at the desired vertical dimension of occlusion.

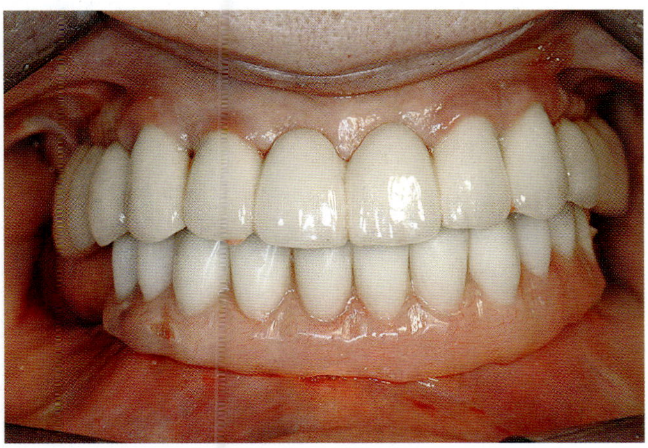

FIGURE 8-21 An increase of clinically appropriate vertical dimension of occlusion is seen in the patient's converted immediate denture.

1. Presence or absence of a composite defect
2. Whether to use a ceramo-metal bridge or a profile prosthesis
3. Aesthetic confirmation of the intended treatment by evaluating the transition zone
4. Radiographic studies to evaluate the position of the mental foramen and the anterior loop of the inferior alveolar canal, preparing the implant team to initiate the surgical procedure

This surgical procedure can be performed in the office under local anesthesia as well as under general anesthesia in the operating room. Usually it is performed under intravenous sedation in the office setting. One hour prior to the surgical procedure, patients are premedicated with 2 g of amoxicillin or 600 mg of clindamycin.

Criteria for immediately loading the edentulous mandible are:

1. Use of single-threaded, regular platform (RP) implants.
2. The osteotomy is undersized to a minimum of 2.8 mm and a maximum of 3 mm for placement of 4-mm diameter implants in most cases. Individual evaluation of bone density should be made, however, as in the severely atrophic mandible; predominance of cortical bone may at times warrant using the bone tap prior to insertion of the implants.
3. Implant insertion torque is 40 Ncm.
4. Immediate cross-arch splitting of all implants is performed.
5. Use of 0° to 5° denture teeth in group function.
6. The prosthesis is not electively removed until completion of the 3-month waiting period, before the fabrication of a final prosthesis with a metal substructure.

SURGICAL PROTOCOL AND TECHNIQUE

The surgical protocol begins with the administration of local anesthetic. Lidocaine 2% with 1:100,000 epinephrine is used. After adequate time is allowed for the local anesthetic to take effect, a crestal incision is made to expose the alveolus. The incision extends approximately to the mesial aspect of the second molar region. Blunt dissection is used to identify the mental foramen (Figure 8-22). Once the mental foramen has been identified, a minimum distance of 5 mm measured anteriorly is allowed for the loop of the inferior alveolar nerve before its termination as the mental nerve. To create a visual guideline prior to preparation of the osteotomy, a straight line is taken superiorly

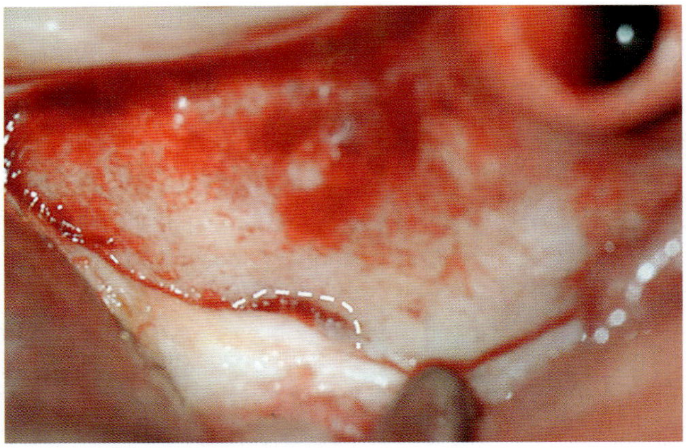

FIGURE 8-22 Blunt dissection identifies the mental foramen.

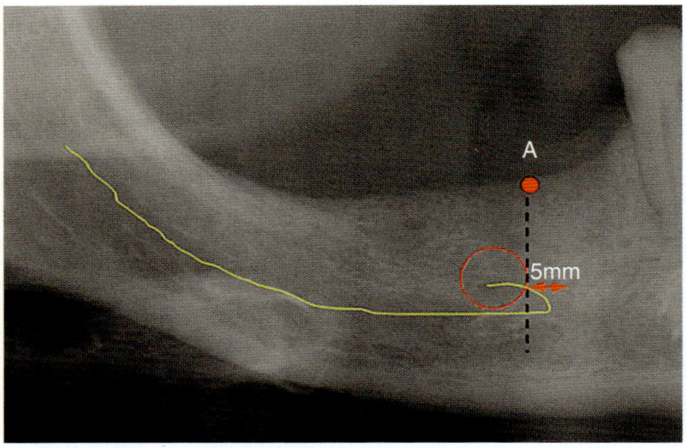

FIGURE 8-23 Point *A* demarcates the anterior-most extension of the mental foramen. The loop of the inferior alveolar nerve extends approximately 5 mm anterior to point *A*.

from the anterior-most aspect of the mental foramen to its corresponding position on the crest of the mandible; this is point A (Figure 8-23). A second point, point B, is marked on the mandibular crest 9 mm anterior to point A (Figure 8-24). A third straight line is dropped vertically from point B to point C at the level equal to the midpoint of the anterior wall of the mental foramen (Figure 8-25). The position of point D is picked to allow the most distal placement of the implant platform (Figure 8-26). Point D is determined by inclining line C–D posteriorly. The posterior inclination of line C–D cannot not exceed 45° from line B–C (Figure 8-27). The rational for the maximum 45° tilting is as follows: Two adjacent implants may be divergent by 15°, yet the framework will still "draw" using the straight multiunit abutments. Mechanical limitations of abutment fabrication allow for production of angulated abutments with the maximum angulation of 30°. Therefore, the addition of 15° to the correction potential of the 30° abutment allows the distal implant to be 45° divergent

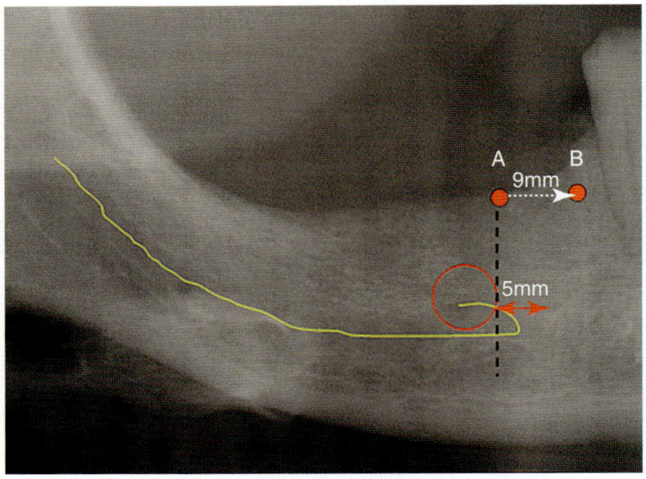

FIGURE 8-24 Point *B* demarcates a point 9 mm anterior to point *A*.

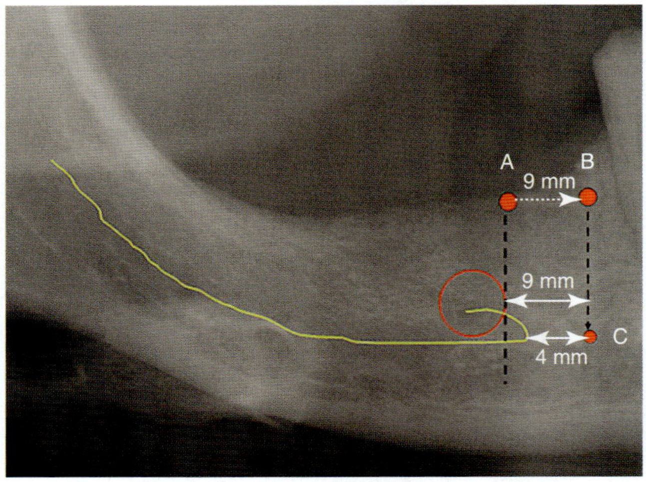

FIGURE 8-25 Point *C* is the inferior extension of point *B*, demarcating a point 4 mm anterior to the anterior-most portion of the inferior alveolar loop.

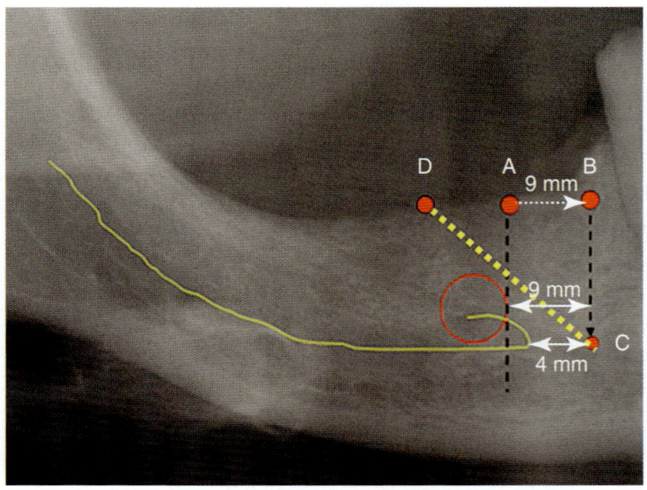

FIGURE 8-26 Point *D* demarcates the most posterior position from the mental foramen possible while drawing a line that connects point *D* and point *C*.

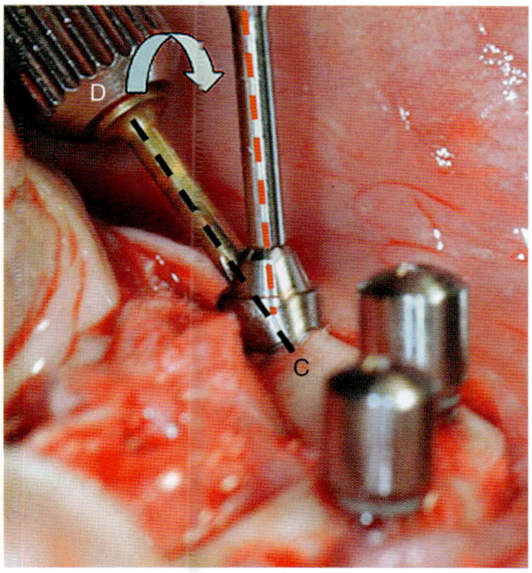

FIGURE 8-27 *Line D–C* may not extend beyond 45° from the vertical axis because the greatest correction abutment available is 30°.

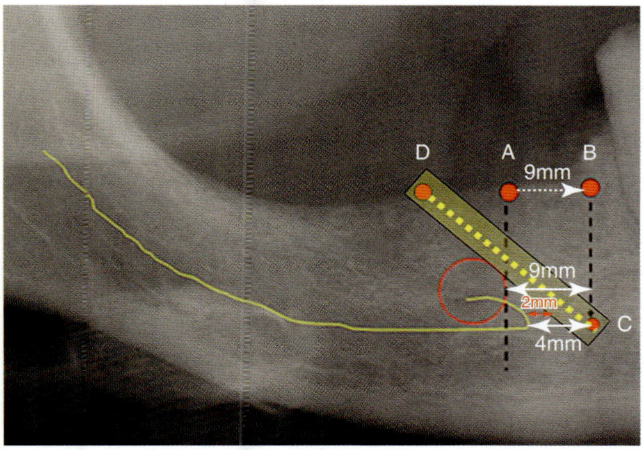

FIGURE 8-28 The guideline *D–C* represents the central axis of the proposed implant.

from the anterior axial implant. With the use of the 30° multiunit abutment, the framework will still draw.

At this time, the surgeon is ready to initiate the osteotomy using the 2-mm pilot drill. The 2-mm pilot drill connects and bisects point D with point C. This guideline represents the central portion of a 4-mm diameter RP implant (Figure 8-28). By following this guideline, the final tilted implant position will be 2 mm anterior to the loop of the mental nerve (Figure 8-29).

The same protocol is followed to identify the contralateral mental foramen and to place the second tilted implant. To allow ease of orientation and inclination of the axial as well as the tilted implants, a surgical guide is available with vertical grooves etched onto its surface; these grooves function as reference guides

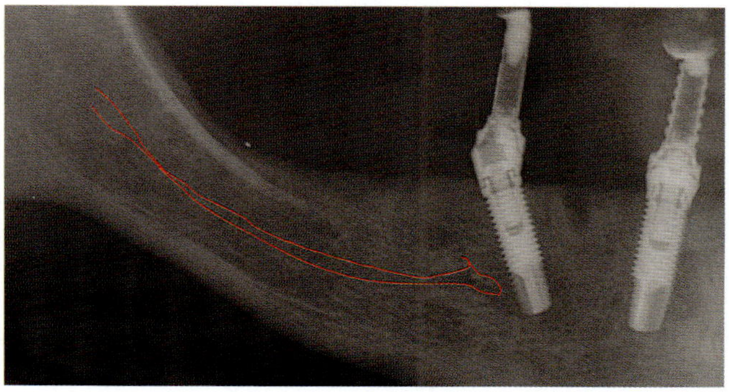

FIGURE 8-29 The final implant position is 2 mm anterior to the anterior-most portion of the loop of the inferior alveolar nerve.

(Figure 8-30, *A*). Using a 2-mm drill in the mandibular midline, the drill guide is stabilized to the mandible (Figure 8-30, *B*). To initiate the tilted implant position, the 2-mm drill is tilted a maximum of 45° from the reference line on the drill guide (Figure 8-30, *C*). The surgical stent is used at this point to guide the surgeon in placement of the two anterior axial implants. These implants are placed in a position as far anterior to the two posterior implant platforms as possible. The surgeon must take into consideration the position of the anterior teeth, keeping the axis of the implant and therefore the implant platform at the level of the cingulum or slightly lingual to the cingulum of the anterior teeth (Figure 8-30, *D*). Respecting prosthetic needs permits use of screw-retained abutments and attachment of temporary cylinders for conversion of the immediate denture into an immediate provisional profile prosthesis.

The osteotomy is completed for most cases using a final 2.8-mm drill (in severely resorbed ridges and very dense bone, a 3- or 3.2-mm final osteotomy drill with or without a bone tap may be used) (Figure 8-31). The single-threaded implants (Figure 8-32) are placed with the implant handpiece motor set at 20 Ncm. As the resistance during placement of the implant increases and stalls the handpiece, the insertion torque is increased to 40 Ncm. It may be necessary to hand-torque implants into their final seating if the insertion torque exceeds the 40-Ncm setting of the handpiece motor (Figure 8-33).

The posterior implant axis is corrected by the placement of 30° multiunit abutments, which are torqued to 20 Ncm. Two temporary abutments are placed on the anterior implants until indexing of the denture is completed, determining whether straight or 17° angulated abutments should be used (Figure 8-34). This completes the surgical procedure. Temporary plastic caps are placed on the 30° abutments and the soft tissues are adapted to all four abutments (Figure 8-35).

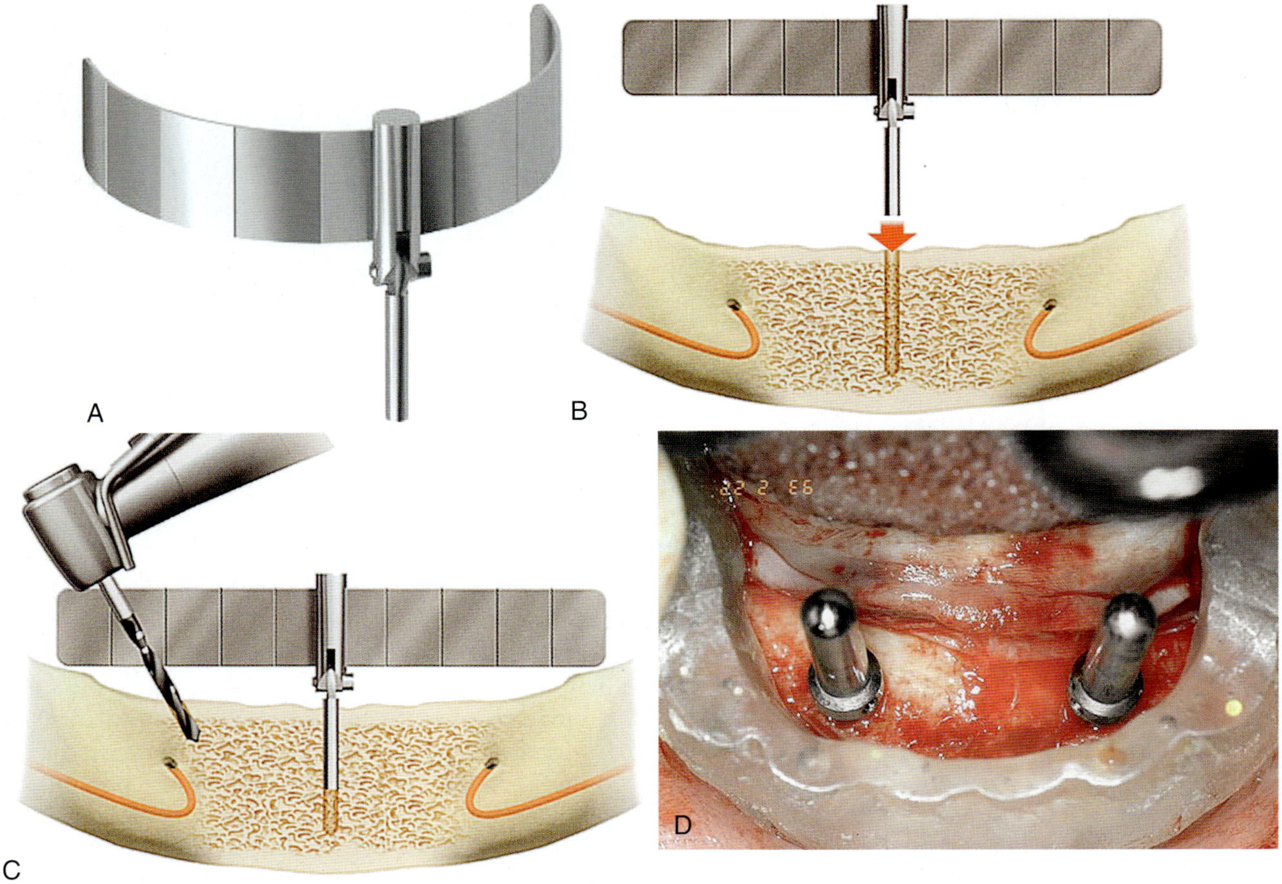

FIGURE 8-30 **A,** A malleable guide is available to allow easier drill orientation during preparation of the tilted and axial implants. **B,** The malleable guide is secured to the mandible by preparing a 2-mm wide osteotomy in the central portion of the edentulous alveolus and securing the fixation pin of the guide within the osteotomy. **C,** The vertical orientation guidelines on the malleable guide are used to orient the drill prior to initiating the osteotomy for distal tilted implants. **D,** The position of the anterior axial implants is in line with the cingulum of the anterior teeth or lingual to them. *(A–C courtesy of Nobel Biocare, Yorba Linda, Calif.)*

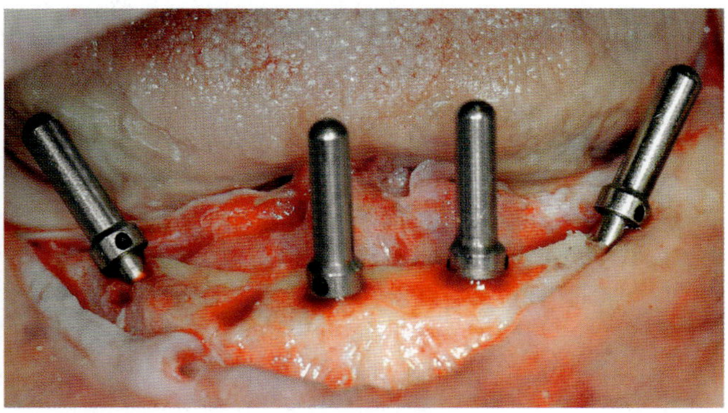

FIGURE 8-31 The paralleling pins demonstrate the distribution of the proposed implants.

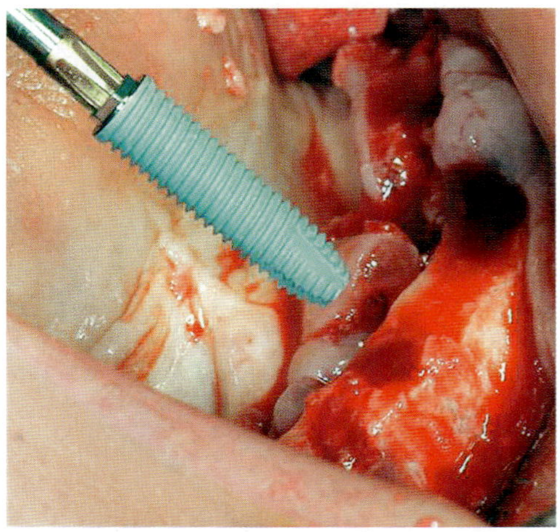

FIGURE 8-32 Parallel-wall or tapered-wall implants are used depending on the density of the bone observed during the preparation of the osteotomy sites.

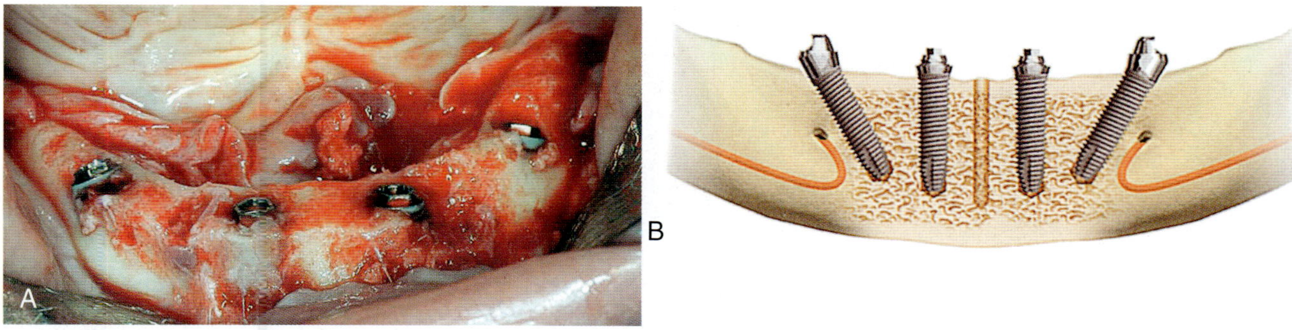

FIGURE 8-33 **A,** Final positioning of the implants with the implant platforms at the crest of the edentulous mandibular alveolus. **B,** The final implant positions place the distal implants at least 2 mm anterior to the inferior loop and the anterior implants as far forward as possible to maintain the greatest anterior-posterior distribution. *(B courtesy Nobel Biocare, Yorba Linda, Calif.)*

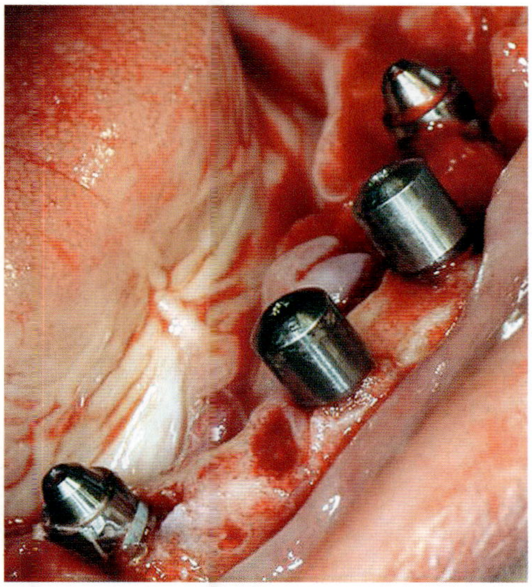

FIGURE 8-34 Temporary healing abutments are placed on the anterior implants prior to indexing the position of the implants onto the intaglio surface of the patient's denture during the conversion process.

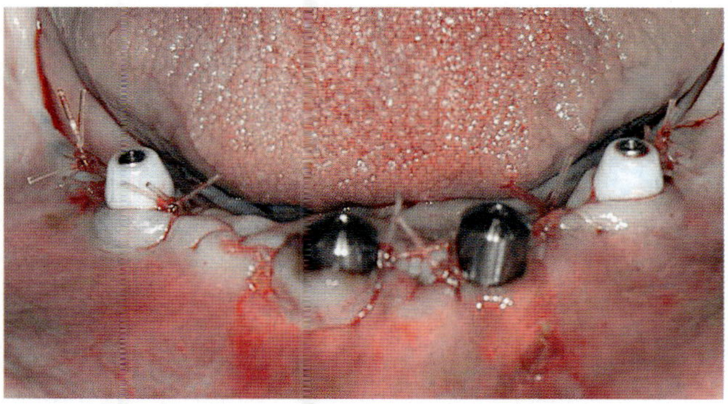

FIGURE 8-35 Multiunit abutments of 30° or 17° are placed on the distal implants with their associated healing cap prior to suturing the soft tissues.

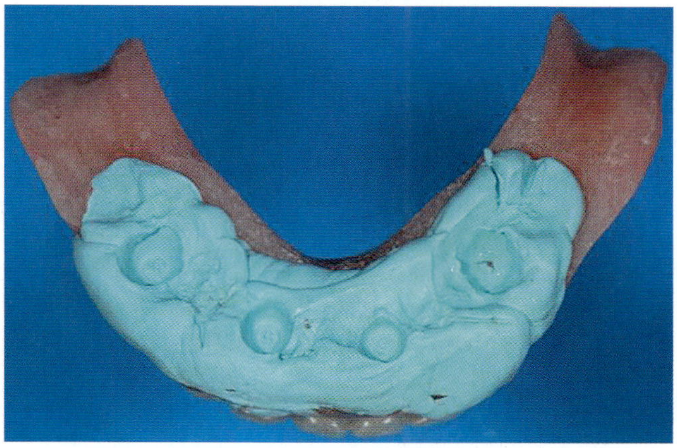

FIGURE 8-36 Registration material transfers the position of the implants to the intaglio surface of the mandibular denture.

PROSTHETIC CONVERSION

Prosthetic conversion follows the same protocol as described in earlier publications.[27] Indexing material of the practitioner's choice, such as polyvinylsiloxane, is used to imprint the position of the abutments on the intaglio surface of the mandibular denture (Figure 8-36). Once this registration material has set, the denture is removed and a small-diameter laboratory bur is used to transfer the position of the abutments to the denture base (Figure 8-37). As is evident in Figure 8-38, straight, multiunit abutments were selected for this case and placed on the anterior implants. The abutments were torqued to 35 Ncm. To begin the attachment of the mandibular denture to the implants, temporary titanium cylinders are screwed into the multiunit abutments (Figure 8-39). The denture is placed over the temporary cylinders, ensuring complete circumferential clearance of the acrylic from the titanium cylinders (Figure 8-40). The operator may choose to lute each cylinder individually to the denture, to lute all four cylinders, or to lute any combination

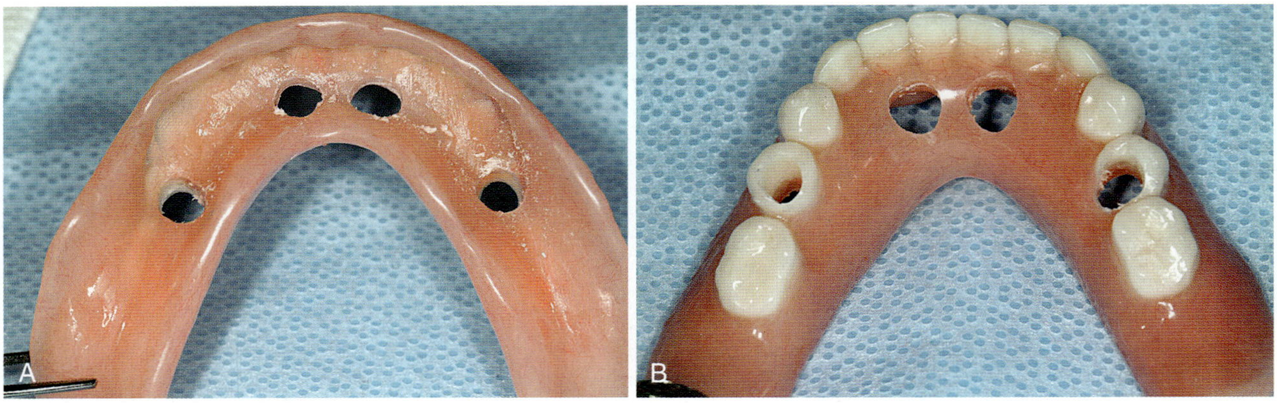

FIGURE 8-37 A, A small-diameter acrylic bur is used initially to perforate through the denture base. B, A larger acrylic bur enlarges the implant positions of the denture base. Note the position of the anterior implant openings, which will allow the use of straight multiunit abutments.

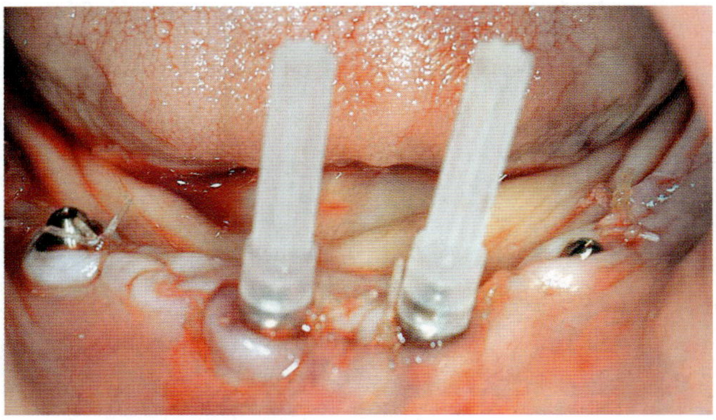

FIGURE 8-38 Straight multiunit abutments are secured to anterior implants.

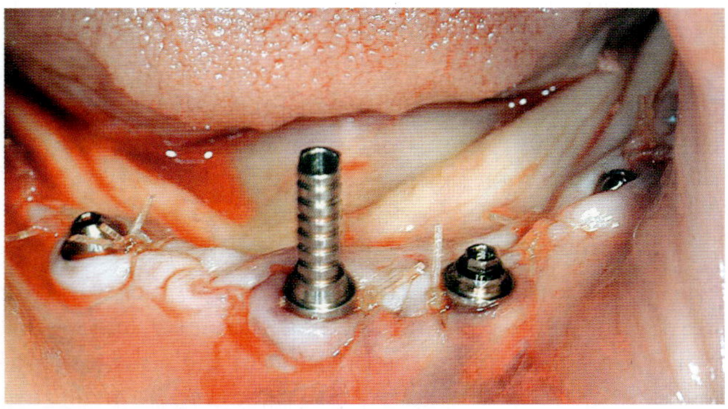

FIGURE 8-39 Temporary titanium cylinders secured to the abutments begin the luting step of the conversion protocol.

(Figure 8-41). The goal prior to luting the cylinders is to make sure that the denture seats over the titanium cylinders without any acrylic binding and that the occlusal plane and the dental midlines are in concert with each other (Figure 8-42). Once the initial luting of the cylinders has been accomplished (Figure 8-43), the

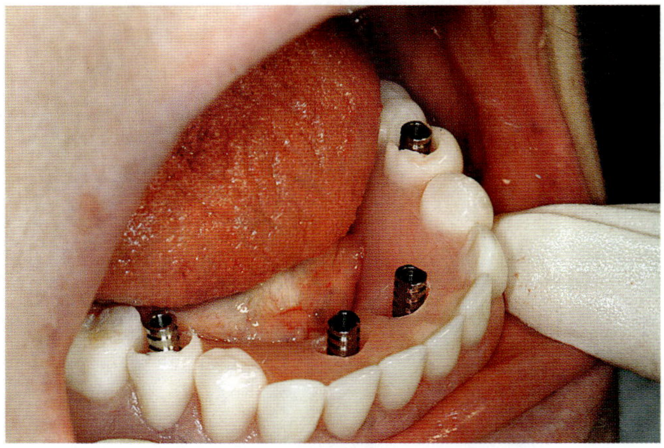

FIGURE 8-40 Confirmation of a circumferential clearance around all titanium cylinders is made prior to luting to the denture base.

prosthesis is carefully removed and the intaglio surface is evaluated and filled with quick-setting acrylic (Figure 8-44). Care must be taken not to cover the 2-mm collar of the temporary cylinders. Figure 8-45 demonstrates the correct height of the acrylic as it meets the titanium cylinder collar. The incorrect height of the acrylic as shown on the left cylinder may lead to soft tissue irritation and should be carefully removed before securing the prosthesis to the abutments. Once all four cylinders have been connected to the denture base, the flange and the distal extension borders are removed (Figure 8-46). The final provisional prosthesis is polished and secured to the patient (Figure 8-47). The occlusion is adjusted to allow bilateral equal occlusion. A postoperative radiograph is evaluated to ensure complete seating of all abutments onto the implant platforms, as well as complete seating of all temporary cylinders onto the abutments (Figure 8-48).

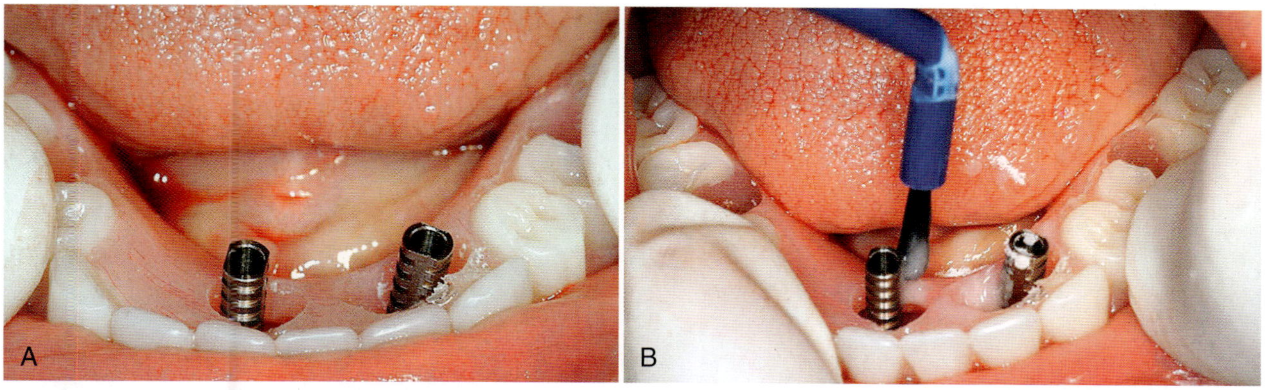

FIGURE 8-41 A, The anterior cylinders in position are ready for luting to the denture base. B, A "salt and pepper" technique is used to secure the titanium cylinders to the denture base.

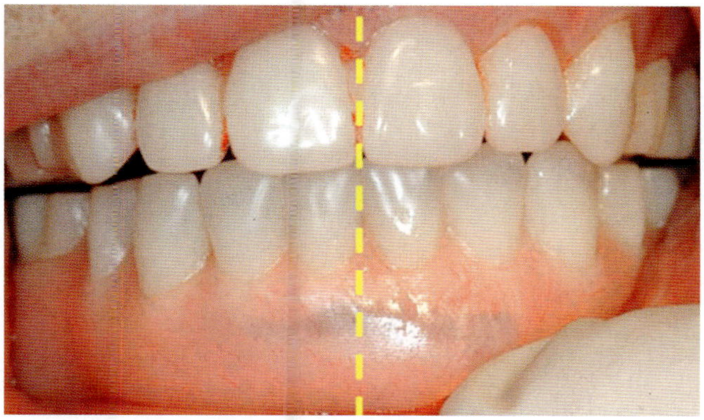

FIGURE 8-42 The proper occlusal and midline positions of the mandibular denture to the opposing teeth must be maintained during the conversion process.

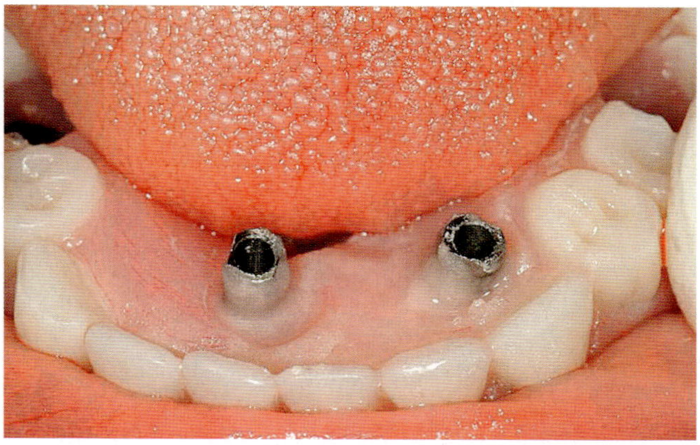

FIGURE 8-43 On completion of the luting of the anterior implant's occlusal surface, the prosthesis is carefully removed from the patient's mouth.

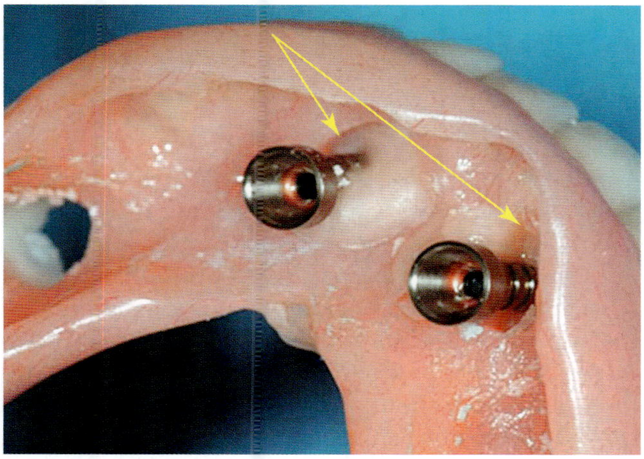

FIGURE 8-44 The intaglio surface of the titanium cylinders is filled with quick-setting acrylic to fully secure the cylinders to the denture base.

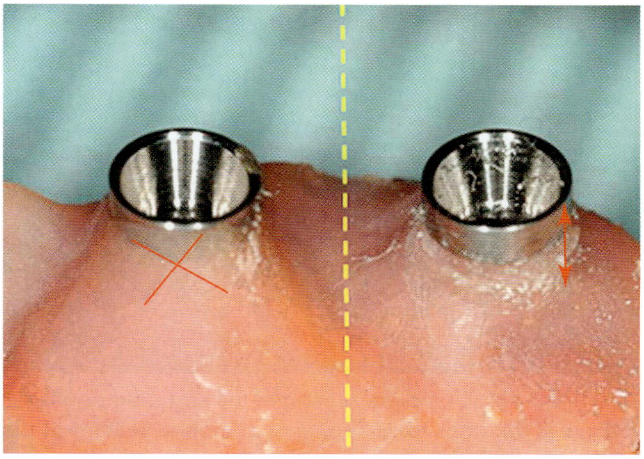

FIGURE 8-45 Care must be taken not to cover the intrasulcular collar of the intaglio surface of the titanium temporary cylinder.

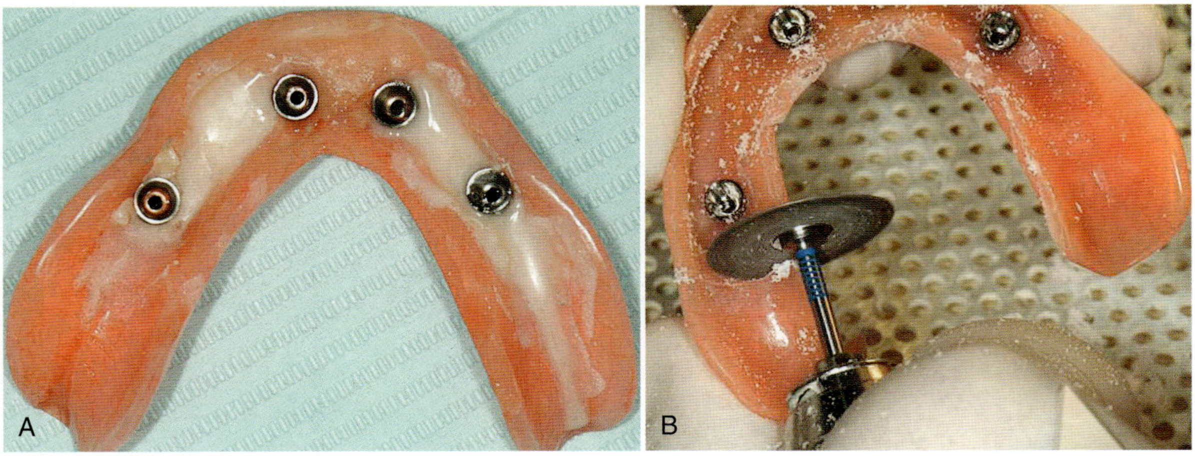

FIGURE 8-46 A, All implants are fully secured to the titanium cylinders prior to reshaping the denture into a provisional profile prosthesis. B, The distal extensions and the flange of the mandibular denture are removed and recontoured to the shape of the profile prosthesis.

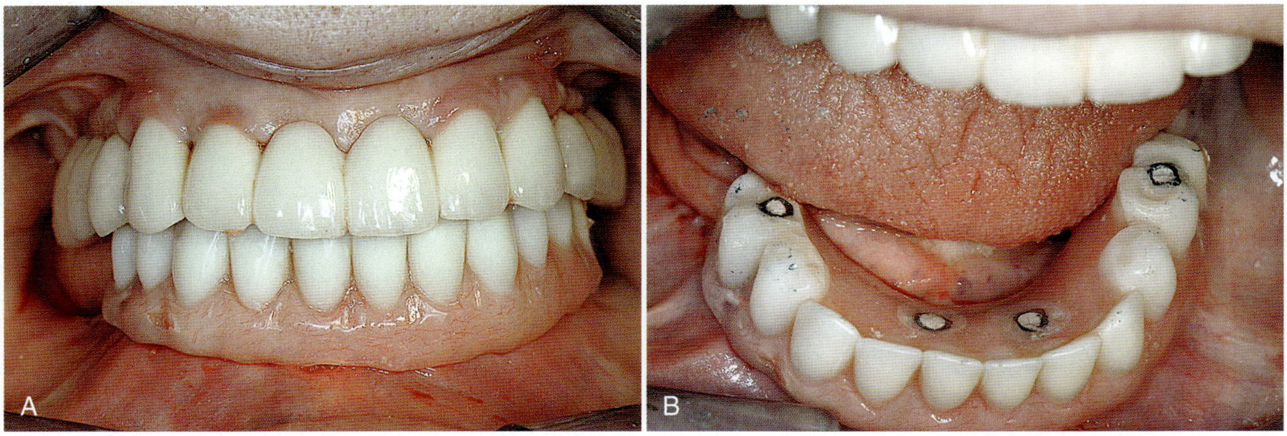

FIGURE 8-47 A, Completed provisional prosthesis in appropriate centric occlusion with midline in line. B, The screw axis holes of the provisional prosthesis are closed using a temporary material of the practitioner's choice to prevent food impaction.

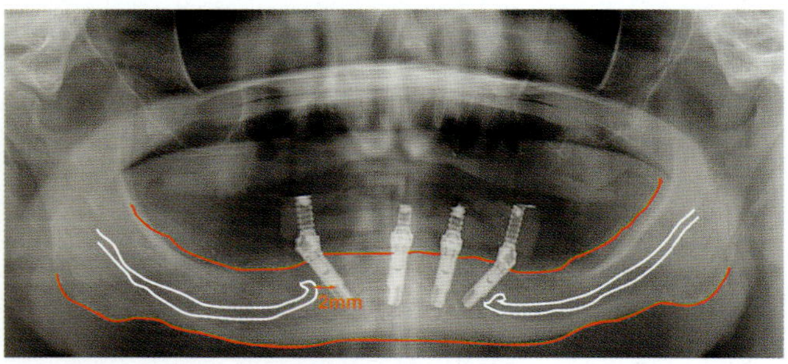

FIGURE 8-48 Complete seating of the abutments onto the implant platform is observed, as is complete seating of the titanium cylinders onto the abutment platform.

POSTOPERATIVE CARE

Immediately after this procedure, patients are able to chew all food types; however, they are cautioned to avoid foods that require significant forces for incising or chewing before ingestion. Noncompliance with these instructions may lead to nonosseointegration of the implants or fracture of the acrylic provisional prosthesis. Therefore patients are advised to eat a soft diet; food consistency should be no harder than that of well-cooked chicken or fish.

Postoperative medications are amoxicillin 500 mg four times daily or clindamycin (Cleocin) 150 mg three times daily for 1 week, as well as an analgesic of the patient's choice as needed. A 0.12% chlorhexidine rinse is used every night at bedtime for 6 months during osseointegration.

The patient's occlusion is checked at the 1-week postoperative appointment. Group function with bilateral, equal centric occlusion is the goal for the next 3 months of osseointegration. Patients are advised to call immediately if they feel that they are biting more heavily on one side than the other. They are also advised to report any swelling, pain, or mobility of the prosthesis encountered at any time after surgery.

PHASE II APPOINTMENT

At the phase II appointment in 3 months, the prosthesis is removed (Figure 8-49), all abutments are checked by applying the torque driver (20 Ncm for angulated abutments and 35 Ncm for straight abutments) (Figure 8-50). Lack of screw loosening, implant immobility, and pain-free upon application of the torque driver confirm osseointegration. At this point, the prosthesis is reconnected to the abutments using the prosthetic retaining screws. Cotton pellet and cavit is applied to seal the screw access holes and the patient is referred to a restorative dentist for fabrication of a definitive profile prosthesis.

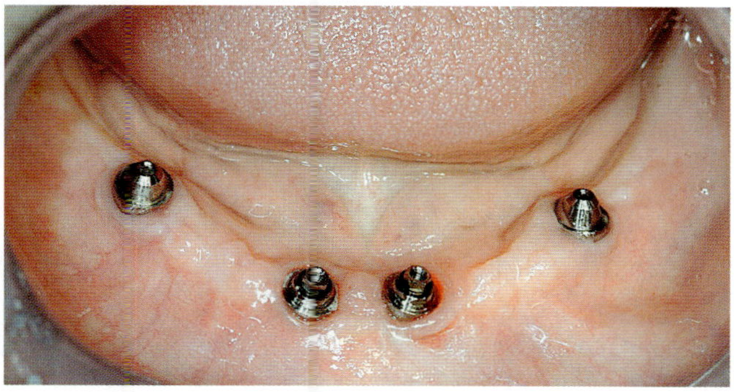

FIGURE 8-49 After 3 months of osseointegration, the mandibular provisional prosthesis is removed.

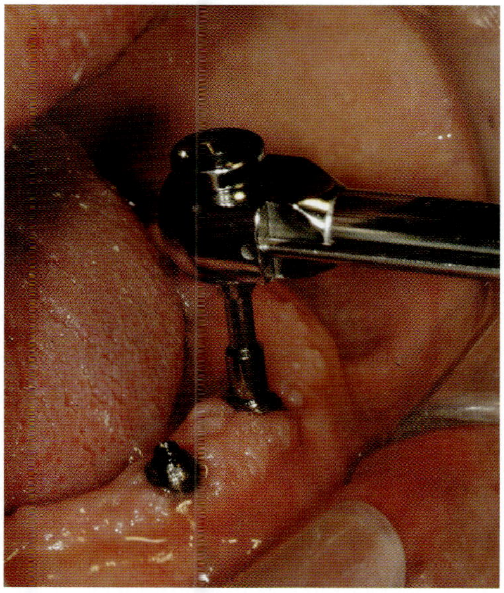

FIGURE 8-50 The stability of the straight and angulated multiunit abutments is checked by applying 35 Ncm and 20 Ncm of torque respectively.

Final Prosthesis

The final profile prosthesis is fabricated using a metal framework (Figure 8-51) of gold or titanium in conjunction with pink acrylic and plastic teeth or pink porcelain and porcelain teeth (Figure 8-52). The final radiograph demonstrates complete seating of all components (Figure 8-53). The patient's transition line is hidden during animation, allowing for a natural and aesthetic clinical presentation of the profile prosthesis (Figure 8-54).

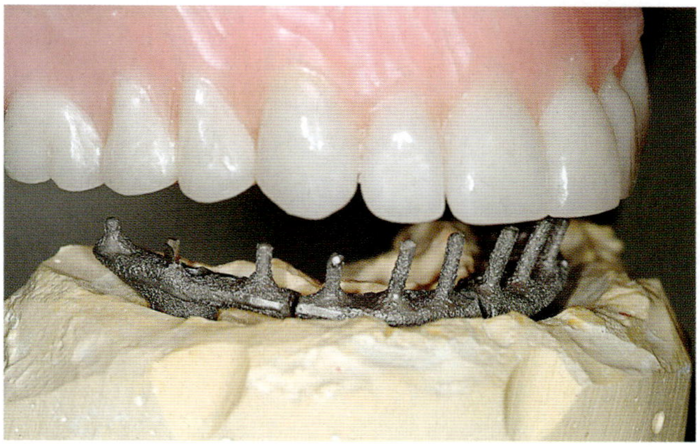

FIGURE 8-51 The metal framework is fabricated ready for clinical evaluation of its passive fit.

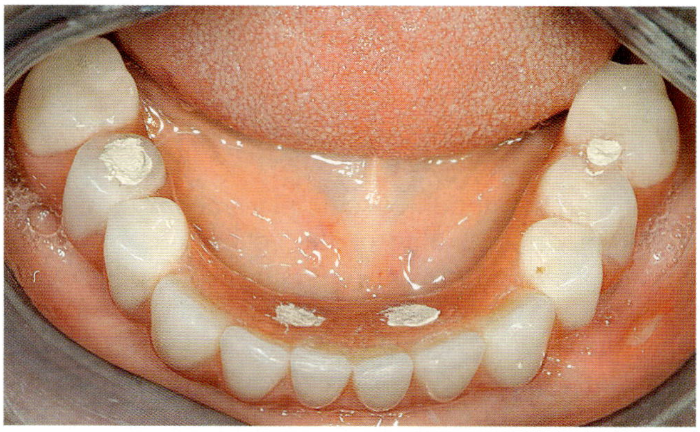

FIGURE 8-52 The final mandibular profile prosthesis delivered.

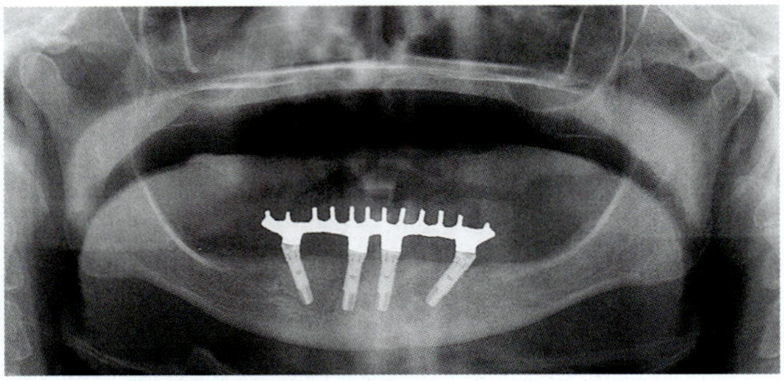

FIGURE 8-53 The final panoramic radiograph illustrates complete seating of the abutments and final framework.

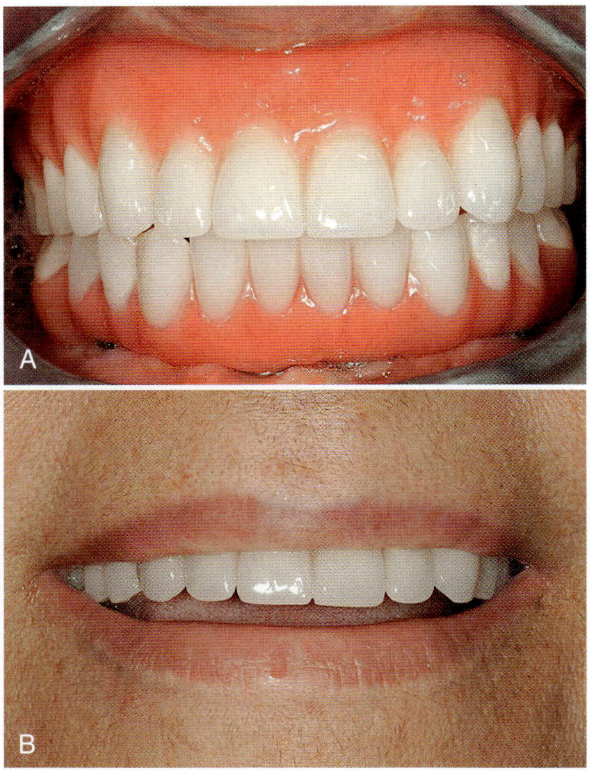

FIGURE 8-54 A, A favorable contour of the base of the profile prosthesis with the edentulous mandibular soft tissues. B, An aesthetic final lower-lip drape and overall smile.

DISCUSSION

This treatment option permits placement of implants and immediate loading of the edentulous mandible without bone grafting in one surgical appointment. The ability to negotiate the loop of the inferior alveolar nerve and place the platform of the distal implants posteriorly permits a favorable AP distribution for immediate loading with a fixed prosthesis. This single-stage procedure is applicable to fully edentulous patients, patients with periodontally involved teeth, and patients with existing implants who have peri-implantitis. The fear of having to wear a denture is removed, allowing patients to participate fully and attentively in their own comprehensive treatment planning.

REFERENCES

1. Schnitman PA, Wohrle PS, Rubenstein E, et al: Ten year results for Brånemark implants immediately loaded with fixed prostheses at implant placement. *Int J Oral Maxillofac Implants* 12:495-503, 1997.
2. Balshi TJ, Wolfinger GJ: Immediate loading of Brånemark implants in edentulous mandibles: A preliminary report. *Implant Dent* 6:83-88, 1997.
3. Brånemark PI, Engstrand P, Ohrnell LO, et al: Brånemark Novum: A new treatment concept for rehabilitation of the edentulous mandible. Preliminary results from a prospective clinical follow-up study. *Clin Implant Dent Relat Res* 1:2-16, 1999.
4. Chow J, Hui E: Immediate loading of Brånemark system fixtures in the mandible with a fixed provisional prosthesis. *Appl Osseointergration Res* 2:30-35, 2001.
5. Brånemark PI: Introduction to Brånemark Novum concept. In Brånemark PI, editor: *The Brånemark Novum protocol for same day teeth. A global perspective,* Berlin, 2001, Quintessence.
6. Duyck J, Van Oosterwyck H: Magnitude and distribution of occlusal forces on oral implants supporting fixed prosthesis: An in vivo study. *Clin Oral Implants Res* 11:465-475, 2000.
7. Krekmanov L, Kahn M, Rangert B, et al: Tilting of posterior mandibular and maxillary implants for improved prosthesis support. *Int J Oral Maxillofac Implants* 15:405-414, 2000.
8. Van Steenberg D, Molly L, Jacobs R, et al: The immediate rehabilitation by means of a ready-made final fixed prosthesis in the edentulous mandible: A 1-year follow-up study of 50 consecutive patients. *Clin Oral Implant Res* 15:360-365, 2004.
9. Maló P, Rangert B, Nobre M: "All-on-4" immediate-function concept with Brånemark system implants for completely edentulous mandibles: A retrospective study. *Clin Implant Dent Relat Res* 5(Suppl 1):2-9, 2003.
10. Brånemark PI,. Hansson BO, Adell R, et al: Osseointegrated implants in the treatment of the edentulous jaw. Experience from a 10-year period. *Scand J Plast Reconstr Surg* 11(16):1-32, 1977.
11. Schroeder A, Pohler O, Sutter F: Geweb reaktion auf ein Titan-Hohlzylinder-Implantat mit Titan-S ritz-schichtoberfache. *Schweiz Monatschr Zahnheilkd* 86:713-727, 1976.
12. Schroder A, Stich H, Straumann F, et al: Uber die Anlagerung Osteocement an eine belasteten Implantat-kbrper. *Schweiz Monatschr Zahnhe lk* 88:1051-1058, 1978.
13. Brånemark PI: Introduction to osseointegration. In Brånemark PI, Zarb G, Albrektsson T, editors: *Tissue-integrated prosthesis-osseointegration: Clinical dentistry,* Chicago, 1985, Quintessence.
14. Bedrossian E: Fixed-prosthetic implant restoration of the edentulous maxilla: A systematic pretreatment evaluation method. *J Oral Maxillofac Surg* 66:112-122, 2008.
15. Skalak R: Biomechanics of osseointegration. In Brånemark PI, Rydevik BL, Skalak R, editors: *Osseointegration in skeletal reconstruction and joint replacement,* Chicago, 1997, Quintessence.

16. Brunski JB, Skalak R: Biomechanical considerations. In Worthington PH, Brånemark PI, editors: *Advanced osseointegration surgery. Applications in the maxillofacial region*, Chicago, IL, 1992, Quintessence.
17. Schackleton JL, Carr L, Slabbert JCG, et al: Survival of fixed implant-supported prosthesis related to cantilever lengths. *J Prosthet Dent* 71:23-26 1994.
18. Naert I, Quirymen M, van Steenberg D, et al: A study of 589 consecutive implants supporting complete fixed prosthesis. Part II: Prosthetic aspects. *J Prosthet Dent* 68:949-956, 1992.
19. Rosenquist BO: Is there an anterior loop of the inferior alveolar nerve? *Int J Periodontics Restorative Dent* 16(1):40-45, 1996.
20. Arzouman MJ, Otis L, Kipris V: Observation of the anterior loop of the inferior alveolar canal. *Int Oral Maxillofac Implants* 8:295-300, 1993.
21. Bavitz JB, Horn SD, Hansen CA: An anatomical study of mental neurovascular bundle-implant relationships. *Int J Oral Maxillofac Implants* 8:563-567, 1993.
22. Misch CE, Crawford EA: Predictable mandibular nerve location—A clinical zone of safety. *Dent Today* 9(9):32-35, 1990.
23. Kaya Y: Retrospective radiographic evaluation of the anterior loop of the mental nerve: Comparison between panoramic radiography and spiral computerized tomography. *Int J Oral Maxillofac Implants* 23:919-925, 2008.
24. Sicher H: *Oral anatomy*. St Louis, 1949, Mosby.
25. Alsaad K, Lee TC, McCartan B: An anatomical study of the cutaneous branches of the mental nerve. *Int J Oral Maxillofac Surg* 32:325-333, 2003.
26. Yosue T, Brooks SL: The appearance of mental foramina on panoramic radiographs. 1. Evaluation of patients. *Oral Surg Oral Med Oral Pathol* 68:360-364, 1989.
27. Bedrossian E: Immediate function with the zygomatic implant: A graftless solution for the patient with mild to advanced atrophy of the maxilla. *Int J Oral Maxillofac Implants* 21(6):937-942, 2006.

CHAPTER 9

Conversion Technique for Immediate Loading

To provide a surgical patient with a fixed provisional prosthesis immediately after the procedure, conversion of the patient's existing full denture or conversion of the newly fabricated immediate denture is undertaken.[1-12] The preoperative denture should be at the proper vertical dimension of occlusion, as well as at the proper tooth position.[9-11] Once the implants have been placed with 40 Ncm insertion torque, attachment of the abutments begins, as does soft tissue closure. For the two anterior implants, as described in Chapter 8, it is advisable to connect temporary abutments, indexing the position of the abutments as they relate to the teeth in the patient's denture, prior to committing to the final abutment. This is important because in many cases it may be necessary to use a 17° angulated abutments to increase the distance between the screw access hole and the cingulum of the anterior teeth, allowing for greater acrylic packing volume to support the teeth on the metal substructure (Figure 9-1). The larger the separation, the more acrylic or porcelain is necessary between the lingual aspect of the anterior teeth and the screw access holes, limiting the potential of "popping" teeth under function. Therefore, prior to suturing, temporary healing abutments are connected to the two anterior implants, allowing closure of the soft tissues using 3-0 gut sutures (Figure 9-2). The heights of the healing abutments are chosen so that after suturing the crestal incision, 1 mm of the healing abutment is above the soft tissue line. When using the tilted-implant protocol, 30° multiunit abutments are placed on the two posterior implants. Likewise, when using the zygoma protocol, two regular straight multiunit abutments are placed on the distal implants. Because the use of the final abutments is known for the posterior implants, the final abutment of choice may be placed and the healing cap attached prior to suturing the soft tissues (Figure 9-3). The patient's denture is relieved to allow passive seating without interference from the anterior temporary healing abutments or the final abutments placed on the distal implants. Polyvinylsiloxane bite registration is flowed into the denture as it is seated in the mouth, ensuring proper occlusion with the apposing dentition as well as proper midline orientation (Figure 9-4). The positions of the healing abutments are imprinted into the polyvinylsiloxane as it sets (Figure 9-5). An acrylic bur is used to perforate the denture base, marking and relating the positions of the implants with the denture acrylic (Figure 9-6). Care must be taken not to make excessive holes or to fracture the denture base. The denture with the prepared holes is once again seated in the mouth in the proper position. Relating the position of the temporary healing abutments to the holes in the denture base allows the practitioner to determine whether straight or 17° multiunit abutments will be used on the two anterior implants for fabrication of the screw-retained provisional profile prosthesis. Once the abutments are chosen and seated onto the implants, reconfirmation of the screw access holes is made by properly seating the denture in the patient's mouth (Figure 9-7). The abutments are torqued to 35 Ncm for straight multiunit abutments and 20 Ncm for 17° or 30° abutments. To fabricate this fixed prosthesis, temporary multiunit titanium cylinders are used (Figure 9-8, *A*). Passive fit of all temporary abutments with the denture is checked prior to luting the temporary abutment to the denture base (Figure 9-8, *B*). The temporary titanium cylinders are cold-cured to the denture base using quick-setting denture repair acrylic (Figure 9-9). After the acrylic hardens of the acrylic, the denture is removed from the patient's mouth by unscrewing the retaining screws. The voids on the tissue surface of the

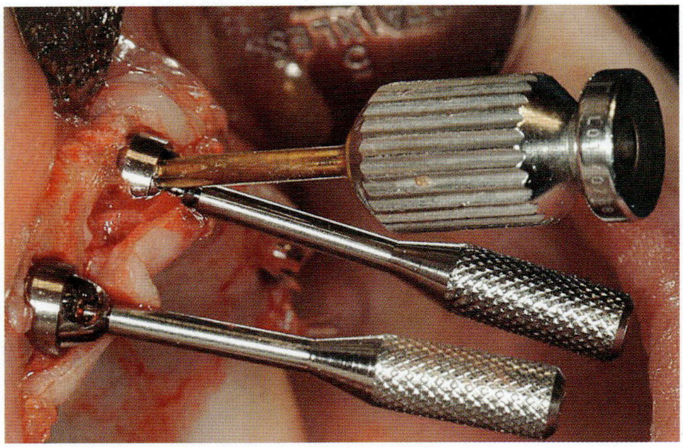

FIGURE 9-1 In selected cases, the use of 17° multiunit abutments allows for a thicker volume of pink acrylic needed to support denture teeth.

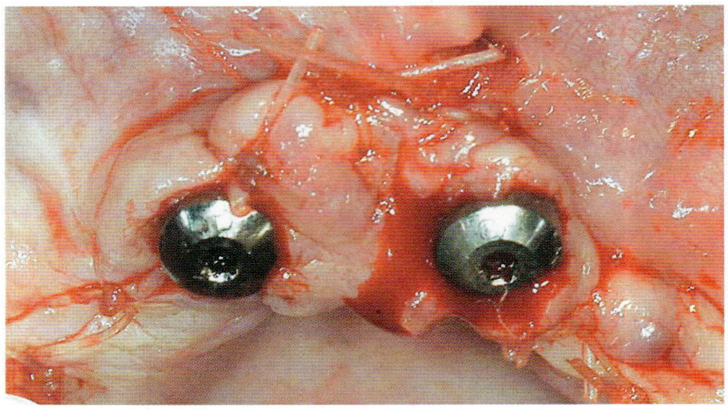

FIGURE 9-2 Prior to indexing the implant positions, temporary healing abutments are placed onto the anterior implants, which allows the practitioner to choose an appropriate abutment once the implant position has been transferred to the intaglio surface of the patient's denture.

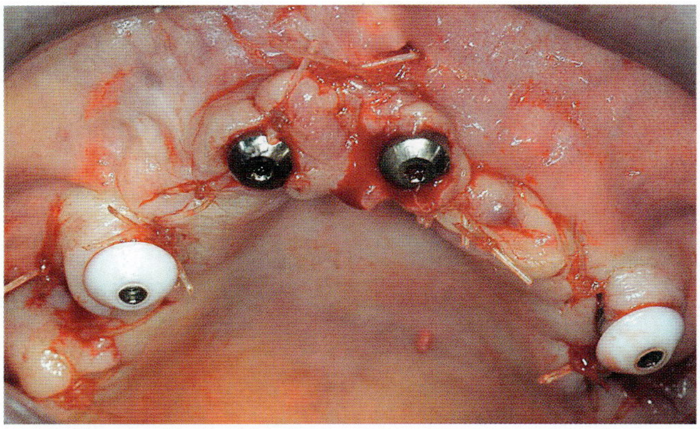

FIGURE 9-3 Prior to indexing of the implants, 17° or 30° multiunit abutments are placed onto the posterior implants.

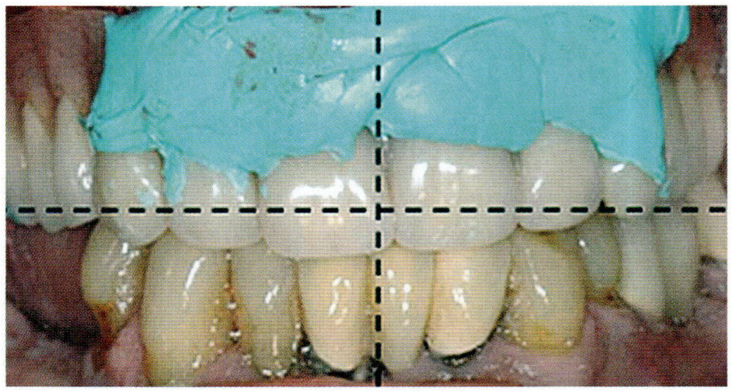

FIGURE 9-4 Proper occlusion and midline position of the prosthesis is maintained while the registration material is set.

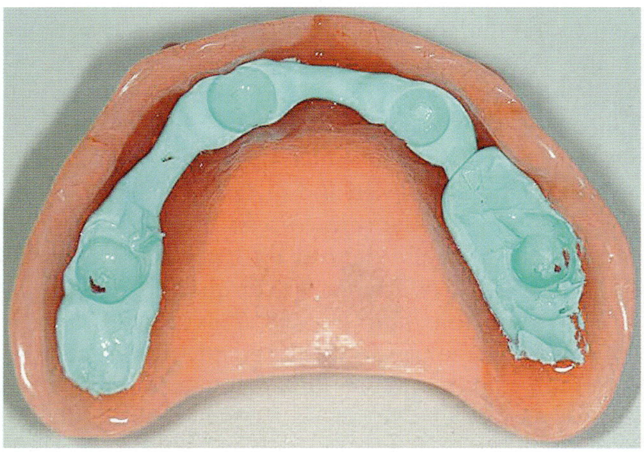

FIGURE 9-5 The position of the implants is registered onto the intaglio surface of the prosthesis.

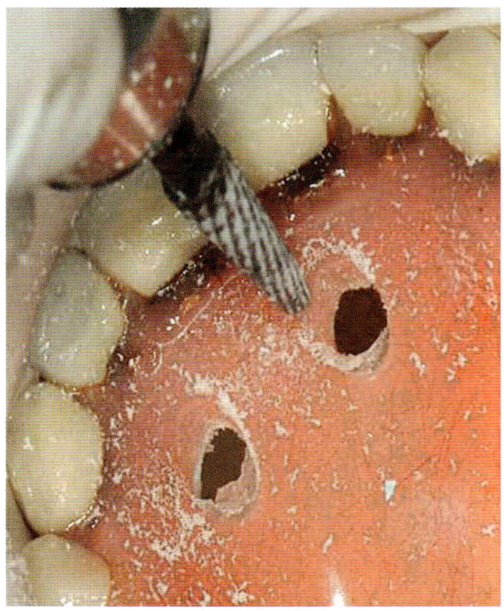

FIGURE 9-6 An acrylic bur is used to perforate the positions of the implants through the denture base.

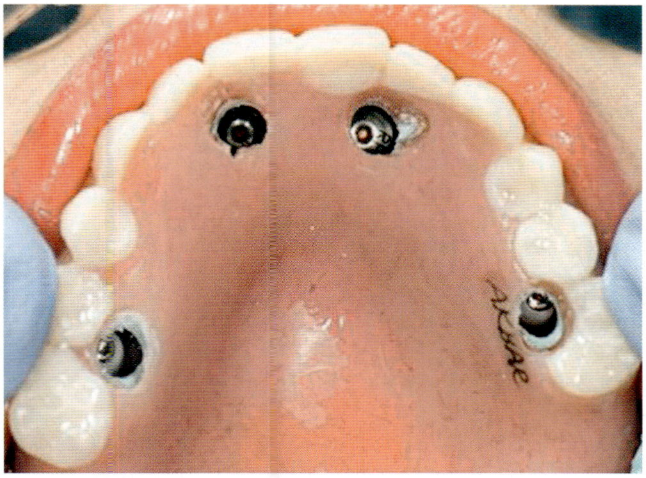

FIGURE 9-7 The proper opening of the access holes through the denture base is confirmed intraorally.

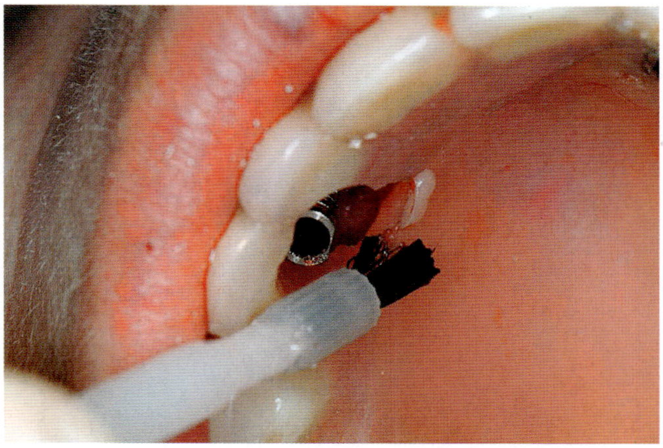

FIGURE 9-9 The salt and pepper technique is used to lute the temporary cylinders to the denture base.

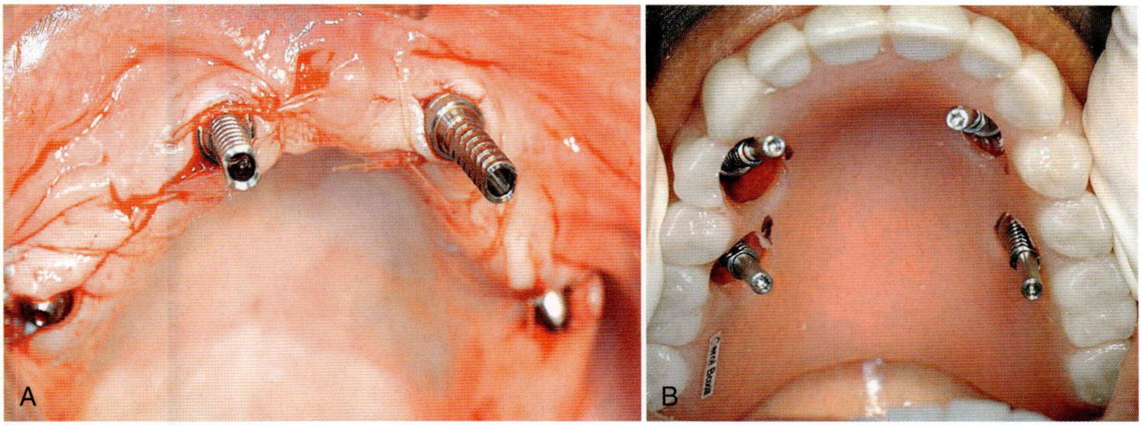

FIGURE 9-8 A, Temporary multiunit titanium cylinders are connected to the abutments. B, To maintain proper position of the denture base on the soft tissues, circumferential clearance of the denture base with the temporary cylinders is confirmed.

denture base around the temporary titanium cylinders are further reinforced with quick-setting acrylic; the practitioner must be careful not to introduce any acrylic into the seating surfaces of the cylinders (Figure 9-10). The palate and denture flanges are removed (Figure 9-11). Recontouring the acrylic on the intaglio side of the prosthesis is completed in an attempt to remove all concavities that may trap food. The patient's occlusion is checked to ensure group function and uniform loading across the entire prosthesis in centric occlusion.[13,14] To avoid bending moments, teeth close to 0° are used to fabricate this provisional prosthesis (Figure 9-12). A temporary material of the practitioner's choice is used to cover the retaining screw holes. In cases in which four premaxillary implants and two posterior implants have been placed, the same sequence is followed. The implants are indexed with polyvinylsiloxane (Figure 9-13). The desired abutments are attached and torqued, and the temporary cylinders are then connected (Figure 9-14). Passive fit of the prosthesis in relation to the temporary cylinders is confirmed prior to luting with quick-set acrylic (Figure 9-15). To maintain soft tissue health, the 2-mm collar of the temporary cylinder should be left exposed, as demonstrated in Figure 9-16 by the temporary cylinder on the right.

POSTOPERATIVE INSTRUCTIONS

Patients are instructed to maintain a soft-food diet. Food consistency should not exceed that of well-cooked chicken or fish. A soft-food diet is necessary to minimize stress placed at the implant-bone interface, as well as to prevent fracture of the all-acrylic provisional prosthesis.

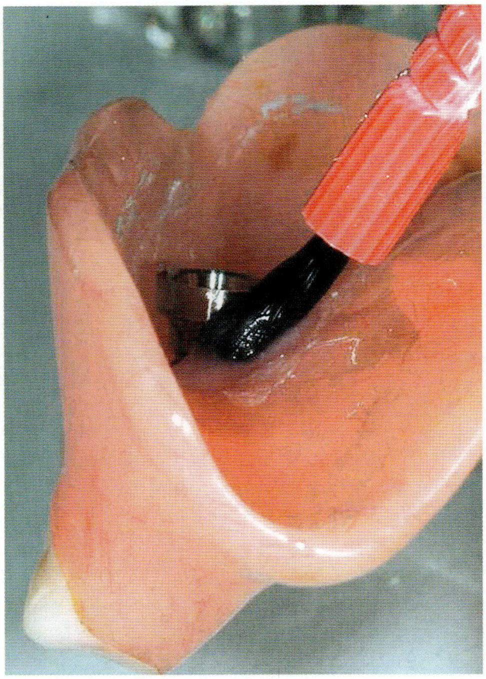

FIGURE 9-10 The intaglio surface of the titanium cylinder is also secured to the denture base using quick-setting acrylic.

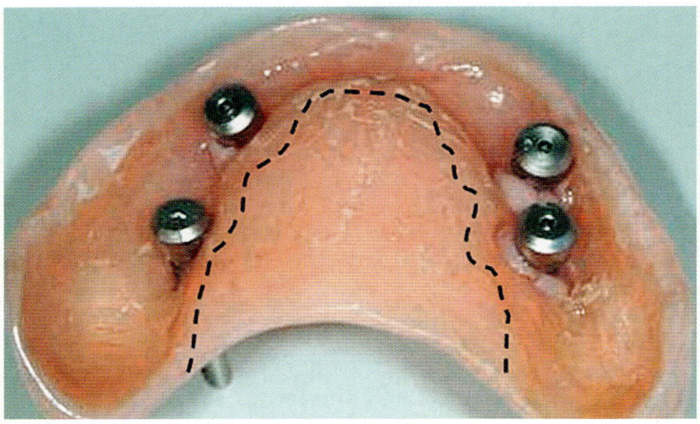

FIGURE 9-11 The palate of the denture is removed after securing all temporary cylinders to the denture base.

Daily oral hygiene includes use of a soft brush to clean the provisional prosthesis. A 0.12% chlorhexidine rinse before bedtime is prescribed for the first month. After 1 month, use of a one-use syringe or a oral water jet appliance will further allow maintenance of good oral hygiene.

It is equally important to check and recheck the patient's occlusion on a regular basis. Success of this type of treatment is in part due to bilateral, balanced occlusion using 0° to 5° denture teeth. Patients are advised to report any changes in their occlusion immediately. The patient's occlusion is checked at the 1-week, 1-month, and 3-month postoperative appointments.

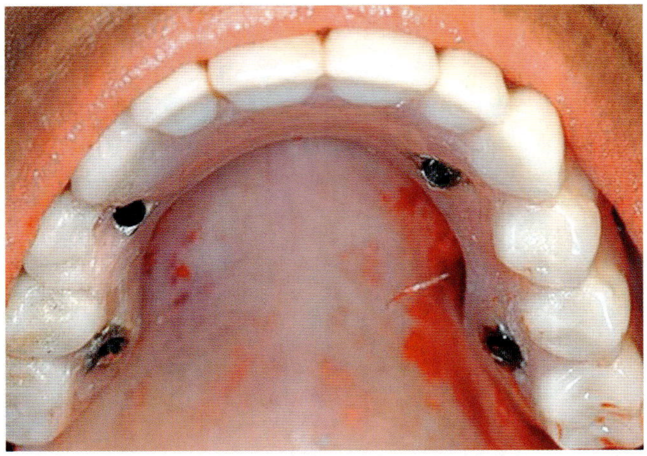

FIGURE 9-12 The denture teeth used are 0° to 5° for the profile provisional prosthesis.

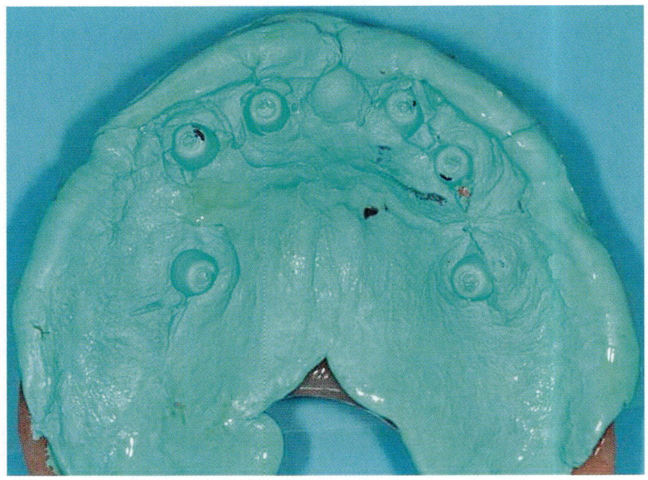

FIGURE 9-13 The position of the six implants is indexed using polyvinylsiloxane registration paste.

Practitioners often believe they need to remove the appliance for inspection of the abutments and soft tissue interface or to clean the intaglio surface. This should be avoided if possible. Glauser et al. reported the implant stability quotient (ISQ) values of implants using frequency resonance analysis.[15,16] They documented the ISQ value of the implants at the time of insertion. The ISQ values of the implants were monitored at regular intervals of 1, 4, 8, 12, and 25 weeks postoperatively (Figure 9-17). The ISQ values fell during the first 4 weeks after placement, with week 4 demonstrating the lowest measurement. This is consistent with the bony remodeling during the first 4 to 6 weeks after preparation of the osteotomy and placement of the implant. The ISQ values began to rise at week 8 and continued to rise through week 25,

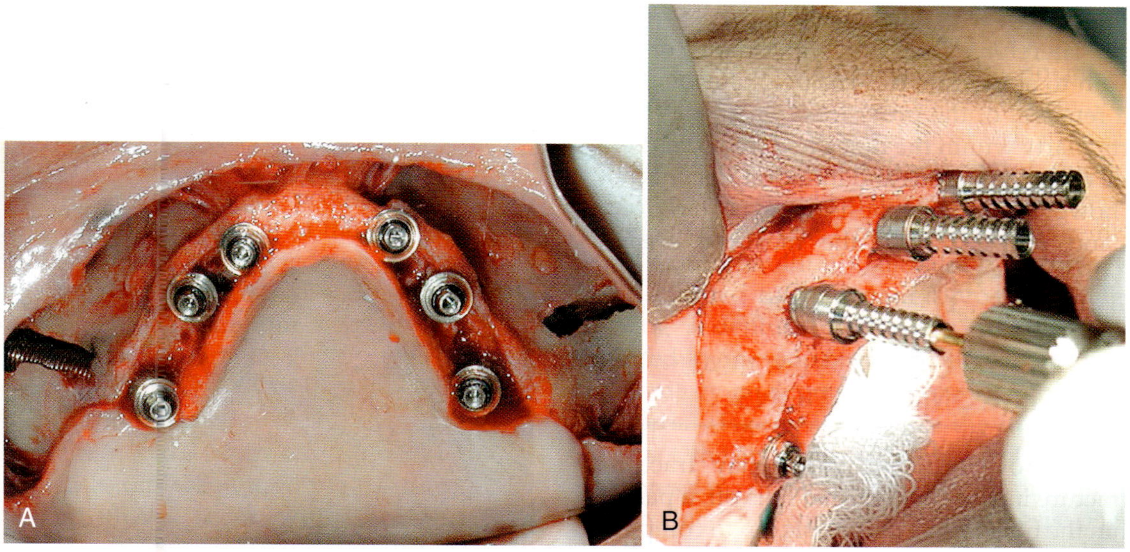

FIGURE 9-14 A, Straight multiunit abutments are chosen for all six implants for this patient. B, Temporary titanium cylinders are connected to all six implant abutments.

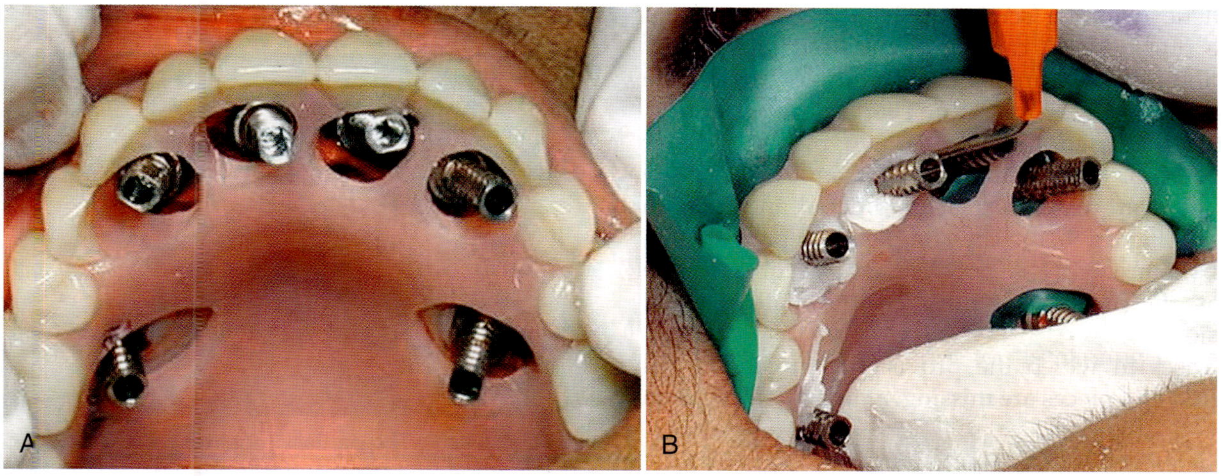

FIGURE 9-15 A, With the titanium cylinders connected to all six abutments, the passive seating of the denture base is confirmed. B, Quick-set acrylic may be used in a syringe to lute the cylinders to the denture base.

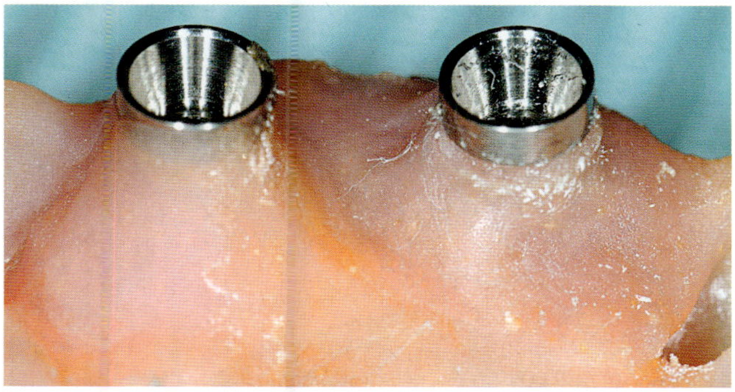

FIGURE 9-16 The 2-mm intrasulcular collar of the temporary cylinder should not be covered by acrylic as shown on the right cylinder.

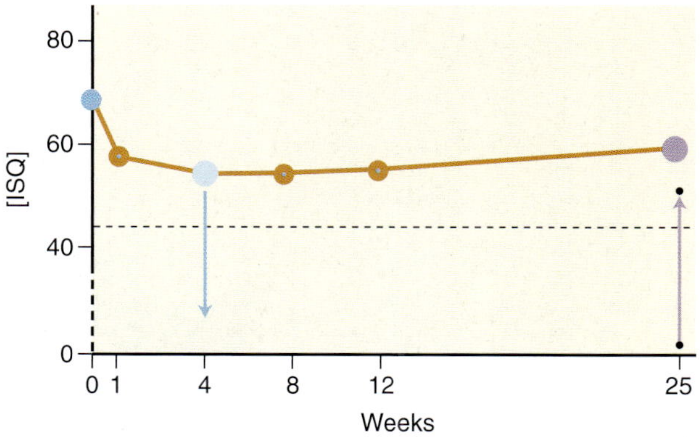

FIGURE 9-17 The period of weakest bone-to-implant stability is between 4 and 6 weeks postoperative. Elective removal of the provisional prosthesis should be avoided.

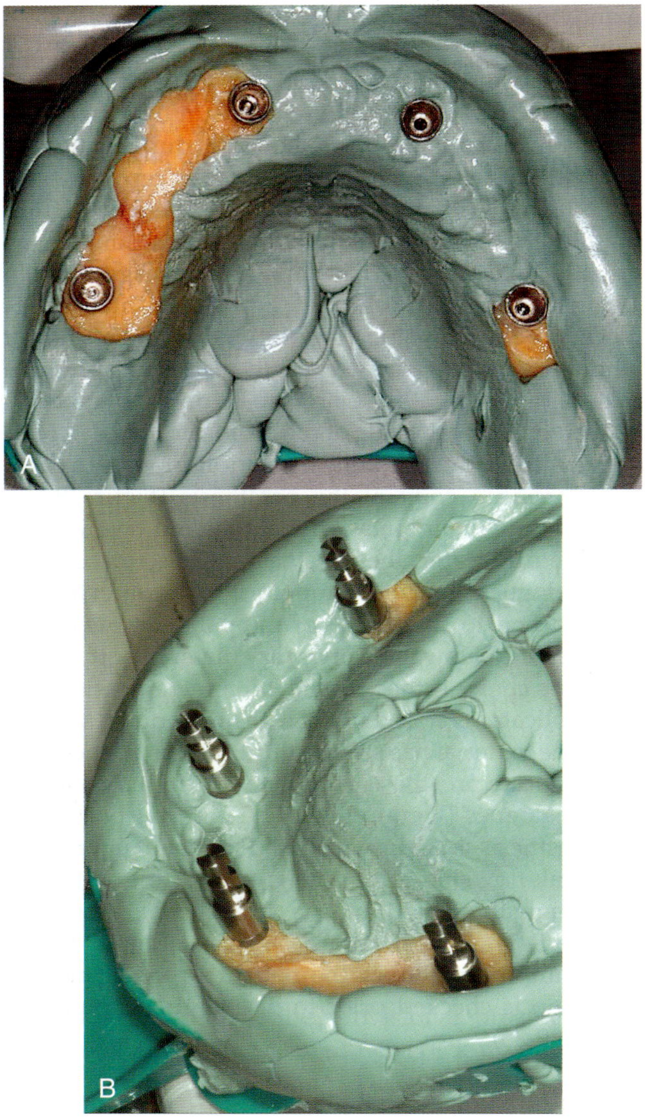

FIGURE 9-25 A, The impression is inspected to ensure proper pickup of all components. B, Multiunit laboratory analogues are secured to the temporary titanium cylinders of the fractured provisional bridge.

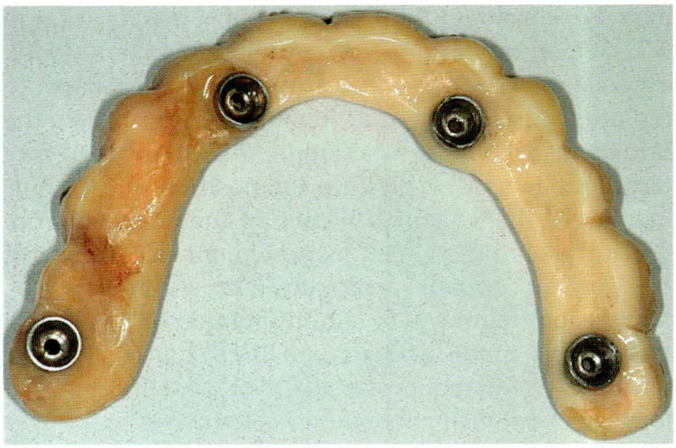

FIGURE 9-26 The laboratory-cured and repaired provisional prosthesis.

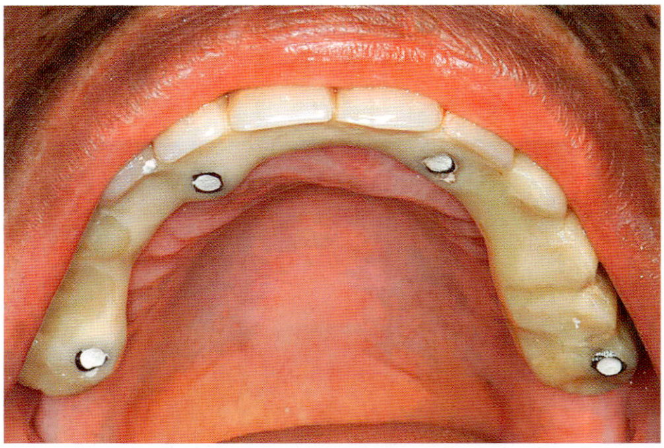

FIGURE 9-27 Repositioning the repaired prosthesis is required to ensure a passive fit and proper occlusion.

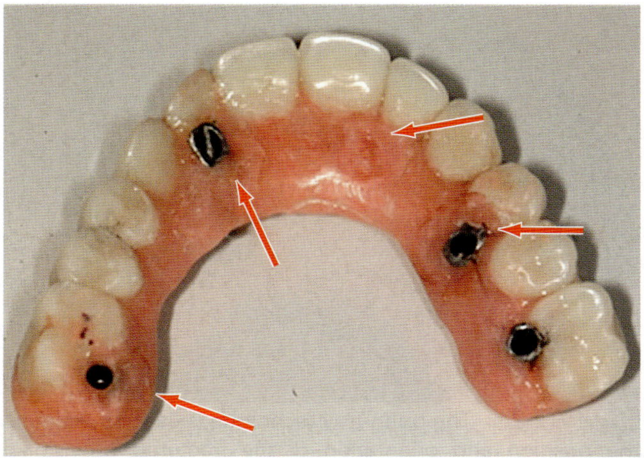

FIGURE 9-28 This provisional prosthesis has experienced multiple fractures and has been repaired several times.

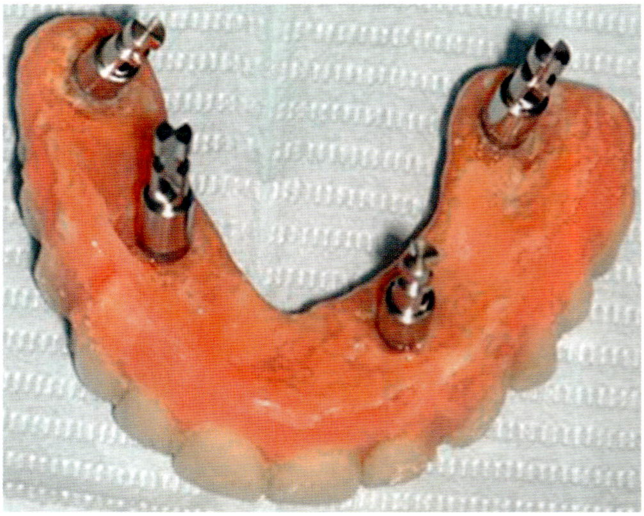

FIGURE 9-29 After intraoral repair and luting of the fractured prosthesis, it is removed and laboratory analogues are attached.

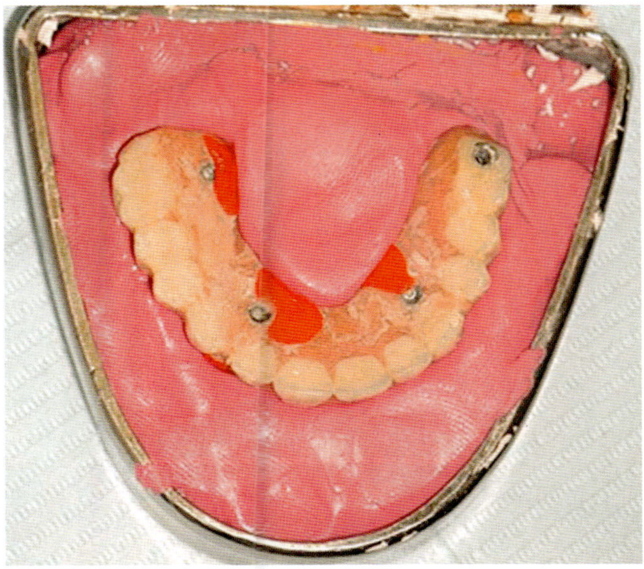

FIGURE 9-30 Duplicating the intaglio surface of the repaired provisional prosthesis begins with insertion of the attached laboratory analogues into a polyvinyl impression material placed in a denture duplicator.

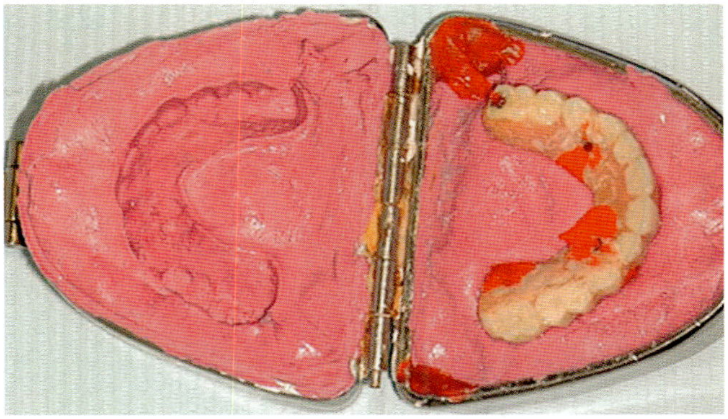

FIGURE 9-31 Once the impression material has set, the opposite chamber of the denture duplicator is filled with polyvinyl impression material and closed to duplicate the occlusal portion of the provisional prosthesis.

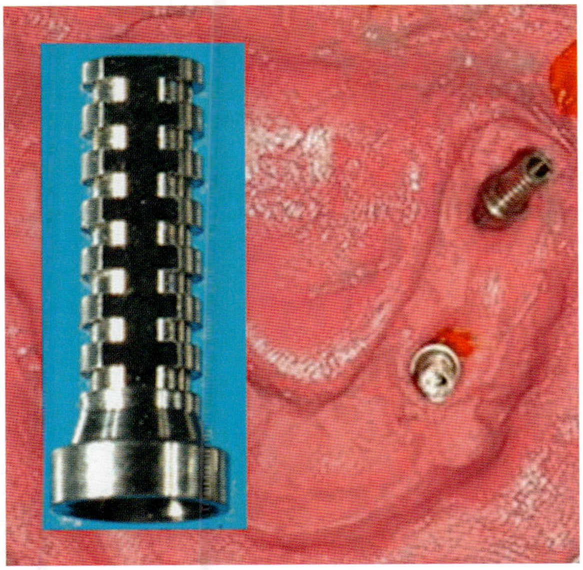

FIGURE 9-32 Once the provisional prosthesis is unscrewed from the laboratory analogues, a new set of temporary titanium cylinders are secured to the laboratory analogues.

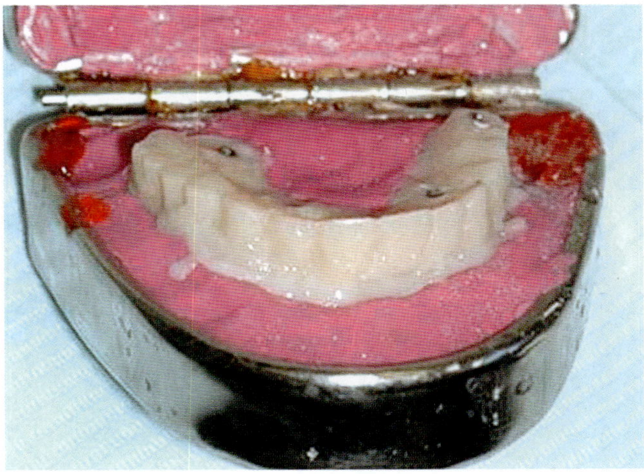

FIGURE 9-33 Temporary acrylic material is mixed and poured into the duplicated provisional prosthesis mold.

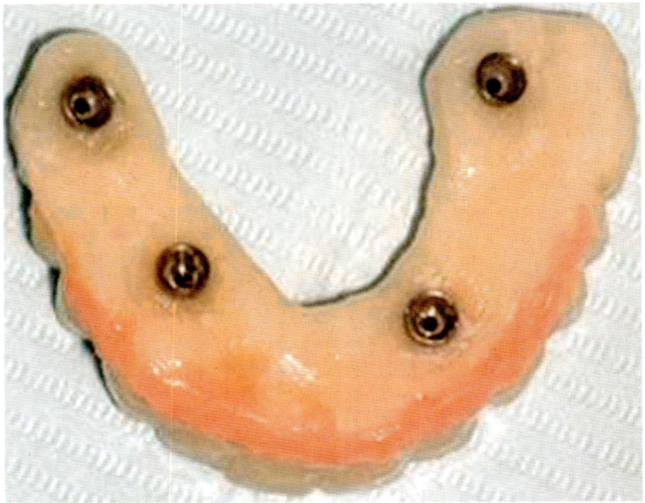

FIGURE 9-34 After the acrylic material has set, the duplicated provisional prosthesis is removed and trimmed, and the buccal gingival area is veneered with soft tissue–colored material for proper aesthetics.

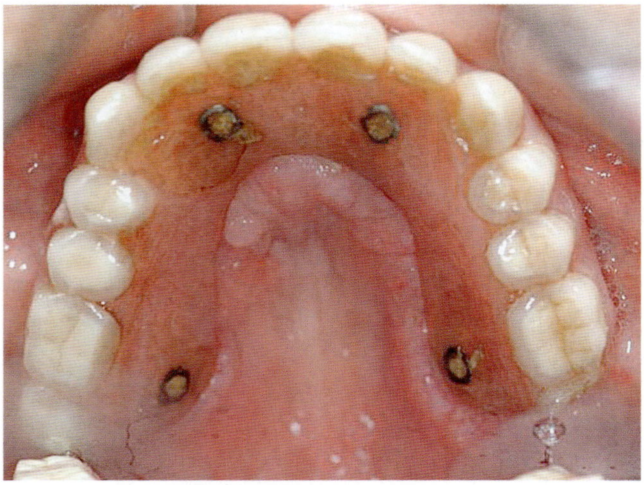

FIGURE 9-35 The newly duplicated provisional prosthesis is secured to the patient's abutments ensuring passive fit and proper occlusion.

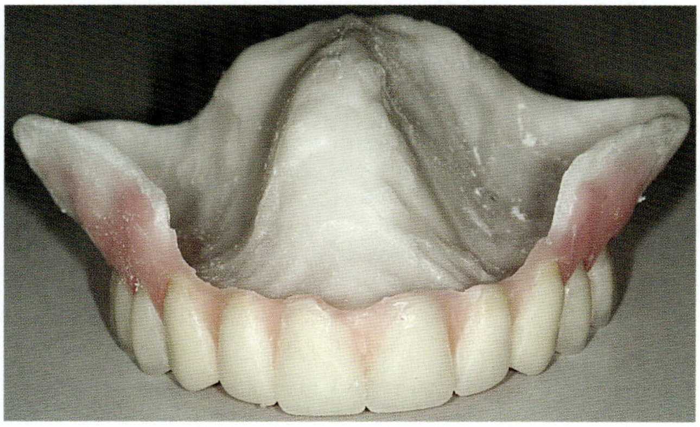

FIGURE 9-36 To confirm the presence of a tooth-only defect, the flange of the provisional denture is removed prior to intraoral placement for clinical confirmation.

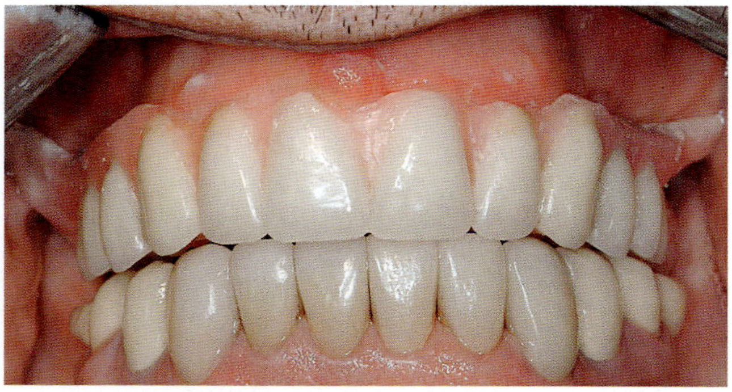

FIGURE 9-37 Lack of space between the cervical position of the denture teeth and the patient's edentulous soft tissues confirms the presence of a tooth-only defect.

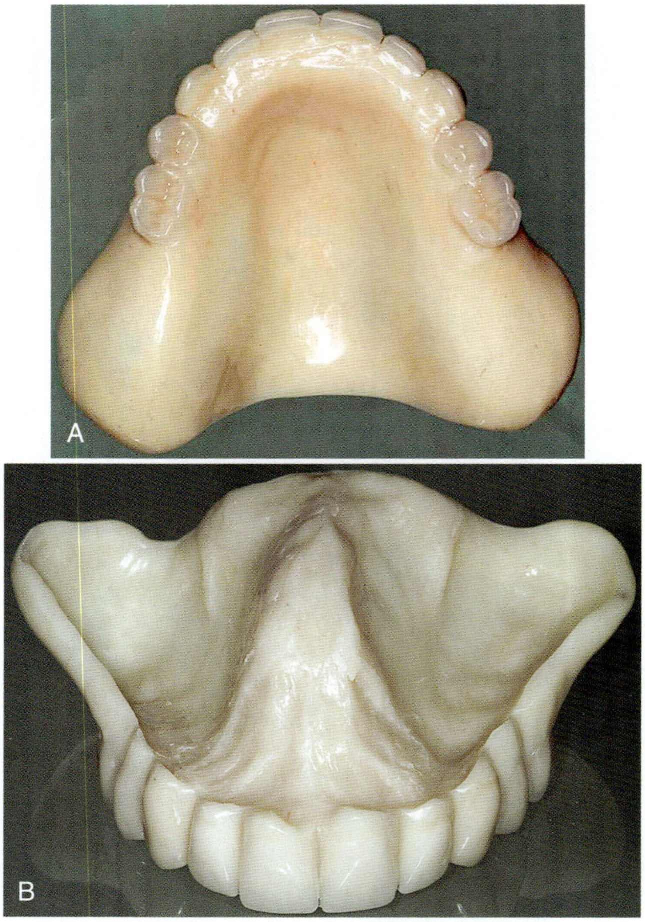

FIGURE 9-38 A, The white denture permits stabilization of the prosthesis during the conversion process into a fixed, tooth-only provisional bridge. B, The palatal portion, tuberosity coverage, and posterior flanges of the white denture allow proper orientation of the provisional prosthesis during luting to the temporary titanium cylinders.

"WHITE DENTURE": TOOTH-ONLY DEFECT

On occasion, the edentulous alveolus is not resorbed despite many years of denture wear. In these patients, the lack of composite defect is confirmed by removing the buccal flange from cuspid to cuspid on a diagnostic set-up (Figure 9-36). Clinical confirmation of a tooth-only defect (Figure 9-37) dictates fabrication of a final ceramo-metal bridge. To provisionally load this group of patients, a "tooth-only" prosthesis is needed. To stabilize the tooth-only provisional prosthesis, it is prudent to add a palate and tuberosity coverage and flanges in the maxilla to allow stabilization of the provisional prosthesis during the conversion steps (Figure 9-38). After placing the implants, indexing the implant positions in the intaglio surface of the white denture, and torquing the appropriate abutment, the temporary

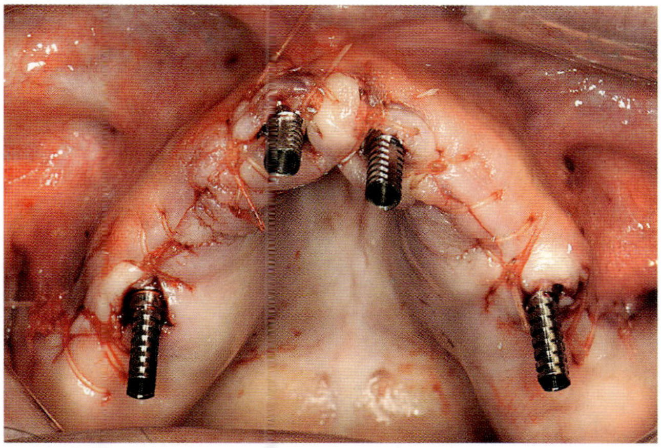

FIGURE 9-39 After implant placement and indexing the white denture, the appropriate abutments are placed and torqued; then the temporary titanium cylinders are connected to the abutments.

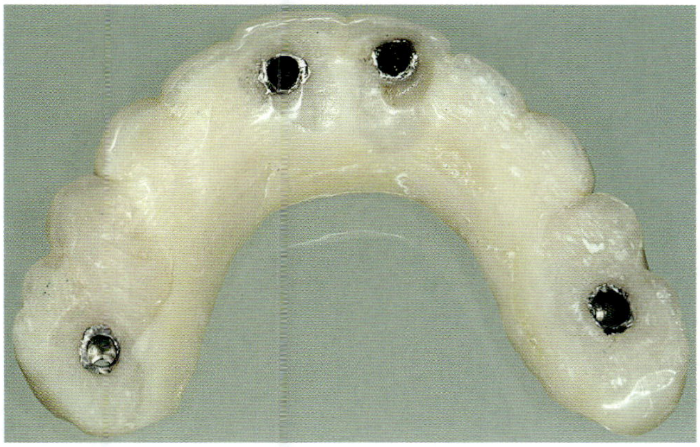

FIGURE 9-40 After completion of the conversion protocol, the palate, the tuberosity coverage, and the flange of the provisional white denture are removed to convert the provisional prosthesis to a tooth-only provisional prosthesis contour.

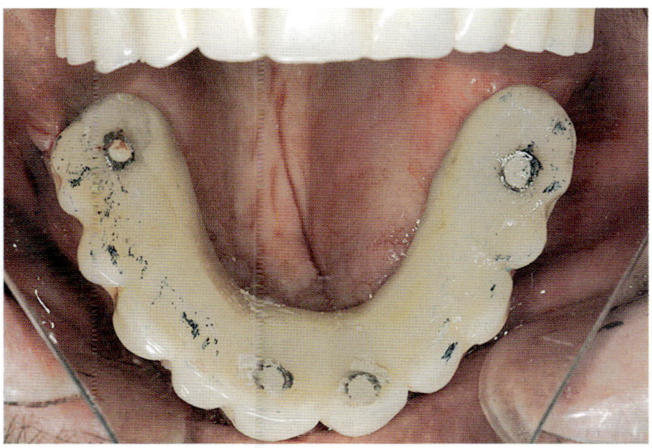

FIGURE 9-41 The provisional prosthesis is connected to the patient's abutments, and group function and occlusion are established.

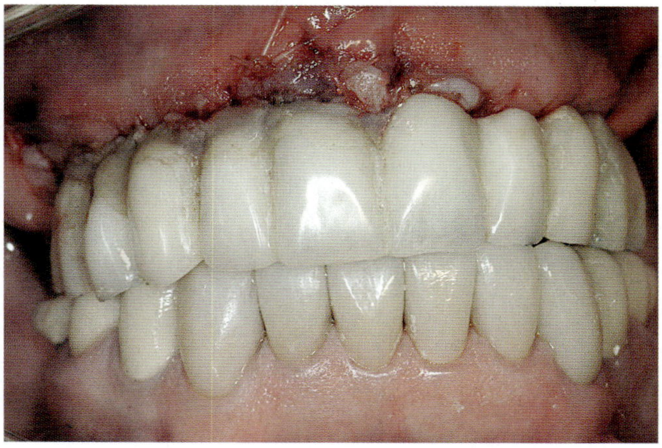

FIGURE 9-42 The midline and the occlusal relationship with apposing dentition is checked.

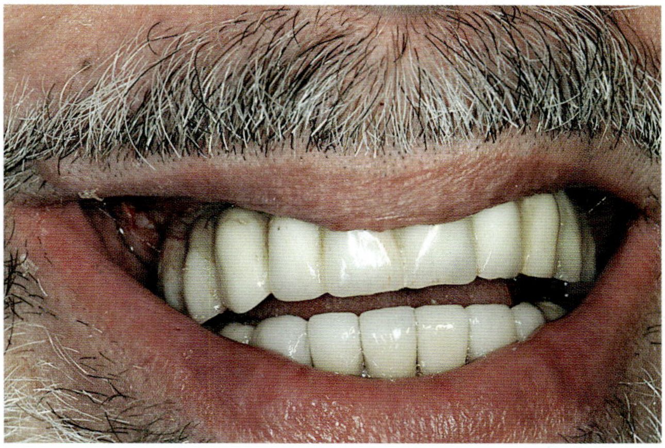

FIGURE 9-43 The 2-month postoperative animation illustrates an aesthetic transition line.

cylinders are attached to the abutments (Figure 9-39). The immediate-load prosthesis (Figure 9-40) is contoured (Figure 9-41) and fixated to the patient using prosthetic screws (Figure 9-42). The provisional white denture simulates the ceramo-metal final prosthesis, restoring this "tooth-only" patient (Figure 9-43).

As described earlier, the prosthesis should not be removed during the 3- to 6-month osseointegration phase unless necessary. If fractures of the prosthesis are noted, it must be removed and repaired and a critical evaluation of the patient's occlusion, including the potential for parafunctional habits, must be made.

REFERENCES

1. Bedrossian E, Rangert B, Stumpel L, et al: Immediate function with the zygomatic implant—A graftless solution for the patient with mild to advanced atrophy of the maxilla. *Int J Oral Maxillofac Surg* 21:1-6, 2006.

2. Nkenke E, Hahn M, Lell M, et al: Anatomic site evaluation of the zygomatic bone for dental implant placement. *Clin Oral Implants Res* 14:72-79, 2003.
3. Weingart D, Schilli W, Strub JR: Preprosthetic surgery and implantology. *Schweizer Monatsschrift Zahnmedizin* 102:1075-1082, 1992.
4. Bedrossian E, Tawfilis A, Alijanian A: Veneer grafting: A technique for augmentation of the resorbed alveolus prior to implant placement. A critical report. *Int J Oral Maxillofac Implants* 15:853-858, 2000.
5. Chow J, Hui E, Lee P, et al: Zygomatic implants—Protocol for immediate loading: A preliminary report. *J Oral Maxillofac Surg* 64:804-811, 2006.
6. Brånemark PI: *Surgery and fixture installation. Zygomaticus fixture clinical procedure,* Gothenburg, Sweden, 1995, Nobel Biocare.
7. Bedrossian E, Stumpel L: Immediate stabilization at phase II of zygomaticus fixtures: A simplified technique. *J Prosthet Dent* 86(1):10-14, 2001.
8. Zhao Y, Skalak R, Brånemark PI: Analysis of a dental prosthesis supported by zygomatic fixtures. The Institute for Applied Biotechnology, Gothenberg, Sweden, unpublished.
9. Swerdlow H: Vertical dimension literature review. *J Prostht Dent* 15:241-247, 1965.
10. Frush J, Fisher R: Introduction to dentogenic restorations. *J Prosthet Dent* 11:586-595, 1955.
11. Rothman R: Phonetic considerations in denture prosthesis. *J Prosthet Dent* 11:214-223, 1961.
12. Balshi TJ: *The Biotes conversion prosthesis: A provisional fixed prosthesis supported by osseointegrated titanium fixtures for restoration of the edentulous jaws,* Chicago, 1985, Quintessence Int.
13. Gapski R, Wang HL, Mascarenhas P, et al: Critical review of immediate implant loading. *Clin Oral Implants Res* 14:515-527, 2003.
14. Van Steenberghe D, Naert I, Anderson M, et al: A custom template and definitive prosthesis allowing immediate implant loading in the maxilla: A clinical report. *Int J Oral Maxillofac Implants* 17(5):663-670, 2002.
15. Glauser R, Portmann M, Ruhstaller P, et al: Stability measurements of immediately loaded machined and oxidized implants in the posterior maxilla. A comparative clinical study using resonance frequency analysis. *Appl Osseointegration Res* 2(1):27-29, 2001.
16. Glauser R, Sennerby L, Merideth N, et al: Resonance frequency analysis of implants subjected to immediate or early functional occlusal loading: Successful vs failing implants, *Clin Oral Implant Res* 15:428-434, 2004.

CHAPTER 10

Computer-Guided Surgery

The growing interest in flapless surgery in conjunction with immediate loading for edentulous patients has led to the development of software programs that assists treatment planning, fabrication of a surgical template, and production of a prosthesis that can be secured to the patient immediately following implant placement. The protocol for the two-scan technique[1] and use of the NobelGuide software has been described in recent literature.[2-4]

It is critical that the implant team cooperate in this treatment concept to minimize errors and to allow for correction of minor discrepancies during treatment. Understanding each others' responsibilities leads to more predictable outcomes.

MATERIAL AND METHOD

Computer-guided surgery software has three uses. The software can be used as a diagnostic and planning tool only, or as a surgical template for flapless surgery. Using the software to its fullest capability includes the laboratory steps, which are needed for production of the master cast and fabrication of the provisional immediate-load prosthesis before surgery. A practitioner may choose to use this technology with all of its components or only as a diagnostic and planning tool. This chapter discusses various uses of computer-guided surgery software. To fully appreciate this concept, understanding scanning protocols is paramount.

Scanning Protocol

To visualize the relationship of the patient's prosthesis to the edentulous ridge, the "two-scan" technique is used.[5] To begin this protocol, radiopaque markers are added to the patient's denture; these will be recognized by the computed tomography (CT) scanner.

After confirming proper fit, proper vertical dimension of occlusion, and proper anterior-posterior tooth position, gutta-percha markers are added to the patient's denture (Figure 10-1). A minimum of six gutta-percha markers are "staggered" (Figure 10-2). Each marker is approximately 2 mm in diameter and 1 mm deep. Bite registration material is used to ensure uniform and reproducible seating of the denture onto the edentulous ridge during the scanning procedure (Figure 10-3). The initial CT or cone beam CT scan is performed with the patient wearing the denture and occluding into the bite registration material (Figure 10-4). The second scan is of the denture only (Figure 10-5). Figure 10-6 demonstrates the schematic of the two scans. The raw data is referred to as *Digital Imaging and Communications in Medicine (DICOM) files,* which are then copied onto a compact disc and labeled as "patient DICOMs" and "denture DICOMs." These two-dimensional DICOM files are imported for analysis and treatment planning within the guided surgery program of choice. The first scan, the patient DICOM file, is imported into the guided surgery software and is converted to a three-dimensional representation (Figure 10-7). The second scan, the denture-only DICOM file, is also imported and converted into three-dimensional format (Figure 10-8). The two three-dimensional scans are merged and superimposed onto each other by overlaying the gutta-perch points of the first scan with the corresponding gutta-percha points on the second scan, relating the patient's edentulous jaw to the denture, which can be visualized on the same screen (Figure 10-9).

The next sections summarize the uses of computer-guided software as a:

1. Planning tool
2. Tool to fabricate a surgical template
3. Tool to fabricate a provisional immediate-load prosthesis

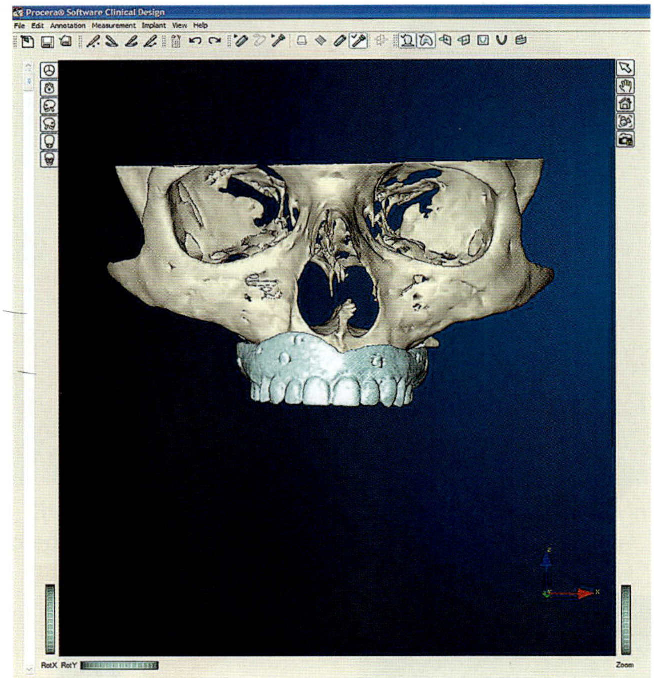

FIGURE 10-9 The third step of the NobelGuide software merges the two scans, placing the patient's denture onto the patient's edentulous jaw.

Step 1: Planning

Once the patient and denture DICOM files have been imported and converted to three-dimensional images, the comprehensive analysis of the patient's bony topography can be made by manipulating the image (Figure 10-10). The virtually planned implant position has been studied and compared with the transfer-planned position (the final surgical position), and has been found to be remarkably accurate and predictable.[6] To begin planning implant placement within the remaining bony housing of the alveolus, a two-dimensional window is opened, allowing visualization of the remaining horizontal bony topography (Figure 10-11). A systematic visualization of the posterior alveolus, including the maxillary sinus in the maxilla and the inferior alveolar nerve in the mandible, can be made (Figure 10-12). The premaxilla and the mandibular symphysis can be evaluated for remaining alveolar bone volume (Figure 10-13). The practitioner can click off the image of the patient's prosthesis, and the implant is positioned in the desirable surgical position (Figure 10-14). The practitioner can click on the image of the patient's denture to see the position of the planned implant axis (Figure 10-15). If the surgical position complements the prosthetic position, the next implant is planned. However, if a conflict exists, the practitioner clicks off the image of the prosthesis, and the implant is manipulated as many times as necessary to coincide with the desired prosthetic emergence profile. The same protocol is followed for planning mandibular implants (Figure 10-16) as well as for planning the position of zygomatic implants (Figure 10-17).

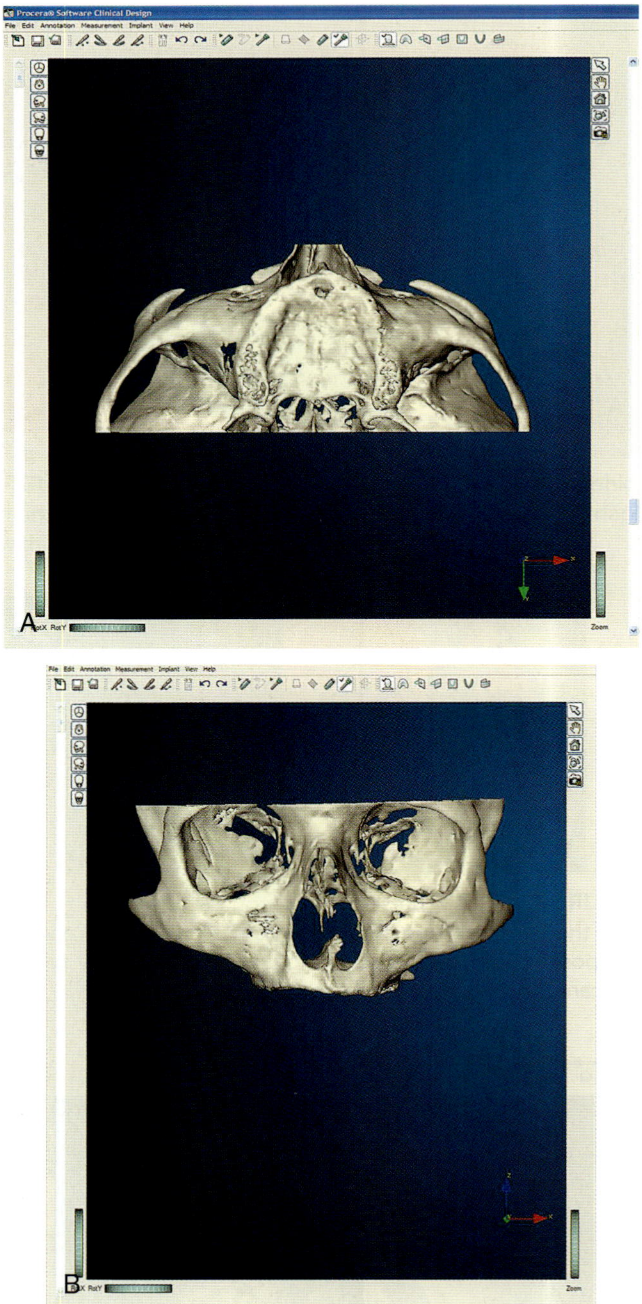

FIGURE 10-10 A, The patient's three-dimensional model may be manipulated to allow study of the anatomic topography. B, The premaxillary contour of edentulous patients can be enlarged or reduced, allowing a critical analysis of anatomic landmarks.

Computer-guided surgery software is effective as a communication tool between the surgeon, the restorative doctor, and the laboratory technician. Implant

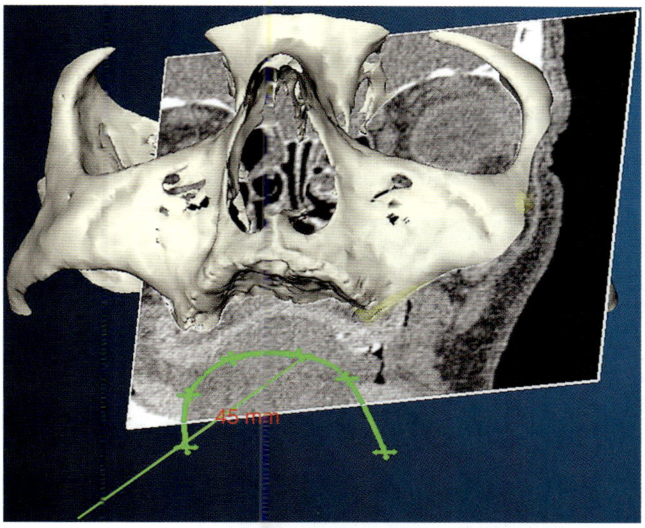

FIGURE 10-11 A two-dimensional cross-section window can be opened and moved across the entire three-dimensional scan, allowing the practitioner to study areas of interest.

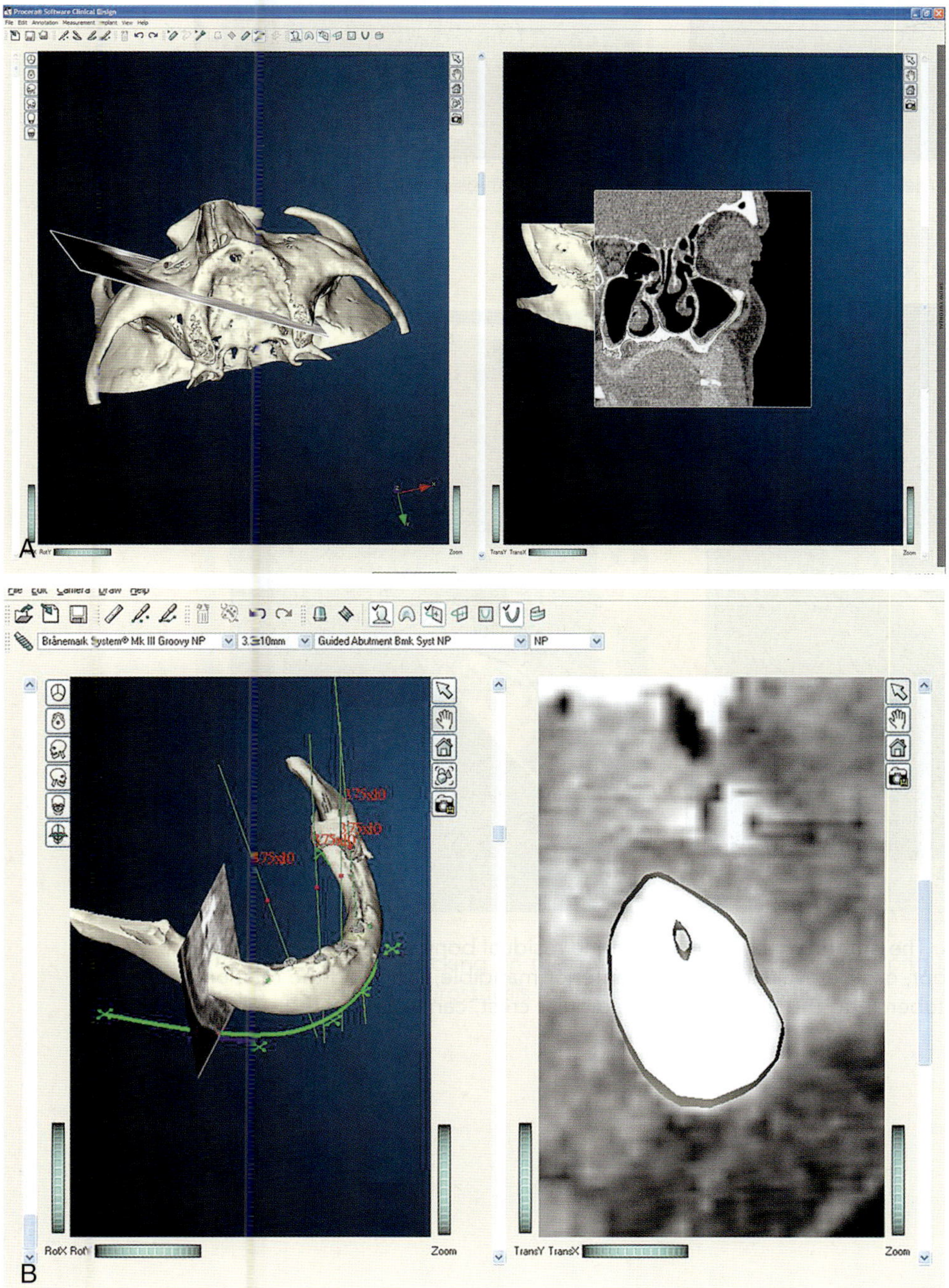

FIGURE 10-12 A, The posterior maxilla, including the maxillary sinus topography and the body of the zygomatic bone, can be evaluated. B, The posterior mandible, including the inferior alveolar canal and the mental foramen, can be evaluated.

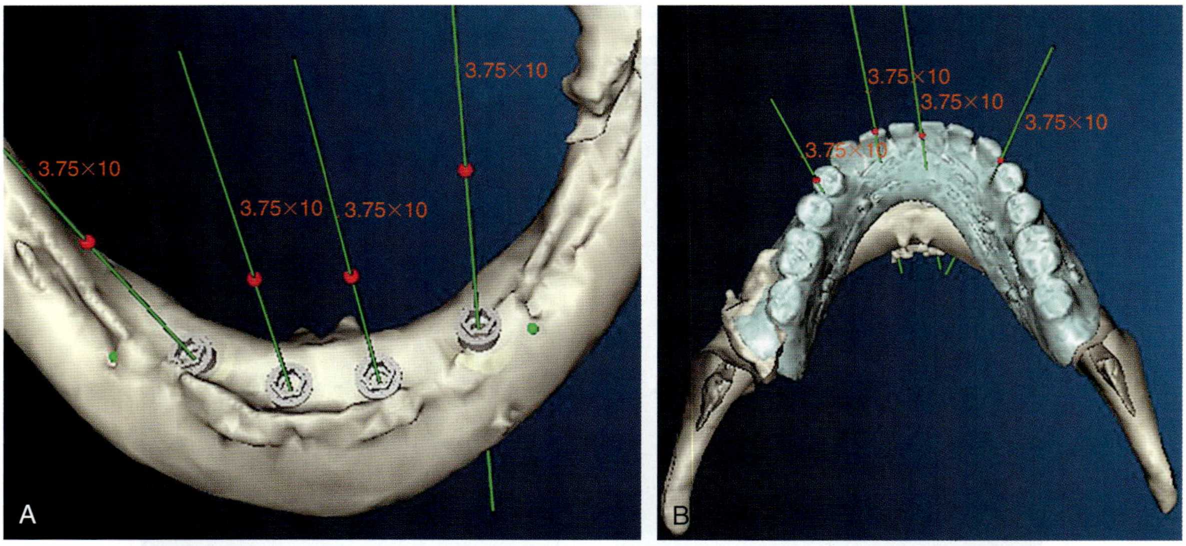

FIGURE 10-16 A, The long axis of the planned mandibular implants can be visualized and manipulated in the three-dimensional bony model. B, The axis of the implants as they relate to the mandibular prosthesis can be visualized by "turning on" the image of the mandibular prosthesis within the software.

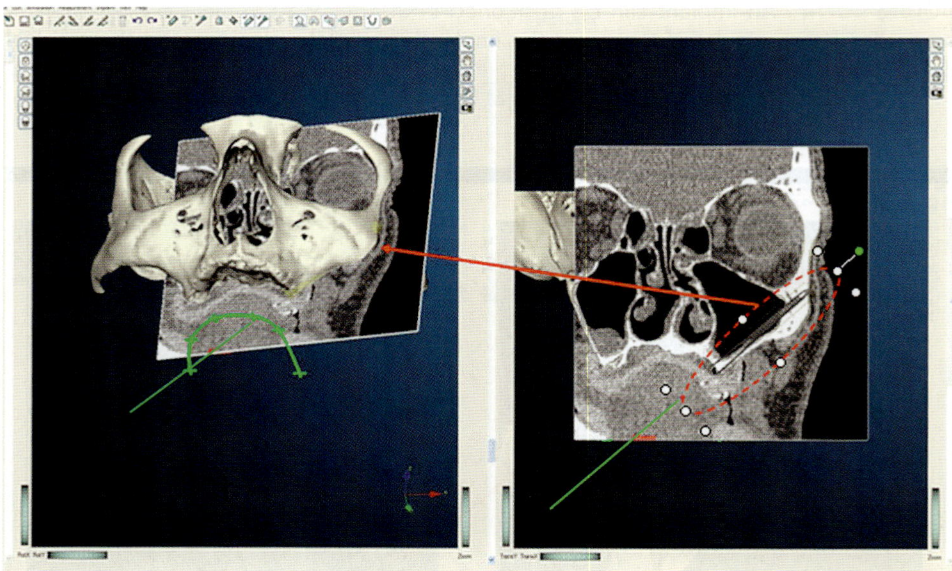

FIGURE 10-17 In computer-guided zygoma implant treatment, the alveolar and apical portions of the zygomatic implant may be visualized and manipulated for optimal implant placement.

surgery is preprosthetic surgery, and any input by the restorative and laboratory team members lends to predictable outcomes.

The next step in the use of computer-guided surgery software is fabrication of a surgical template for implant placement using the flapless approach.

Step 2: Fabrication of Surgical Template

Once the virtual planning of the implants has been completed (Figure 10-18), surgical template planning is initiated (Figure 10-19). Stabilization of the surgical template to the patient is achieved by use of anchor pins. This essential step must be performed before initiation of the osteotomies to allow for the execution of the virtual planned implant positions to the patient. Once the implant positions as they relate to the edentulous alveolus and the prosthesis have been completed and are satisfactory to all team members, position planning for anchor pins begins (Figure 10-20). Three to four anchor pins are strategically placed between the planned implant positions (Figure 10-21), keeping in mind the axial projection of the existing implants. Anchor pin depths are controlled to ensure that the anchor pin sleeves do not project

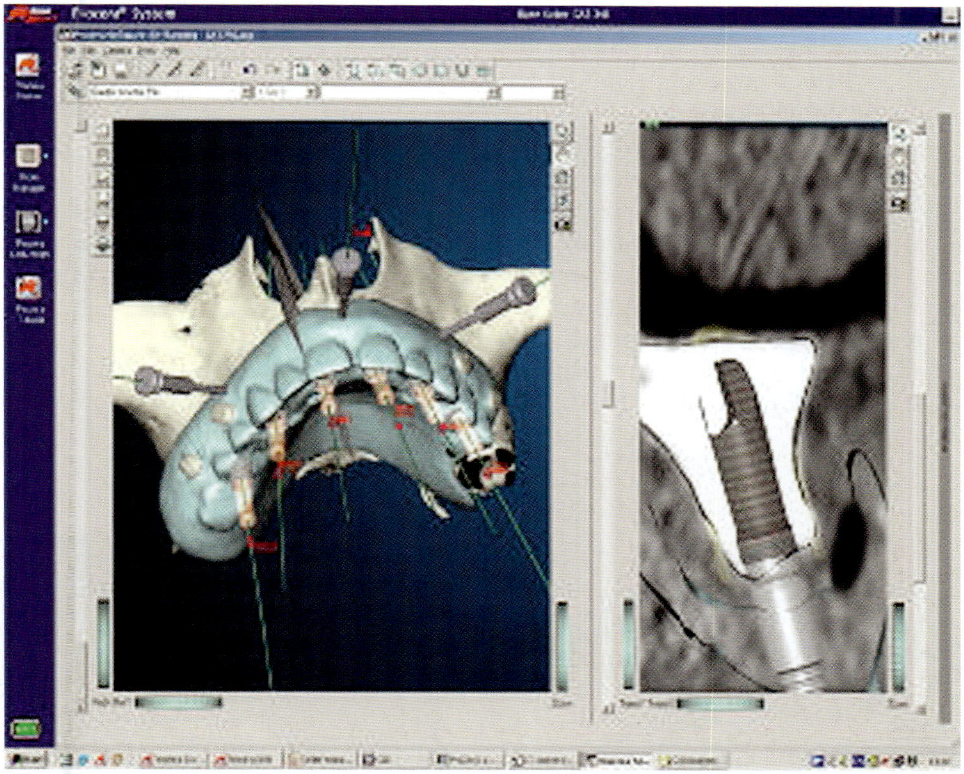

FIGURE 10-18 Completed "virtual" planning, demonstrating the position of the implants and anchor pins.

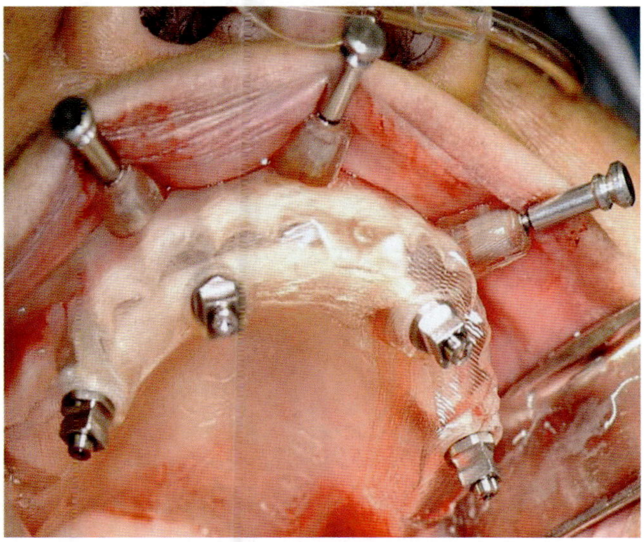

FIGURE 10-19 A surgical template created from virtual planning; the template is stabilized by three anchor pins with all four implants placed.

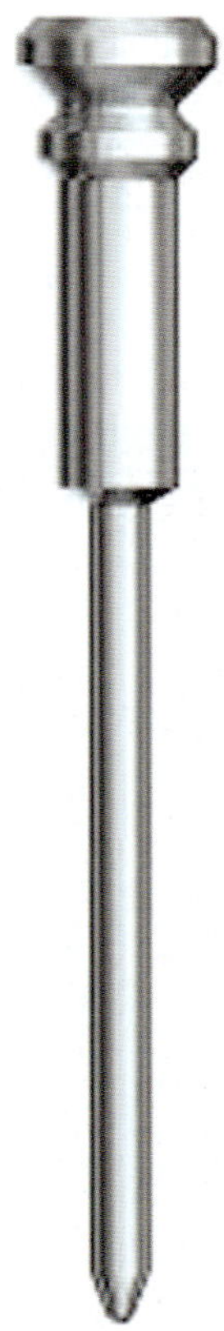

FIGURE 10-20 The anchor pins are planned in strategic positions, allowing stabilization of the surgical template to the patient's edentulous jaw during the surgical procedure. *(Courtesy Nobel Biocare, Yorba Linda, Calif.)*

beyond the intaglio surface of the denture (Figure 10-22). Improper anchor-pin placement can potentially prevent proper seating of the denture onto the edentulous ridge. Prior to completion of this planning phase, the bony window is "turned off" to visualize the relationship of the implants with the anchor pins to ensure that they do not collide (Figure 10-23). Once the proper depth of the anchor pin sleeves into the flange of the denture and the depth of the anchor pin itself into the patient's bone are confirmed, a template is produced by proceeding to the next step in the software. The completed surgical plan is sent for fabrication of the surgical template (Figures 10-24, 10-25, and 10-26).

Computer-guided surgery software can be used for treatment of the mandible as well as the maxilla. The treatment alternatives available for the maxilla include the following:

1. Placement of axial implants
2. Tilted treatment concept using four implants
3. Zygoma treatment concept using either two or four premaxillary implants (Figures 10-27 through 10-30)

For the mandible, the tilted concept is used to support a mandibular fixed-profile prosthesis (Figure 10-31).

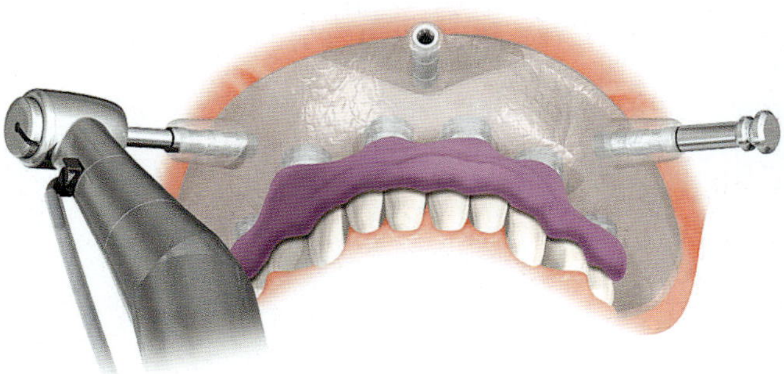

FIGURE 10-21 A minimum of three anchor pins stabilize the surgical template during preparation of the osteotomies. *(Courtesy Nobel Biocare, Yorba Linda, Calif.)*

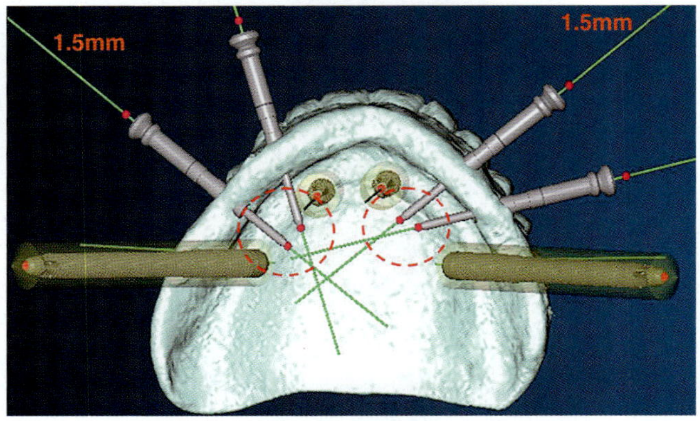

FIGURE 10-23 To avoid collision of the anchor pins with the proposed implant positions, the bony window of the NobelGuide software may be turned off to allow evaluation of the anchor pins and implants.

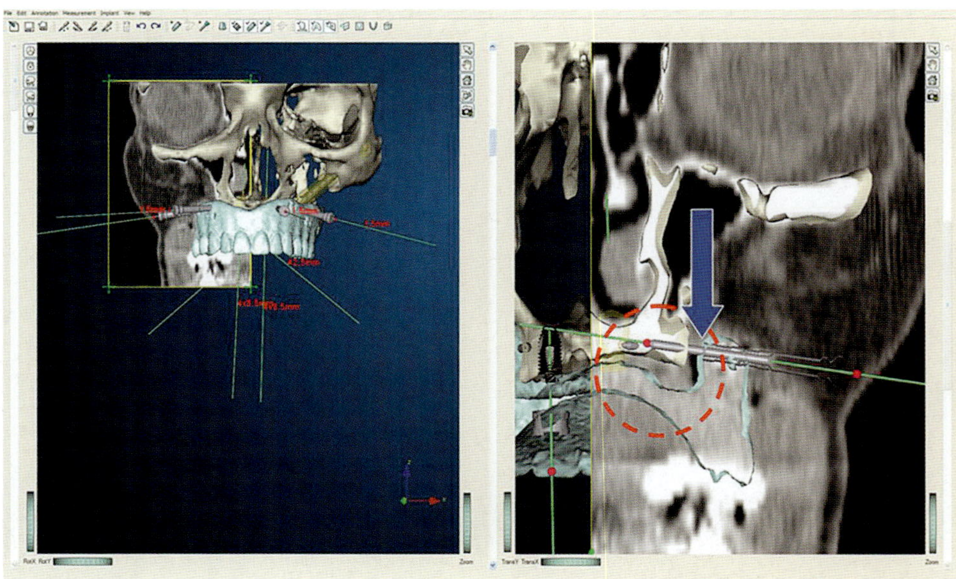

FIGURE 10-22 To ensure proper seating of the surgical template, the sleeves of the anchor pins must not protrude beyond the intaglio surface of the surgical template during the planning phase.

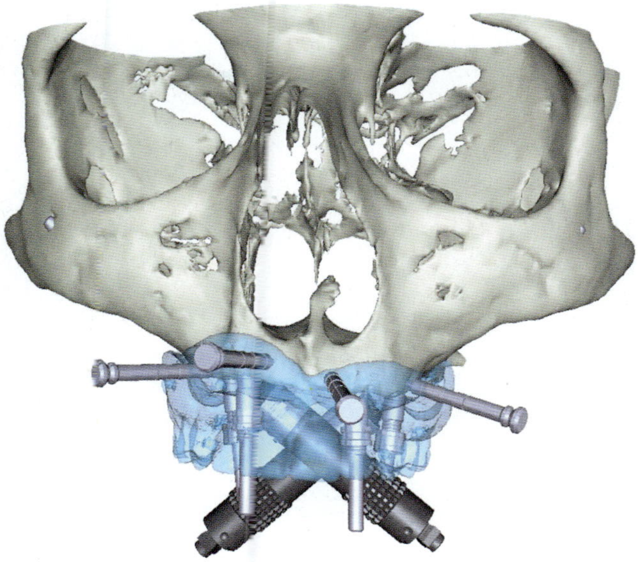

FIGURE 10-24 Completed surgical planning of the edentulous maxilla.

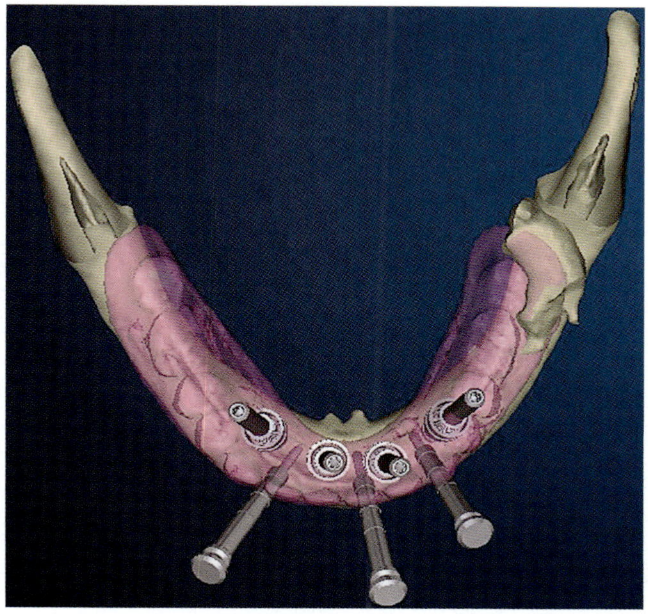

FIGURE 10-26 Completed planning of the computer-guided tilted mandibular protocol.

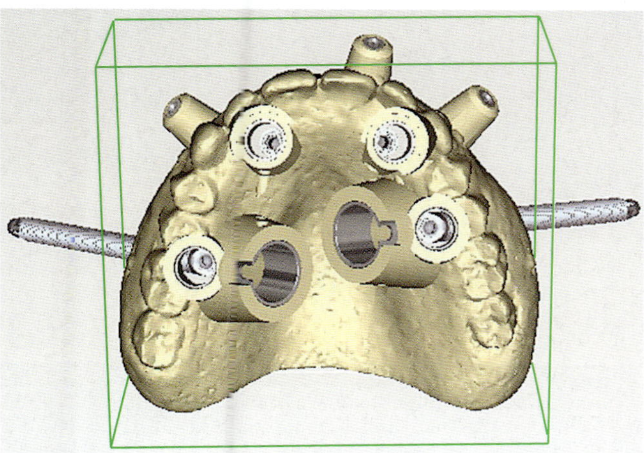

FIGURE 10-25 Completed surgical template of a computer-guided zygoma protocol.

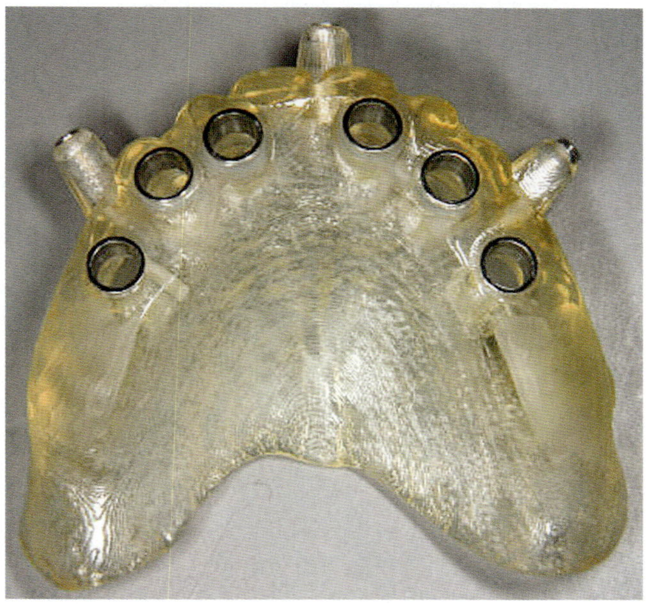

FIGURE 10-27 Surgical template for a six-axial computer-guided procedure.

If the practitioner chooses, after implant placement, temporary healing abutments may be placed during a soft reline of the patient's full denture. The implants will be allowed to osseointegrate for 3 to 6 months before proceeding with fabrication of the final prosthesis. If the practitioner chooses to immediate-load the implants after placement with the guided template, the analogue techniques described in Chapters 6, 7, or 8 can be used (Figure 10-32). The following section describes the steps needed to prepare a prefabricated immediate-load prosthesis.

Step 3: Fabrication of Provisional Immediate-Load Prosthesis

Complete use of computer-guided surgery software includes preoperative fabrication of an immediate-load prosthesis. Fabrication of the prosthesis begins after receiving the surgical template (Figure 10-33).

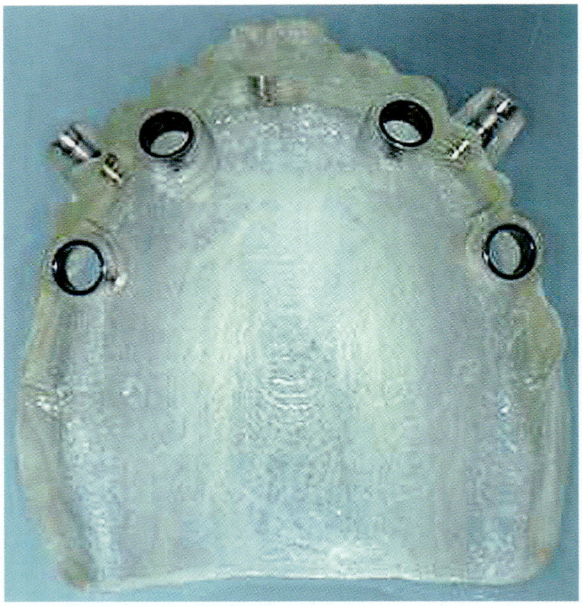

FIGURE 10-28 Surgical template for a tilted four-implant maxilla procedure.

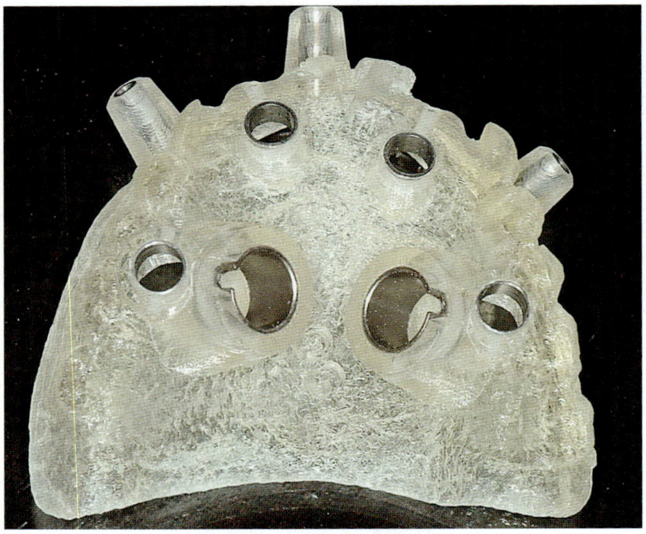

FIGURE 10-29 Surgical template for a guided zygoma procedure.

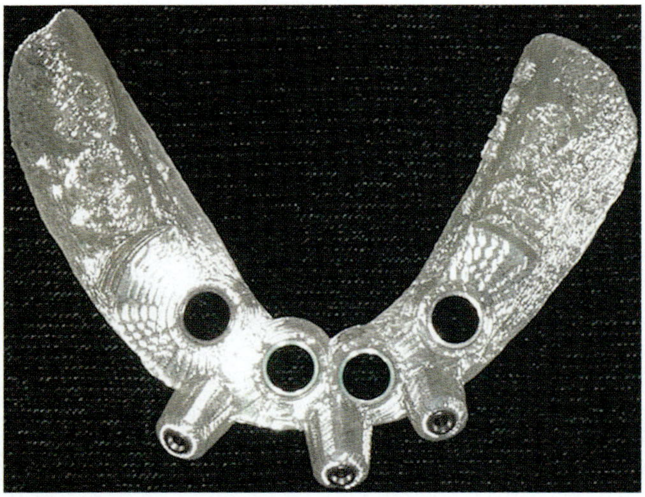

FIGURE 10-30 Surgical template for a tilted four-implant mandibular procedure.

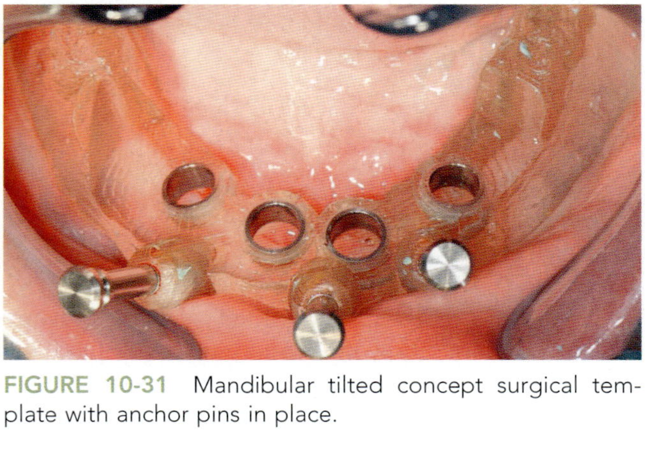

FIGURE 10-31 Mandibular tilted concept surgical template with anchor pins in place.

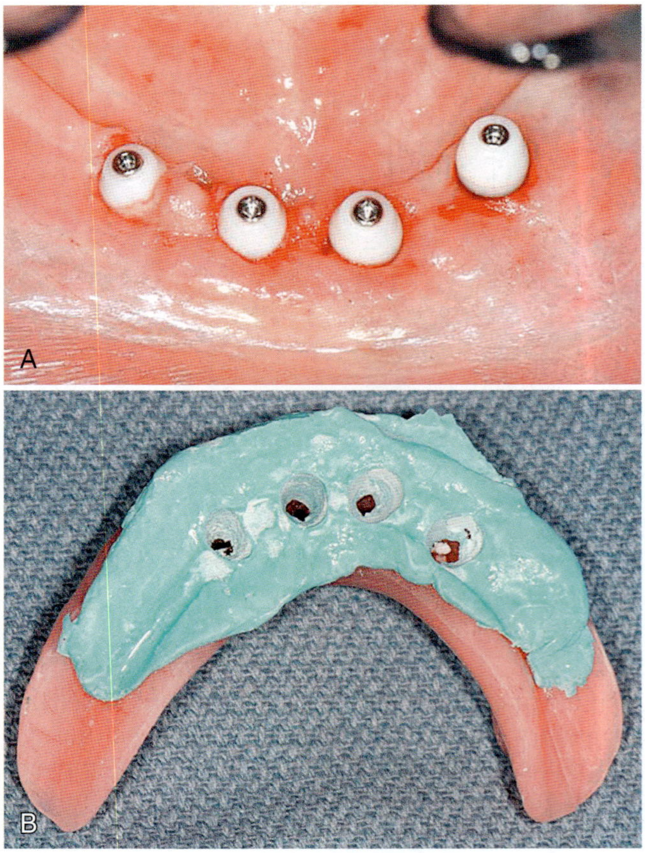

FIGURE 10-32 A, The computer-guided protocol may be used for implant placement and in combination with chairside conversion of the provisional immediate-load prosthesis alone. B, Chairside conversion protocol: Indexing the implants placed using the computer-guided surgical template.

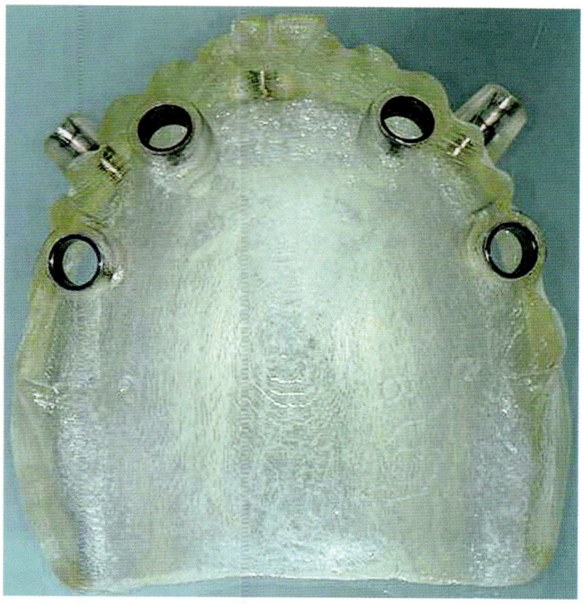

FIGURE 10-33 The completed surgical template is used to begin the laboratory protocol for fabrication of the immediate-load prosthesis.

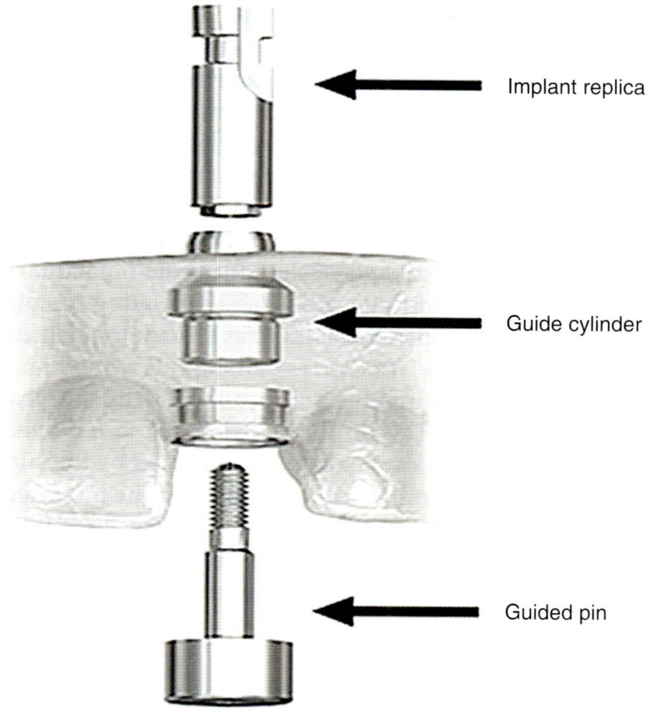

FIGURE 10-34 Fixture-level laboratory analogues are secured to the surgical template, initiating the fabrication process for the master model. *(Courtesy Nobel Biocare, Yorba Linda, Calif.)*

The surgical template, a stone model of the apposing arch and a duplicated denture of the edentulous jaw planned for implant placement, is sent to the laboratory. The next section describes the steps taken in the laboratory: pouring the master model and fabricating the provisional immediate-load prosthesis.

Laboratory Steps

Delivery of the completed surgical template to the laboratory technician begins the next phase of treatment with computer-guided surgery. The initial step in the laboratory process is fabrication of a master cast. To pour the master model, special components are needed; these are the guided sleeve, the guided pin, and the implant replicas (Figure 10-34). The guided sleeves duplicate the platform position of the fixture-level implant replica to the surgical template. It is important for the laboratory technician to accurately position and completely seat the three fixation pins within the surgical template prior to pouring the master model (Figure 10-35). The fixation pins orient the position of the surgical template to the master model and in turn dictate the position of the provisional prosthesis in three dimensions. The same three fixation pins are used to stabilize the surgical template to the patient during the surgical procedure (Figure 10-36). Accuracy in management of the fixation pins is critical to ensure proper orientation and occlusion of the provisional prosthesis in the patient's mouth

A

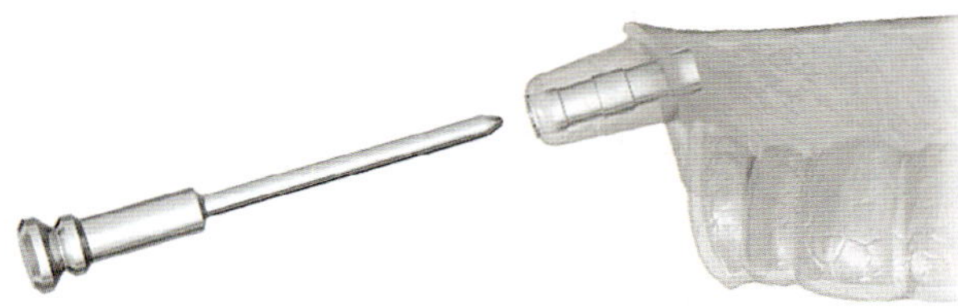

B

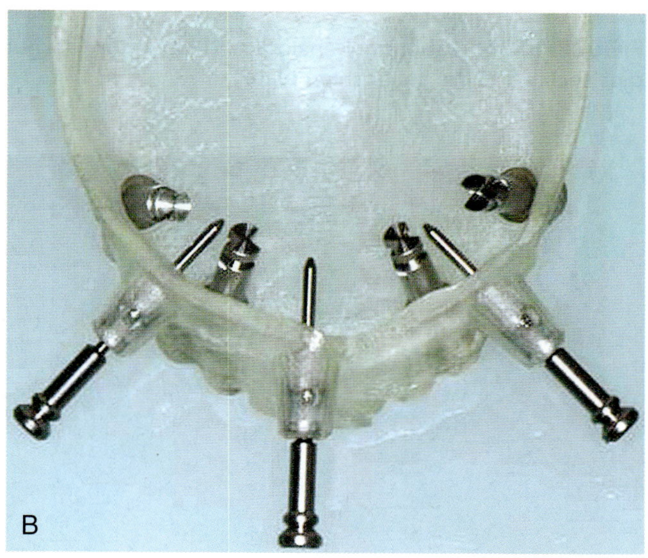

FIGURE 10-35 Laboratory anchor pins are placed through the anchor pin sleeves of the surgical template. *(B courtesy Nobel Biocare, Yorba Linda, Calif.)*

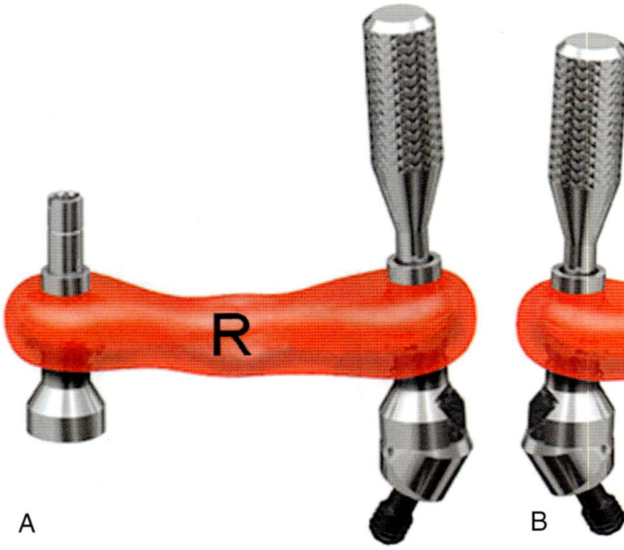

FIGURE 10-50 To eliminate confusion during surgery, the jig for the patient's right side is marked with an *R* and the left side with an *L*. *(Courtesy Nobel Biocare, Yorba Linda, Calif.)*

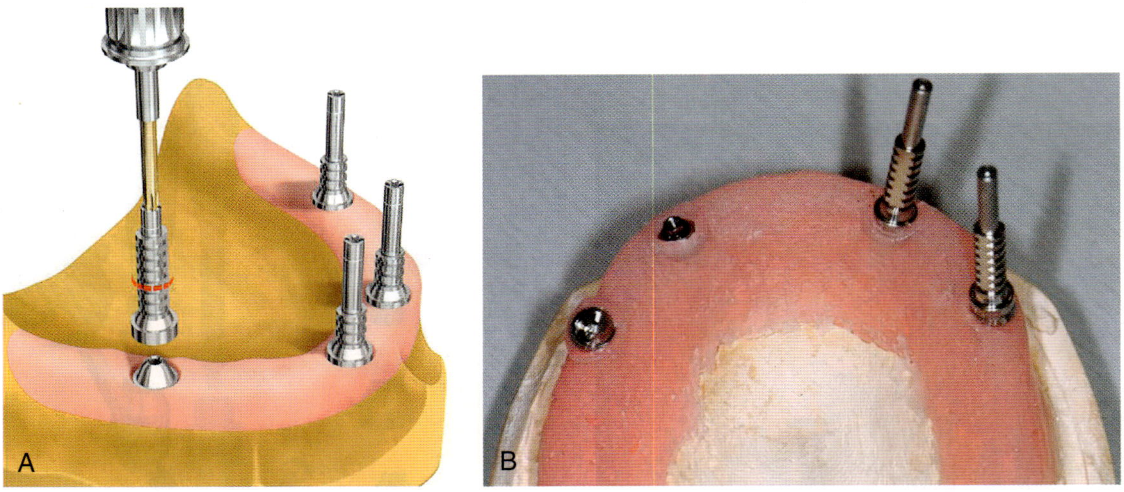

FIGURE 10-51 Multiunit temporary titanium cylinders are connected to the abutments, initiating fabrication of the provisional prosthesis. *(A courtesy Nobel Biocare, Yorba Linda, Calif.)*

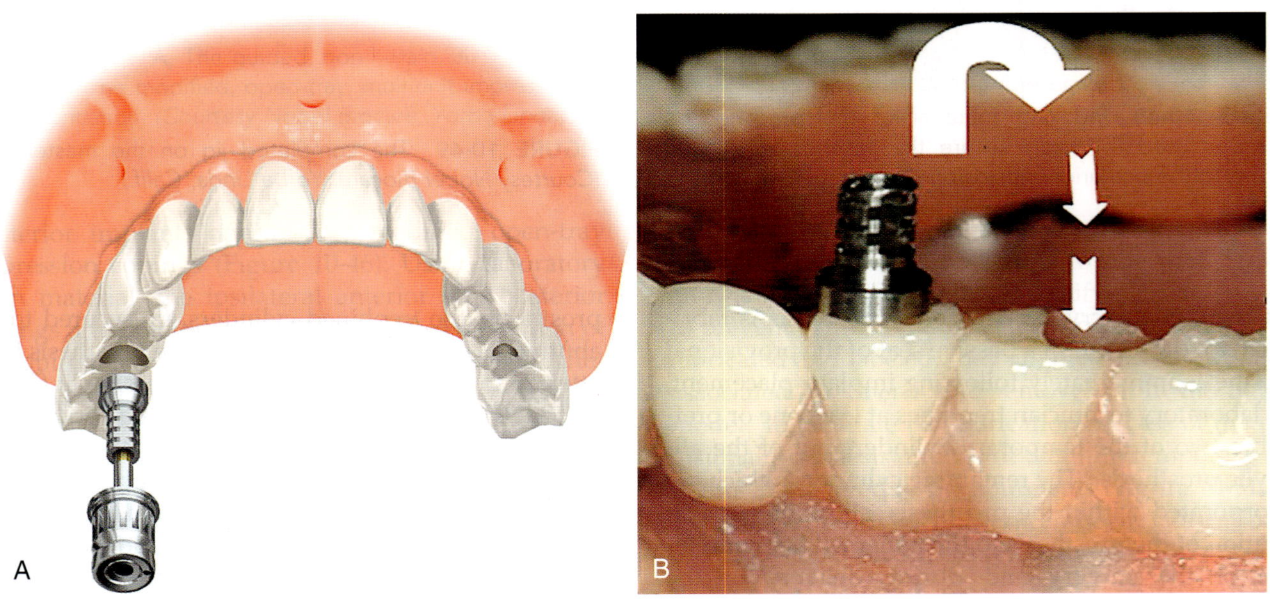

FIGURE 10-52 To assist in a passive fit of the provisional prosthesis, one or two of the temporary cylinders may be trephined out of the completed provisional prosthesis and directly luted intraorally after completion of the surgical phase of the procedure. *(A courtesy Nobel Biocare, Yorba Linda, Calif.)*

from the master model, the fabricated jigs are screwed back onto the abutments, which are still secured to the master model. First, the abutment screw of the 30° abutment is loosened and removed. This leaves the 30° abutment securely attached to its impression coping. Then the open-tray impression coping screw of the anterior implant abutment is removed. The "jig" at this point is composed of the open-tray impression coping anteriorly and the modified open-tray impression coping secured to the 30° abutment posteriorly. The jigs are packed carefully to prevent breakage. The straight multiunit abutments are now removed from the anterior implants and packaged separately.

The laboratory delivers the final prosthesis, including the trephined titanium temporary cylinders, the right and left jigs, the two abutments for the anterior implants, the surgical templates with the three fixation pins, and the surgical bite registration, to the implant team.

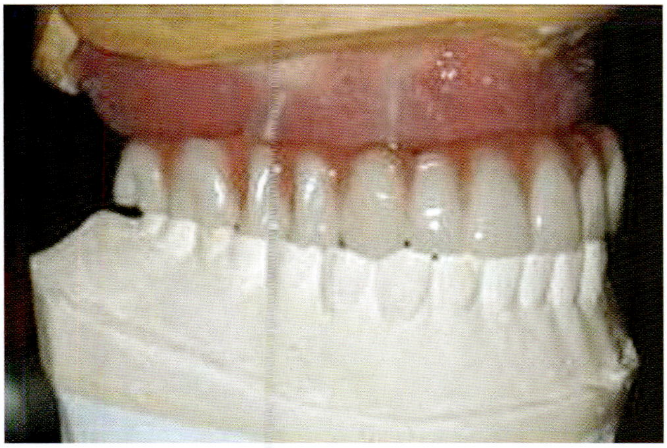

FIGURE 10-53 The completed immediate-load provisional prosthesis.

COMPUTER-GUIDED SURGICAL PROTOCOL FOR TILTED IMPLANTS: MAXILLA

The guided surgical armamentarium includes two kits. The first kit contains the anchor pins, implant mounts, template abutments, and drills needed to complete the osteotomies (Figure 10-54). The second kit contains drill guides specific for each drill (Figure 10-55). For ease of handling during the surgical procedure, a handle for the drill guides is available (Figure 10-56). Besides the NobelGuide surgical armamentarium required for implant placement, the patient's immediate-load prosthesis (Figure 10-57), the surgical

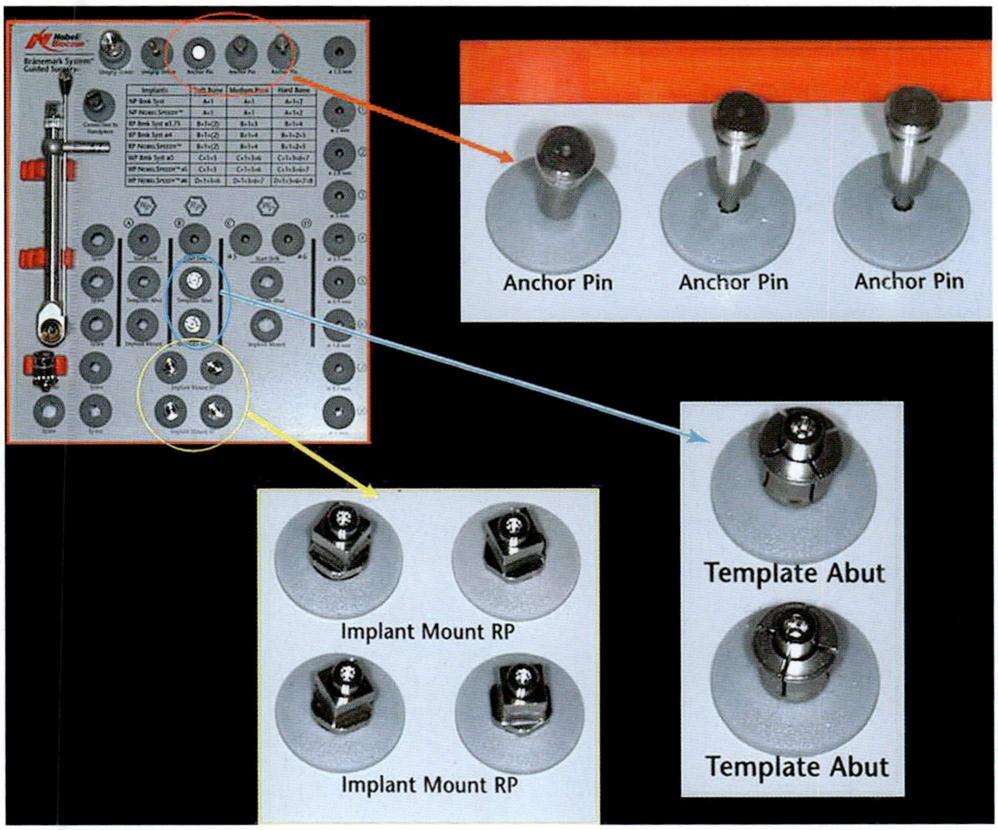

FIGURE 10-54 First surgical kit includes surgical anchor pins, fixture mounts, and template abutments.

template including the surgical bite registration (Figure 10-58), and the right and left jigs (Figure 10-59) are needed prior to initiation of the procedure. Because this protocol usually takes less than 45 minutes, the patient may elect not to be sedated, instead choosing to have the procedure performed under local anesthesia.

The surgical procedure begins with administration of local anesthetic. Bilateral maxillary buccal infiltration and bilateral greater palatine nerve blocks using 2% lidocaine with 1:100,000 epinephrine are sufficient. After adequate time has elapsed for the local anesthetic to take effect, the surgical template is seated and oriented onto the patient's edentulous ridge with the aid of the surgical bite registration (Figure 10-60). Using the 1.5-mm drill, the osteotomy for the fixation pins is completed, followed by pin placement (Figure 10-61). The surgical bite registration is now removed from the patient's mouth and the stability of the attachment between the template and the patient is confirmed by clinical evaluation (Figure 10-62). To initiate the osteotomy, the "start drill" (Figure 10-63), a

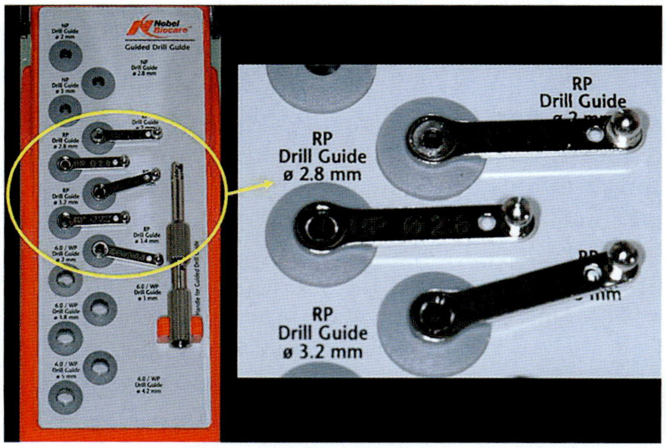

FIGURE 10-55 The second computer-guided surgical kit contains drill guides.

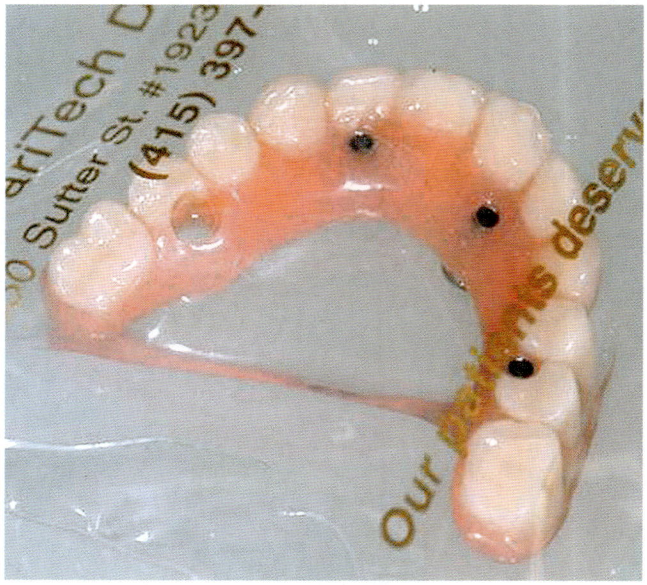

FIGURE 10-57 The immediate-load provisional prosthesis is sterilized and packaged ready for surgery.

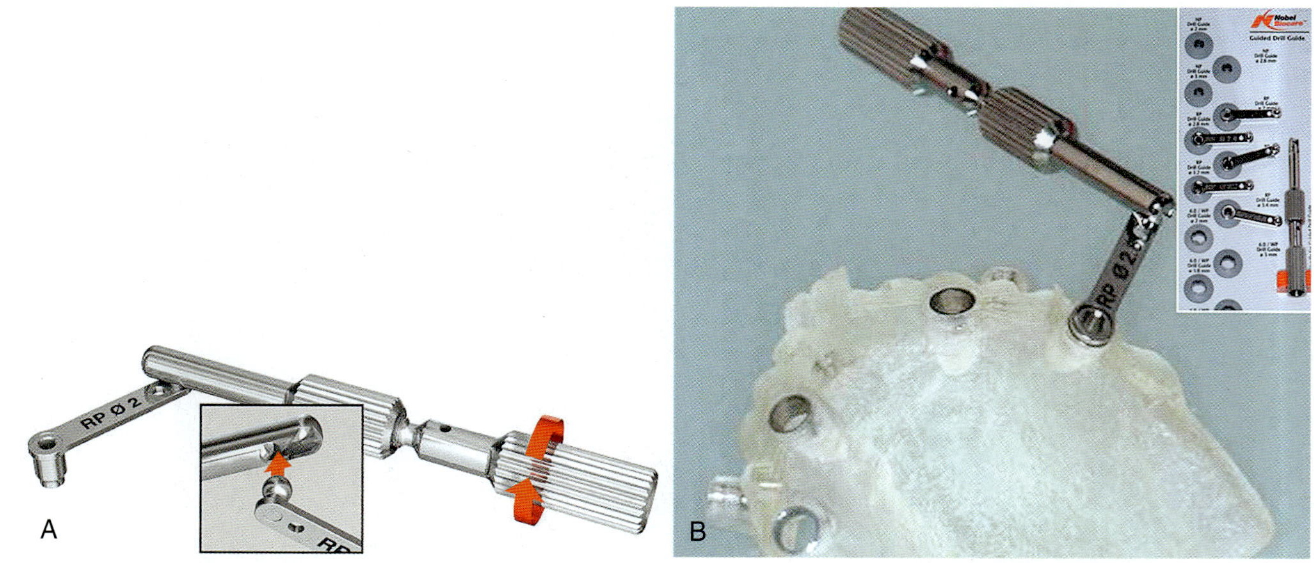

FIGURE 10-56 A, A handle is available for ease of handling of the drill guides. B, Illustration of the mounted drill guide handle and the drill guide placed into the surgical template. *(A courtesy Nobel Biocare, Yorba Linda, Calif.)*

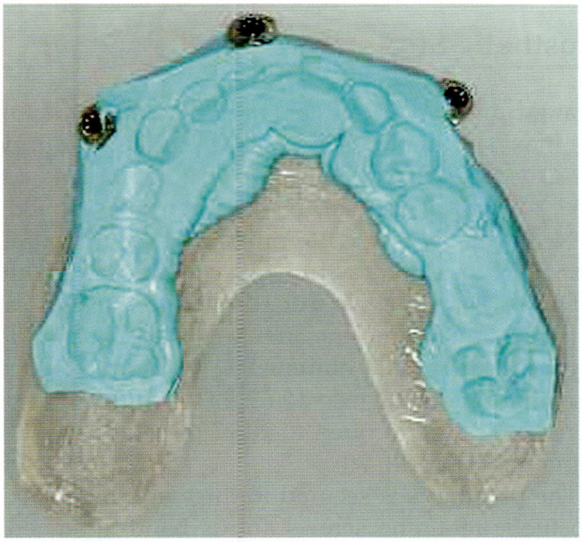

FIGURE 10-58 The surgical template and the surgical bite registration are ready for surgery.

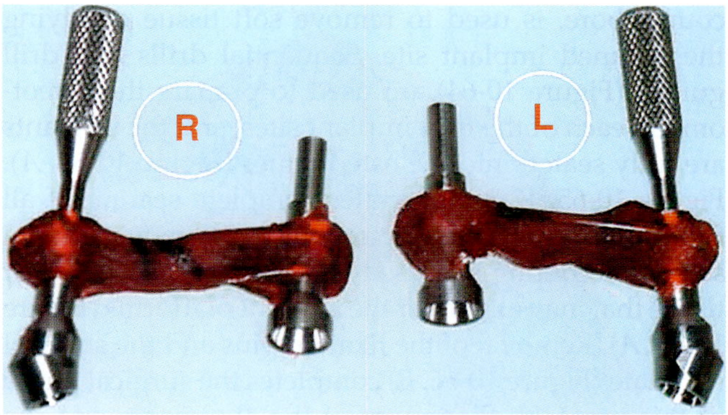

FIGURE 10-59 The right and left jigs are ready for surgery.

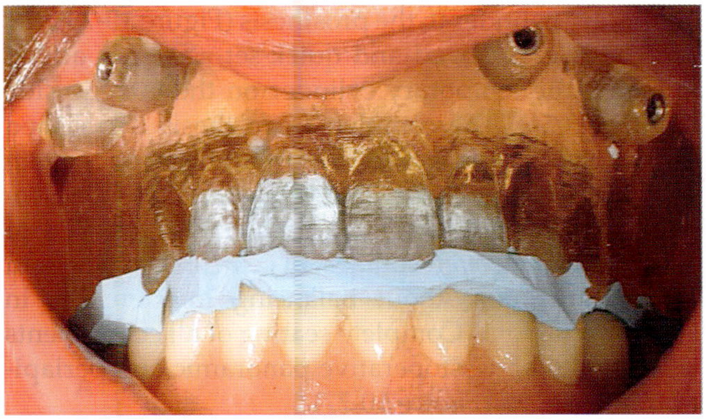

FIGURE 10-60 The surgical template is stabilized uniformly against the edentulous ridge by the surgical bite registration.

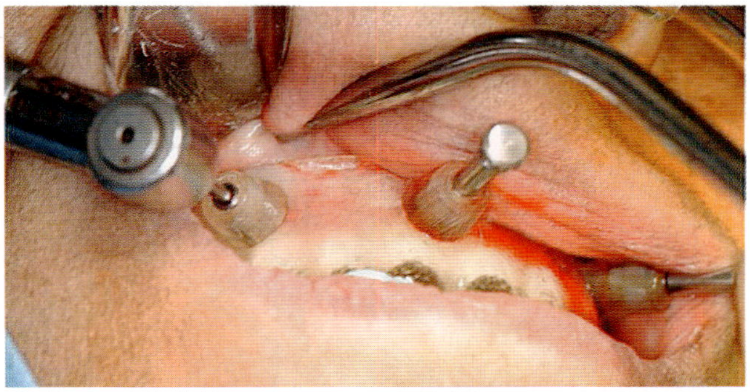

FIGURE 10-61 A 1.5-mm guided drill is used to prepare the osteotomy for insertion of the anchor pins.

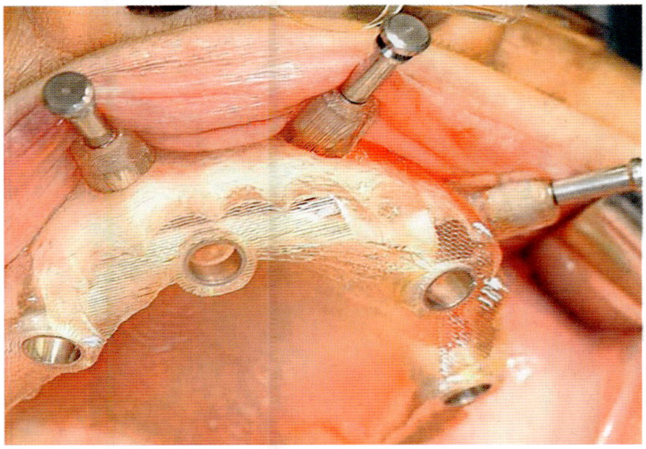

FIGURE 10-62 All anchor pins in place and the surgical bite registration removed. Evaluation of a uniform blanching of the crestal soft tissues is made.

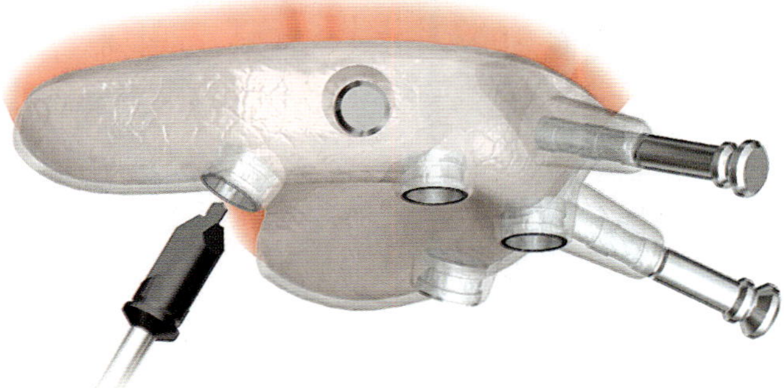

FIGURE 10-63 A counterbore drill is used to remove the crestal soft tissues prior to initiation of the osteotomy. *(Courtesy Nobel Biocare, Yorba Linda, Calif.)*

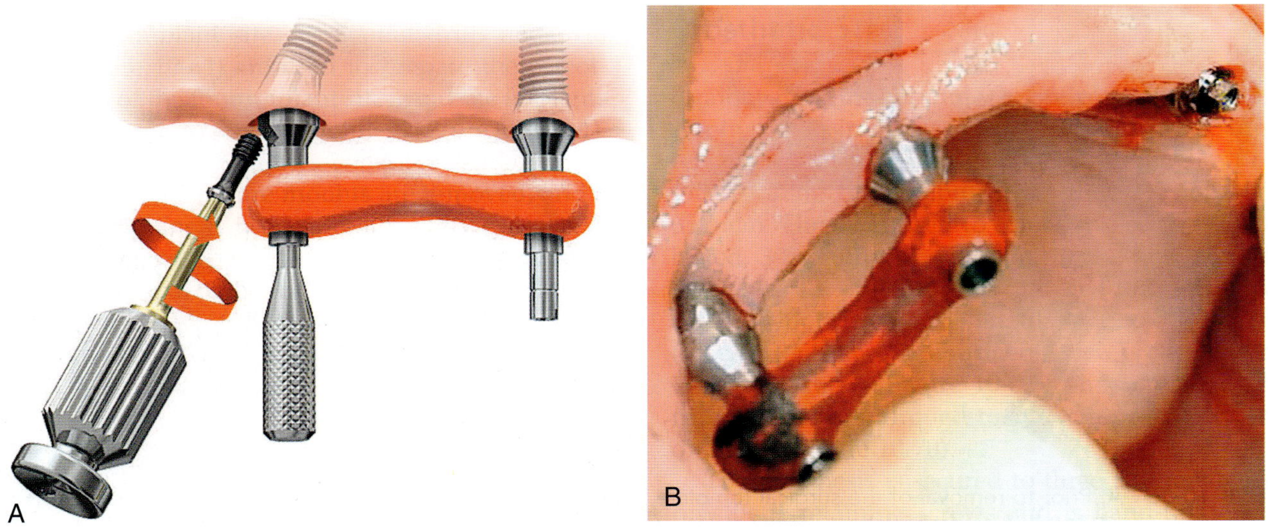

FIGURE 10-69 **A,** The abutment screw of the non-hexed, 30° multiunit abutment is secured to the posterior tilted implants. **B,** After securing the jig to the anterior multiunit abutments, the abutment screw of the non-hexed, 30° multiunit abutment is torqued to 20 Ncm. *(**A** courtesy Nobel Biocare, Yorba Linda, Calif.)*

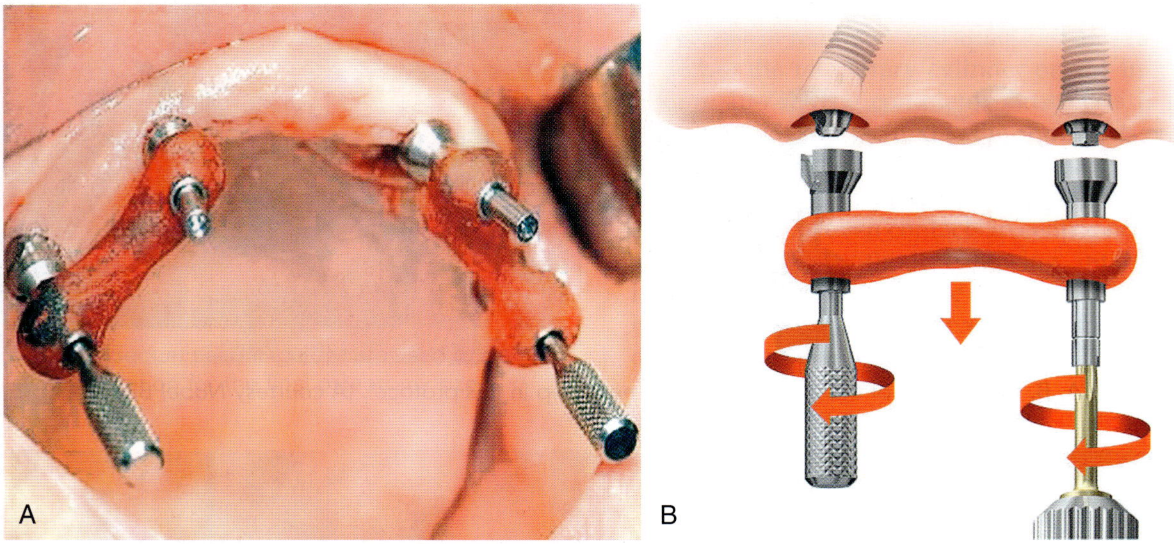

FIGURE 10-70 **A,** The contralateral jig is secured and the posterior abutment torqued. **B,** The open-tray impression coping screws are loosened, allowing removal of the jigs after both tilted implant abutment screws are torqued to 20 Ncm. *(**B** courtesy Nobel Biocare, Yorba Linda, Calif.)*

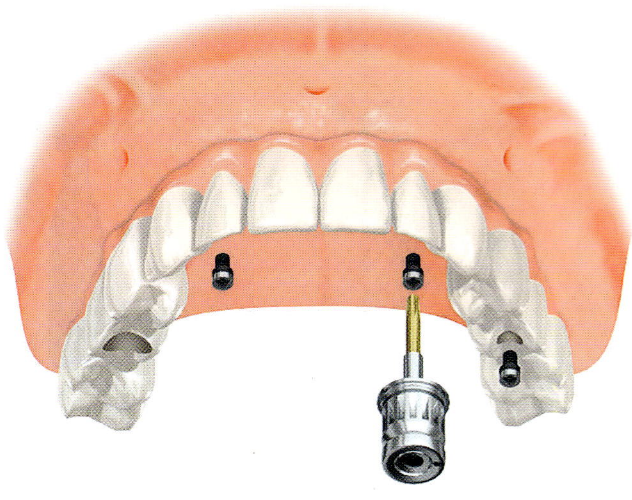

FIGURE 10-71 The provisional prosthesis is secured to the three implants by the prosthetic retaining screws. *(Courtesy Nobel Biocare, Yorba Linda, Calif.)*

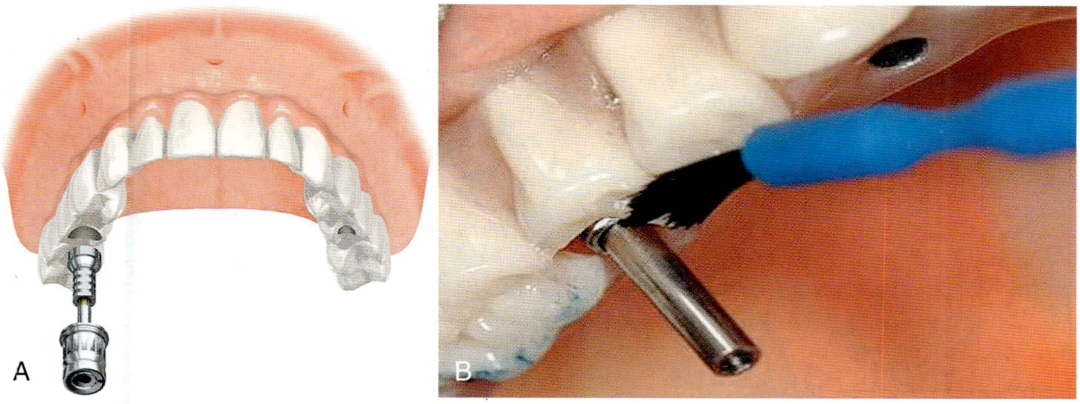

FIGURE 10-72 A, The forth titanium cylinder is placed through the trephined opening of the prosthesis and secured to the abutment using prosthetic retaining screws. B, The titanium cylinder is directly "salt and peppered" using quick-set acrylic, attaching it to the prosthesis. *(A courtesy Nobel Biocare, Yorba Linda, Calif.)*

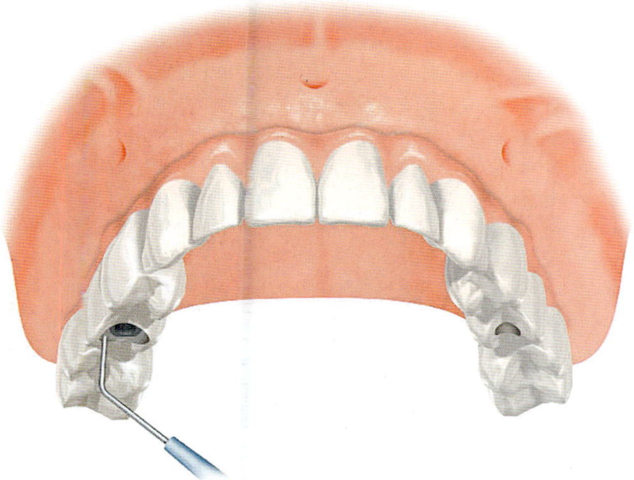

FIGURE 10-73 Additional quick-set acrylic is added prior to removal of the prosthesis. *(Courtesy Nobel Biocare, Yorba Linda, Calif.)*

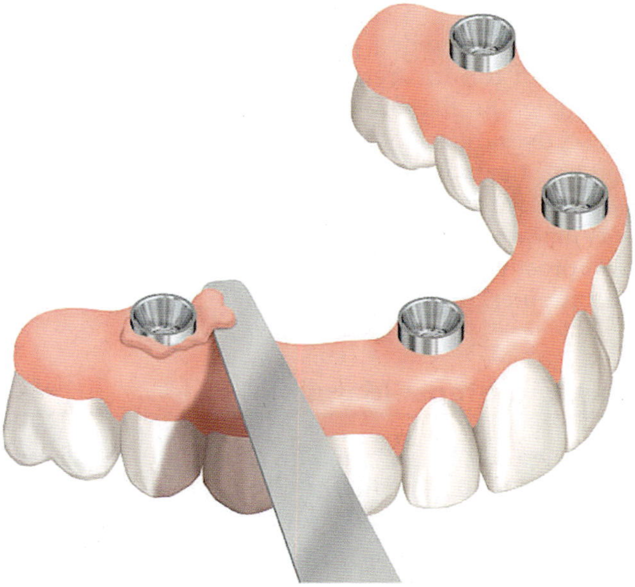

FIGURE 10-74 The intaglio surface of the forth titanium cylinder is also luted to the prosthesis using quick-set acrylic. *(Courtesy Nobel Biocare, Yorba Linda, Calif.)*

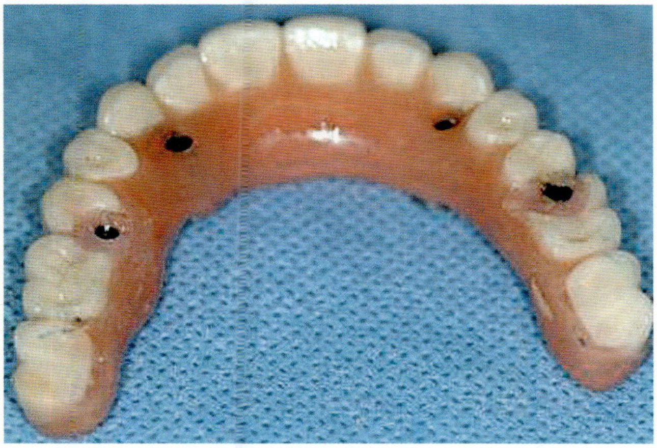

FIGURE 10-75 The completed provisional immediate-load prosthesis.

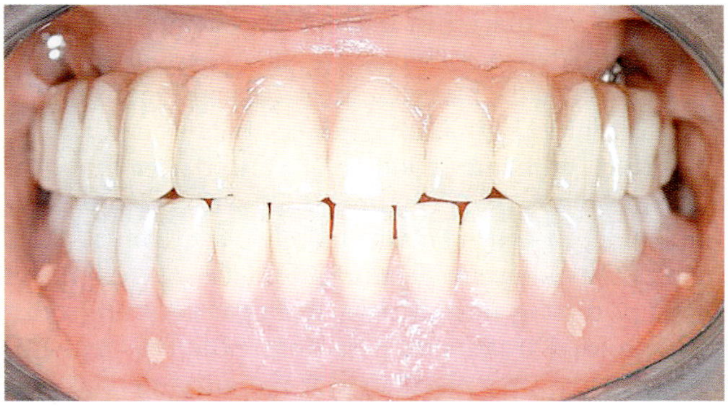

FIGURE 10-76 The provisional prosthesis is secured to the abutments using prosthetic retaining screws and hand-tightened to 10 Ncm. Proper interdigitation and midline position may be established by minor occlusal adjustments as needed.

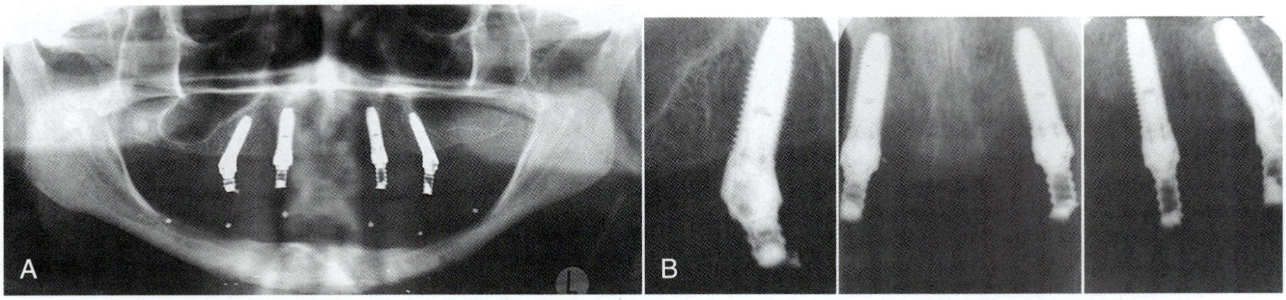

FIGURE 10-77 A, Postoperative radiograph confirming the position of the proposed implants. B, Complete seating of the abutments and the prosthesis may be confirmed using periapical radiographs.

COMPUTER-GUIDED SURGICAL PROTOCOL FOR TILTED CONCEPT: MANDIBLE

The computer-guided protocol may also be used in part or in full for treatment of the fully edentulous mandible. In the following sections, the planning phase, the surgical template, and the computer-guided flapless treatment concept are discussed. For the patient used as an example in this section, the decision was made to convert the denture into an immediate-load prosthesis chairside, illustrating the versatile uses of computer-guided treatment.

Planning Steps: Mandible

The lateral cephalometric film (Figure 10-78) demonstrates adequate mandibular symphysis width for placement of implants. The panoramic radiograph (Figure 10-79) allows visualization of the existing tilted-concept protocol used to treat the patient's maxilla as well as the topography of the patient's edentulous mandible. To begin the scanning protocol for treatment of the edentulous mandible using the computer-guided treatment software, the gutta-percha markings are placed in the mandibular denture. The six gutta-percha markings are staggered for ease of recognition by the NobelGuide software (Figure 10-80). The clinical examination of the patient's mandible is consistent with moderate to advanced resorption of the edentulous ridge (Figure 10-81) with minimal vestibular depth and resultant inability to retain a stable mandibular denture, leading to lack of functional capacity during mastication. To begin planning computer-guided treatment, a radiographic bite registration is made after placement of the gutta-percha pins in the patient's mandibular denture (Figure 10-82) and the patient is scanned. After importing the patient's mandibular DICOM files and the mandibular denture DICOM files into the NobelGuide software, the data is converted into a three-dimensional format, allowing visualization of the patient's edentulous mandible as well as the patient's denture. Systematic evaluation of the two-dimensional window superimposed onto the three-dimensional date (Figure 10-83) allows

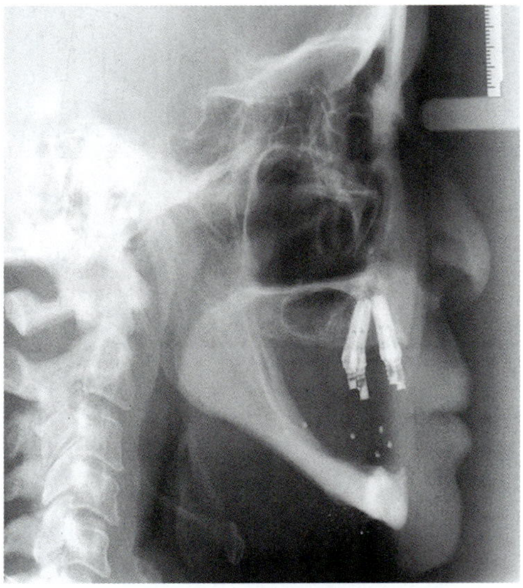

FIGURE 10-78 Lateral cephalometric radiographs may be used to study the topography of the mandibular symphysis region.

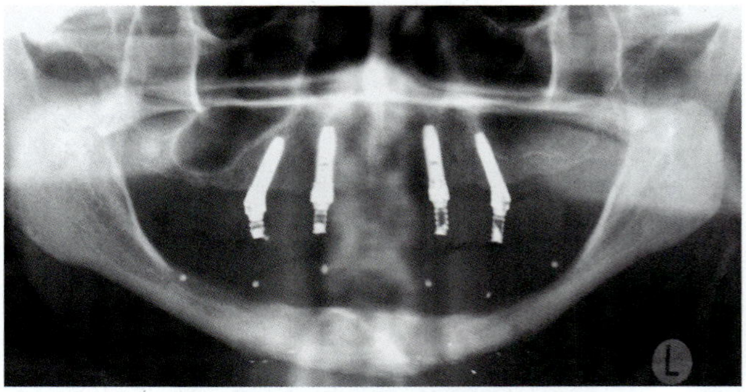

FIGURE 10-79 The panoramic radiographic study is useful to evaluate the path of the inferior alveolar nerve and the positions of the mental foramina.

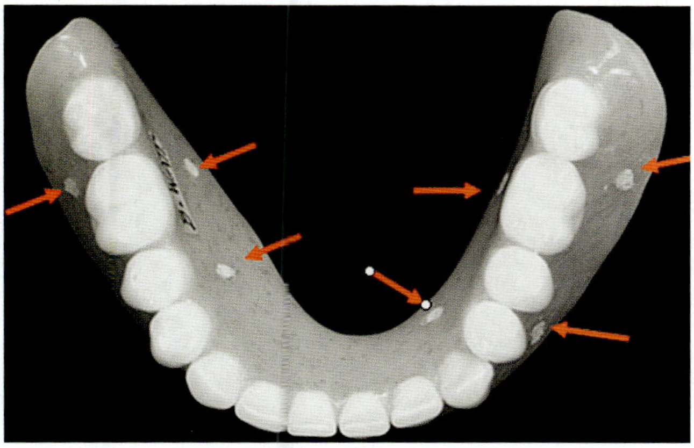

FIGURE 10-80 Six to eight gutta-percha markers may be used as radiographic markers before scanning the patient using the NobelGuide software for computer-guided implant placement.

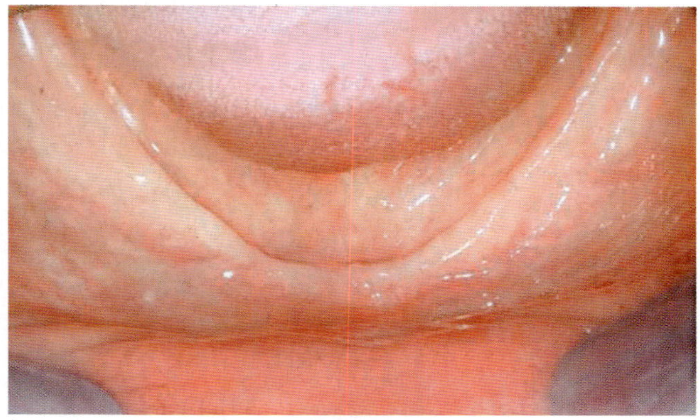

FIGURE 10-81 Moderate resorption of the edentulous mandible with loss of vestibular depth.

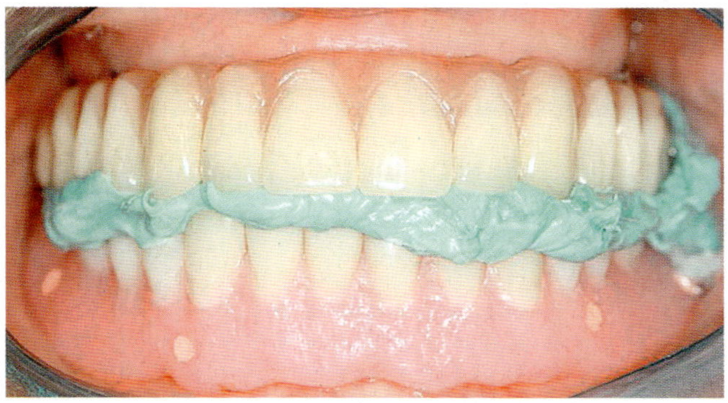

FIGURE 10-82 Polyvinylsiloxane is used to fabricate the radiographic bite registration.

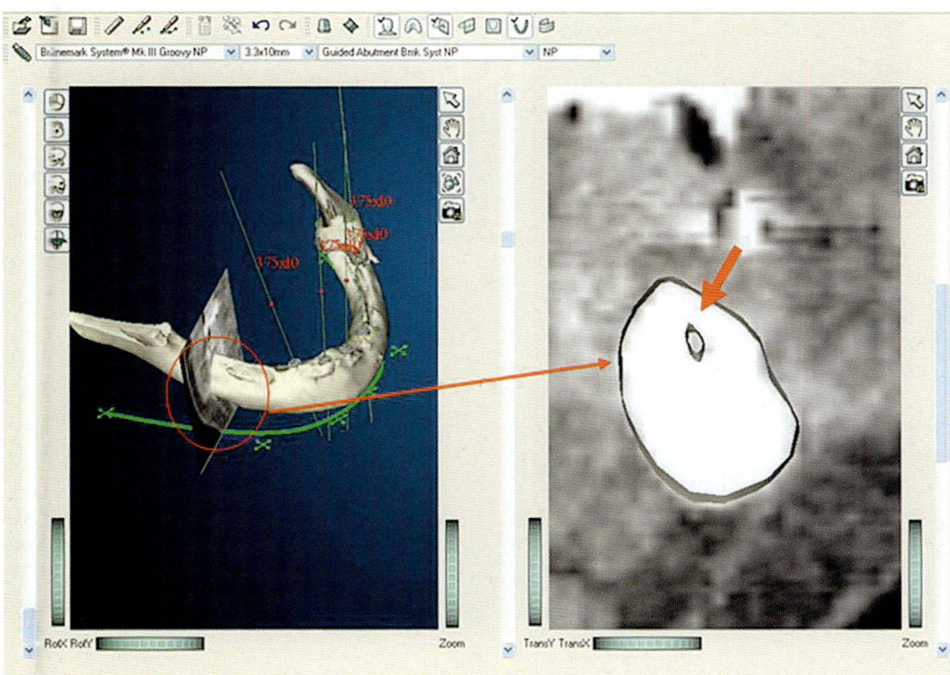

FIGURE 10-83 The cross-sectional window permits evaluation of the topography and vital structures from the three-dimensional radiograph.

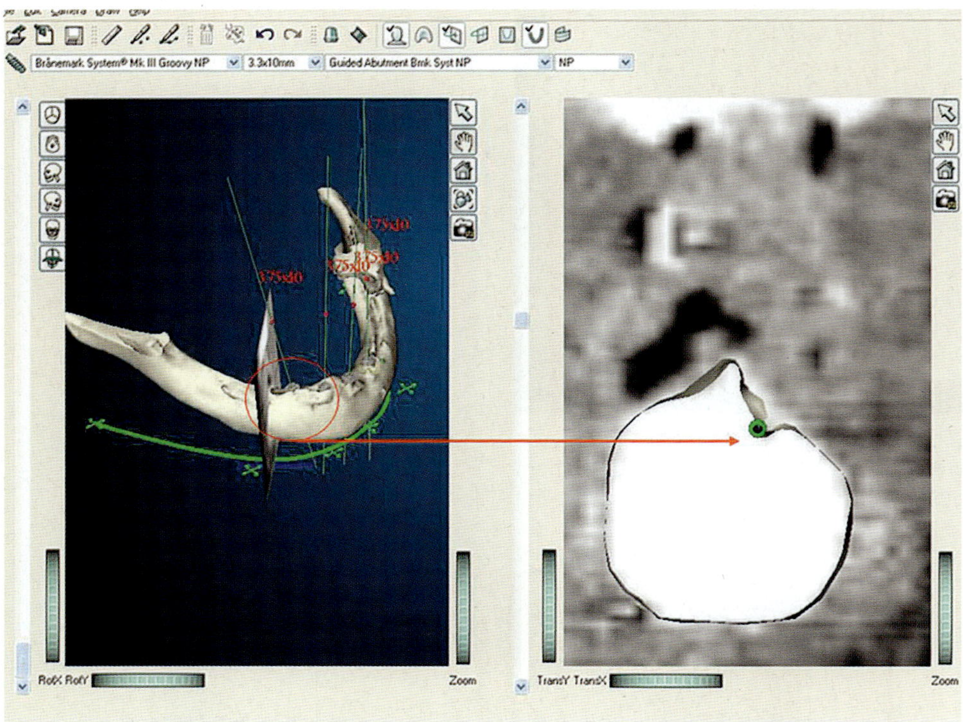

FIGURE 10-84 Visualization of the right mental foramen.

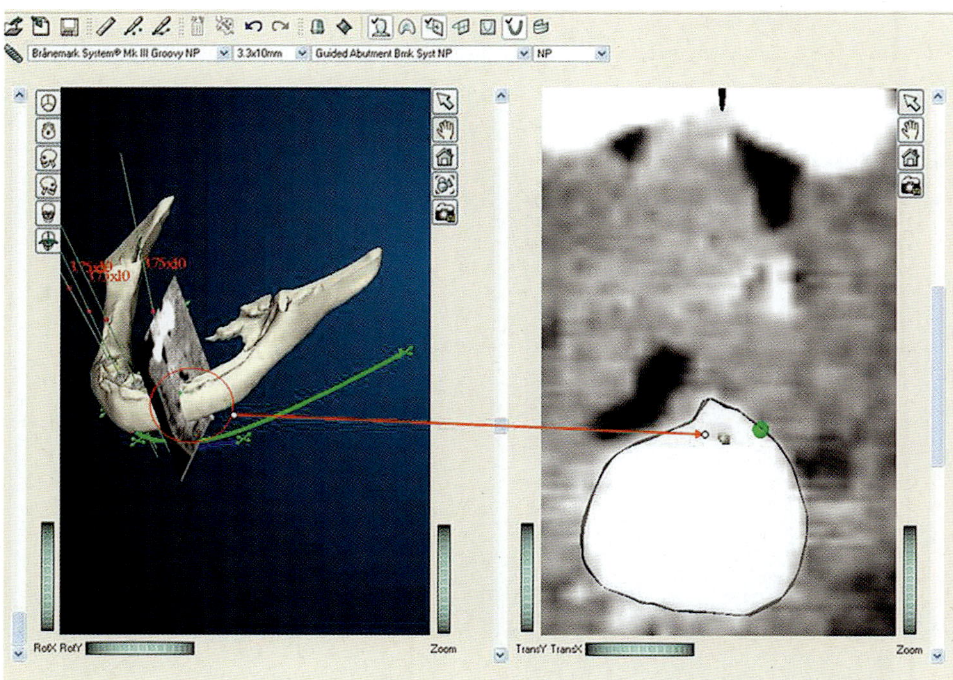

FIGURE 10-85 Visualization of the inferior alveolar nerve at the left mental foramen area.

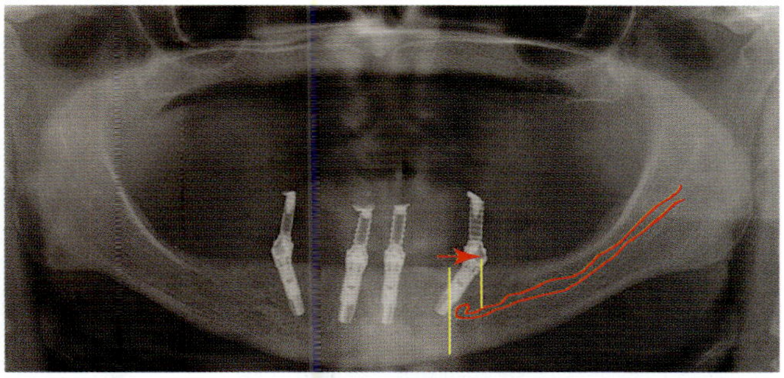

FIGURE 10-86 Availability of alveolar bone superior to the mental foramen allows tilting of the distal implant.

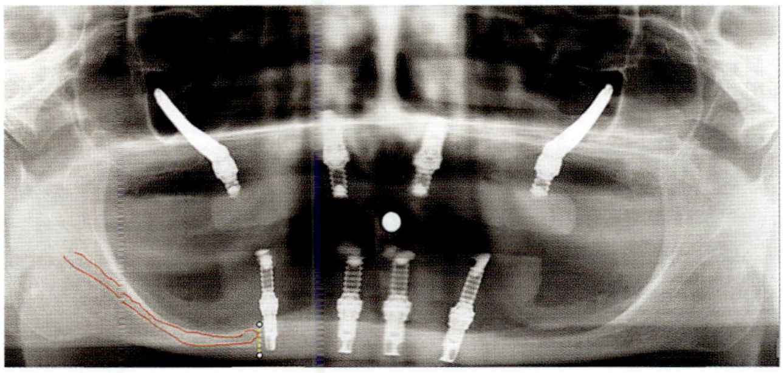

FIGURE 10-87 As the availability of alveolar bone superior to the mental foramen is reduced, tilting of the distal implant is also limited.

visualization of the inferior alveolar canal within the body of the mandible, consistent with the moderate-to-severe posterior mandibular atrophy appreciated during clinical examination. Cross-sectional evaluation of the bilateral mental foramen areas (Figures 10-84 and 10-85) show minimal alveolar bone above the mental foramen. In cases in which adequate bone exists over the mental foramen (Figure 10-86), the posterior implant platforms are tilted distally. In patients in whom the roof of the mental foramen is near or at the crest of the edentulous ridge (Figure 10-87), the posterior implants are placed in an axial inclination. Further evaluation of this patient reveals that the mental foramen is very close to the crest of the edentulous ridge (Figure 10-88). Therefore, the posterior implants are minimally tilted (Figure 10-89) almost in the same axial plane as the anterior implants (Figure 10-90). By "turning on" the prosthesis, the axes of the implants are related to the prosthesis and coincide with the desired prosthetic positions (Figure 10-91). The surgical template is designed (Figure 10-92) and processed (Figure 10-93).

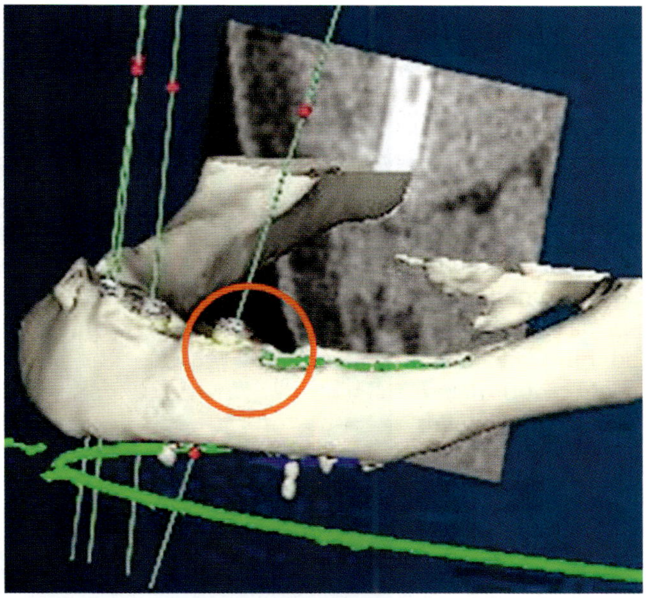

FIGURE 10-88 The NobelGuide software allows visualization of the mental foramen and its relationship to the proposed tilted implant platform.

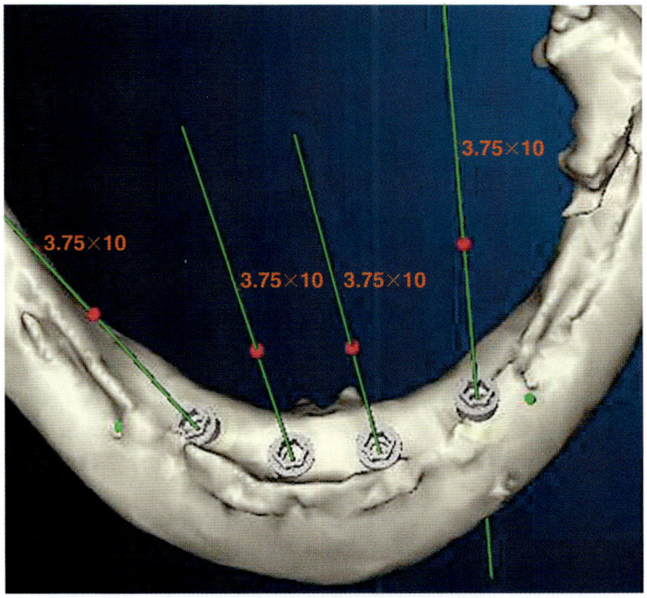

FIGURE 10-89 Because of the extraosseous presentation of the mental nerve, the distal implants are tilted minimally.

Laboratory Steps: Mandible

In this particular case, the decision was made to convert the prosthesis using the chairside conversion technique as described in Chapter 9. If a prefabricated prosthesis is desired, however, the laboratory protocol for tilted maxillary cases is followed. Prior to surgery, the patient's casts are mounted and a surgical bite registration is fabricated (Figure 10-94).

registration is removed from the template (Figure 10-97). Drill stops are available and can be fixated to the drills at the depth that coincides with the length of the chosen implant (Figure 10-98). Using drill guides (Figure 10-99), the osteotomy is initiated using the 2-mm drill (Figure 10-100). Generally, 4-mm, regular platform, single-thread implants are placed. Therefore, depending on the bone density appreciated at the time of the osteotomy, the practitioner may choose to undersize the osteotomy, stopping at the 2.8-mm drill. Or the osteotomy may be enlarged to 3 mm and at times to 3.2 mm to accommodate the regular platform implant. After completion of the osteotomy with the final drill size of choice, the guided fixture mount is secured to the implant (Figure 10-101). Using the implant guide (Figure 10-102), the implant is directed into the osteotomy site with the handpiece torque set at 20 Ncm. When the handpiece "stalls," the torque setting is increased to 40 Ncm (Figure 10-103) until the guided fixture mount completely seats against the surgical template (Figure 10-104). This protocol is repeated for the remaining three implants until all implants are fully seated at 40 Ncm insertion torque (Figure 10-105). The fixture mounts are removed and the soft tissue trephine is used to remove any excess soft tissues from the implant platforms (Figure 10-106). Prior to removal of the fixation pins and template, the implant platforms are inspected through the opening of the

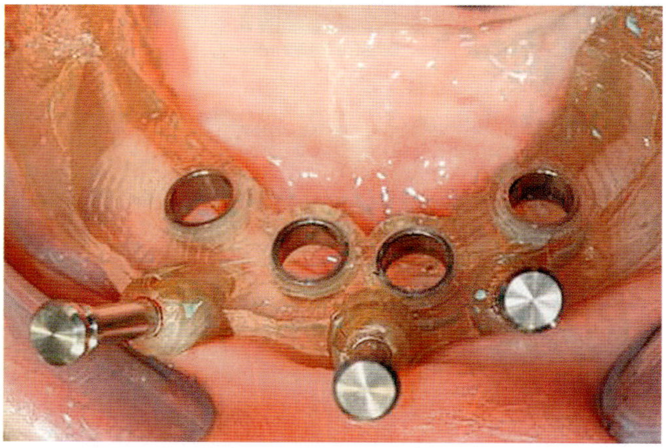

FIGURE 10-97 Uniform blanching of the edentulous soft tissues and the complete seating of all anchor pins permits initiation of the osteotomy for the proposed implants.

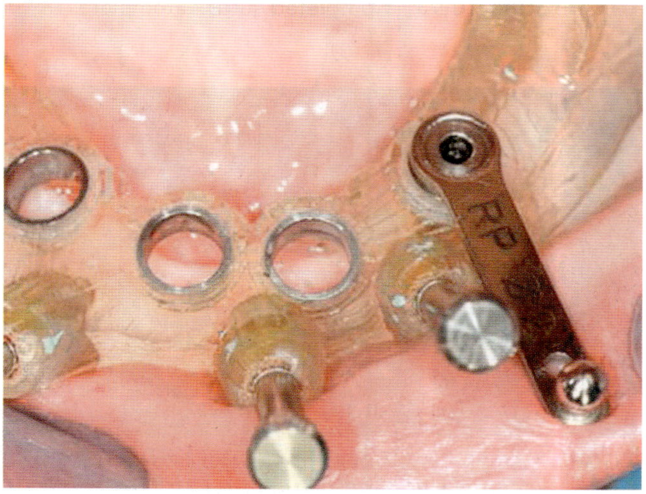

FIGURE 10-99 Sequential drill guides direct the position of the drills during preparation of the osteotomies.

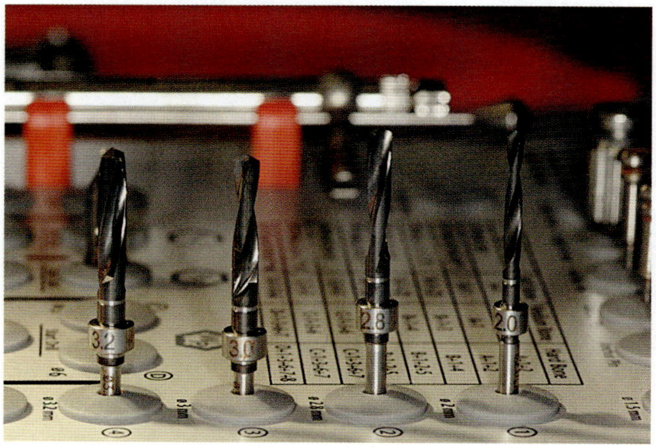

FIGURE 10-98 Drill stops may be used to ensure the desired osteotomy depth.

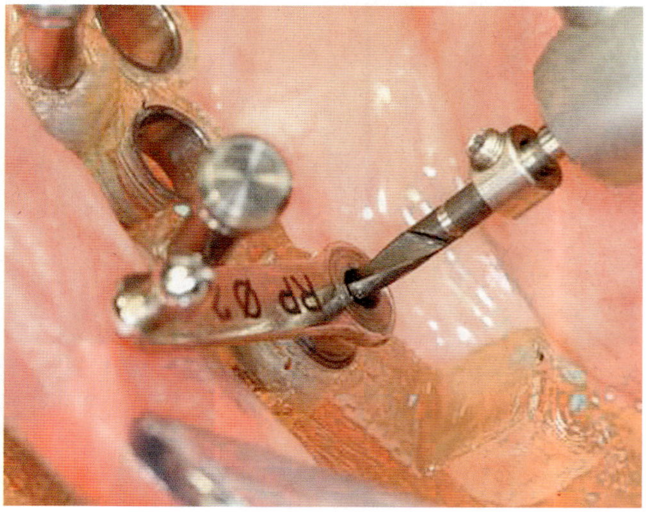

FIGURE 10-100 The 2-mm drill initiates the bony osteotomy after the crestal soft tissues have been removed using the bore drill.

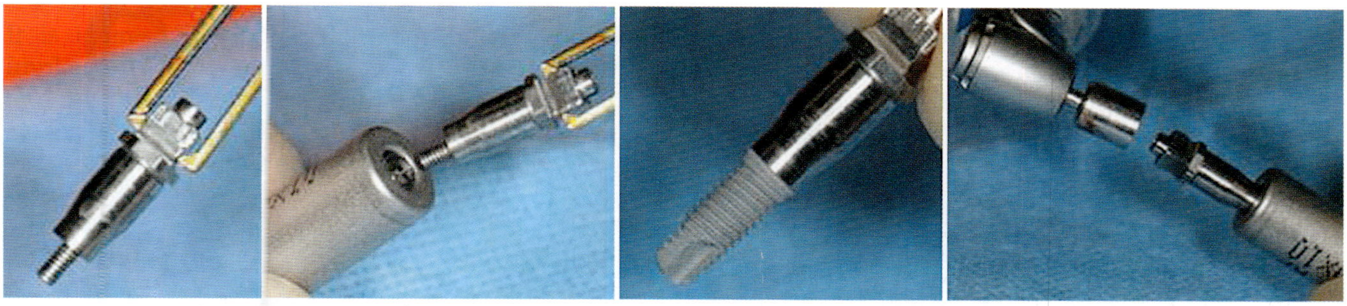

FIGURE 10-101 The guided fixture mount is attached to the implants, allowing them to be picked up by the fixture carrier connected to the handpiece.

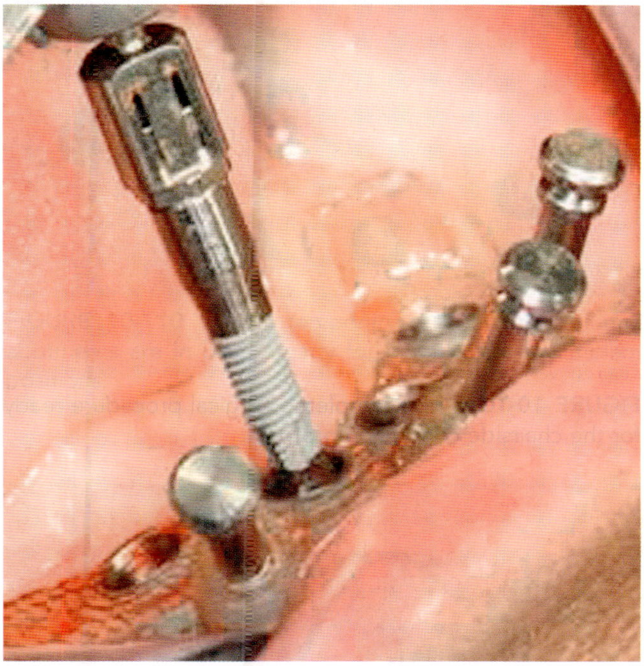

FIGURE 10-102 The surgical template guides the implant placement.

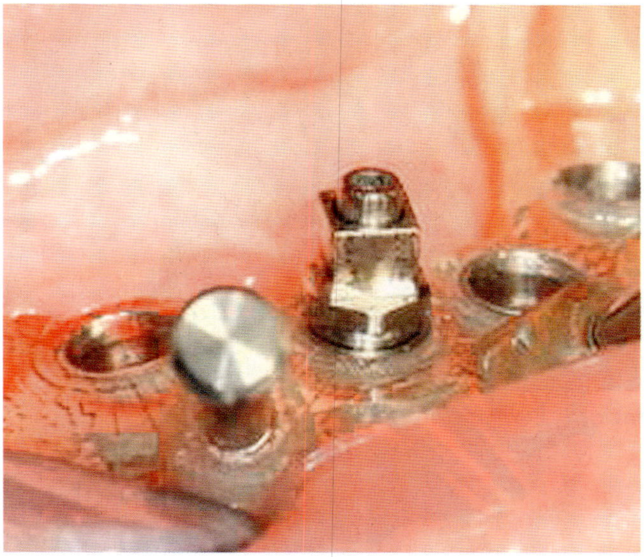

FIGURE 10-104 Complete seating of the flange of the fixture mount against the surgical template must be achieved.

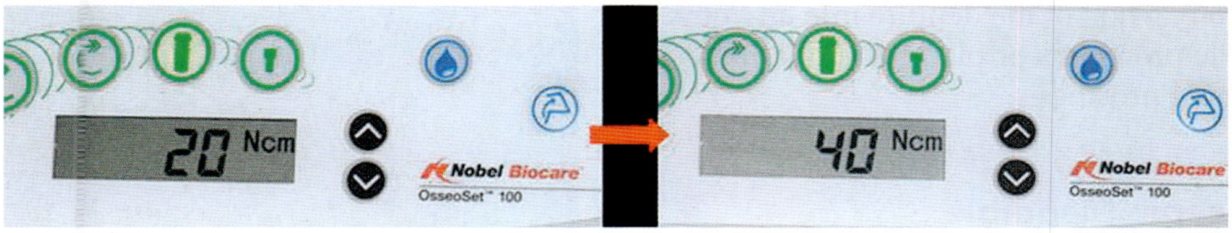

FIGURE 10-103 Initial insertion torque setting is 20 Ncm. When the handpiece stalls, the insertion torque is increased to 40 Ncm to allow complete seating of the implant in its osteotomy.

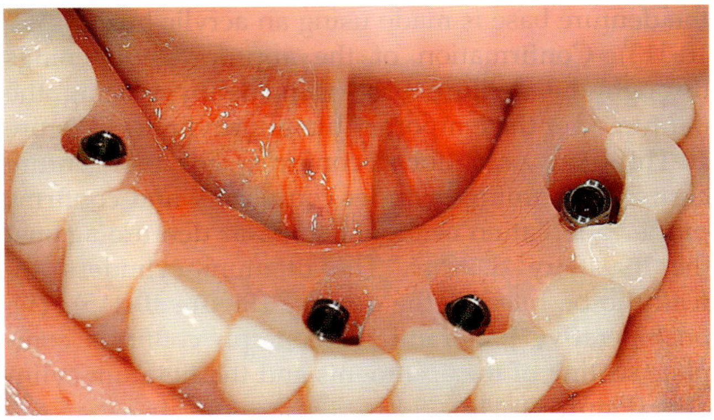

FIGURE 10-114 Passive circumferential seating of the temporary abutments to the access holes of the denture is confirmed prior to luting the titanium cylinders.

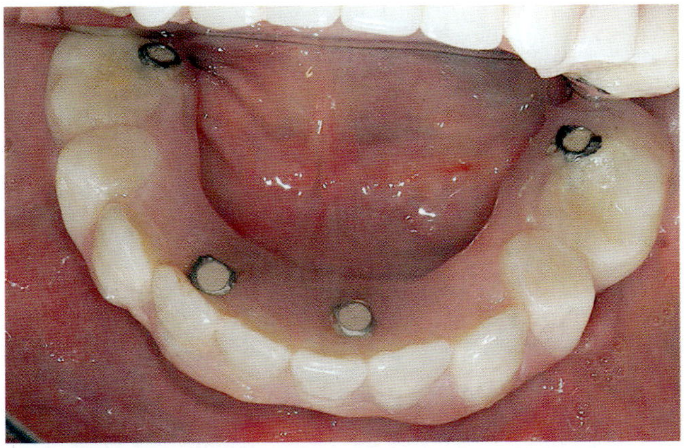

FIGURE 10-115 The completed chairside conversion of the immediate-load provisional prosthesis.

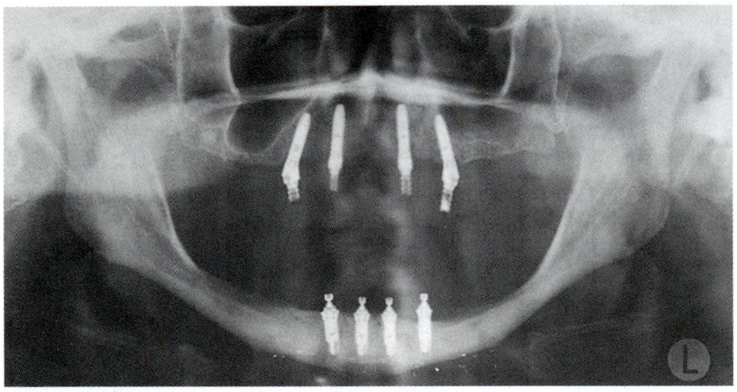

FIGURE 10-116 Immediate postoperative panoramic radiograph illustrates complete seating of the abutments and titanium cylinders.

COMPUTER-GUIDED SURGICAL PROTOCOL FOR ZYGOMA IMPLANTS: AN INVESTIGATIONAL PROCEDURE

Use of computer-guided surgery for implant placement and the accuracy of information transfer from the planning software to the patient has been reported in many previous publications.[9-12] The surgical templates in these studies were fabricated from stone models derived form intraoral impressions. The accuracy of information transfer from the planning software to the patient was not optimal and further development of this technique was warranted. Fiortin et al.[13] in 1995 and Demey and Vrielink[14] in 1999 used surgical templates modeled from three-dimensional computer data and reported a fabrication error of less than 0.5 mm using this technique.

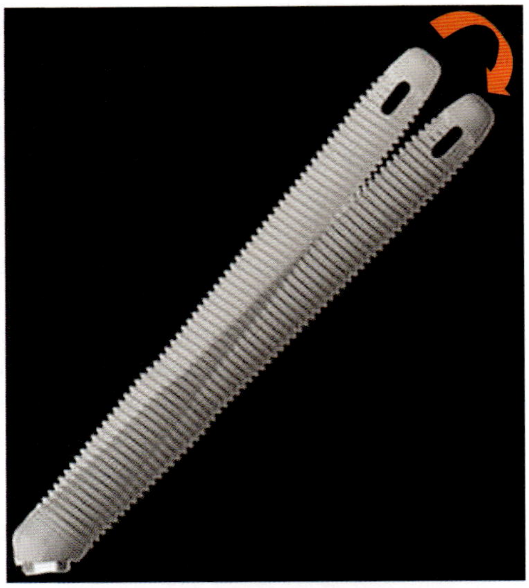

FIGURE 10-117 The potential variation of the trajectory of the zygomatic implants using the computer-guided protocol comparing the virtual versus actual placement. *(Courtesy Nobel Biocare, Yorba Linda, Calif.)*

In 2003 the specific transfer error of the zygomatic implant axis (in all three dimensions) from preoperative planning to the surgical site (Figure 10-117) was studied by van Steenberghe et al.[15] The surgical templates used in these studies were fabricated by stereolithography from three-Dimensional CT scan data. The templates were designed to be placed in intimate contact with the bone, and the surgical protocol for placement of the zygoma implants was modified by eliminating the opening of the lateral maxillary wall,[16,17] as described in the analogue protocol for placement of zygoma implants. Therefore, after raising the soft tissue flap, the surgical template was placed on the superficial bony surface (bone-supported) and the osteotomy for placement of the zygoma implants was initiated through drilling cylinders, which were incorporated in the surgical template. Complete dependence on the surgical guide for trajectory of the zygoma implant was made. Such reliance on the surgical template to guide the axis of the zygomatic implant demands understanding of three-dimensional morphology of the zygomatic bone.

In 2003 Nkenke at al.[18] studied and reported the quantity and quality of zygomatic bone. At the same time, in preparation for their study, van Steenberghe et al. quantified the dimensions of 20 human zygoma bones (10 subjects) using three-dimensional scans. The height, lateral width, and anterior-posterior length of the zygoma bone was measured. Analyzing this data, it was apparent that the height along the proposed implant axis varied from 7.9 to 24.9 mm. The horizontal (coronal) width varied between 11.2 and 28.2 mm, and the anterior-posterior (sagittal) width varied between 6.6 to 11.1 mm.

With this information at hand, six guided zygoma implants were placed in three cadavers. Postoperative CT scans were used to compare the angle of the virtual planned zygoma implants with the actual postoperative position of the zygoma implants. Less than 3° of angle variation were noted in four of the six zygoma implants. The largest deviation, measuring 2.7 mm, was noted at the apical portion (zygoma end) of the planned implant as compared with the postoperative CT scan. Considering the pilot studies reporting on the three-dimensional measurements of the zygoma bone, it is apparent that the anterior-posterior (sagittal) dimension is critical because of the potential existence of an exaggerated concavity of the posterior aspect of the zygoma bone. Immediately posterior to the zygoma body is the infratemporal fossa, which contains vital anatomic structures. Fenestration of the posterior aspect of the zygoma bone could result in damage to muscular and neurovascular content of the infratemporal fossa.

Professor van Steenberghe's conclusion that the complex surgical protocol as well as the wide variation in the anatomy of the zygoma bone warrant further study of the potential use of computer-guided treatment planning for zygoma implant placement is important to recognize.

The use of computer-guided surgery for placement of zygomatic implants is currently the subject of an international, multicenter study. This concept is considered for patients who have zone I alveolar bone only and are missing alveolar bone in zones II and III (Figure 10-118).

Planning Steps

Computer-guided treatment planning for zygoma implant placement begins with the "two-scan" technique, described previously. DICOM files are generated for analysis and treatment planning within the NobelGuide program (Figure 10-119). After reformatting the DICOM files into a three-dimensional model and superimposing the patient's denture onto the bony model, placement of zygoma implants in zone III

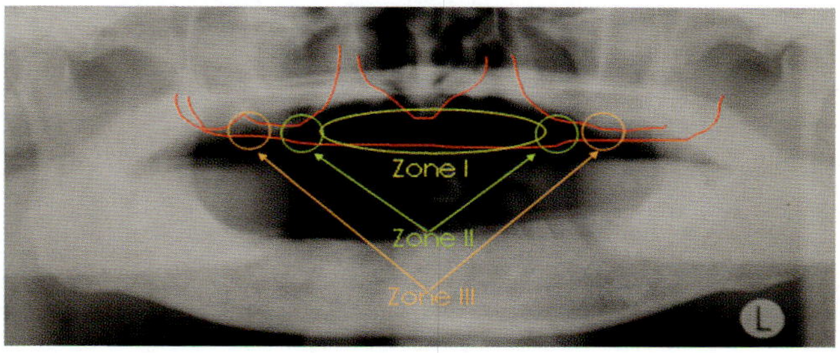

FIGURE 10-118 Edentulous maxilla with zone I bone only.

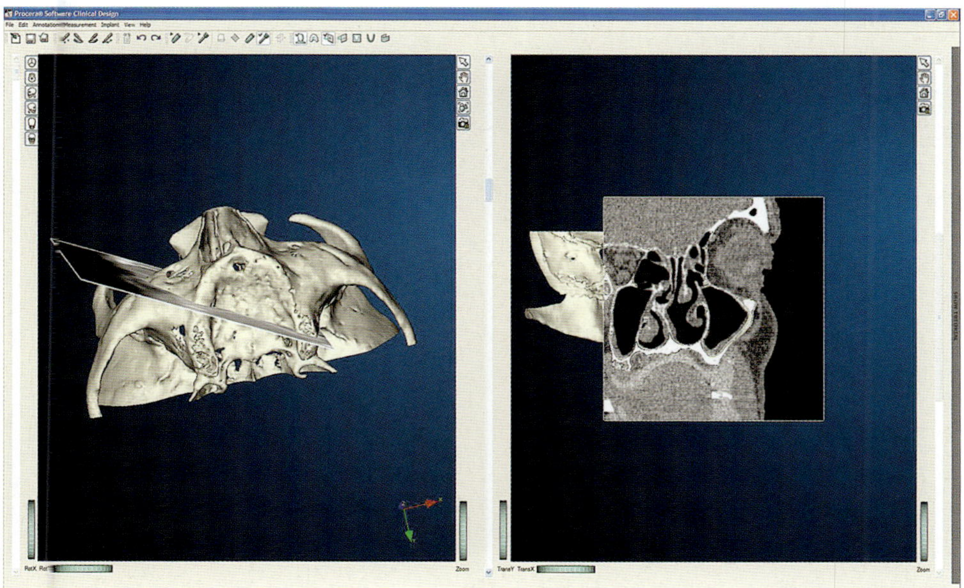

FIGURE 10-119 The NobelGuide software may be used to plan placement of zygomatic implants.

(Figure 10-120) and two anterior maxillary implants in zone I are planned (Figure 10-121).

The surgical template is fabricated and returned to the oral and maxillofacial surgeon (Figure 10-122). Because of the length of the guided sleeves required for placement of the zygomatic implant, "collision" of the sleeves may occur if both guided sleeves are fabricated on a single surgical template (Figure 10-123). Therefore, the two-template (or dual-template) method is adopted to allow guided placement of zygomatic implants (Figure 10-124). In the dual-template protocol, the primary template is used to place the anterior maxillary implants and the left zygomatic implant (Figure 10-125). The template is removed and the secondary template is secured to the patient using template abutments. The right zygomatic implant is now placed (Figure 10-126). After the implant positions are successfully planned, the single-template or dual-template data is transmitted to the laboratory for fabrication of the surgical templates. The laboratory then begins fabrication of a provisional immediate-load profile prosthesis.

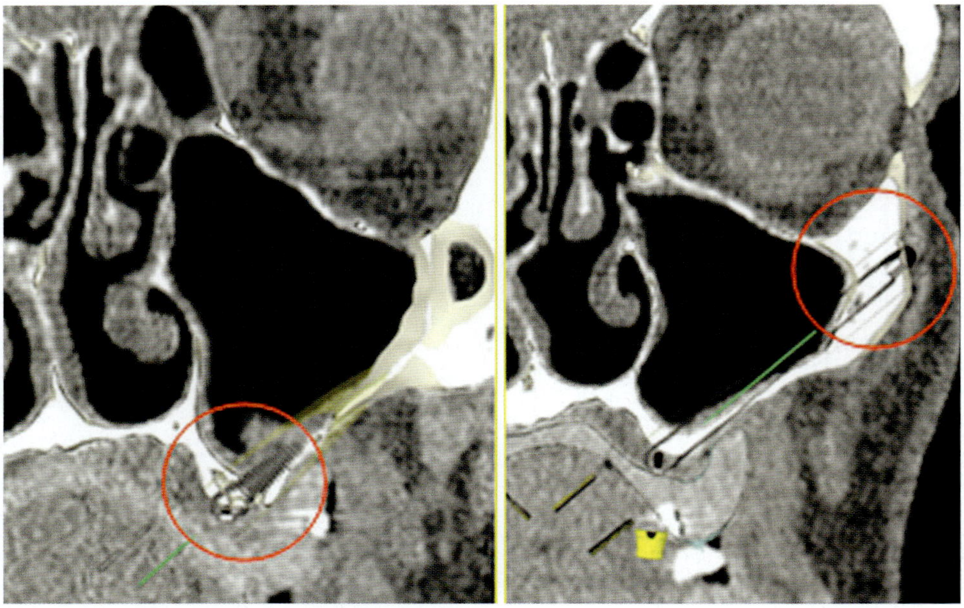

FIGURE 10-120 Virtual placement of the zygomatic implant in zone III.

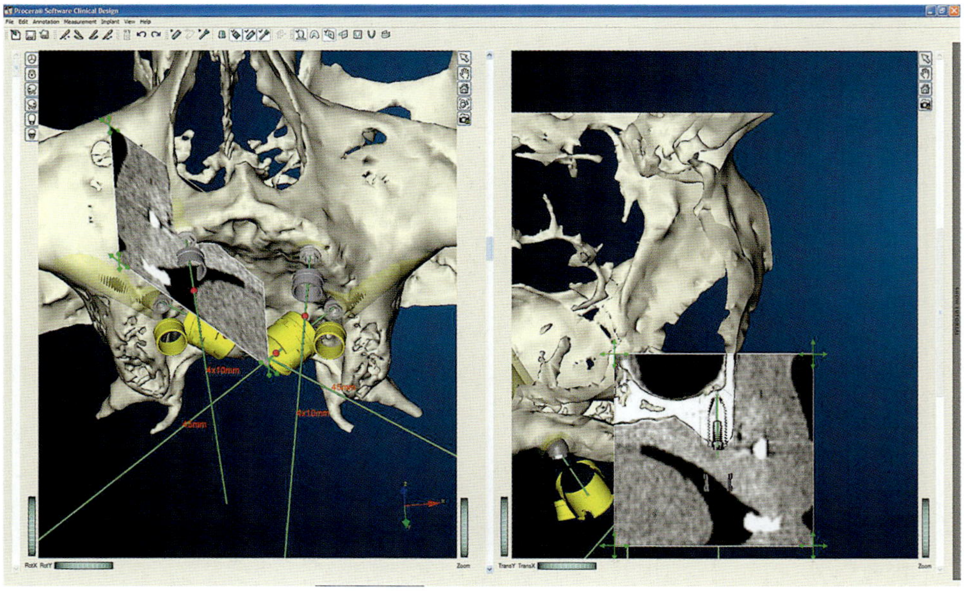

FIGURE 10-121 Virtual placement of axial anterior maxillary implants.

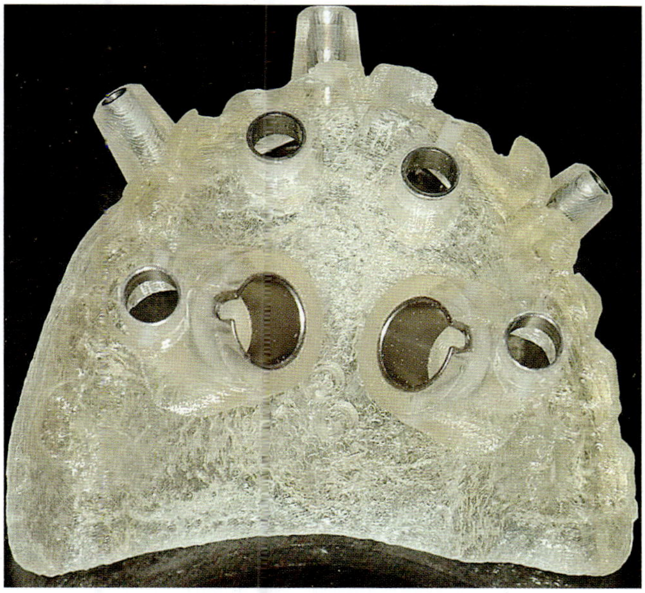

FIGURE 10-122 The completed single-template guided zygoma surgical template.

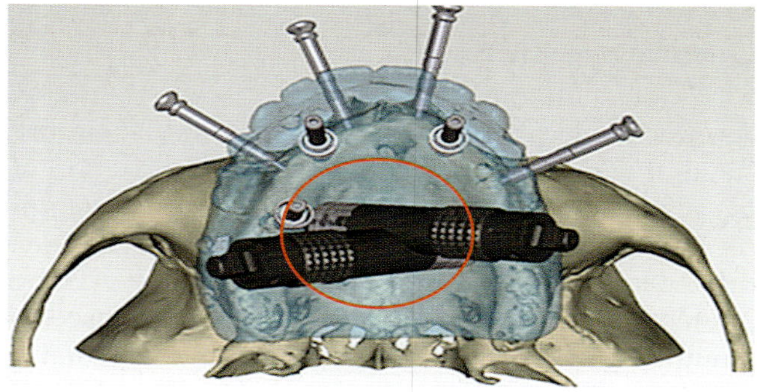

FIGURE 10-123 Collision of the guided zygoma sleeves may be observed during planning.

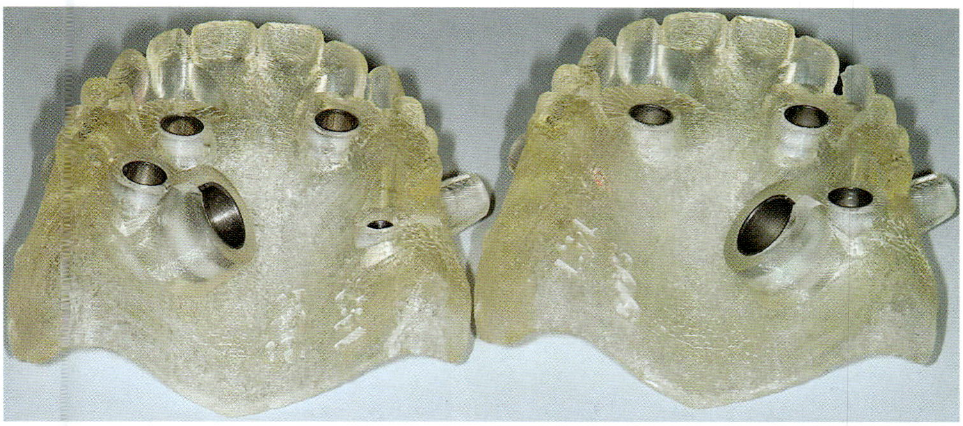

FIGURE 10-124 The completed dual-template guided zygoma surgical templates.

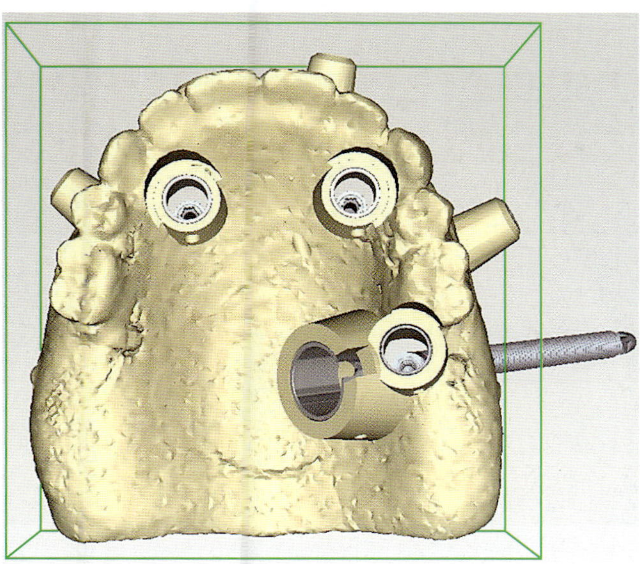

FIGURE 10-125 The primary template is used to place the axial and left zygomatic implants in the dual-template protocol.

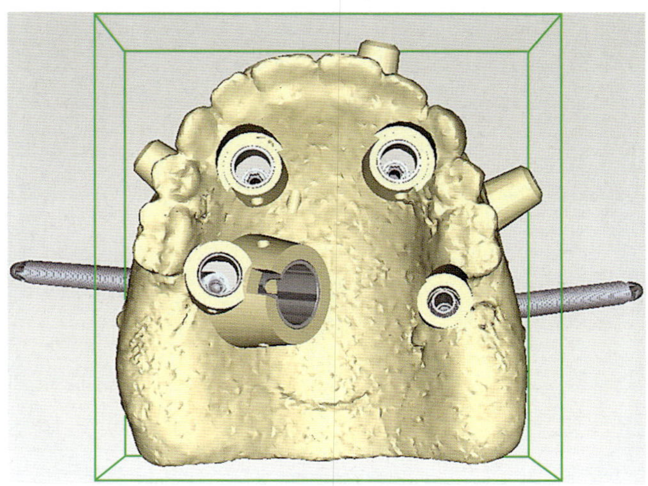

FIGURE 10-126 The secondary template is used to place the right zygomatic implant in the dual-template protocol.

Laboratory Steps

As described earlier, the first step in the laboratory stage of computer-guided treatment is fabrication of the master cast. The computer-guided zygoma surgical template (Figure 10-127) is used to back-pour the master cast (Figure 10-128). As the master cast is being poured, the patient's duplicated dentures are used to mount the preoperative models to the articulator (Figure 10-129). Once the master cast is poured (Figure 10-130), the patient's duplicated denture is used to mount the master cast to the articulator (Figure 10-131). To begin fabrication of the provisional immediate-load prosthesis, abutments have to be chosen and secured to the fixture-level master cast. The abutments used for computer-guided zygoma implant treatment are guided abutments. (Figure 10-132). Laboratory-guided abutments (Figure 10-133) are used along with temporary cylinders to fabricate the immediate-load provisional prosthesis (Figure 10-134). After completion (Figure 10-135), the immediate-load prosthesis is removed from the master cast and the surgical template is substituted using fixation pins (Figure 10-136). Registration material is used to fabricate the surgical bite registration (Figure 10-137), which will be used to properly position the template in the patient's mouth prior to initiation of the osteotomies.

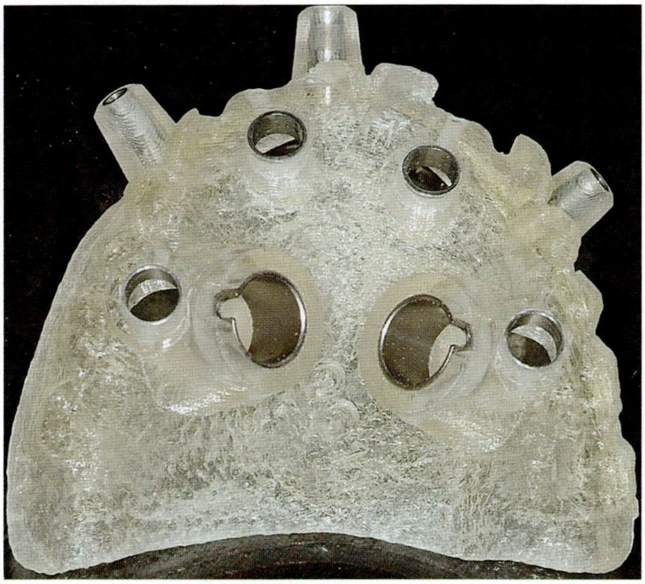

FIGURE 10-127 The computer-guided zygoma template is used to initiate fabrication of the master cast.

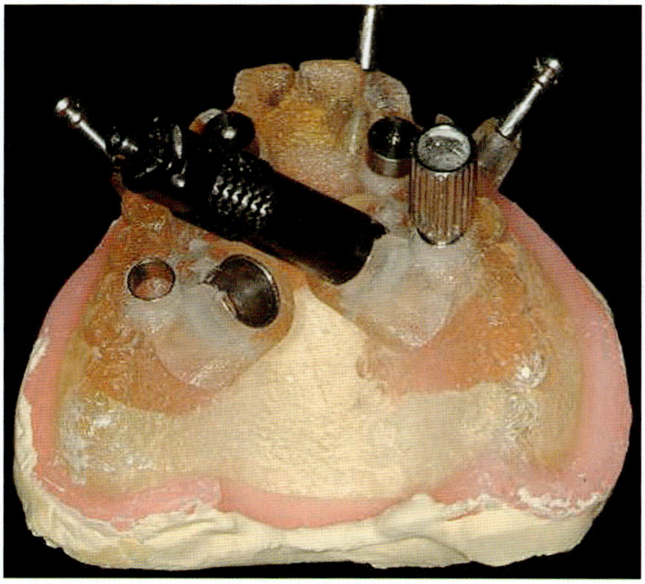

FIGURE 10-128 The fabrication of the stone master cast model.

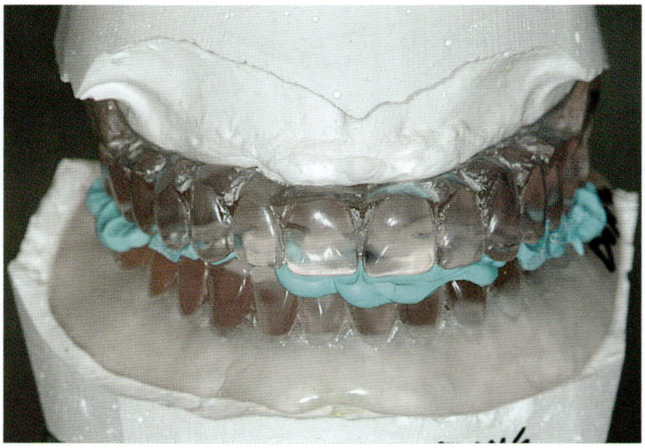

FIGURE 10-129 The duplicate maxillary denture is used to mount the preoperative study casts.

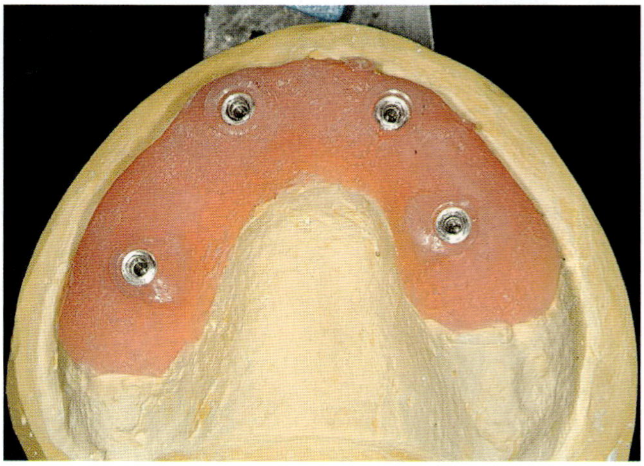

FIGURE 10-130 The completed master cast.

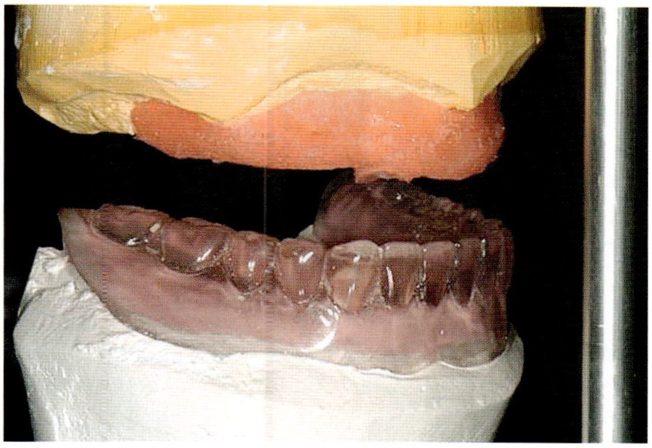

FIGURE 10-131 The master cast is mounted, replacing the preoperative maxillary study model using the duplicated denture.

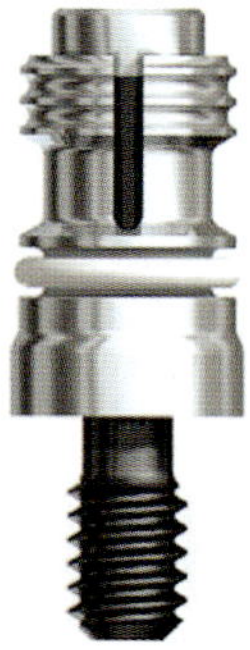

FIGURE 10-132 Guided abutments are used in the computer-guided zygoma protocol. *(Courtesy Nobel Biocare, Yorba Linda, Calif.)*

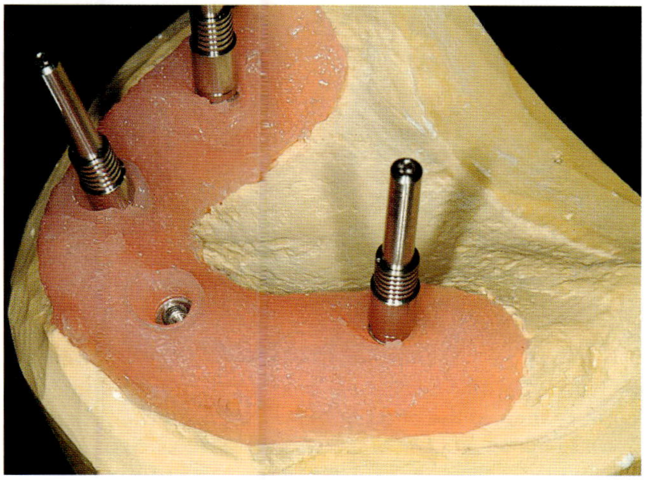

FIGURE 10-133 Laboratory-guided abutments and temporary titanium cylinders are used to initiate fabrication of the provisional immediate-load prosthesis.

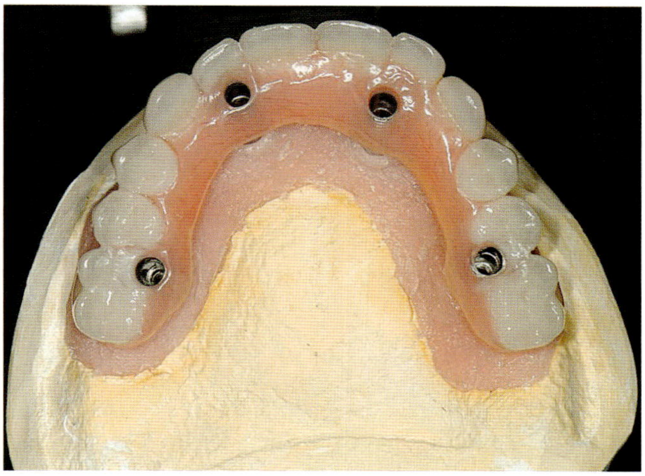

FIGURE 10-134 Completed immediate-load prosthesis.

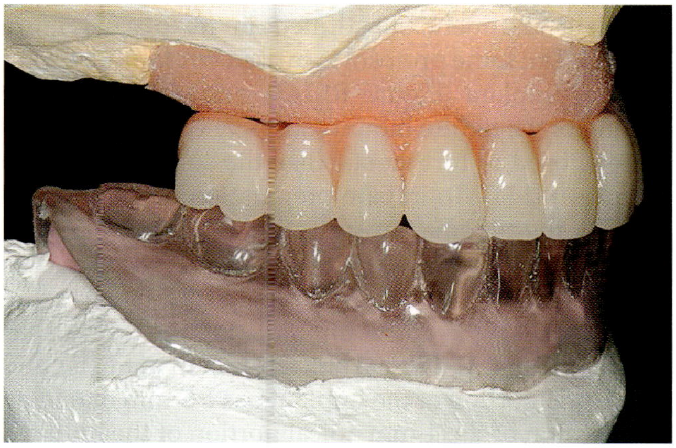

FIGURE 10-135 Completed immediate-load prosthesis articulating against the opposing occlusion.

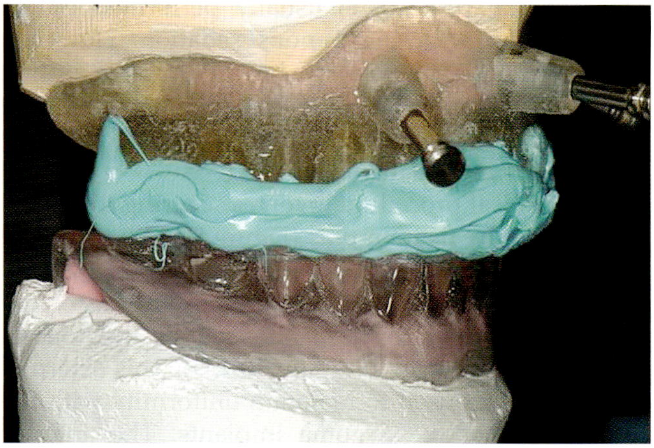

FIGURE 10-136 Fixation pins are used to connect the surgical template to the master cast.

which accepts the 5-mm diameter portion of the implant, can be further enlarged to 4.2 mm or left at 3.5-mm diameter. This decision is made clinically, and is based on the quality and quantity of bone encountered. Once the 3.5-mm osteotomy is completed and the surgeon believes that appropriate expansion of the buccal and lingual plates at the crest of the maxilla can be achieved by insertion of the implant, it is inappropriate to use the 4.2-mm drill. After completion of one of the zygoma implant osteotomies, to guide the zygoma implant in the same position as the preoperative virtual planning site, the computer-guided, implant-mount zygoma is used (Figure 10-148). This surgical component consists of (1) the extension sleeve, (2) the guided screw, and (3) the retention screw, and is used to direct the axis of the zygoma implant. The extension sleeve portion of the computer-guided zygoma implant mount is attached to the surgical template by aligning the notch of the template with the small projection on the extension sleeve (Figure 10-149).

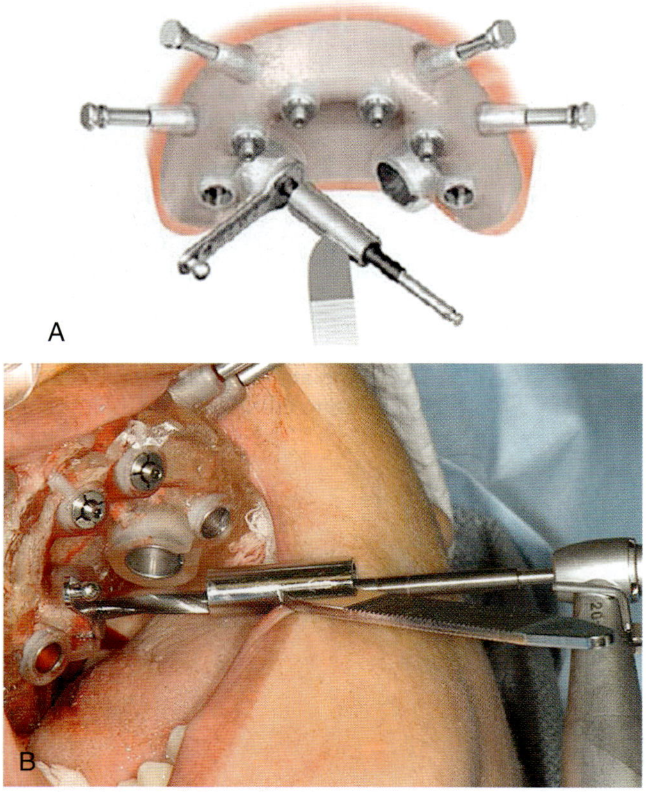

FIGURE 10-147 A, After using the soft tissue counterbore, the 4.2-mm drill guide is used to direct the 4.2-mm drill. B, The 3.5-mm drill guide is used to direct the 3.5-mm drill, completing the osteotomy of the zygomatic bone. *(A courtesy Nobel Biocare, Yorba Linda, Calif.)*

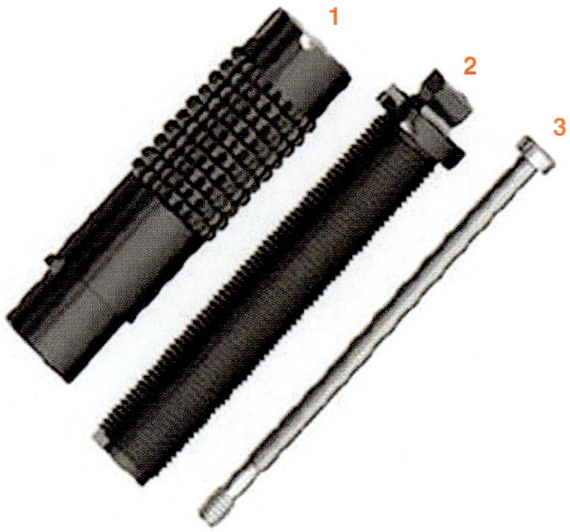

FIGURE 10-148 The computer-guided implant-mount zygoma procedure is used to direct the zygomatic implant though the surgical template. *(Courtesy Nobel Biocare, Yorba Linda, Calif.)*

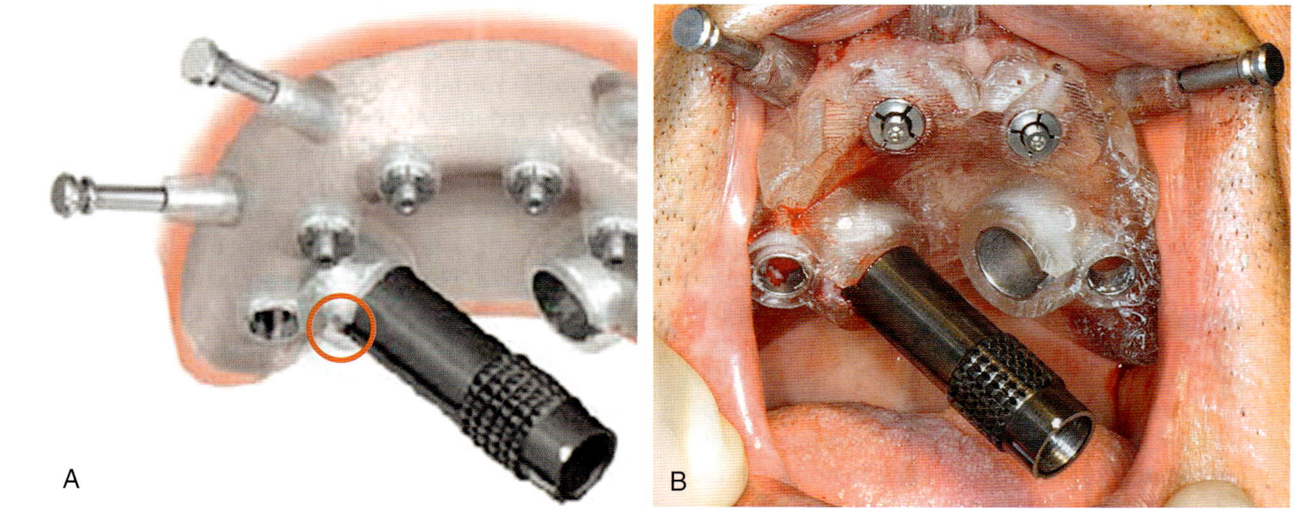

FIGURE 10-149 A, The projection of the extension sleeve portion of the computer-guided implant-mount zygoma must be fully seated into its corresponding notch in the surgical template. B, Complete seating of the extension sleeve with the surgical template. *(A courtesy Nobel Biocare, Yorba Linda, Calif.)*

The 45° platform of the zygoma implant has a premounted fixture mount (Figure 10-150), which "straightens" the implant so that it is ready for insertion into the osteotomy. The retention screw of the computer-guided implant-mount zygoma is used to fix the zygoma implant to the guided screw (Figure 10-151). The guided screw has a flat marking that is lined with the fixture-mount screw of the zygoma implant. Once the guided screw is snapped over the fixture mount, the retention screw is tightened (Figure 10-152). The guided screw–implant complex is carefully inserted into the extension sleeve (Figure 10-153, *A*). The first thread of the guided screw marked by the *red arrow* (Figure 10-153, *B*) is slowly guided until it engages the first threads of the extension sleeve marked by the *yellow arrow*. Once the threads of the guided screw have engaged and guided the sleeve, the projection of the zygoma implant is established. Complete vertical seating of the zygoma implant is confirmed when the vertical leg of the T on the

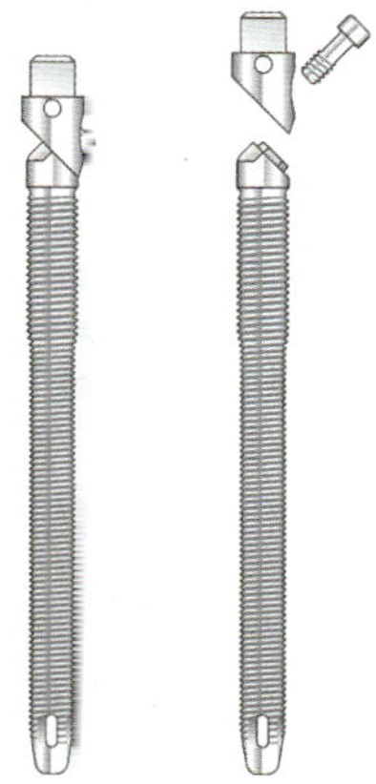

FIGURE 10-150 Premounted fixture mounts straighten the 45° tilted platform of the zygoma implant. *(Courtesy Nobel Biocare, Yorba Linda, Calif.)*

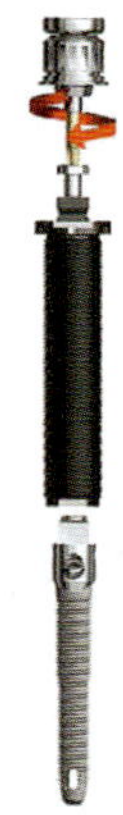

FIGURE 10-151 The retention screw of the guided zygoma mount is secured to the fixture mount of the zygoma implant. *(Courtesy Nobel Biocare, Yorba Linda, Calif.)*

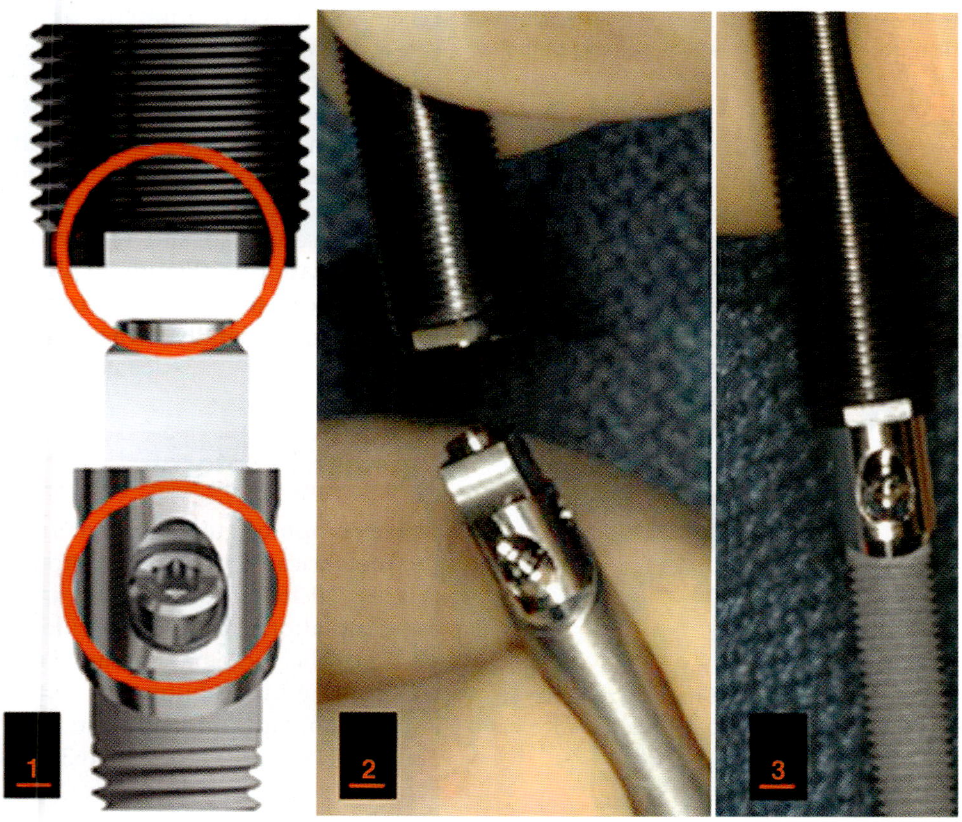

FIGURE 10-152 The flat marking of the guided zygoma mount is lined with the fixture mount of the zygoma implant prior to securing with the retention screw. *(Courtesy Nobel Biocare, Yorba Linda, Calif.)*

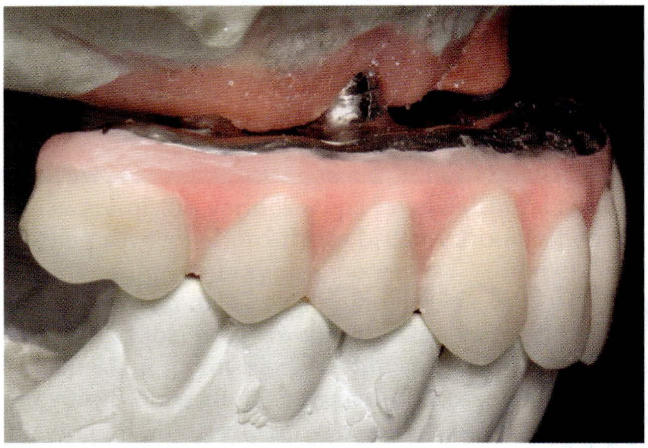

FIGURE 11-1 The maxillary hybrid prosthesis: The existing space between the intaglio surface of the prosthesis and the soft tissues does not allow for proper phonetics in the edentulous maxillary arch.

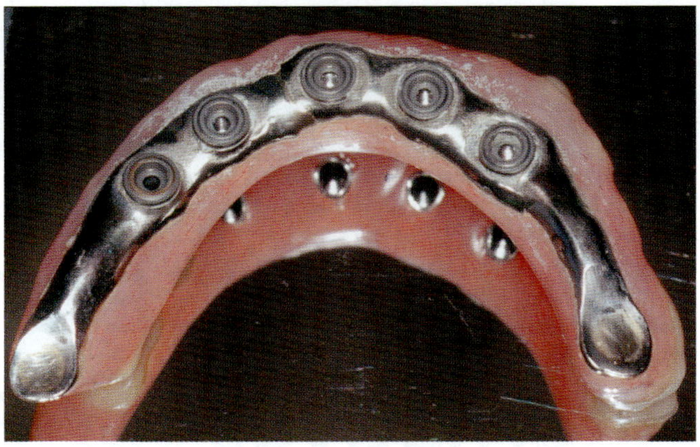

FIGURE 11-2 The intaglio surface of the conventional hybrid prosthesis: The finish line between the metal substructure and the overlying pink acrylic is evident.

The Profile Prosthesis: Gold Framework

The intaglio surface of the profile prosthesis has a cross-section similar to a pontic tooth in a conventional fixed partial denture. Pink acrylic surrounds a metal substructure and meets the soft tissue crest with pinpoint contact. This seals the gap, and phonetics in the maxillary profile prosthesis are acceptable.

An important feature of the profile prosthesis is the design of the metal substructure. Whether gold or titanium framework is used, extension of the framework to support the overlying pink acrylic and teeth is crucial. To allow the laboratory technician to design a metal substructure with adequate extensions in both the anterior-posterior (AP) and lateral dimensions, the initial step in profile prosthesis design involves setting acceptable denture teeth. Proper extension of the metal framework permits well-supported occlusal loads, which prevents teeth from "popping off" during function.

The following section demonstrates the various steps in the fabrication of a maxilla and/or mandibular profile prostheses (Figures 11-3 to 11-17).

Text continued on P. 155.

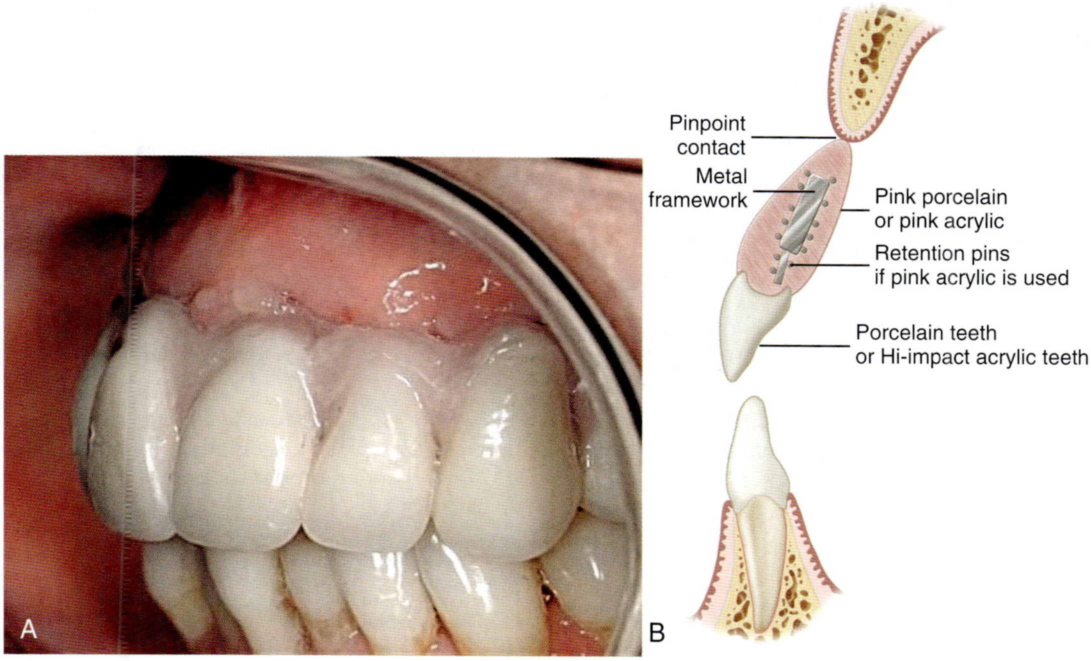

FIGURE 11-3 A, Clinical presentation of the "profile prosthesis" as it relates to the edentulous soft tissues. B, The maxillary profile prosthesis: The interimplant pink acrylic wraps around the metal substructure and is in pinpoint contact with the soft tissue of the maxillary ridge.

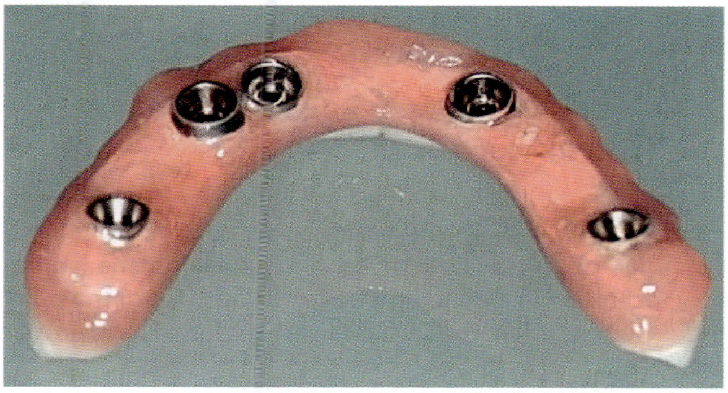

FIGURE 11-4 The pink acrylic completely wraps around the metal substructure of this profile prosthesis.

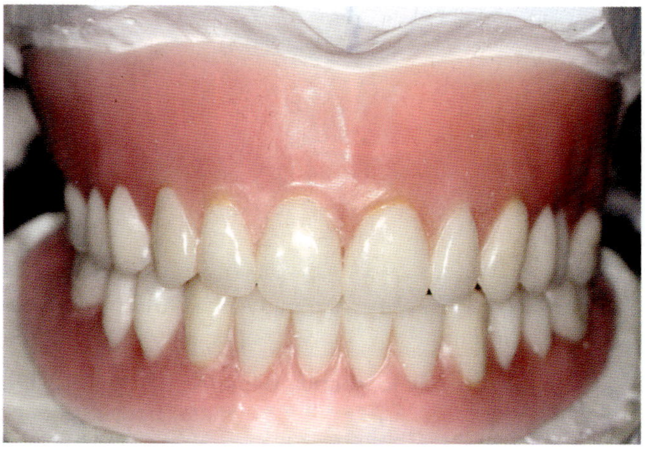

FIGURE 11-5 The initial step involved in fabrication of a profile prosthesis is proper anterior-posterior and proper vertical dimension of occlusion setup. Shown is the first wax try-in.

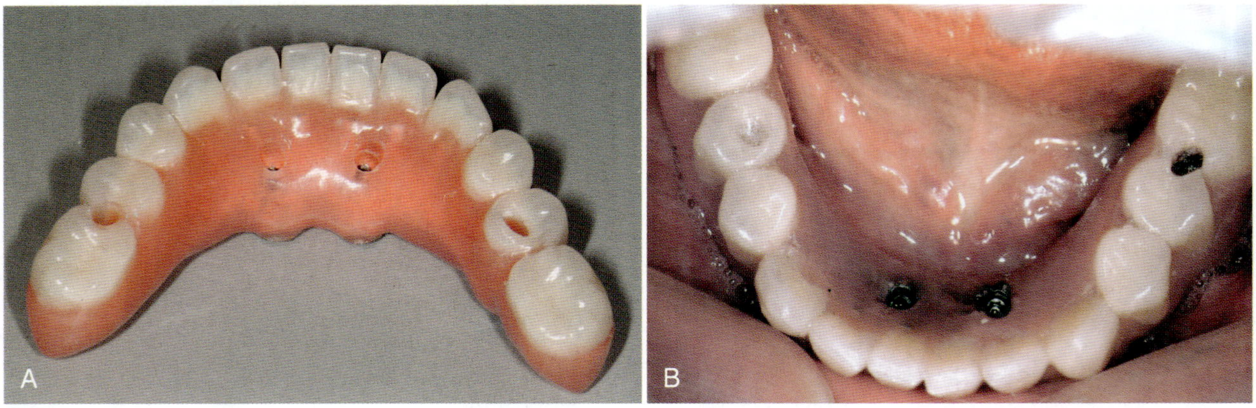

FIGURE 11-14 A, Completed mandibular profile prosthesis. B, Prosthetic screw access holes will be sealed for oral hygiene purposes.

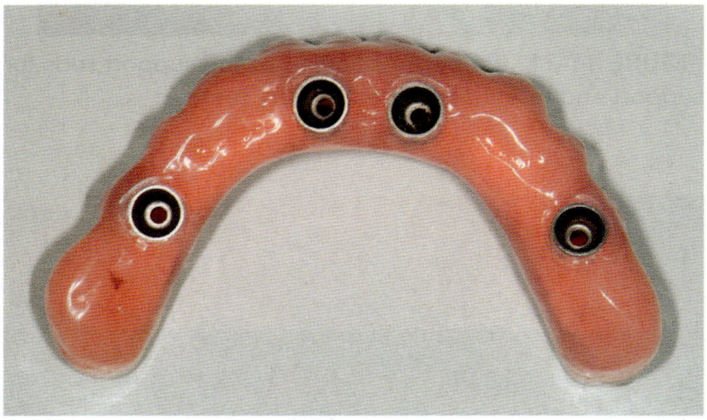

FIGURE 11-15 Intaglio surface of the completed maxillary profile prosthesis: The interimplant acrylic meets the patient's soft tissues with a pontic-like, pinpoint contact.

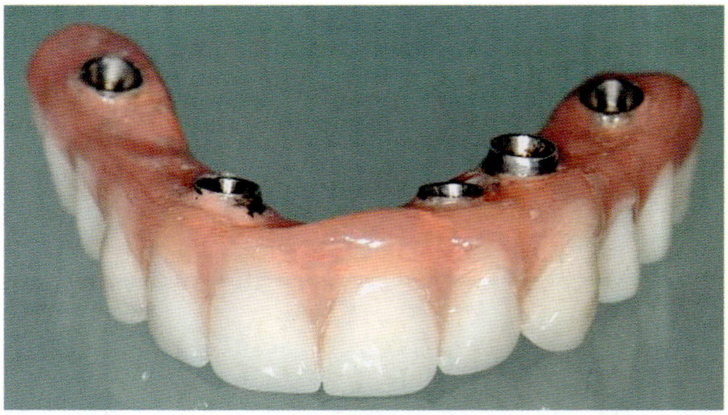

FIGURE 11-16 Completed maxillary profile prosthesis.

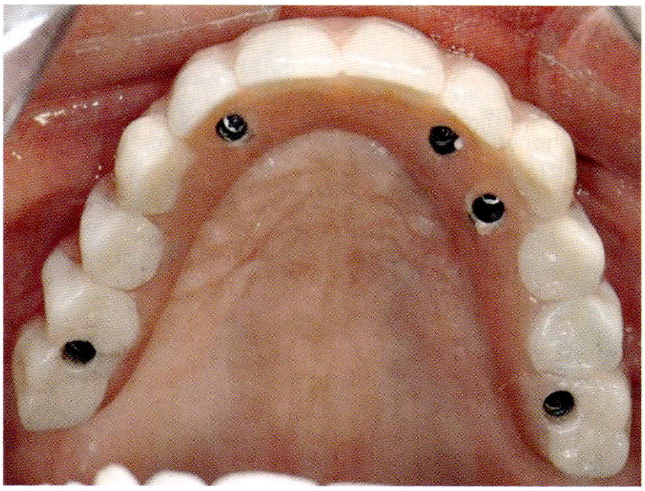

FIGURE 11-17 Delivered maxillary profile prosthesis with proper palatal seal, which allows correct pronunciation of dentoalveolar sounds.

TITANIUM FRAMEWORK: PROCERA IMPLANT BRIDGE

A 43-year-old woman with nonrestorable maxillary dentition presented for definitive treatment of her maxilla with an implant-supported prosthesis. Her clinical evaluation resulted in the following findings:

1. Partial maxillary edentulism
2. Presence of mid-composite defect
3. Favorable transition line
4. Presence of zones I and II on radiographic evaluation

(Figures 11-18 to 11-20)

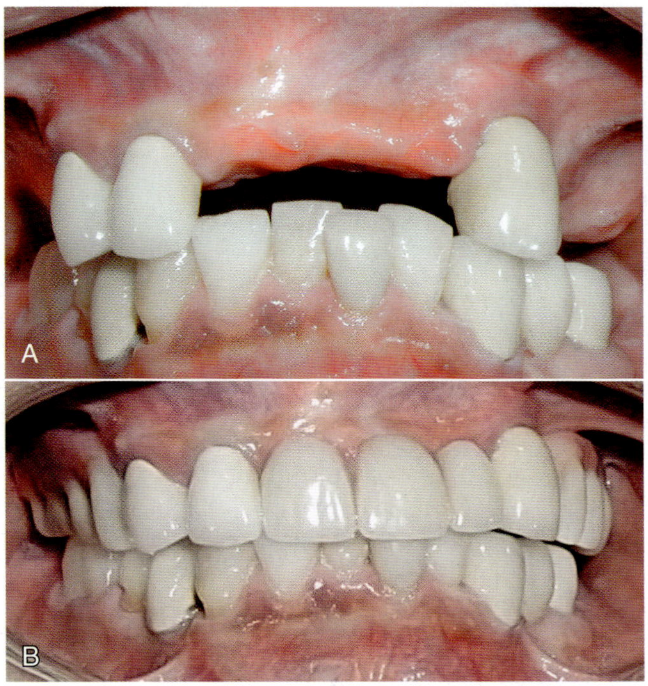

FIGURE 11-18 Partially edentulous maxillary dentition restored with a removable partial denture. Presence of long teeth suggests the existence of mild composite defect.

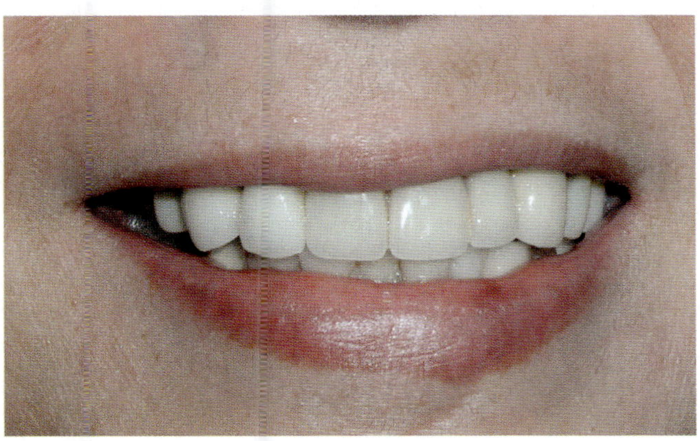

FIGURE 11-19 Hidden transition line during animation suggests a positive outcome for a final profile prosthesis.

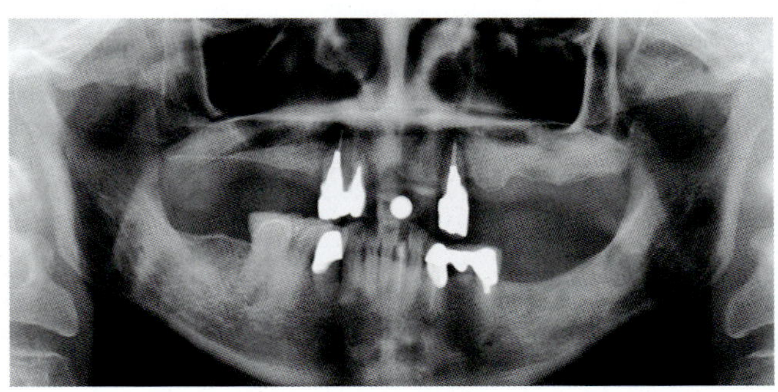

FIGURE 11-20 Presence of zones I and II allows adoption of the tilted implant treatment concept.

Treatment Plan

1. Removal of all remaining maxillary teeth
2. Placement of four premaxillary implants and two tilted posterior implants
3. Immediate-load provisional prosthesis
4. Final Procera titanium framework profile prosthesis

(Figures 11-21 to 11-24)

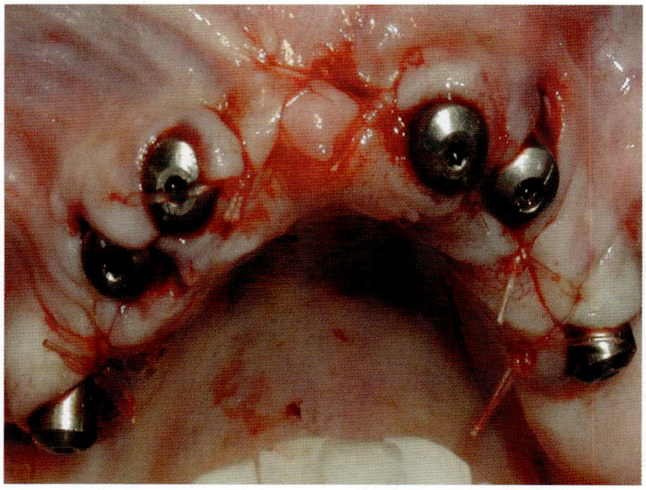

FIGURE 11-21 Removal of the existing maxillary teeth with immediate placement of implants. Immediate loading is considered after reaching 40 Ncm. The decision was made to incorporate four of the six implants into the provisional prosthesis.

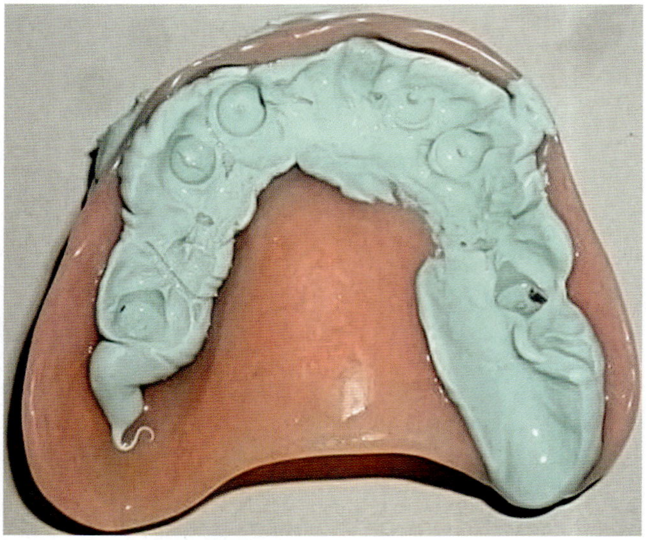

FIGURE 11-22 Indexing the intaglio surface of the denture to transfer the position implants to the full maxillary denture.

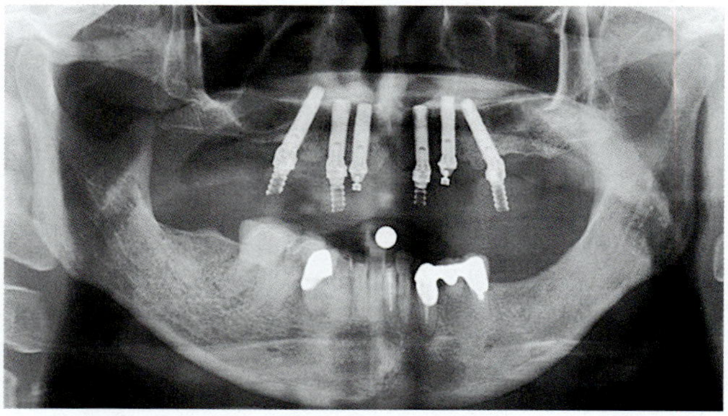

FIGURE 11-23 Immediate postoperative panoramic radiograph demonstrating implant distribution.

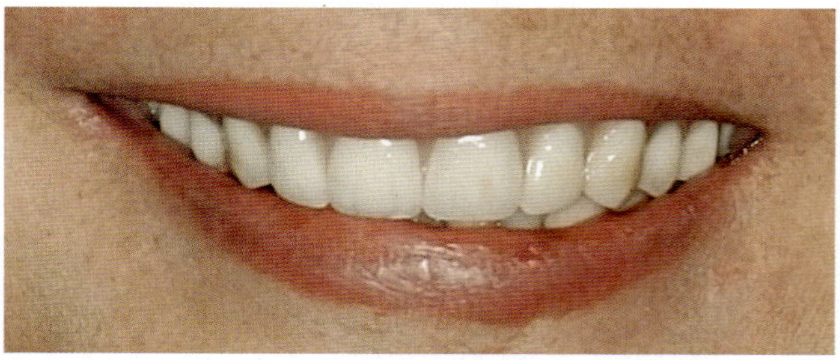

FIGURE 11-24 Six months after implant placement, an aesthetic smile line with hidden transition line is achieved, and it is time to fabricate the final prosthesis.

Appointment Schedule for Fabrication of a Procera Profile Prosthesis

Appointment 1: Impressions are taken.
Appointment 2: Vertical dimension of occlusion (VDO) is established.
Appointment 3: First wax try-in establishes the AP tooth position.
Appointment 4: The resin pattern is indexed.
Appointment 5: Try-in is performed for the titanium framework.
Appointment 6: Second wax try-in is performed and soft tissue impressions are taken.
Appointment 7: The Procera profile prosthesis is delivered to the patient.

(Figures 11-25 to 11-40)

Text continued on P. 162.

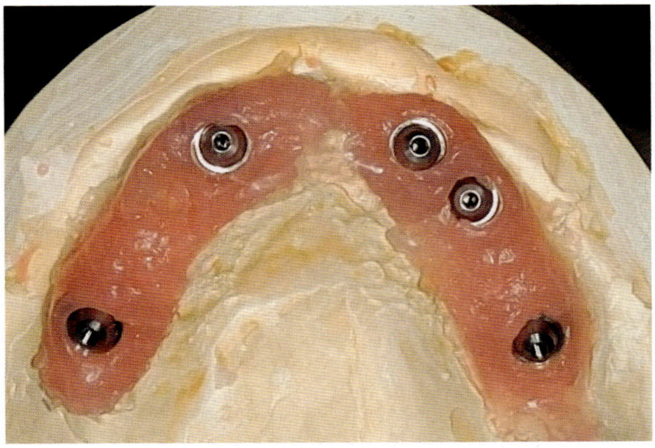

FIGURE 11-25 At the first appointment, multiunit impression copings are used to take the master impression and fabricate a soft tissue model.

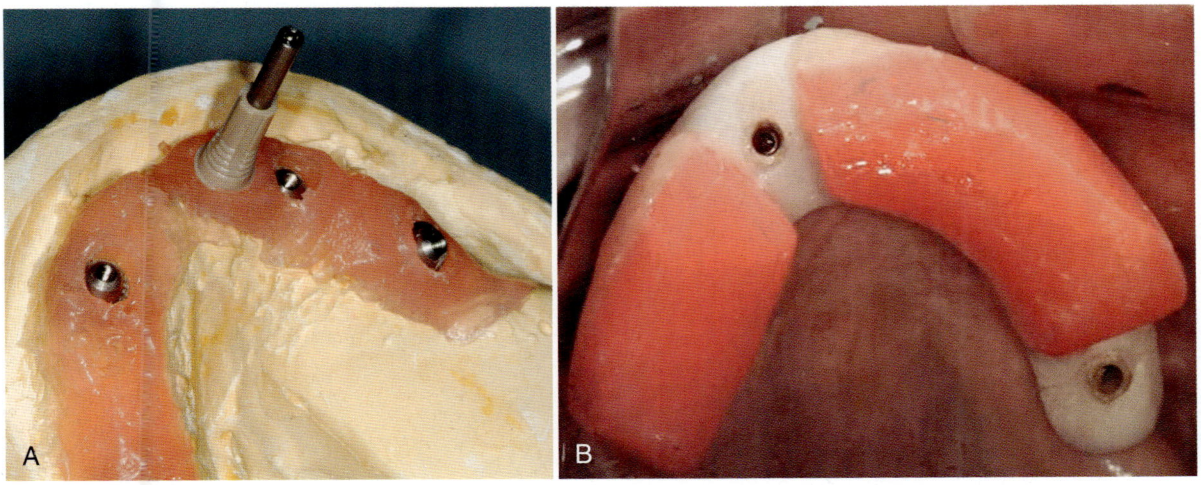

FIGURE 11-26 Plastic or titanium temporary cylinders are connected to the master cast (A) and incorporated into the wax rim (B).

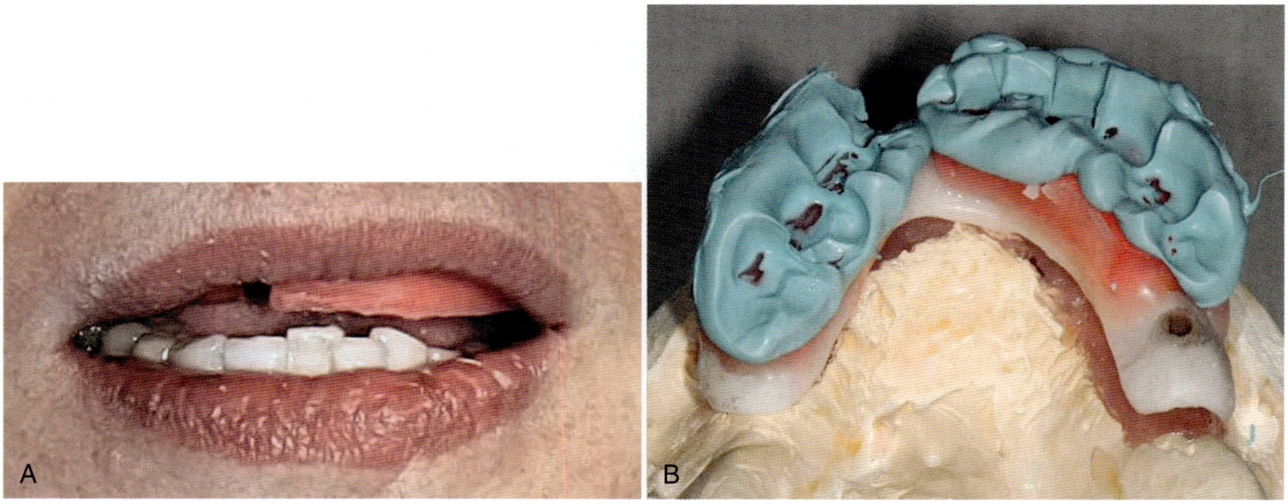

FIGURE 11-27 **A**, Completed screw-retained wax rim. At the second appointment, a clinically stable wax rim allows predictable and efficient record-taking. **B**, A final bite registration allows mounting of the patient's plaster casts.

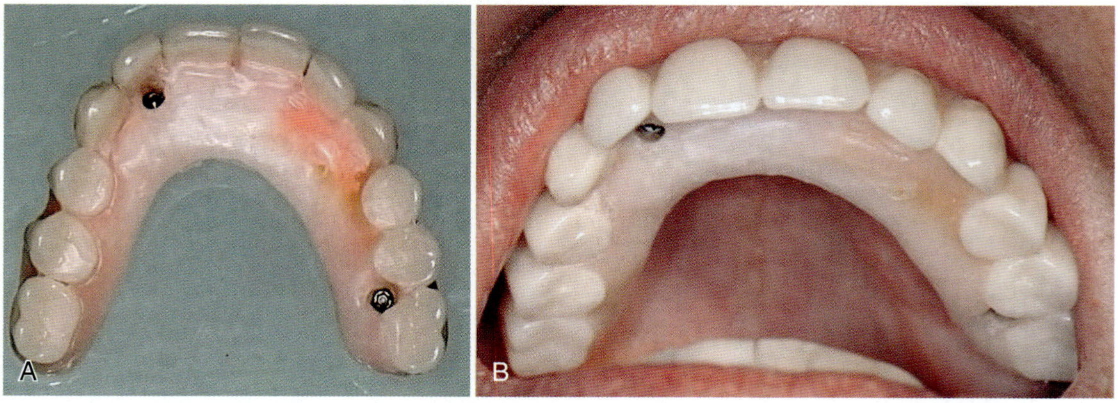

FIGURE 11-28 At the third appointment, the addition of teeth to the wax rim allows establishment of proper anterior-posterior tooth position.

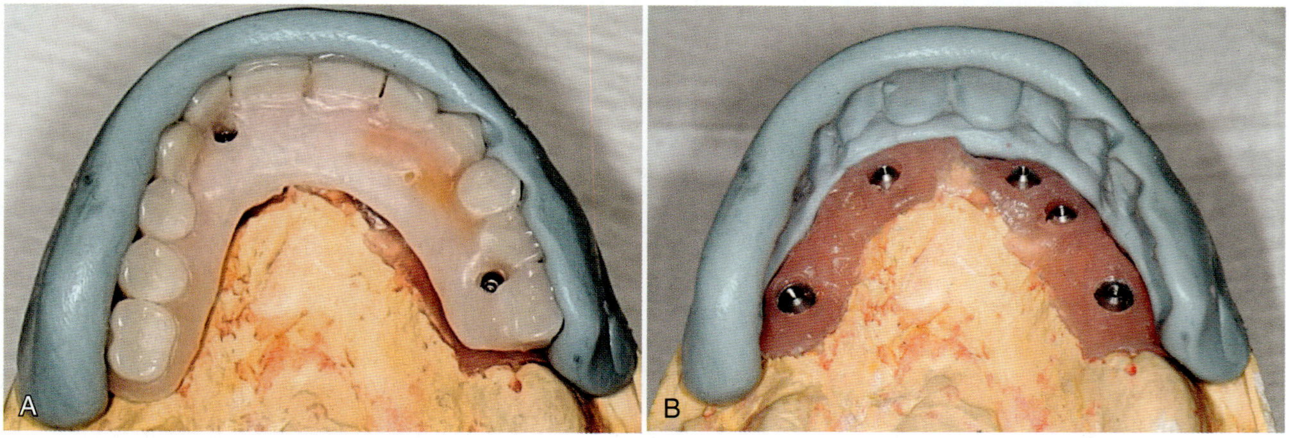

FIGURE 11-29 A putty index of the proper anterior-posterior tooth position allows the laboratory technician to properly extend the dimensions of the framework to support the occlusal loads, preventing acrylic stress fractures and "popping teeth."

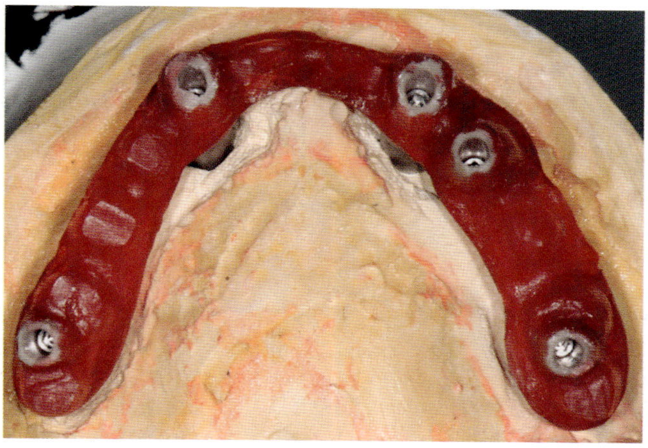

FIGURE 11-30 The completed resin pattern of the Procera titanium framework.

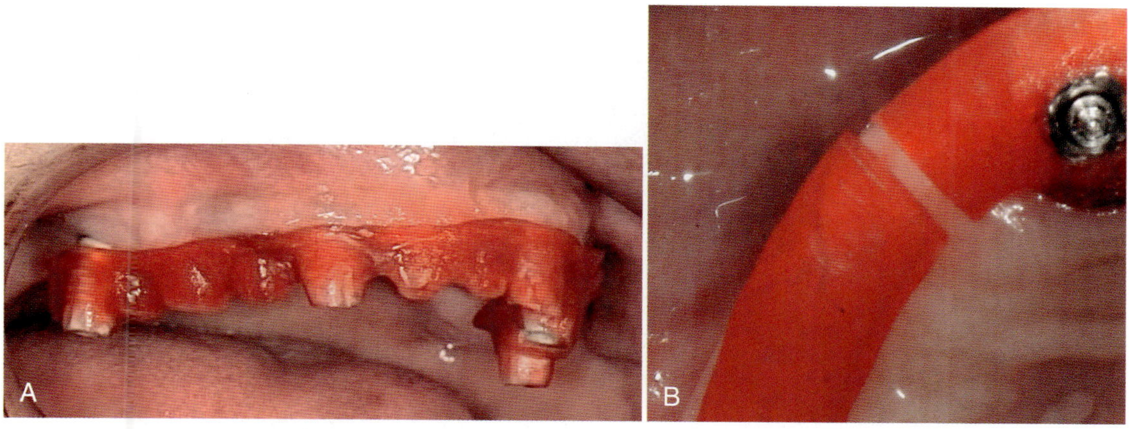

FIGURE 11-31 The framework is secured to only one abutment with one prosthetic screw. If an incomplete passive fit is suspected, the resin pattern is separated and individually secured to the abutments. The salt and pepper technique is used to lute the pattern back together.

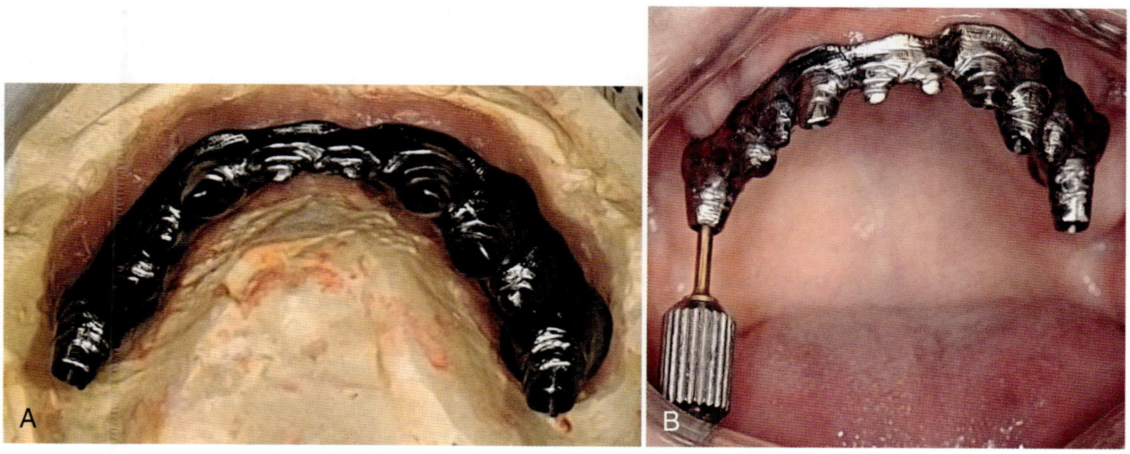

FIGURE 11-32 The resin pattern is scanned and milling of the Procera framework from a titanium block begins. A second framework try-in using a single screw is examined to ensure passive seating of the titanium framework.

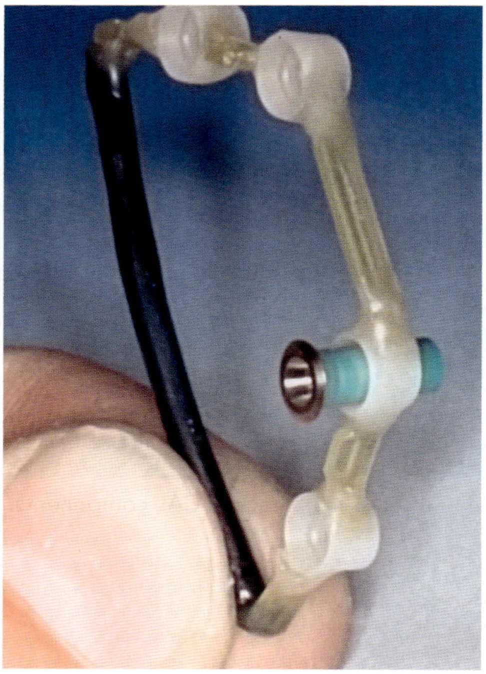

FIGURE 11-45 Clinical attachment level bar ready for investing and casting.

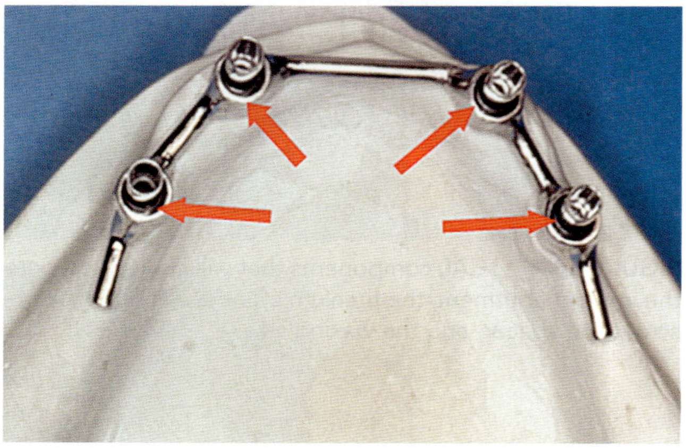

FIGURE 11-46 Casted clinical attachment level bar is placed over the titanium cylinders with the spacers removed. Permanent cement will fill the gaps and connect the bar to the cylinders.

A 67-year-old woman presented with a chief complaint of an inability to function satisfactorily with the existing full maxillary denture. Evaluation of her smile line was consistent with an aesthetic smile and complete fill of the buccal corridors. Animating with the denture removed did not display any maxillary soft tissues, suggesting an aesthetic final outcome if a fixed profile prosthesis were used because the transition line would be hidden. Intraoral examination revealed a flat maxillary vault and shallow vestibule. The preoperative panoramic radiograph demonstrated alveolar bone in zones I and II of the maxilla. Therefore, the decision to adopt the tilted treatment concept was made. For this patient, the computer-guided tilted treatment concept was used; the virtual planning was completed on the NobelGuide software. To begin the NobelGuide protocol, gutta-perch points were placed onto the patient's existing dentures, which were determined to have the proper VDO and AP tooth position. A radiographic bite registration was taken according to NobelGuide planning software dual scan protocol. After planning was complete, the surgical template was manufactured and used to place the four maxillary implants. After completion of the surgical protocol, multiunit abutments were connected and the prefabricated provisional profile prosthesis was connected with good maximum intercuspation and aesthetics (Figures 11-47 to 11-51).

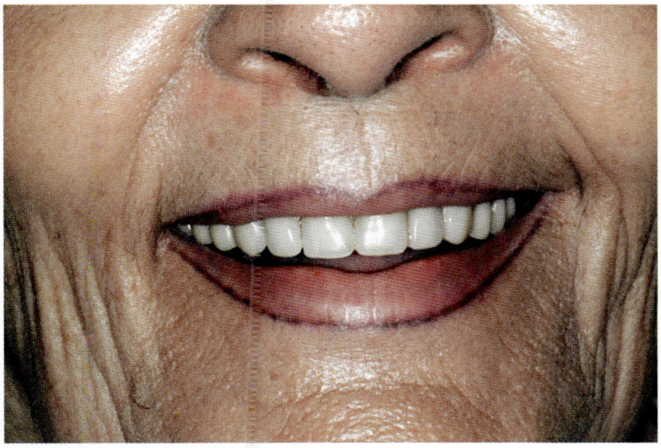

FIGURE 11-47 Preoperative denture has the proper vertical dimension of occlusion and anterior-posterior tooth position, which results in an aesthetic smile line and facial support.

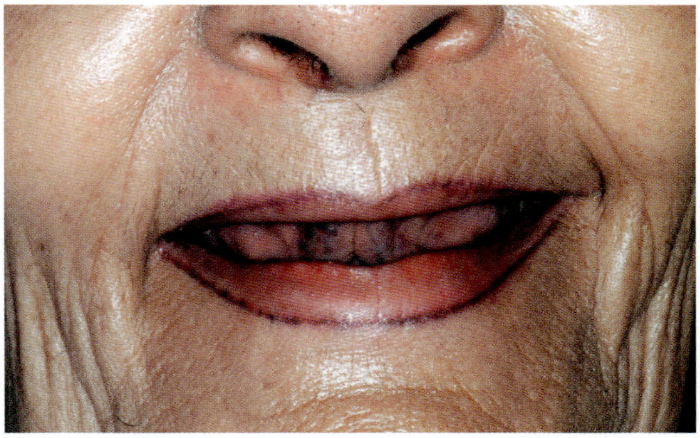

FIGURE 11-48 The absence of maxillary edentulous soft tissue display during animation with the denture removed suggests a hidden transition line.

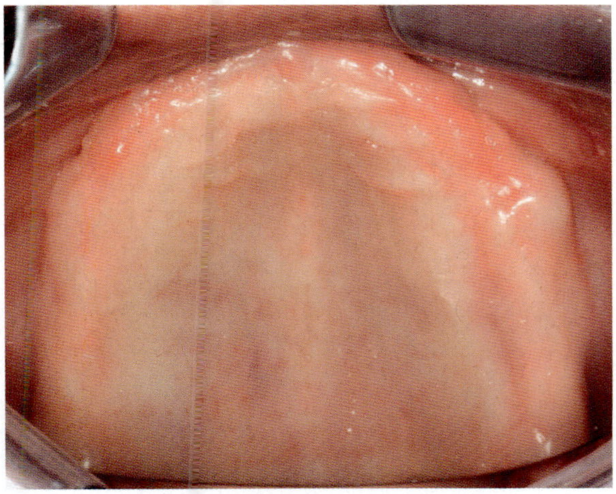

FIGURE 11-49 An existing flat maxillary vault and shallow maxillary vestibule is evident.

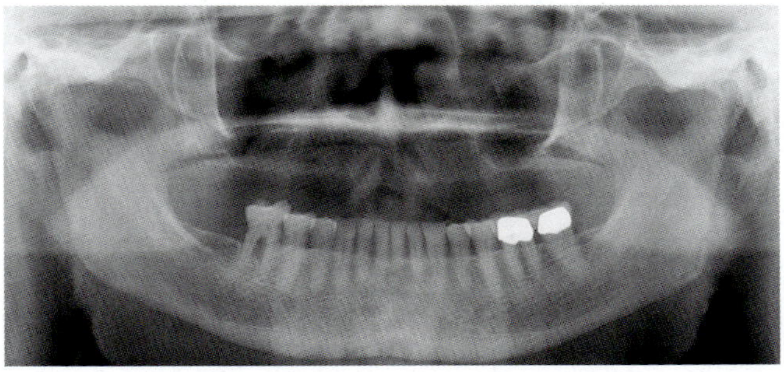

FIGURE 11-50 Preoperative panoramic radiograph demonstrates the existence of zones I and II.

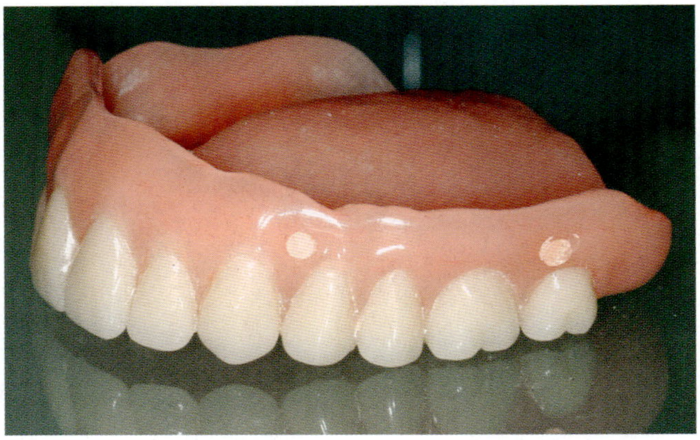

FIGURE 11-51 Placement of six to eight gutta-percha points for the patient's computed tomography scanning appointment.

Treatment Plan

1. NobelGuide tilted implant treatment concept is considered.
2. Gutta-percha points are placed in the maxillary denture.
3. Radiographic bite registration is taken for the NobelGuide scanning protocol.
4. Computed tomography scanning follows the NobelGuide dual scan protocol.
5. The tilted implant treatment concept using four implants is planned virtually.
6. The immediate-load provisional prosthesis is fabricated preoperatively.
7. Computer-guided surgery protocol using the NobelGuide surgical template is followed.
8. The implants are immediately loaded with the prefabricated profile prosthesis.
9. The final profile prosthesis is fabricated using the CAL technique 6 months after surgery.

(Figures 11-52 to 11-58)

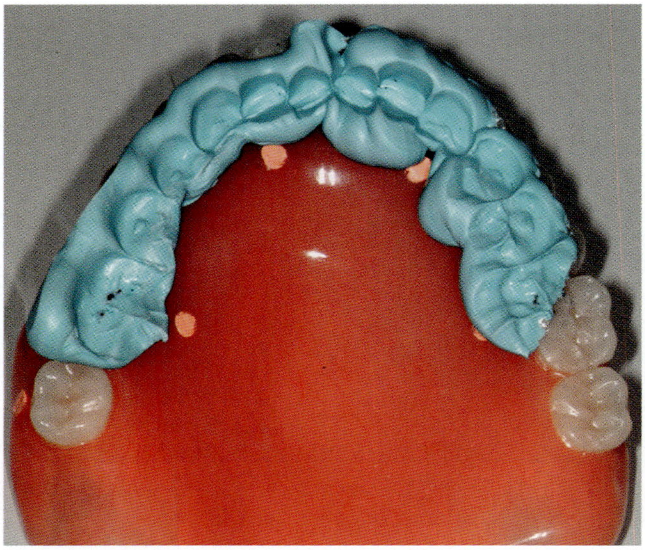

FIGURE 11-52 Radiographic bite registration and the gutta-percha–indexed denture ready for the NobelGuide dual scanning protocol.

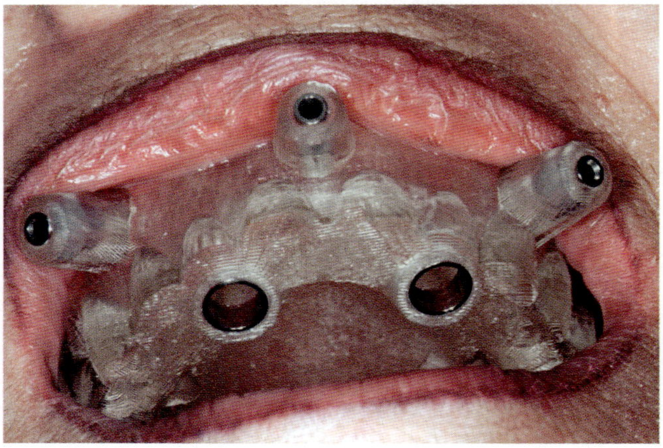

FIGURE 11-53 Placement of surgical template prior to stabilization with three fixation pins to the patient's maxilla.

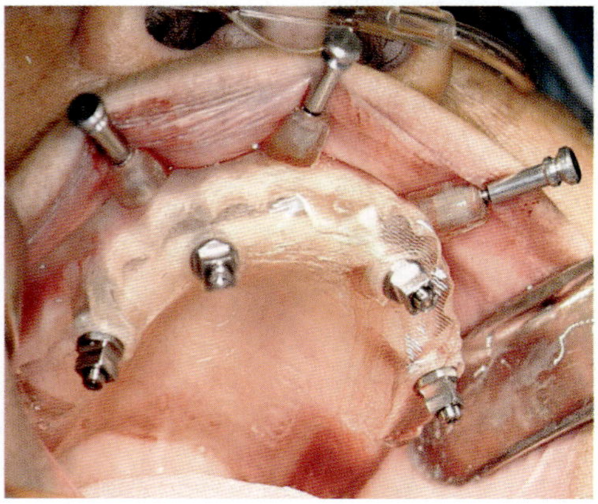

FIGURE 11-54 Complete seating of all four implants.

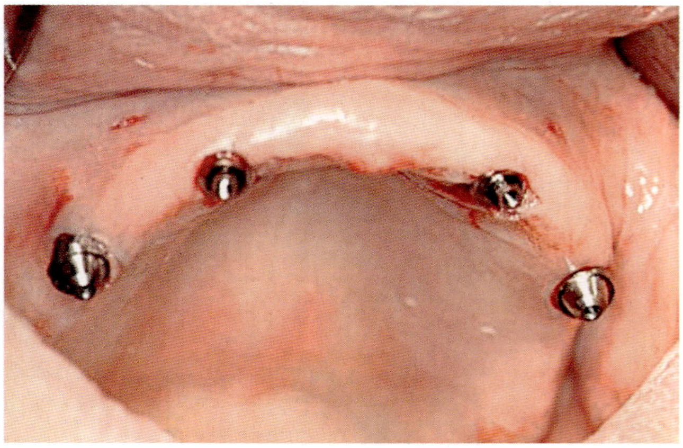

FIGURE 11-55 Connection of multiunit abutments to four implants.

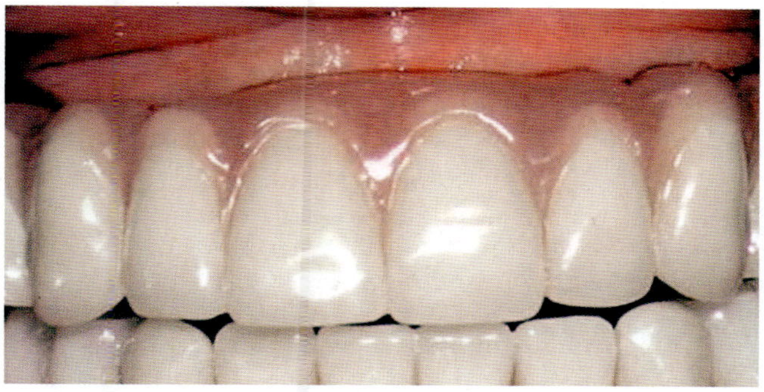

FIGURE 11-56 Delivery and occlusal adjustment of the prefabricated provisional immediate-load profile prosthesis.

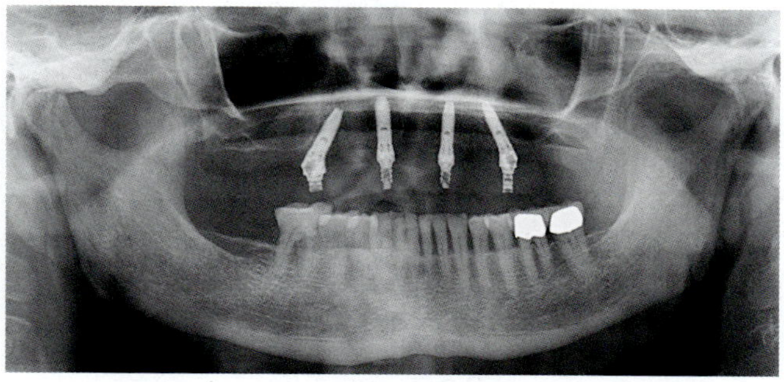

FIGURE 11-57 Immediate postoperative panoramic radiograph demonstrates complete seating of all components.

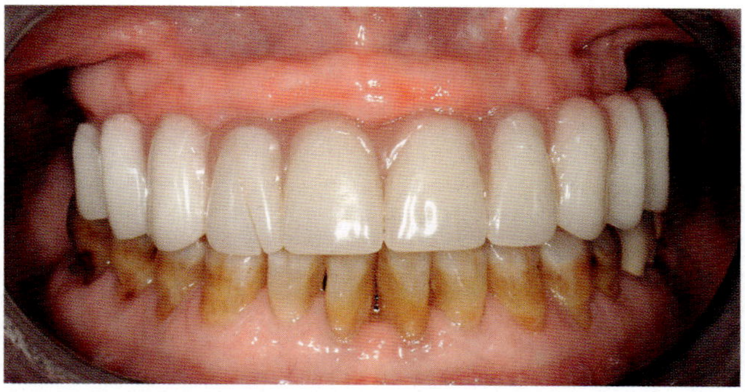

FIGURE 11-58 Six months postoperatively, the patient is ready for fabrication of the final metal-based profile prosthesis using the clinical attachment level technique (CAL technique).

The CAL protocol for fabrication of the final profile prosthesis is performed 6 months after surgery. The acceptable VDO of the provisional prosthesis is duplicated for the final prosthesis. A bite registration is made prior to removal of the provisional prosthesis and osseointegration of the four implants is confirmed. Multiunit laboratory analogues are connected to the provisional prosthesis and the bite registration is used to relate the provisional prosthesis to a stone model of the apposing arch. After mounting the models, the provisional prosthesis is reconnected to the patient's abutments and the patient is discharged. The laboratory technician uses the putty index of the provisional prosthesis to guide the extensions of the CAL bar and uses the CAL technique to fabricate the CAL bar. At the next appointment, the provisional prosthesis is removed and each of the titanium CAL cylinders are connected directly to the abutments with their prosthetic screws; one by one they are luted to the CAL bar to produce a one-piece, passive-fitting, rigid bar. A light-cured block of composite is used to re-establish the desired VDO with the CAL bar in position. A light body wash between the underside of the bar and the soft tissues allows the laboratory technician to pour an accurate soft tissue model. A new bite registration is made and the bar is removed. A new set of multiunit analogues is attached to the CAL bar–soft tissue wash–bite registration complex. Using the apposing stone model, a new mounting of the patient is created. The acrylic teeth are secured to the framework using wax and, at the wax try-in appointment, proper aesthetics and phonetics are confirmed prior to packing and processing the final CAL bar profile prosthesis (Figures 11-59 to 11-70).

Text continued on P. 172.

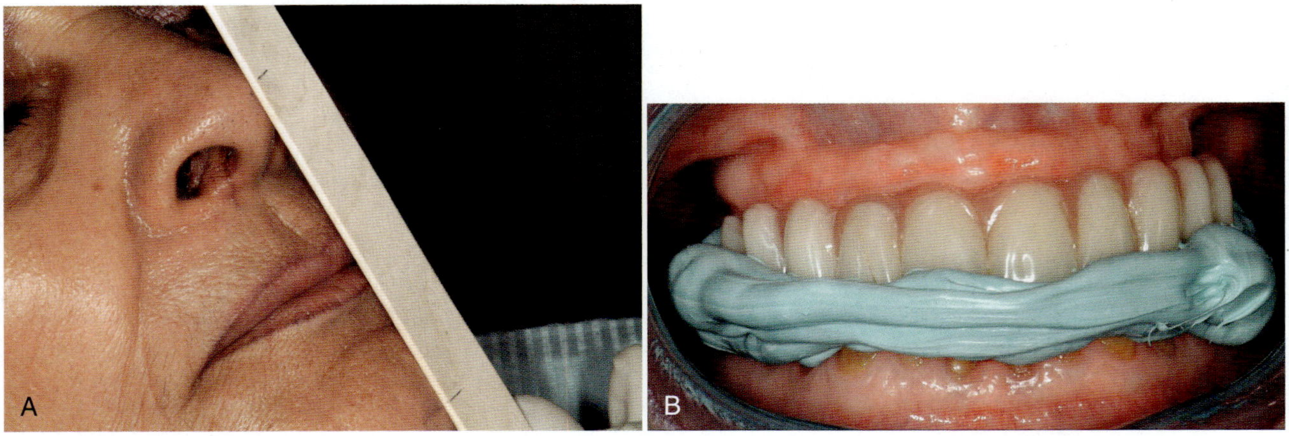

FIGURE 11-59 **A,** The acceptable vertical dimension of occlusion of the provisional prosthesis will be used for fabrication of the final prosthesis. **B,** A new bite registration is made before removal of the profile prosthesis.

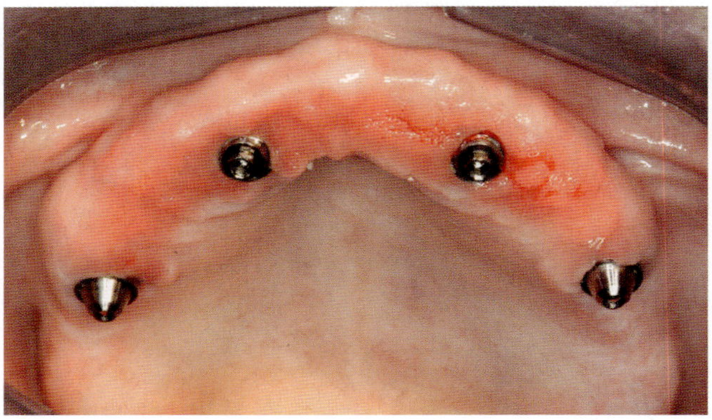

FIGURE 11-60 Each implant-abutment complex is checked by a torque driver to ensure osseointegration.

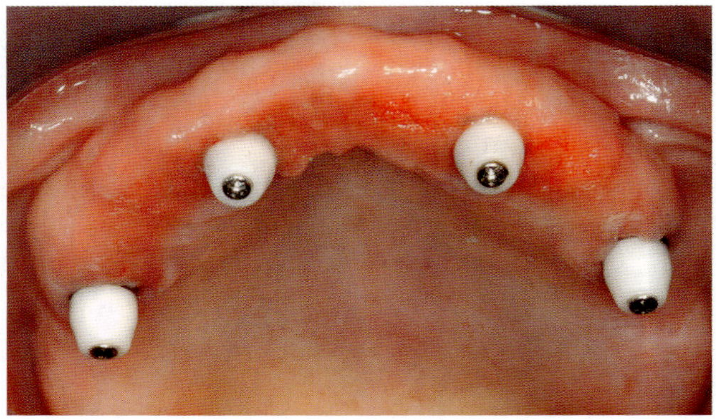

FIGURE 11-61 During the 90-minute laboratory procedure, temporary multiunit abutment caps are placed to maintain the soft tissue contours around each abutment.

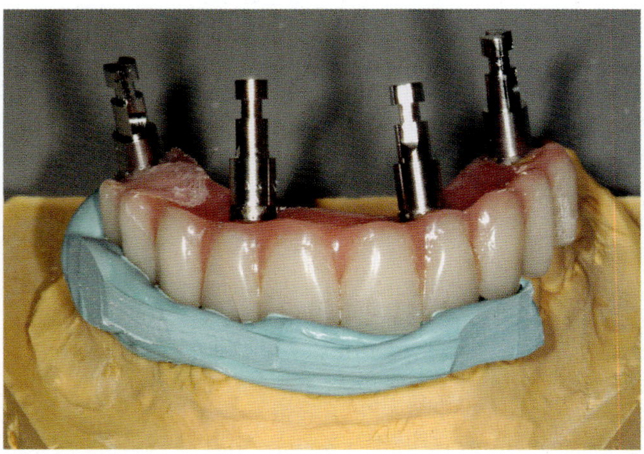

FIGURE 11-62 Multiunit laboratory analogues are attached to the provisional prosthesis and the bite registration is used to relate the provisional prosthesis to the apposing stone model.

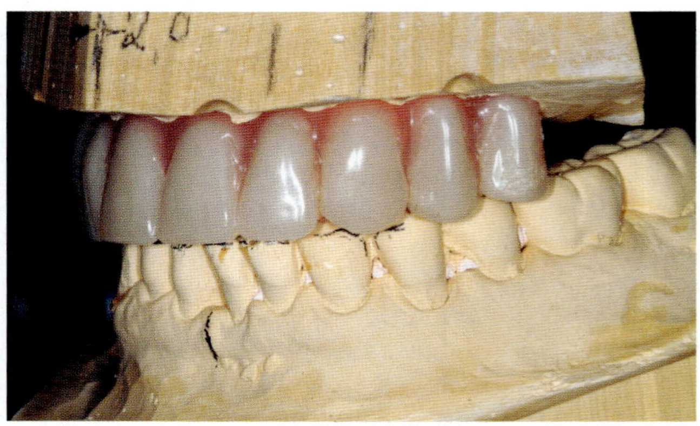

FIGURE 11-63 Mounted models ready for fabrication of the final prosthesis.

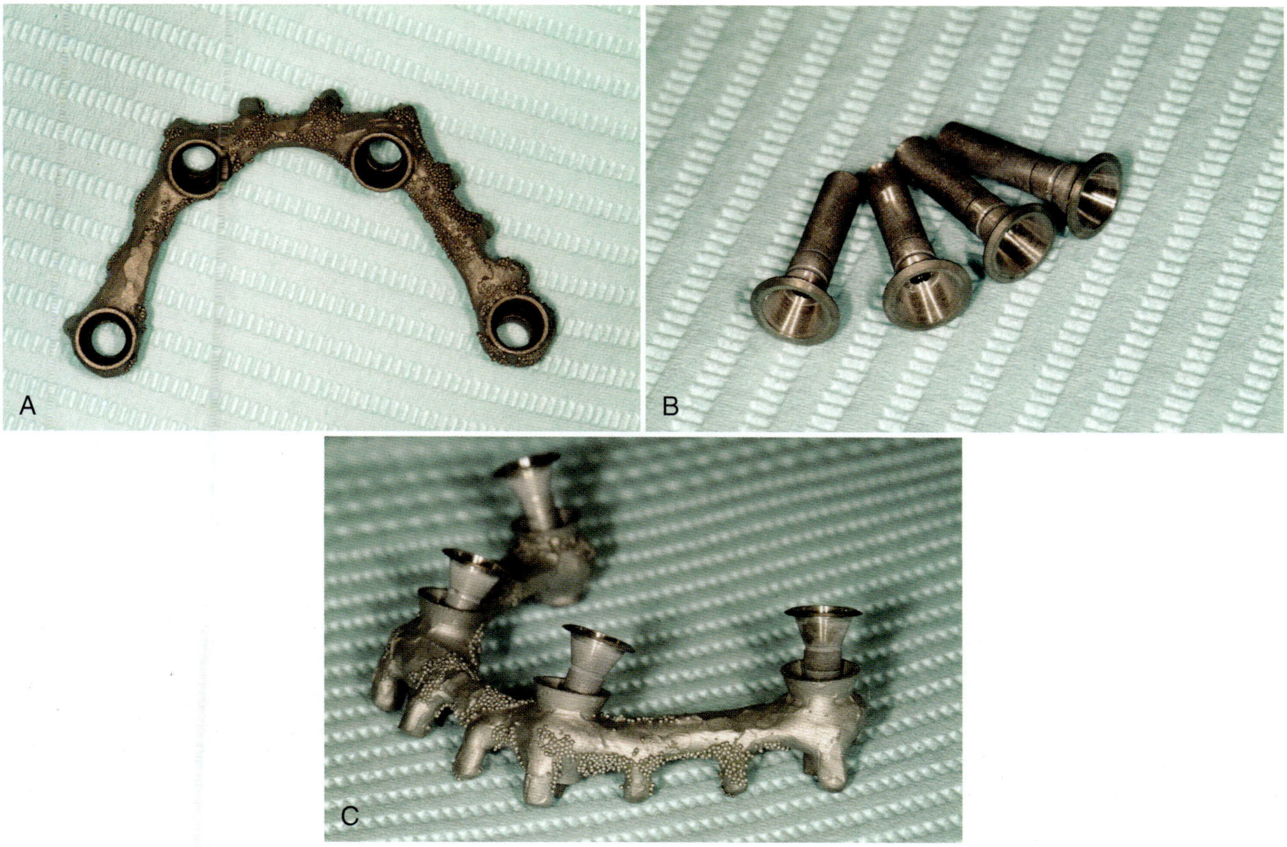

FIGURE 11-64 Completed clinical attachment level (CAL) bar (A) and CAL cylinders (B). Intraorally, after securing the cylinders to the abutments, the bar is placed over the cylinders (C) and they are connected to each other by permanent cement.

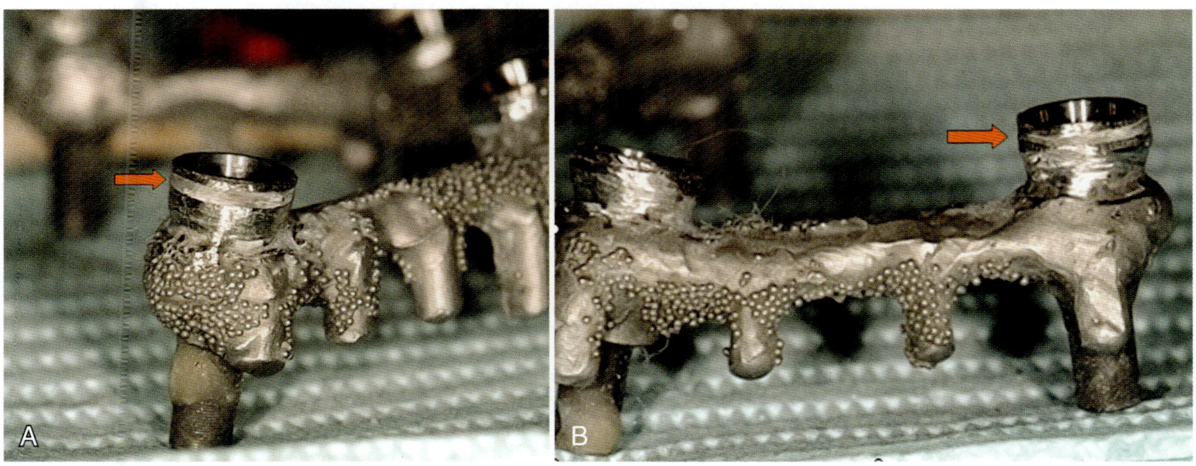

FIGURE 11-65 A, Asymmetric vertical thickness of the cement illustrates the correction of the potential misfit if the bar was cast with the cylinders as one unit. B, The final clinical attachment level bar has a passive fit on all abutments.

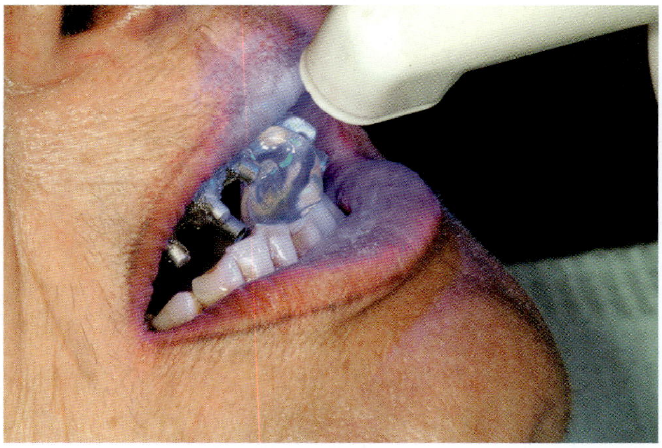

FIGURE 11-66 Light-cured composite cube is used to re-establish the proper vertical dimension of occlusion between the clinical attachment level bar and the apposing arch.

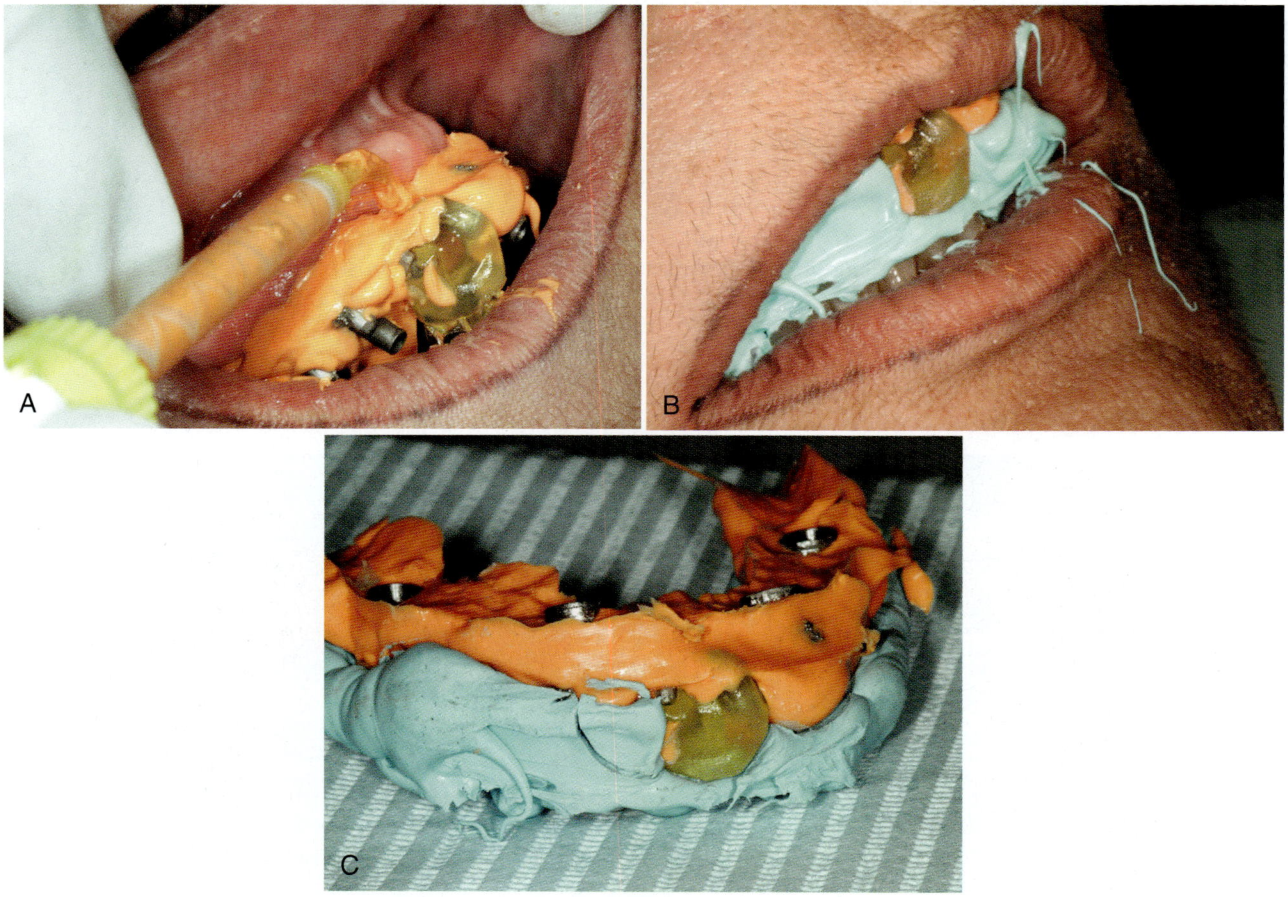

FIGURE 11-67 **A-C,** Prior to removal of the clinical attachment level (CAL) bar, a polyvinyl "wash" of the space between the CAL bar and the soft tissues is made for pouring a new soft tissue model.

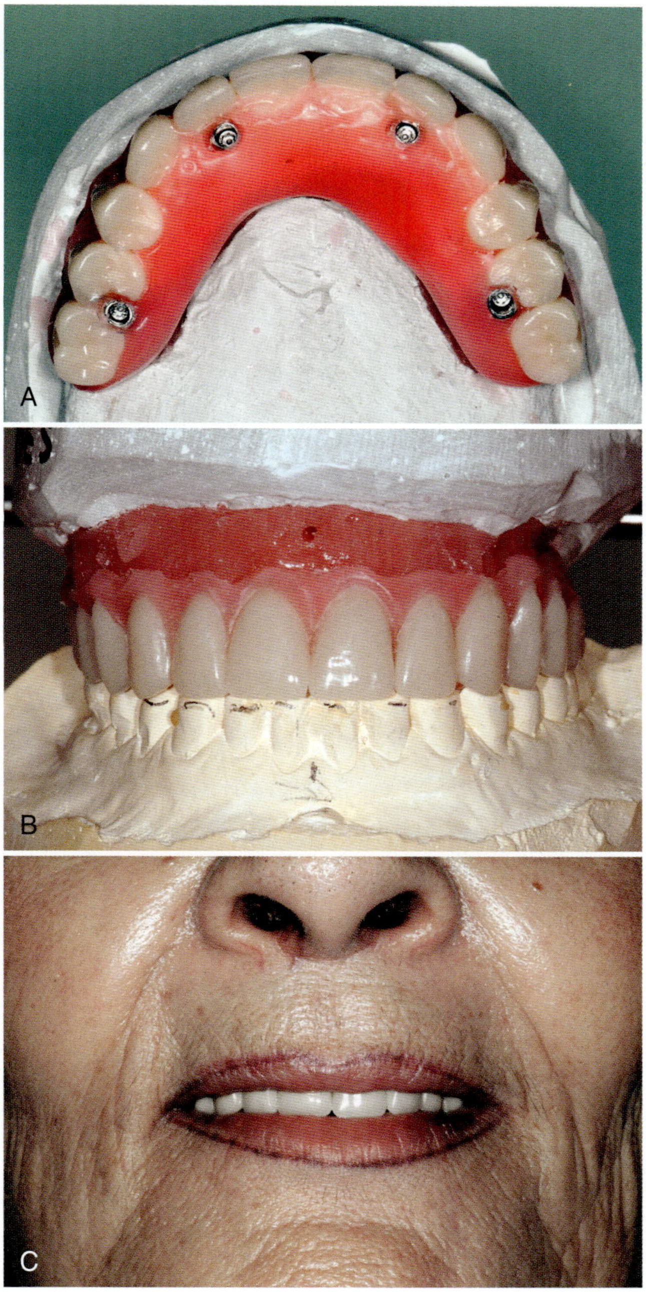

FIGURE 11-68 A-C, Wax try-in of the clinical attachment level bar profile prosthesis, assessing aesthetics and phonetics.

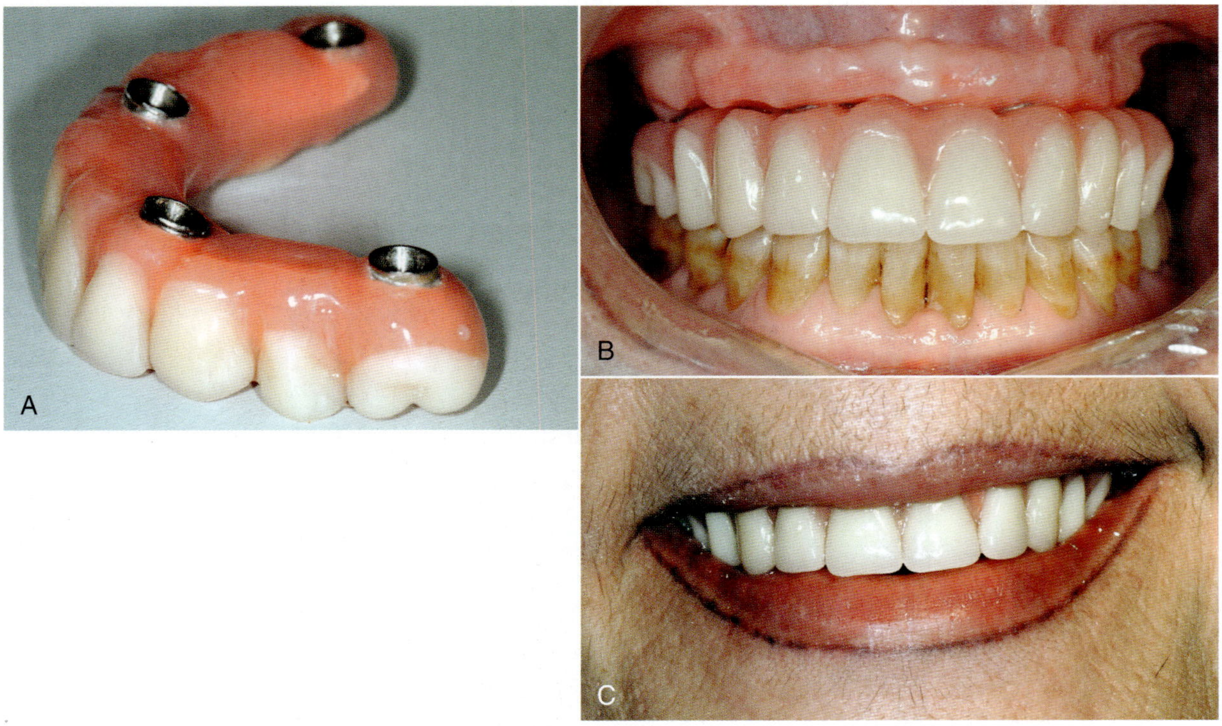

FIGURE 11-69 **A-C,** Processed final profile prosthesis with hidden transition line and aesthetic smile line.

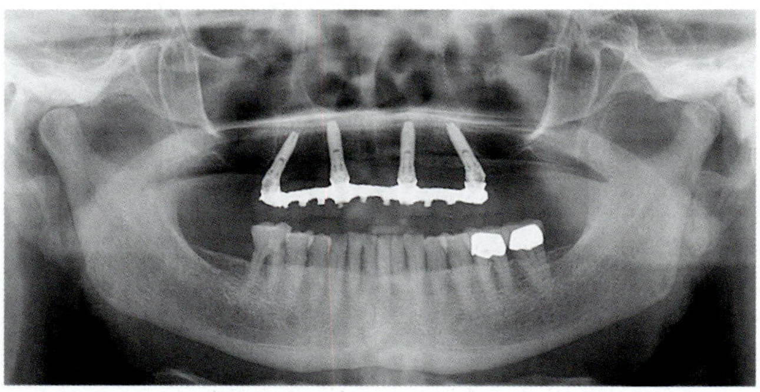

FIGURE 11-70 Final panoramic radiograph with all components fully seated onto the implants.

The three different approaches for the fabrication of the final profile prosthesis allow for a stable and functional long-term treatment plan. Adoption of any one technique is the choice of the practitioner.

CHAPTER 12

CASE PRESENTATIONS: Immediate-Loading Tilted Implants

TILTED TREATMENT CONCEPT: MAXILLA

A 62-year-old woman presented with maxillary full and mandibular partial edentulism. She reported a poor-function maxillary full denture. The patient's primary concern was rehabilitation of her dentition with a fixed maxillary and mandibular prosthesis. Initial evaluation of the patient's smile line demonstrated an unaesthetic buccal corridor in her existing full maxillary denture. With the denture removed and while animating, the patient did not demonstrate edentulous maxillary soft tissues, suggesting that a hidden transition line and therefore an aesthetic outcome would be possible for a fixed, implant-supported maxillary prosthesis. Intraoral examination demonstrated excessive horizontal overlap and visible unaesthetic clasps of the mandibular removable partial dentures. With the maxillary denture removed, the edentulous maxilla had a uniform U shape with a relatively shallow palatal vault (Figures 12-1 to 12-4).

The preoperative radiograph demonstrated zones I and II. Large, pneumatized, bilateral maxillary sinuses restricted the possibility of implant placement in zone III.

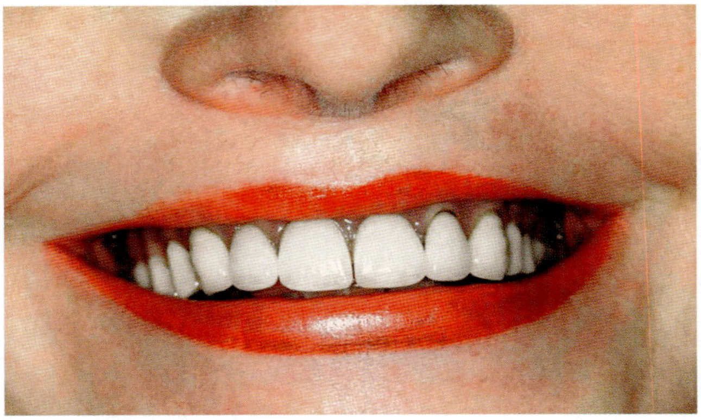

FIGURE 12-1 Existing maxillary full denture with unaesthetic buccal corridors.

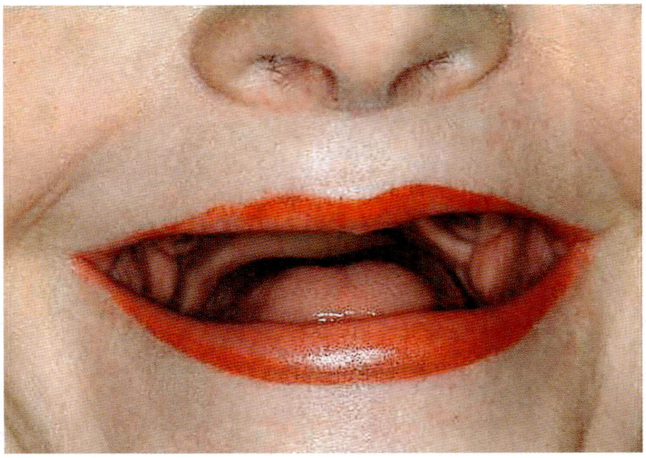

FIGURE 12-2 Hidden transition line is evident; the crestal soft tissues are not visible during animation.

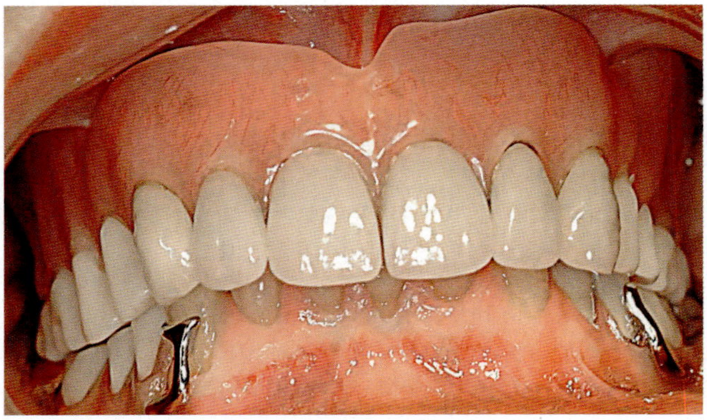

FIGURE 12-3 Excessive horizontal overlap and unaesthetic mandibular removable partial denture clasps.

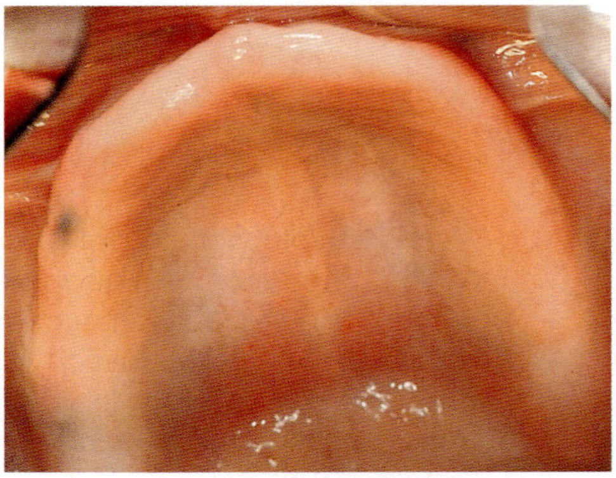

FIGURE 12-4 Shallow maxillary vault with relatively resorbed horizontal alveolar dimension.

Treatment Plan

1. Placement of implants, adopting the tilted treatment concept for the maxilla
2. Immediately loading the maxilla by converting the existing full upper denture into an immediate-load provisional prosthesis
3. Placement of implants in the bilateral posterior mandible at positions 18, 19, 28, 29, and 30 in one stage
4. Final metal-based profile prosthesis for the maxilla
5. Final two-unit fixed implant bridge for implants 18-19
6. Final three-unit fixed, implant-supported bridge for implants 28-30

Treatment planning for the maxilla begins with placement of anterior maxillary implants in positions 7 and 10. The posterior implants are placed as distal as possible, immediately in front of and paralleling the anterior wall of the maxillary sinus bilaterally. This position achieves the maximum anterior-posterior implant distribution, minimizing the need for posterior cantilevering of the final fixed maxillary prosthesis (Figures 12-5 to 12-9).

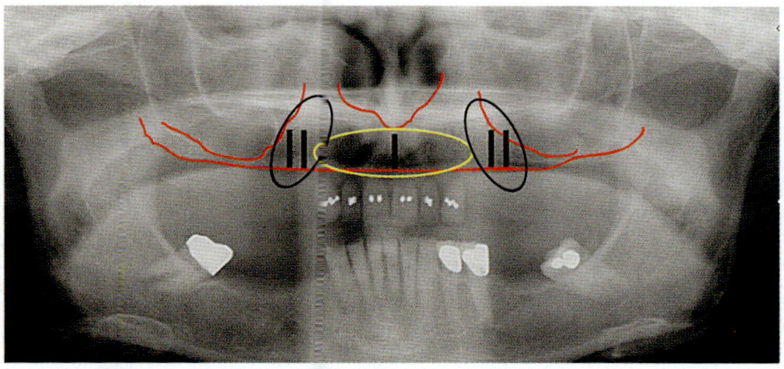

FIGURE 12-5 Preoperative panoramic radiograph demonstrating zones I and II only.

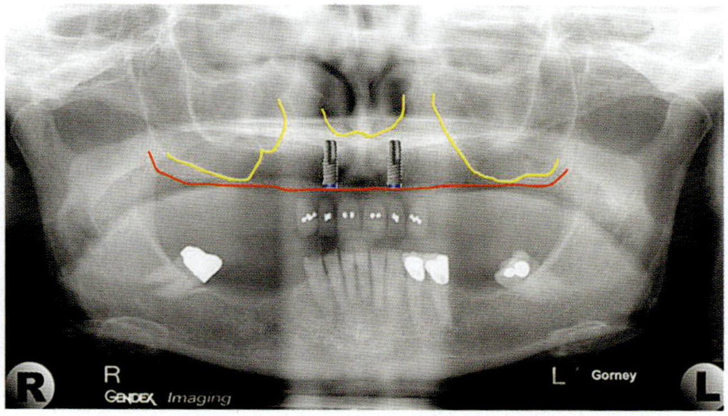

FIGURE 12-6 Placement of the anterior maxillary implants in positions 7 and 10.

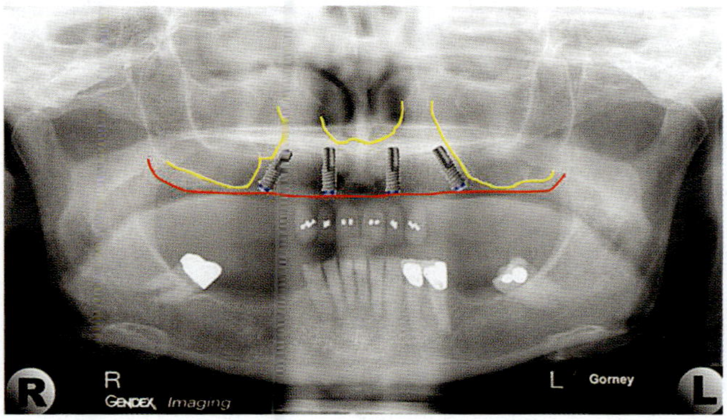

FIGURE 12-7 Posterior maxillary implants, tilted and paralleling the slope of the anterior maxillary sinus walls.

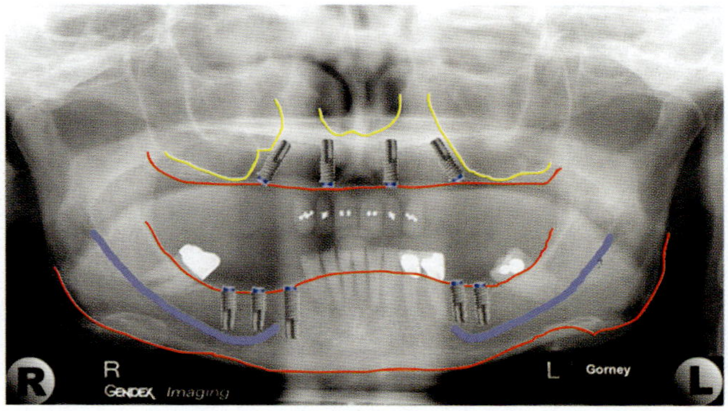

FIGURE 12-8 Placement of implants in the posterior mandible.

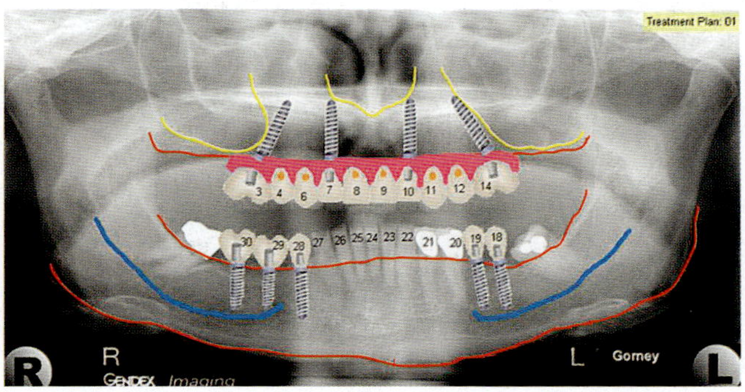

FIGURE 12-9 Schematic of the final treatment plan demonstrating a final maxillary profile prosthesis and fixed, implant-supported mandibular bridges.

Placements of the four maxillary implants are completed after minor recontouring of the maxillary alveolus to achieve a uniform topography of the edentulous ridge. For the posterior tilted implants, 30° multiunit abutments are placed, bringing the prosthetic platform into the occlusal plane. Temporary healing abutments are placed on the anterior implants and temporary abutment covers are placed on the posterior implants, allowing closure of the soft tissues. Registration material placed into the intaglio surface of the existing full upper denture allows transfer of the implant positions to the denture base (Figures 12-10 to 12-13).

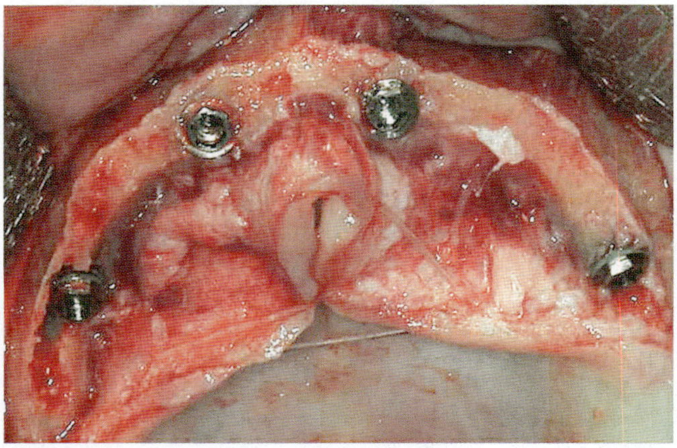

FIGURE 12-10 After establishing a uniform topography of the maxillary alveolar ridge, the implants are placed.

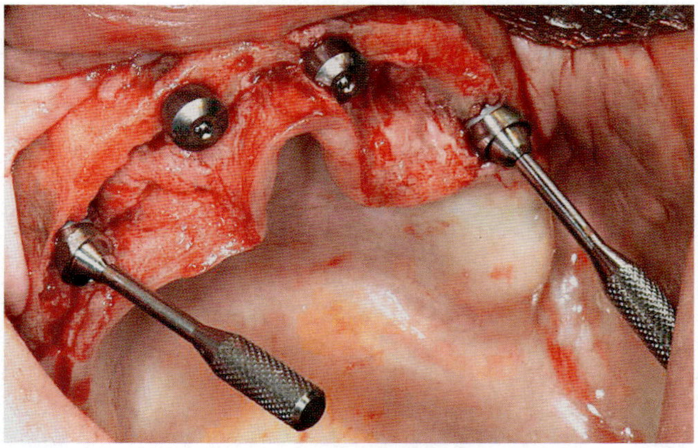

FIGURE 12-11 Multiunit 30° abutments are placed on the posterior tilted implants and torqued to 20 Ncm.

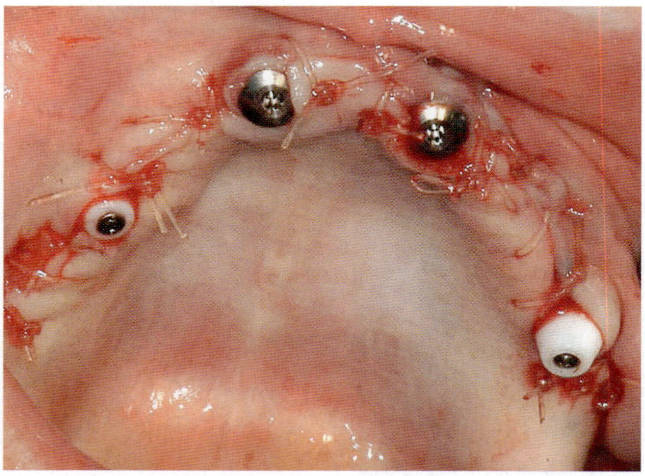

FIGURE 12-12 Placement of temporary healing abutments onto the anterior implants with soft tissue closure.

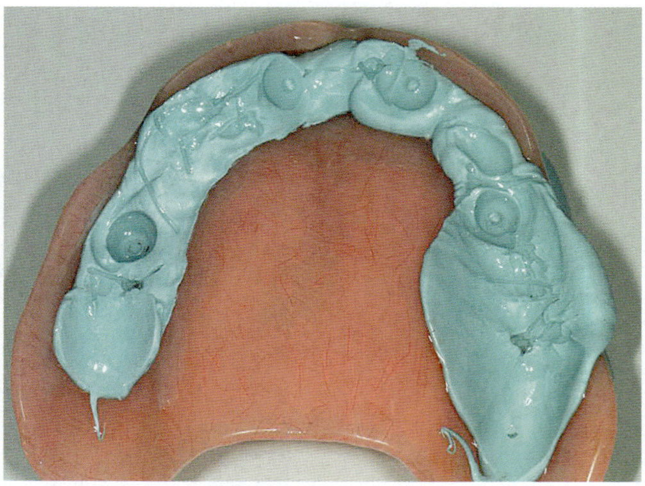

FIGURE 12-13 Transfer of the implant positions to the intaglio surface of the maxillary denture.

The decision was made to place temporary titanium cylinders individually on the posterior abutments and lute them with quick-setting acrylic material to the denture base. After connecting the titanium cylinders to the posterior implants, the anterior portion of the denture is filled with registration paste and the position of the temporary healing abutments is indexed onto the anterior portion of the denture. The decision was made to place 17° multiunit abutments for the anterior implants. The abutments are fully seated and torqued to 20 Ncm. The transferred implant positions are indexed onto the denture base using an acrylic bur. Two titanium cylinders are placed onto the anterior implants and luted to the denture base. Once all four titanium cylinders are connected, the palate and the flanges of the denture are removed. The edges of the prosthesis are contoured to eliminate the concavity of the intaglio surface between the titanium cylinders to permit adequate oral hygiene during osseointegration. The prosthesis is complete (Figures 12-14 to 12-18).

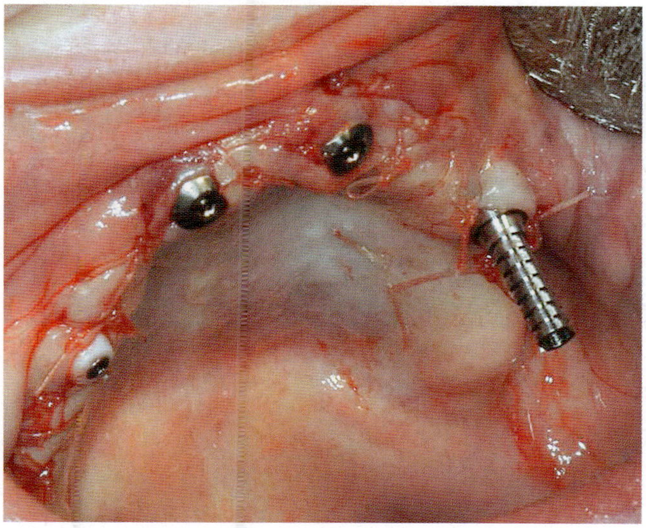

FIGURE 12-14 Temporary titanium cylinder is placed on the posterior implant abutments.

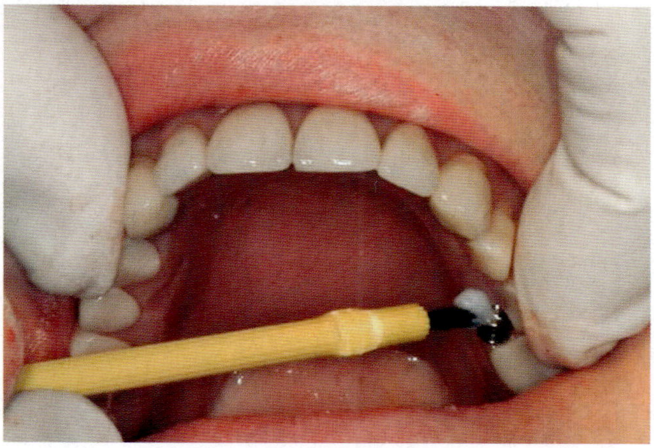

FIGURE 12-15 Quick-setting acrylic material is used to connect the titanium cylinder to the denture base.

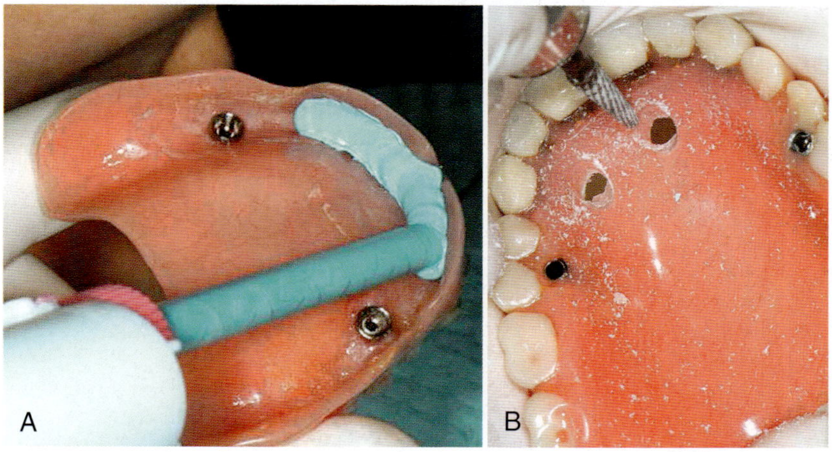

FIGURE 12-16 Reindexing the position of the anterior implants allows for a more accurate opening of the acrylic in the denture base for luting the temporary titanium cylinders.

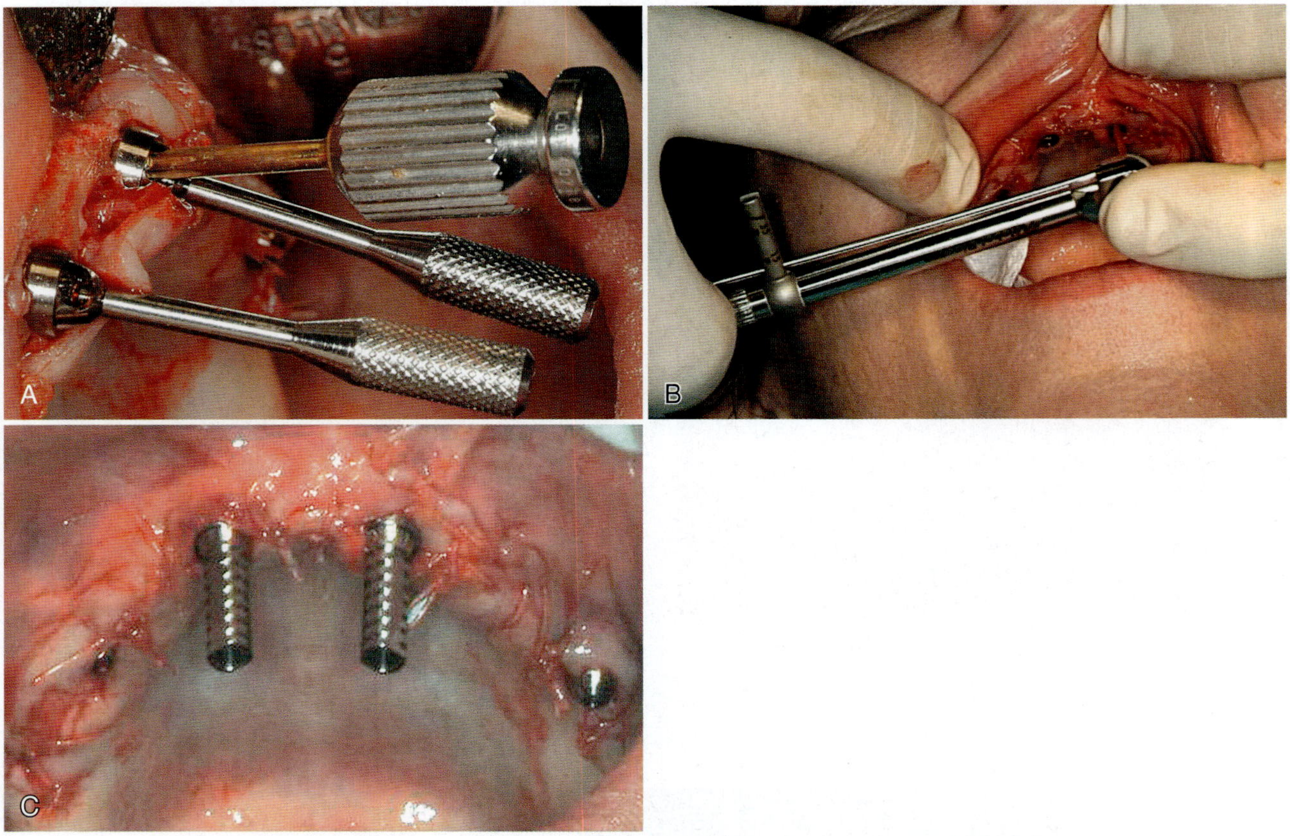

FIGURE 12-17 Angulated 17° multiunit abutments are placed and torqued, and titanium temporary cylinders are connected to the anterior implants.

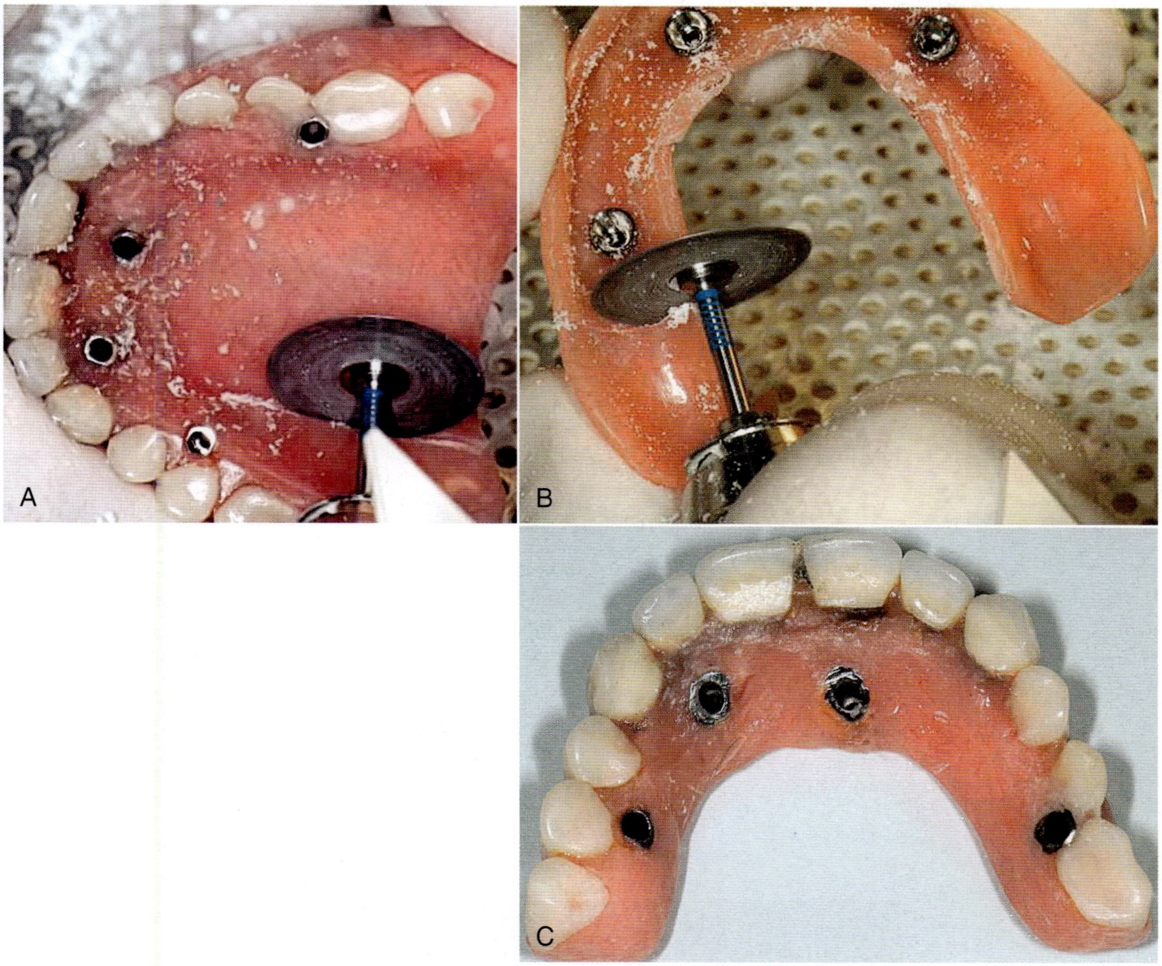

FIGURE 12-18 After luting all titanium cylinders, the palate and the flange of the maxillary denture is removed, converting the denture into a provisional fixed prosthesis.

The positions of the mandibular implants are identified on the mandibular cast and are placed in the posterior mandible bilaterally using the surgical stent (Figures 12-19 and 12-20).

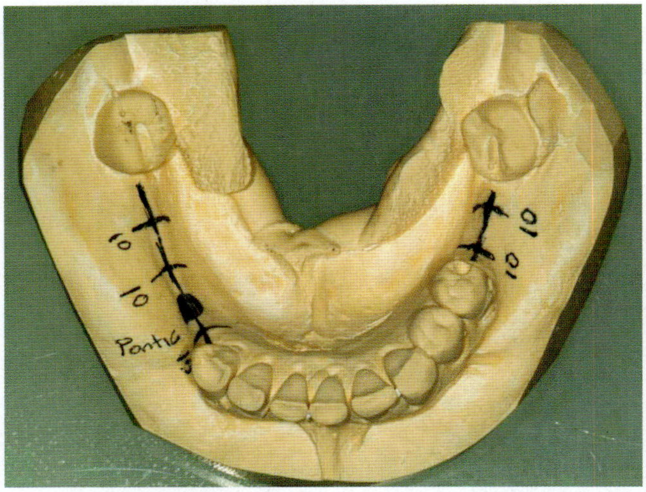

FIGURE 12-19 Intended positions of implants 18, 19, 28, 29, and 30.

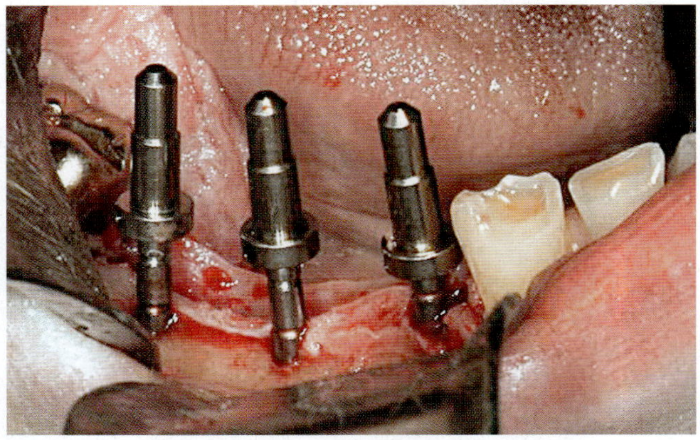

FIGURE 12-20 Paralleling pins demonstrating the positions of the implants in the lower-right quadrant.

After the 6-month osseointegration period, the protocol for fabrication of the final metal-based maxillary profile prosthesis is carried out. Impressions of the mandibular implants are also taken for fabrication of the implant-supported bridges. The final maxillary prosthesis allows exposure of more than 95% of the patient's palate. The stability of the prosthesis allows the patient to have excellent masticatory ability. The cement-retained mandibular bridges allow restoration of the mandibular missing teeth with two implant-supported bridges (Figures 12-21 to 12-25).

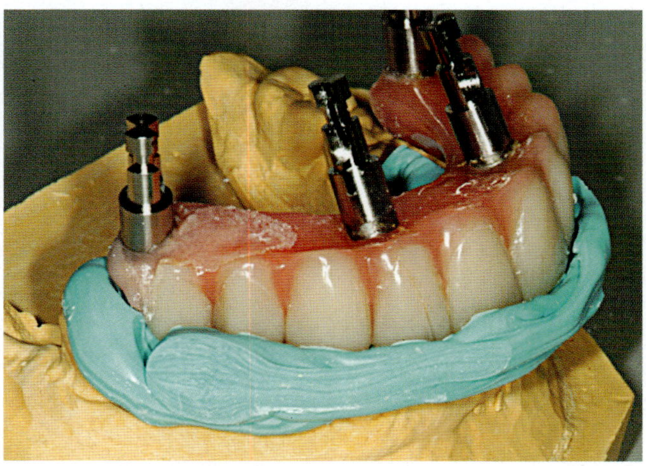

FIGURE 12-21 The final metal-based profile prosthesis is fabricated at 6 months.

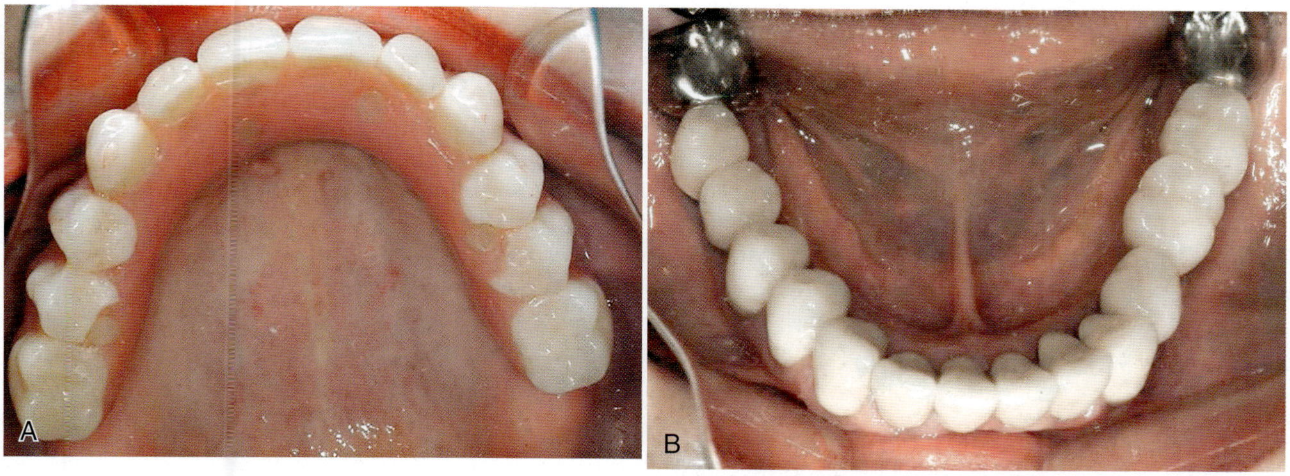

FIGURE 12-22 Completed maxillary profile prosthesis and implant bridges 18-19 and 28-29-30.

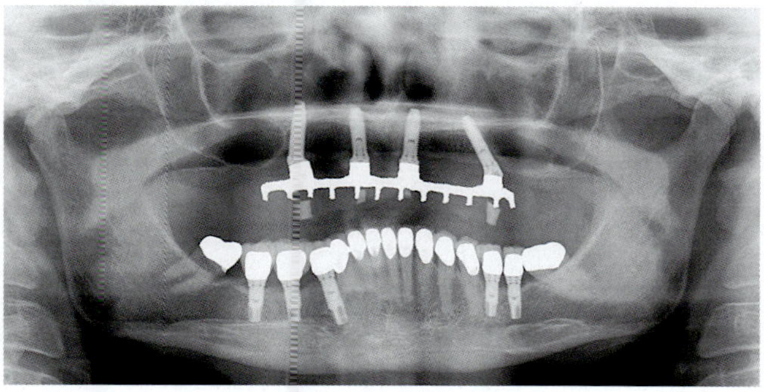

FIGURE 12-23 Final panoramic prosthesis demonstrating complete seating of the abutments onto the implant platforms as well as complete seating of the profile prosthesis.

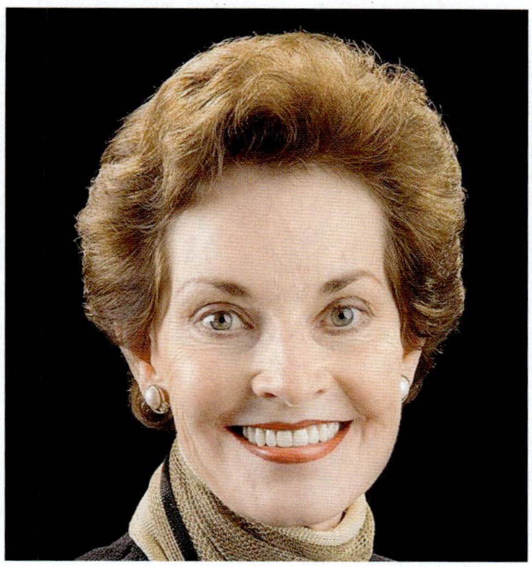

FIGURE 12-24 Completed maxillary profile prosthesis.

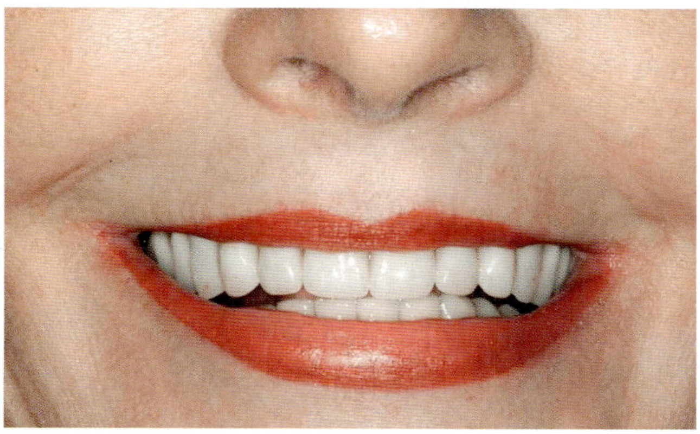

FIGURE 12-25 Hidden transition line and aesthetic bilateral buccal corridors.

TILTED CONCEPT: MANDIBLE

A 57-year-old woman presented with complete maxillary and partial mandibular edentulism. The patient's primary complaint was difficulty chewing with her mandibular removable partial denture. She also wanted to improve the retention and aesthetics of her maxillary full denture. Her preoperative radiograph was consistent with moderate maxillary resorption and mild posterior mandibular resorption with retained mandibular incisor teeth, which have a guarded to poor long-term prognosis (Figure 12-26 and 12-27).

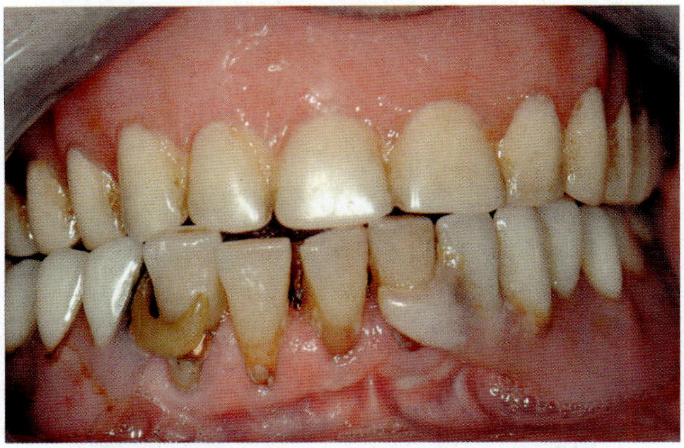

FIGURE 12-26 Preoperative maxillary full denture and mandibular removable partial denture retained by the remaining mandibular incisor teeth.

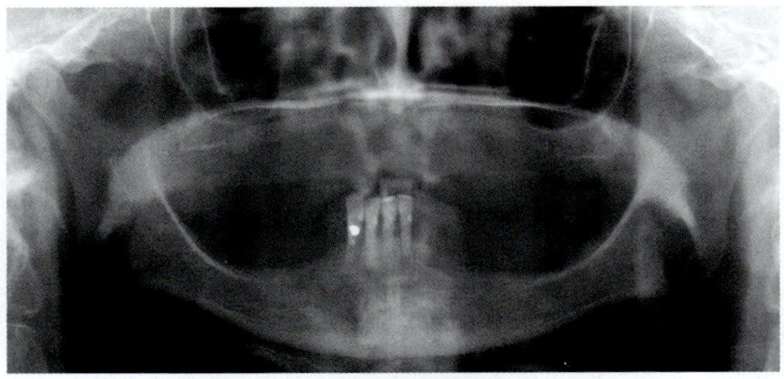

FIGURE 12-27 Preoperative panoramic radiograph.

Treatment Plan

1. Removal of the remaining four mandibular teeth
2. Anterior mandibular alveolectomy to coincide with the posterior mandible, establishing a uniform crestal topography
3. Placement of mandibular implants using the "tilted implant" concept
4. Fabrication of a new full mandibular denture for conversion into an immediate-load provisional prosthesis
5. Immediately loading the mandibular implants with a fixed provisional prosthesis
6. Fabrication of a final new full maxillary denture, with an increase in the patient's vertical dimension of occlusion (VDO) and correction of the dental midline to coincide with the facial midline.
7. Fabrication of a final metal-based mandibular profile prosthesis

(Figures 12-28 and 12-29)

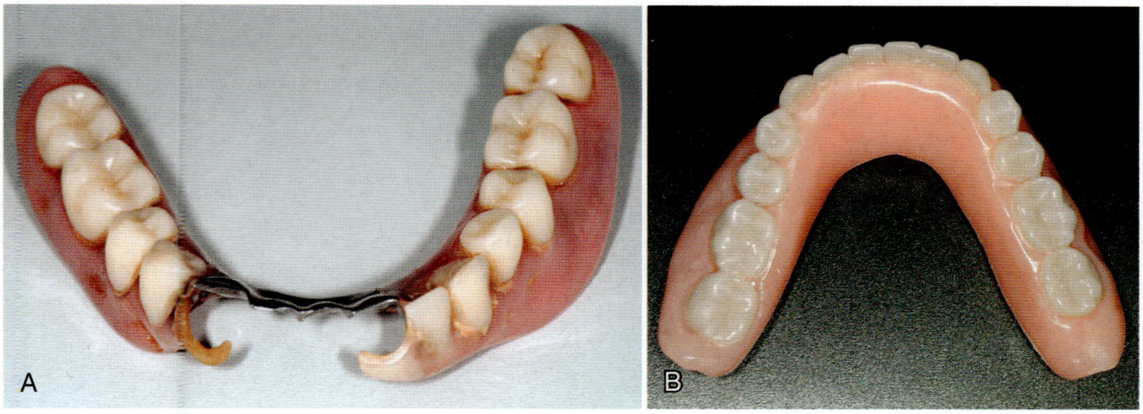

FIGURE 12-28 A, The existing mandibular removable mandibular prosthesis. B, New preoperative full mandibular denture, which will be converted to a fixed, immediate-load prosthesis.

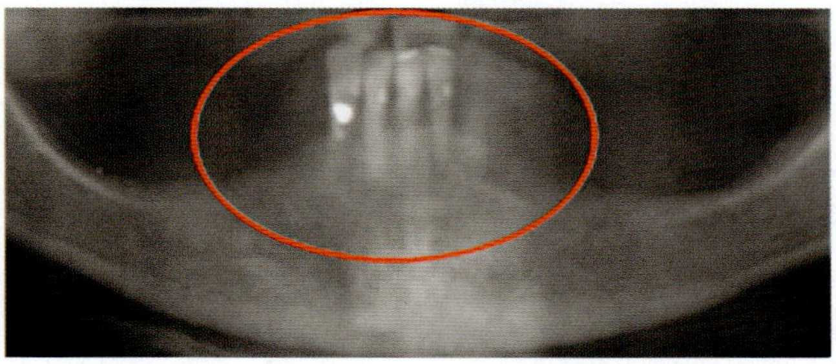

FIGURE 12-29 Planned removal of the four mandibular incisor teeth and anterior mandibular alveolectomy.

Under intravenous sedation, a full-thickness mucoperiosteal flap is developed and the remaining mandibular teeth are removed. A portion of the remaining extraction sockets are removed, creating a uniform topography of the edentulous mandibular crestal bone. Implants are placed using the protocol for the edentulous mandible. After implant placement, the posterior implants receive 30° multiunit abutments, which are placed and torqued to 20 Ncm. For the anterior implants, temporary healing abutments are placed prior to indexing the abutment positions onto the intaglio surface of the mandibular denture. Once the position of the abutments is transferred to the denture, the decision to use straight or 17° multiunit abutments for the two anterior implants is made. Conversion of the preoperative full denture into a fixed, immediate-load provisional prosthesis completes the procedure (Figures 12-30 to 12-36).

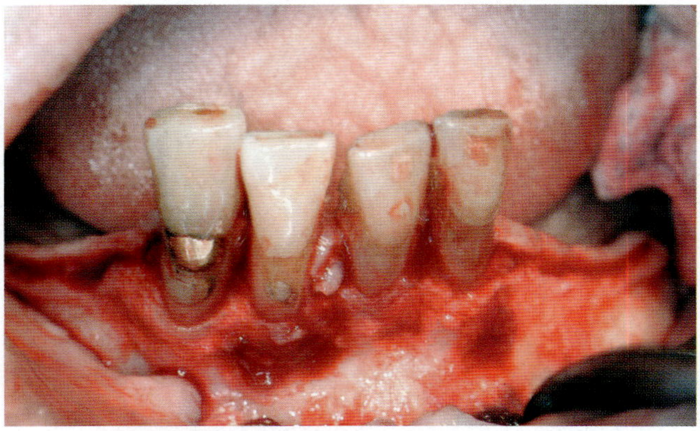

FIGURE 12-30 Full-thickness flap exposing the anterior mandible.

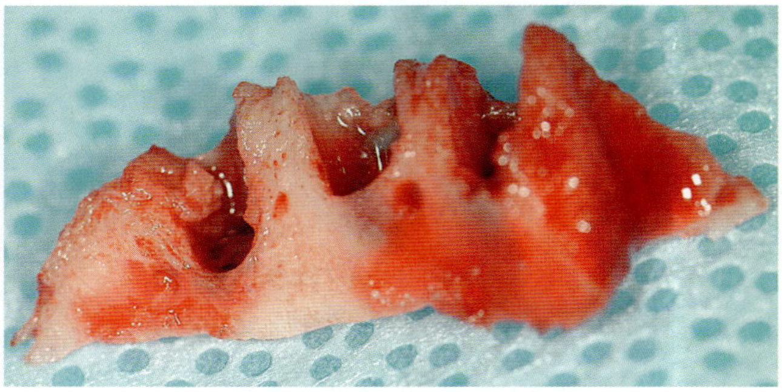

FIGURE 12-31 Removal of a portion of the remaining extraction sockets equaling the posterior mandibular edentulous crest.

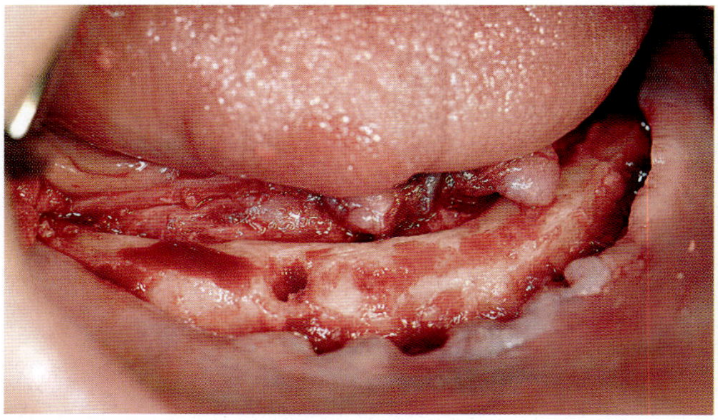

FIGURE 12-32 Confirmation of a uniform mandibular crestal topography prior to implant placement.

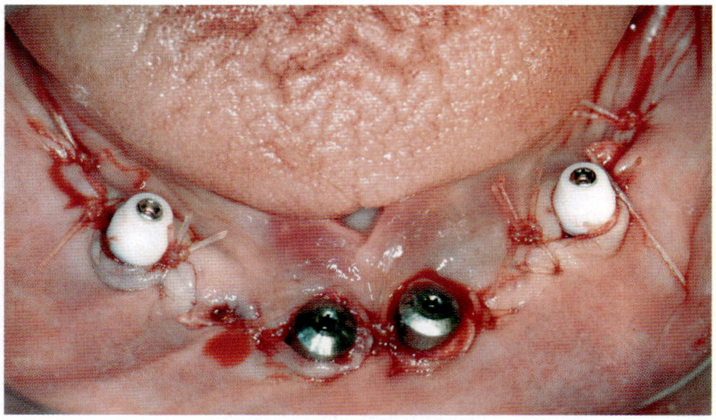

FIGURE 12-33 Completion of implant placement with connection of the abutments.

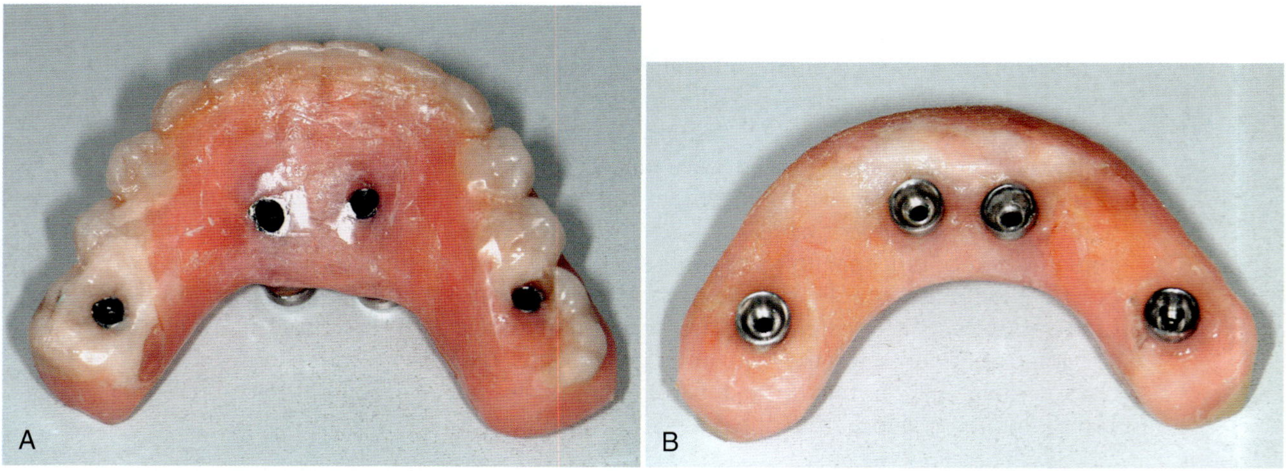

FIGURE 12-34 Completed conversion of the full lower denture into a provisional immediate-load prosthesis.

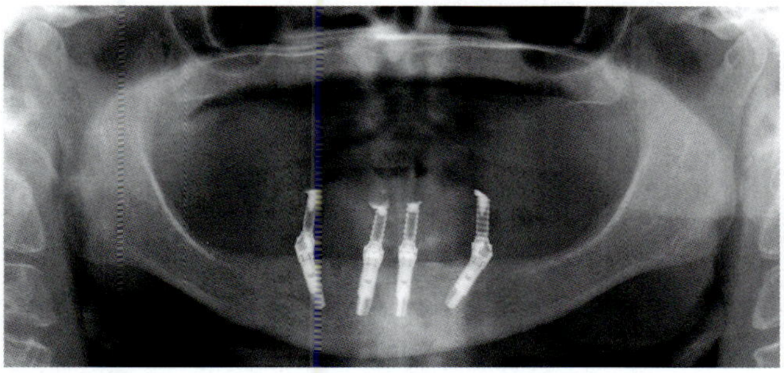

FIGURE 12-35 Panoramic radiograph of the tilted implant concept taken immediately after surgery.

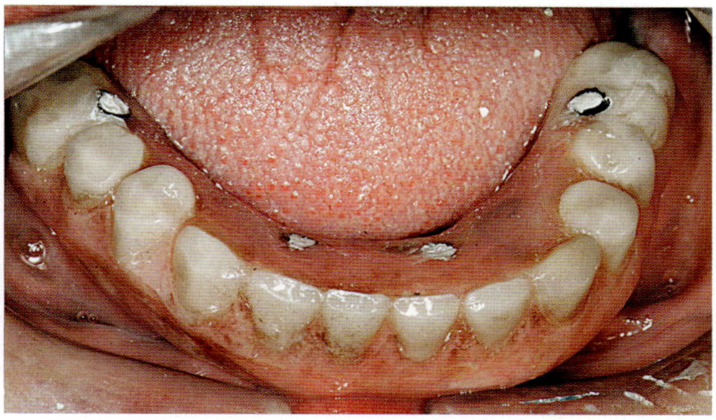

FIGURE 12-36 One-week postoperative view of the provisional prosthesis.

Three months after placement and loading of the mandibular prosthesis, the patient is evaluated to prepare for fabrication of the final maxillary and mandibular prosthesis. To mount the patient's cast, a wash impression of the existing full maxillary denture is made. Registration paste is used to capture the interocclusal record for mounting the prosthesis in the laboratory. The mandibular prosthesis is removed, and implant stability is confirmed by placing 20 Ncm of torque on the angulated abutments and 35 Ncm of torque on the straight abutments. Implant immobility and the absence of pain indicate osseointegration. To prevent collapse of the "sulcular" soft tissues during the 90-minute laboratory model mounting procedure, temporary multiunit caps are placed on the abutments. Four multiunit laboratory analogues are connected to the mandibular provisional prosthesis ready for the laboratory procedure. The full maxillary denture, the occlusal registration, and the mandibular provisional prosthesis are sent to the laboratory to be mounted (Figures 12-37 to 12-43).

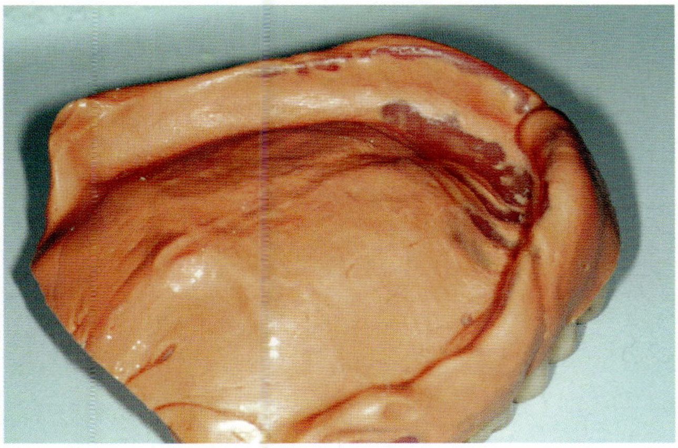

FIGURE 12-37 The patient's existing full upper denture is used as a "custom tray" for creation of the maxillary cast.

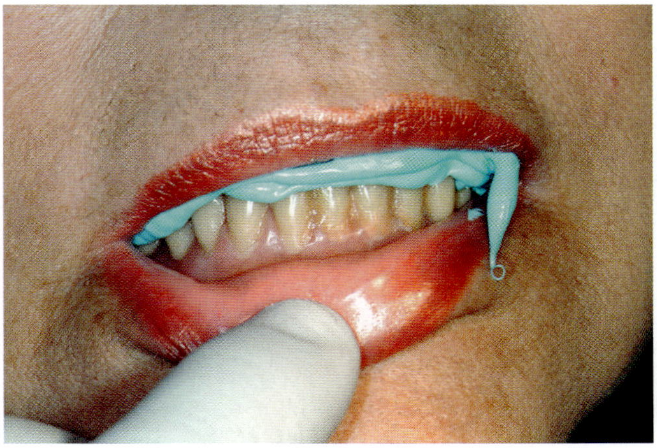

FIGURE 12-38 A bite registration is made after the maxillary denture is stabilized with the polyvinyl wash.

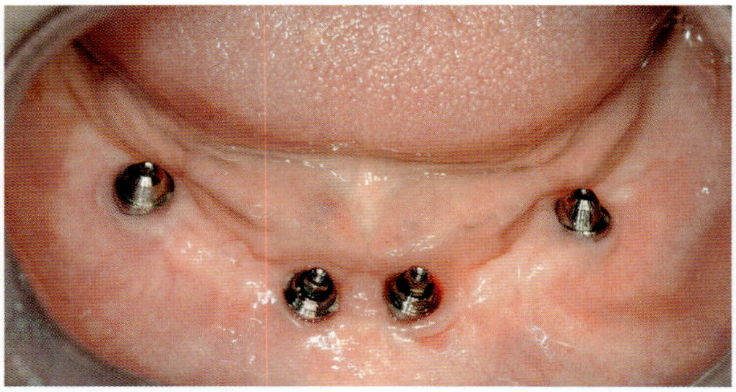

FIGURE 12-39 The mandibular provisional prosthesis is removed, and the health and contour of the soft tissues are evaluated, as is implant stability.

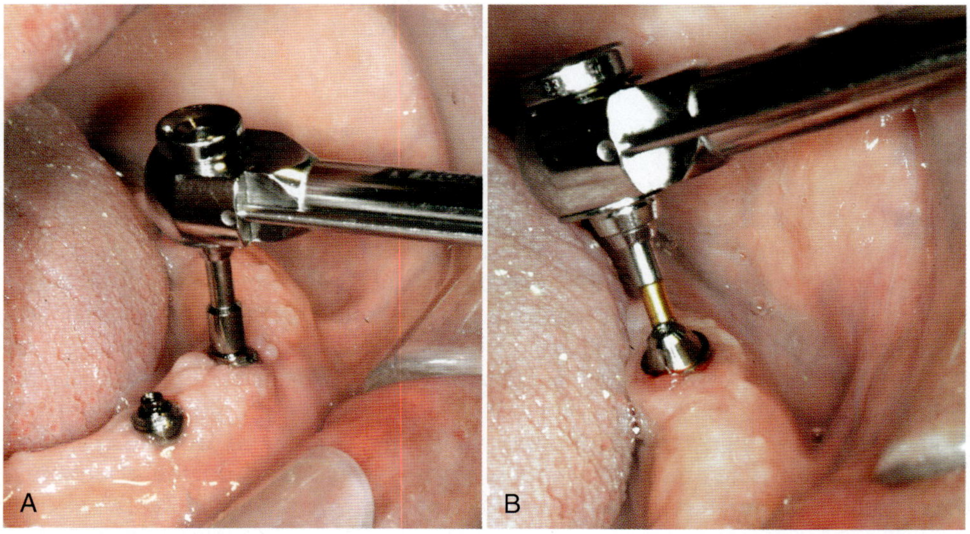

FIGURE 12-40 **A,** Straight multiunit abutments are checked by placing 35 Ncm of torque onto the abutment screws. **B,** The angulated abutments are checked by placing 20 Ncm of torque onto the abutment screws.

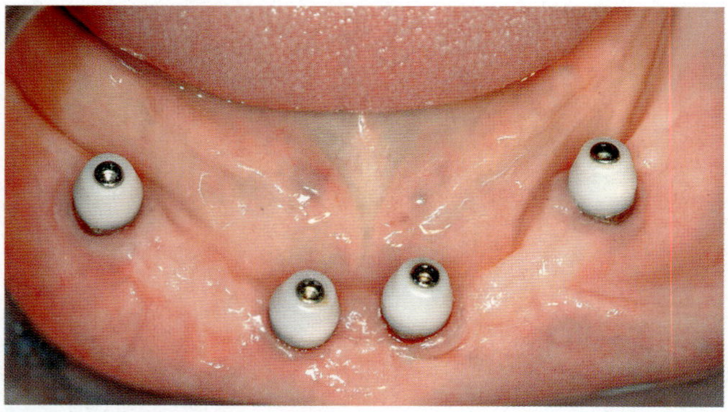

FIGURE 12-41 Temporary abutment caps are placed to maintain the soft tissue contours around the abutments during prosthesis mounting in the laboratory.

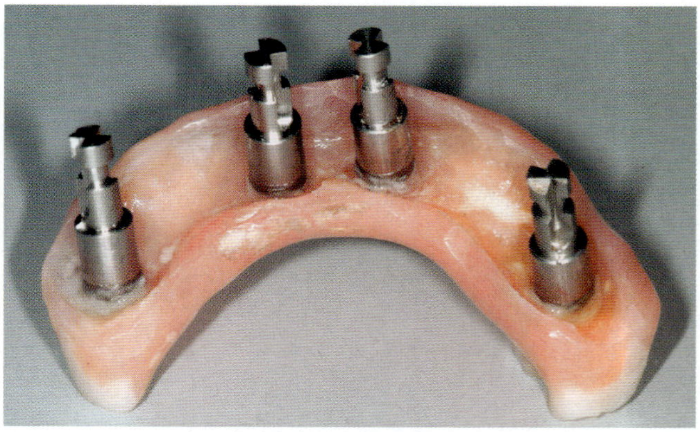

FIGURE 12-42 Multiunit laboratory analogues are connected to the provisional prosthesis.

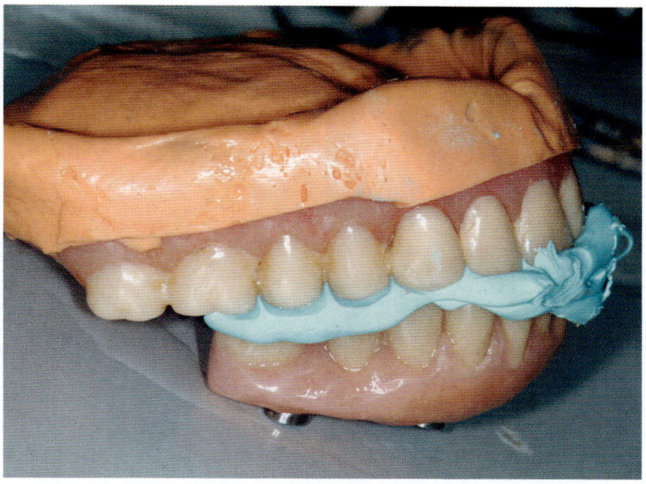

FIGURE 12-43 The maxillary denture, bite registration, and mandibular provisional prosthesis complex is sent to the laboratory.

For most patients, mounting the complex shown in Figure 12-18 establishes proper VDO. For this patient, however, the intention is to increase the VDO of the final prosthesis. Therefore, a wax rim is fabricated and the desired VDO is transferred from the patient to the laboratory, allowing mounting of the maxillary and mandibular casts. The next appointment is the wax try-in. The maxillary denture setup is tissue-supported. The mandibular wax try-in is aided by adding two titanium or plastic cylinders within the mandibular denture base, allowing stabilization of the mandibular prosthesis during the clinical appointments. The tooth-to-lip relationship during animation is evaluated to ensure buccal corridor filling and a smile line acceptable to the patient (Figures 12-44 to 12-47).

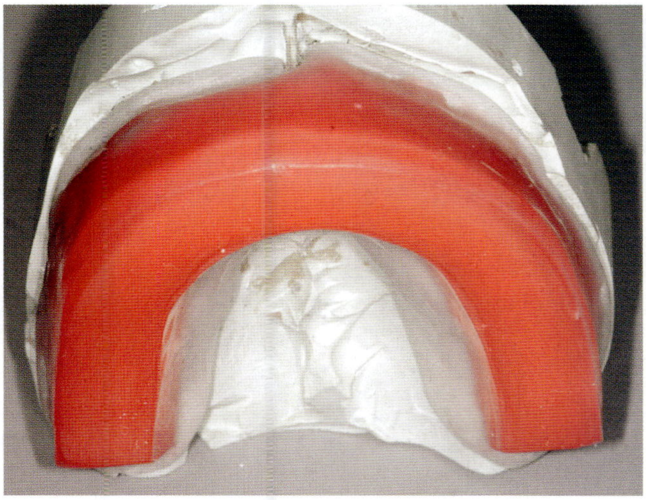

FIGURE 12-44 Maxillary wax rims are ready to establish the increased vertical dimension of occlusion.

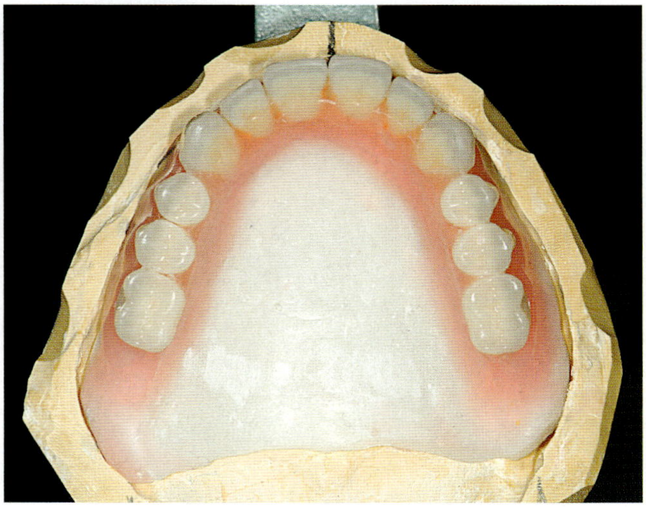

FIGURE 12-45 Wax try-in of the new maxillary denture.

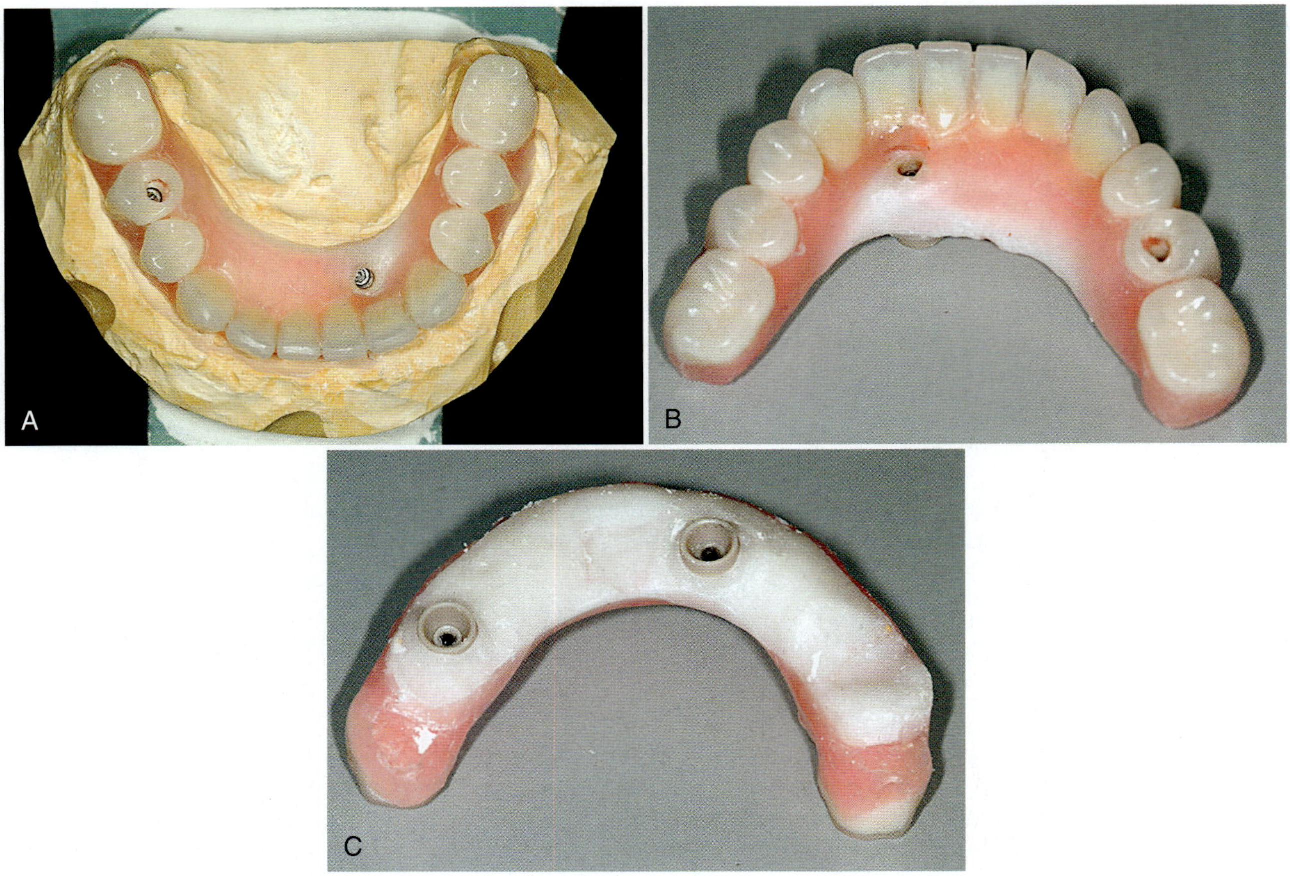

FIGURE 12-46 Wax try-in of the mandibular provisional prosthesis stabilized by plastic temporary cylinders.

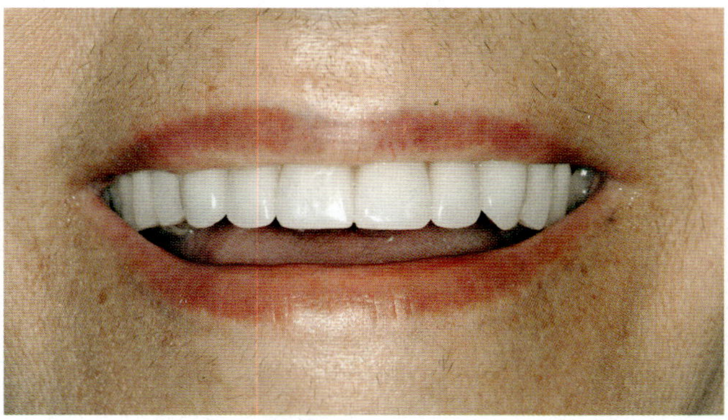

FIGURE 12-47 The patient approves the aesthetics of the maxillary wax mockup.

A putty index of the mandibular teeth position assists the laboratory technician in assessing how far to extend the metal framework to allow proper support for the teeth. The metal framework is waxed and cast. To help the framework fit passively, it is sectioned to be ready for intraoral indexing. Indexing material of the practitioner's choice is used to index framework sections. After careful removal of the indexed framework, additional indexing material is added to the intaglio surface to add rigidity and prevent accidental separation during transport to the laboratory. The indexed framework is soldered, and the next appointment is for a framework try-in. After confirmation of a uniform passive fit, all four screws are attached to the prosthesis and a light body wash of the intaglio surface of the framework is made to allow the laboratory technician to adapt the pink acrylic to a pinpoint contact with the edentulous ridge (Figures 12-48 to 12-54).

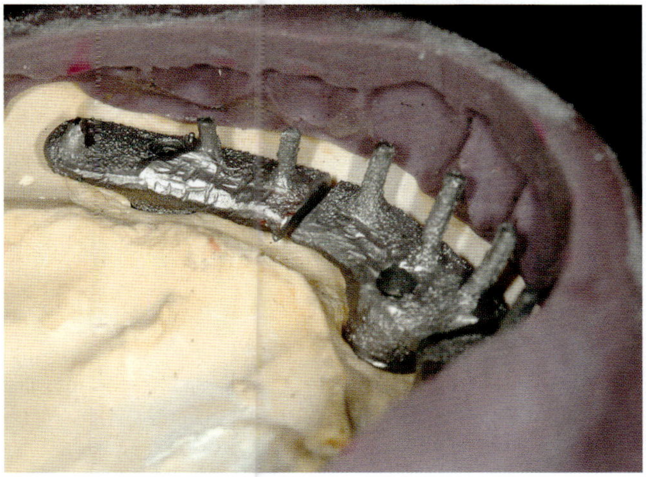

FIGURE 12-48 Putty index of the acceptable denture setup allows proper extension of the metal framework by the technician.

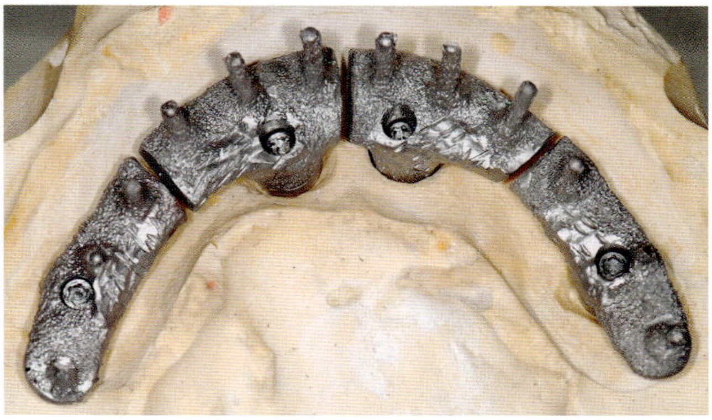

FIGURE 12-49 Casted gold framework, sectioned and ready for intraoral indexing.

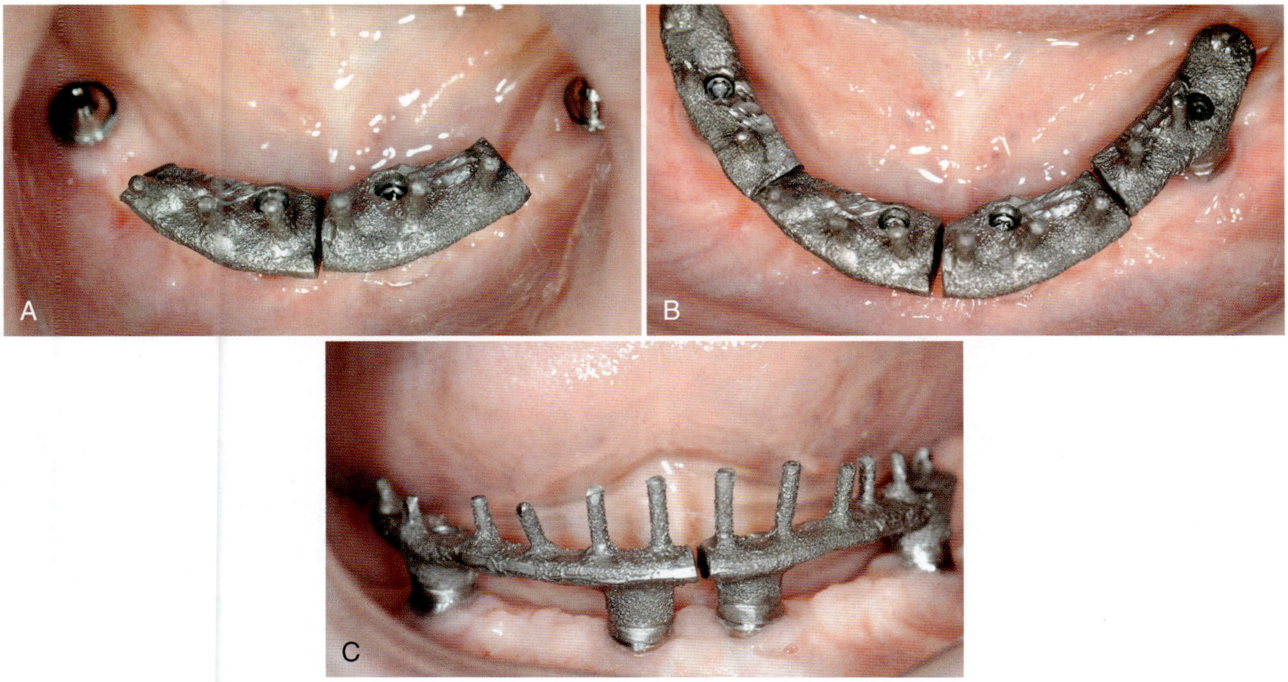

FIGURE 12-50 Transfer of the metal framework intraorally secured by a prosthetic screw.

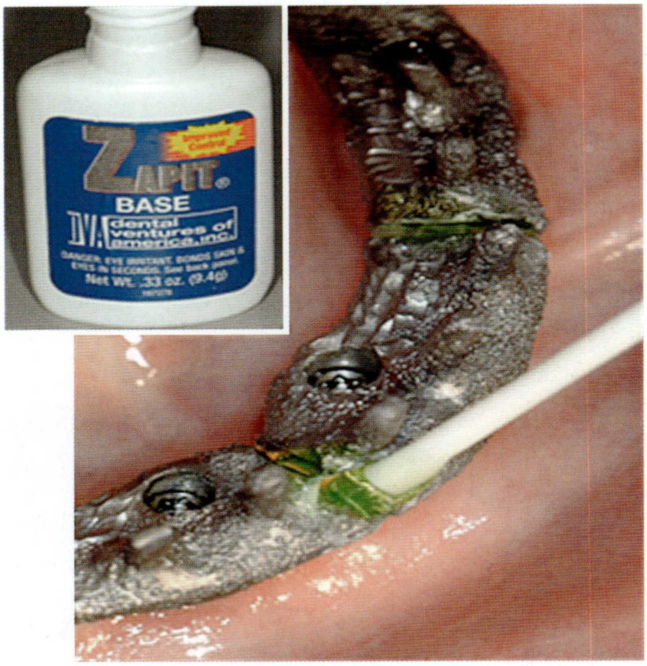

FIGURE 12-51 Indexing the framework.

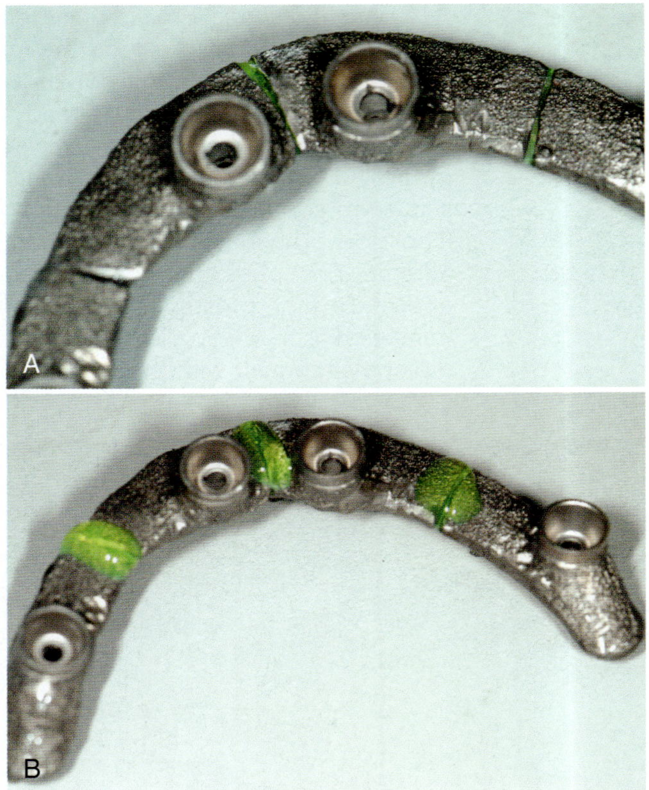

FIGURE 12-52 Indexing material is added to the intaglio surface of the framework to ensure rigidity and prevent accidental separation.

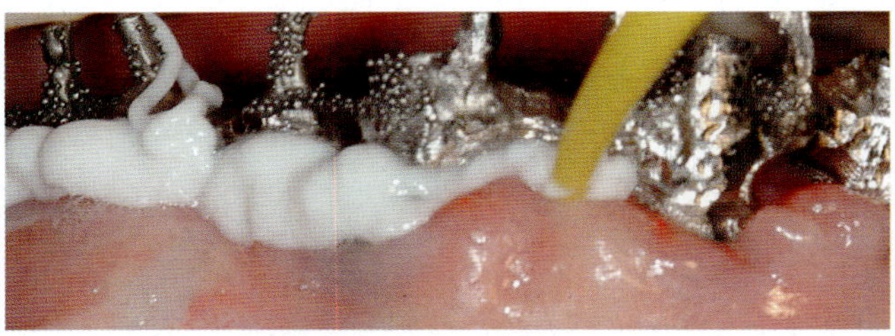

FIGURE 12-53 Light body impression material is carefully placed between the soldered framework and the soft tissues, being careful not to distort the soft tissue topography.

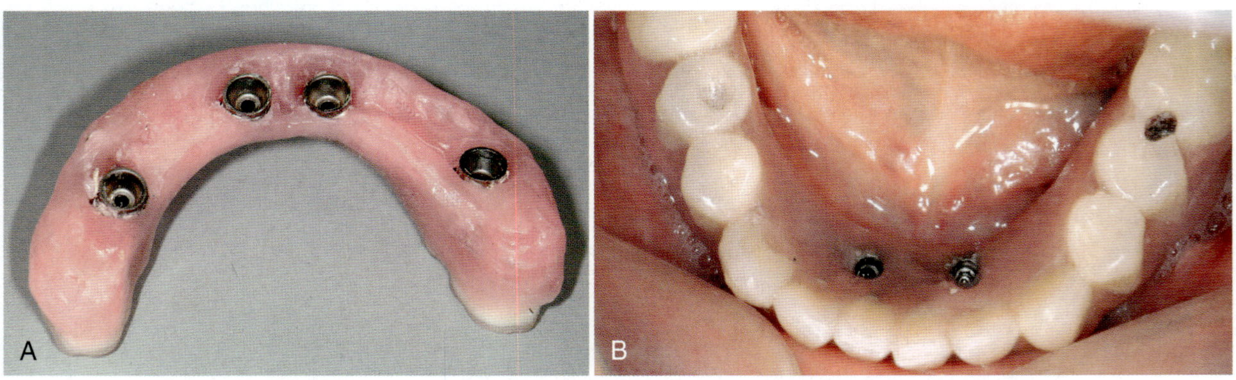

FIGURE 12-54 Second and final try-in prior to processing the mandibular profile prosthesis and the new full maxillary denture.

During the second wax try-in, aesthetics and speech are evaluated. Once the prosthesis is acceptable to the patient, the final prosthesis is produced. The final prosthesis allows for correction of the midline, the proper occlusal plane, and the newly established VDO. The final panoramic radiograph demonstrates complete seating of all abutments onto the implant platform and seating of the framework onto the abutments (Figures 12-55 to 12-57).

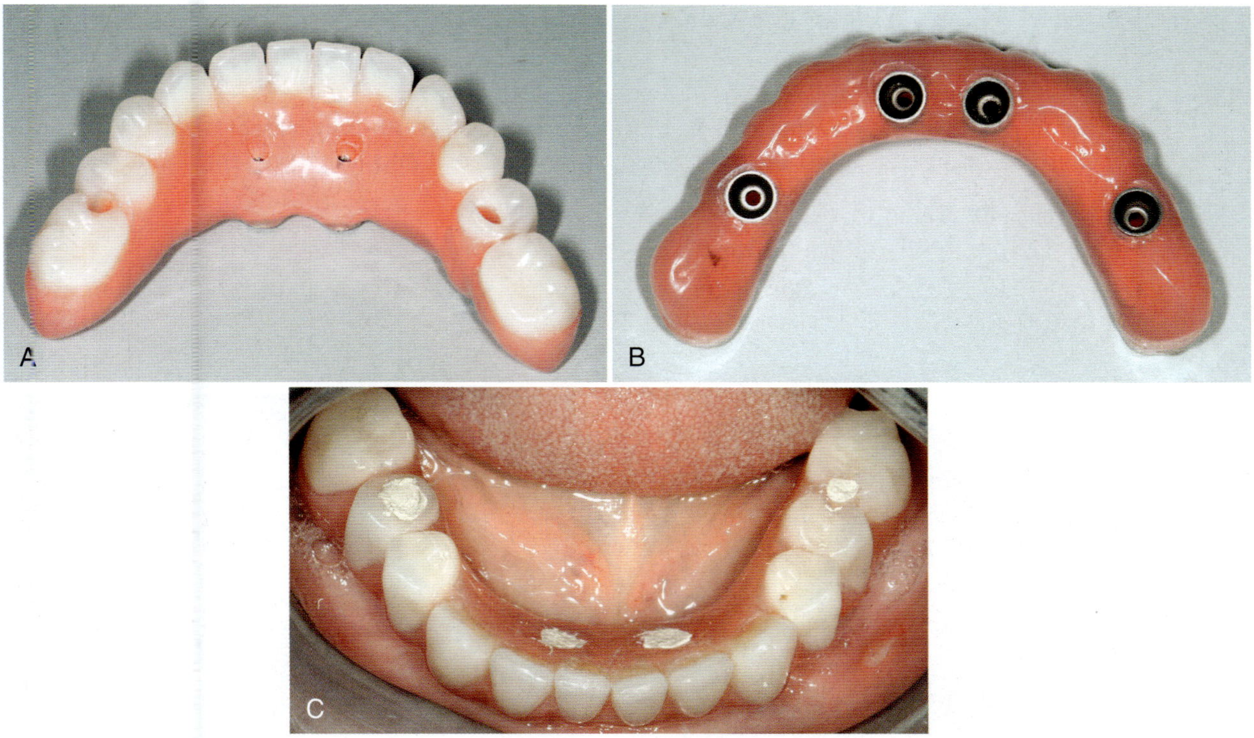

FIGURE 12-55 Final profile prosthesis with extension of the acrylic to a pinpoint contact from the intaglio surface of the prosthesis to the soft tissues.

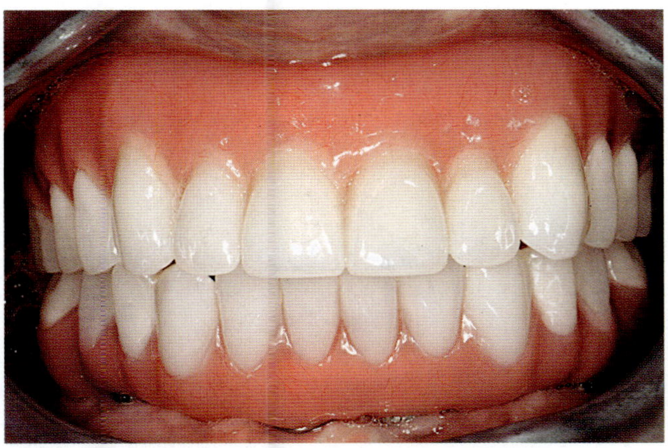

FIGURE 12-56 Completed new maxillary full denture and mandibular profile prosthesis.

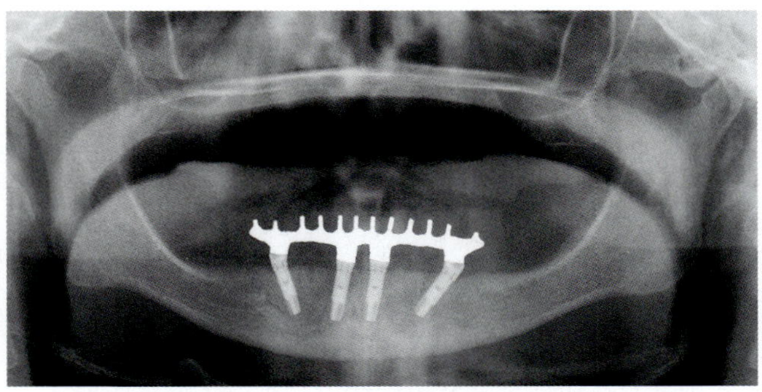

FIGURE 12-57 Final panoramic radiograph.

ALL-ON-4 PORCELAIN FUSED TO METAL BRIDGE

A 57-year-old man has worn maxillary dentures for 18 years. The potential for a fixed prosthesis motivated this patient to seek evaluation for a fixed maxillary implant-supported prosthesis. The patient was evaluated according to the systematic pretreatment evaluation protocol.

Systematic Pretreatment Evaluation

Transition line: Hidden
Composite defect: Absent
Final prosthesis: Ceramo-metal because patient has a tooth-only defect
Surgical protocol: Tilted concept, because only zones I and II are present

(Figures 12-58 to 12-78)

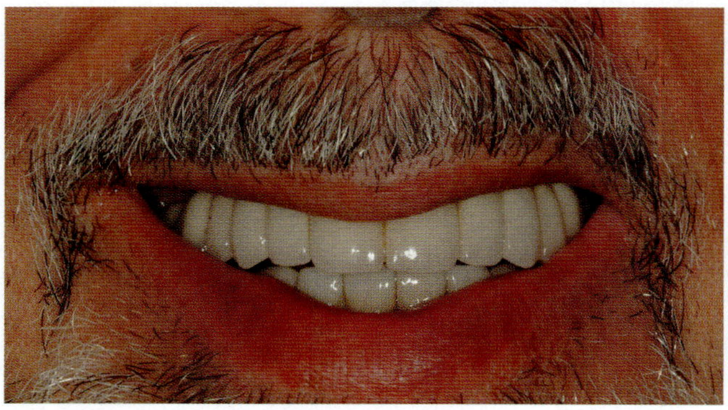

FIGURE 12-58 Preoperative smile line demonstrates a long upper lip without cervical tooth display, suggesting a hidden transition line.

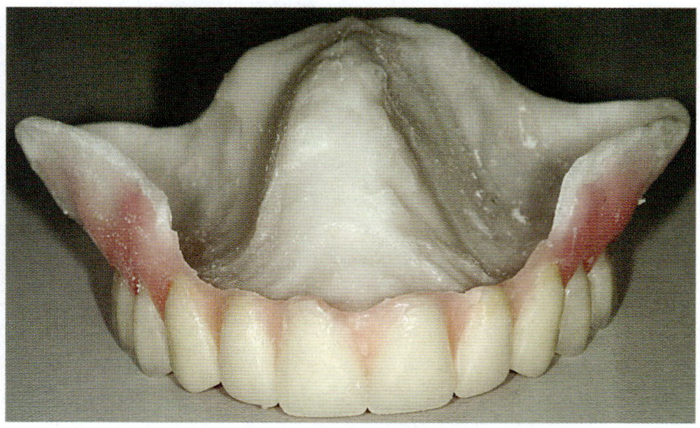

FIGURE 12-59 Patient's diagnostic wax mockup is fabricated without the flange in the anterior sextant.

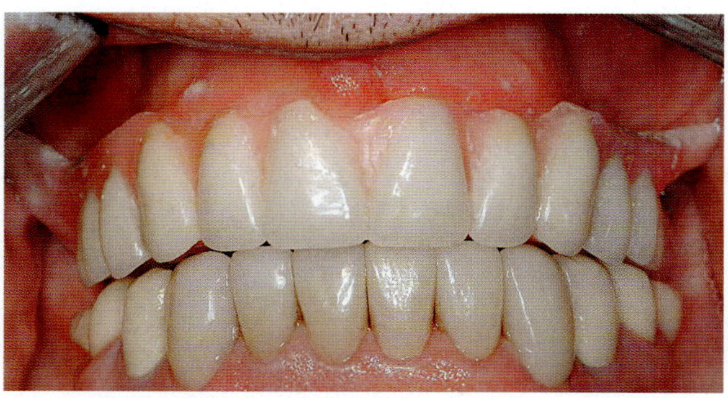

FIGURE 12-60 The cervical portion of the diagnostic teeth rest against the patient's gingival crest, consistent with a tooth-only defect.

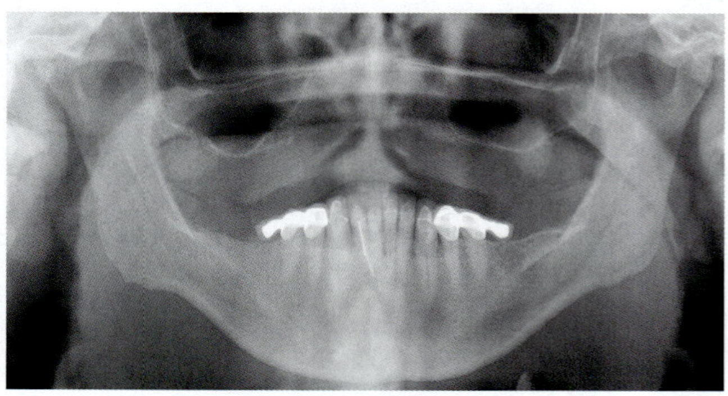

FIGURE 12-61 Evaluation of the zones of the maxilla demonstrates zones I and II. Zone III is missing.

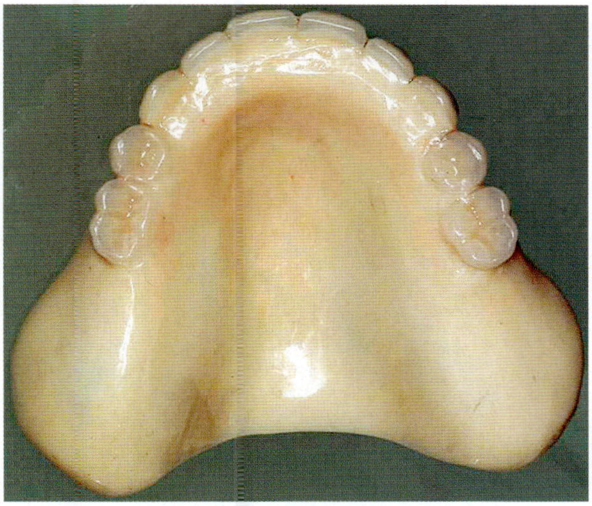

FIGURE 12-62 The immediate-load provisional prosthesis for a tooth-only defect is referred to as a *white denture*.

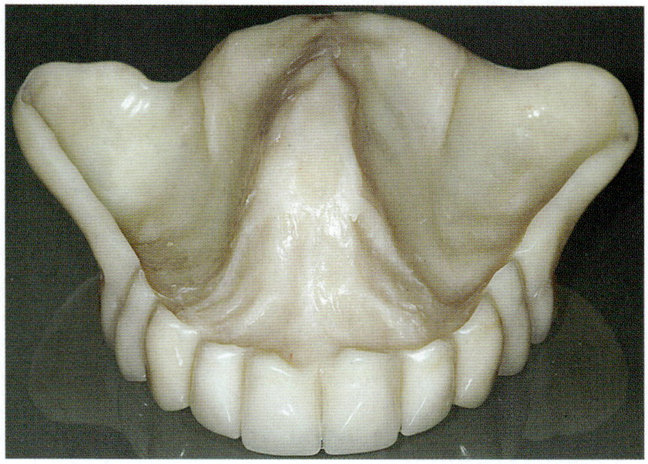

FIGURE 12-63 The palatal portion and posterior flanges of the white denture allow stabilization of the provisional prosthesis during its connection to the temporary cylinders after the implant is placed and the appropriate abutments are secured.

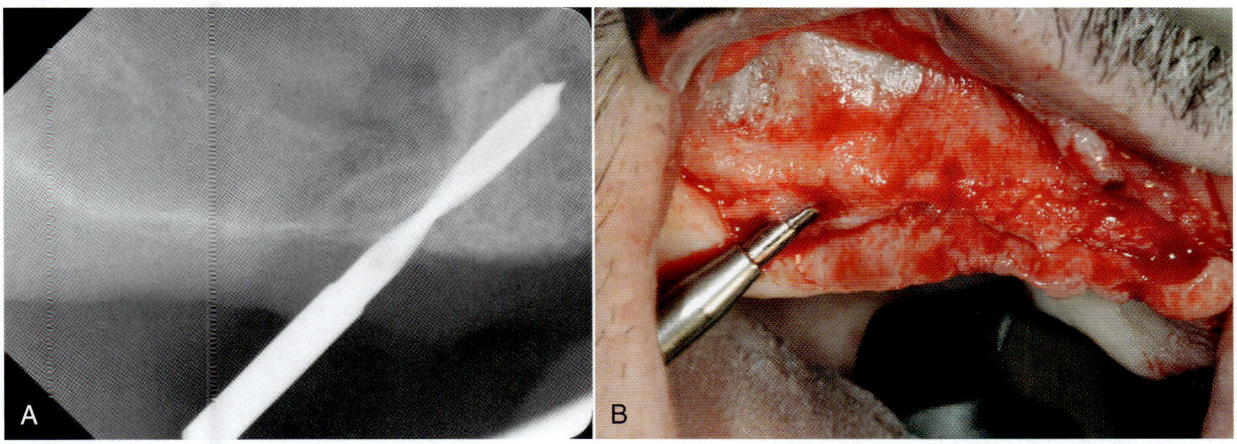

FIGURE 12-64 A, The intraoperative periapical radiograph shows the relationship of the 2-mm drill to the left anterior maxillary sinus wall, confirming favorable angulation of the proposed left posterior tilted implant. B, The right posterior implant is positioned immediately in front of the right anterior maxillary wall.

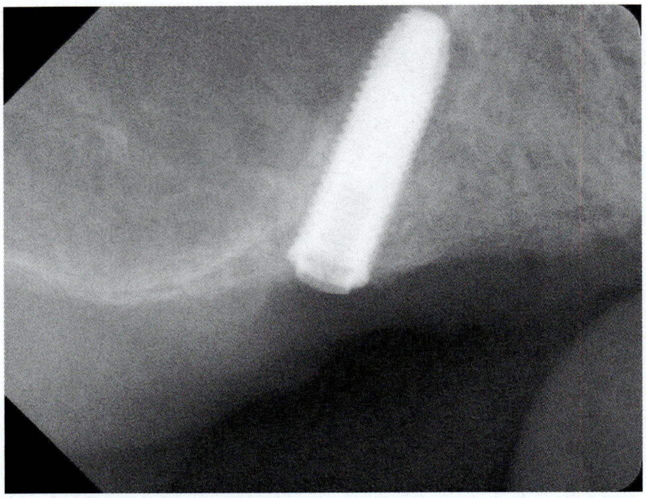

FIGURE 12-65 The final position of the right posterior tilted implant.

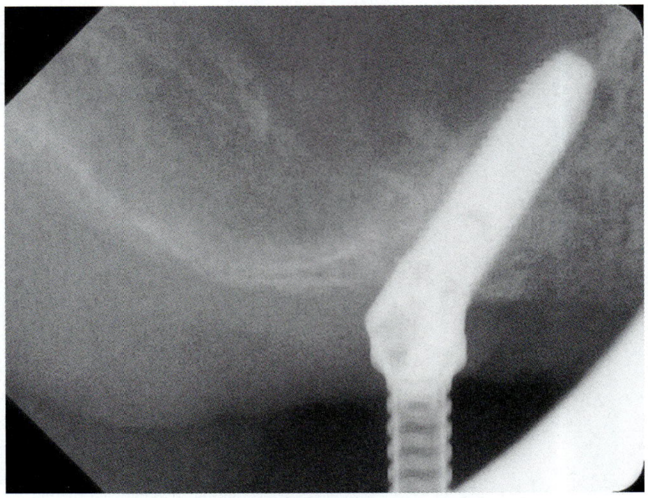

FIGURE 12-66 Complete seating of the 30° angulated multiunit abutment and the titanium cylinder is confirmed.

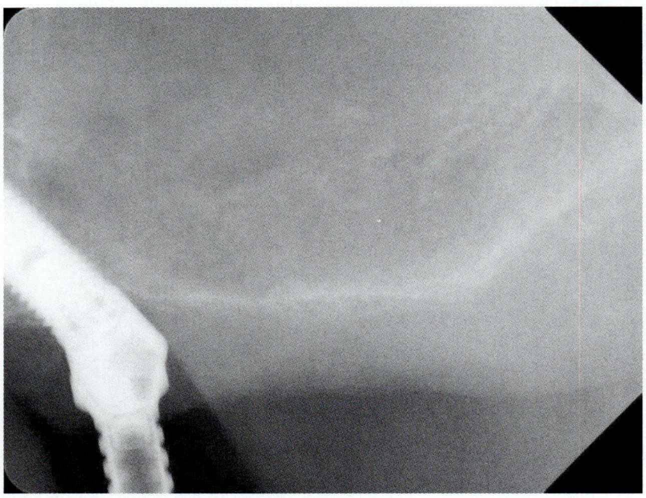

FIGURE 12-67 Complete seating of the 30° angulated multiunit abutment and the titanium temporary cylinder is verified on the left posterior tilted implant.

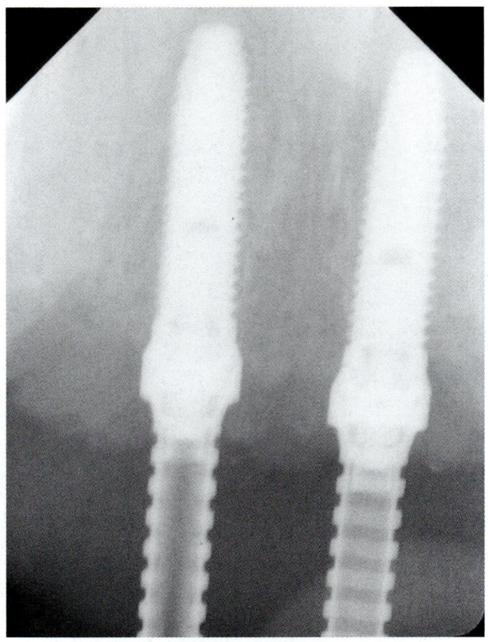

FIGURE 12-68 Complete seating of the temporary titanium cylinders onto the multiunit abutments on the anterior implants is verified before connecting them to the immediate-load prosthesis.

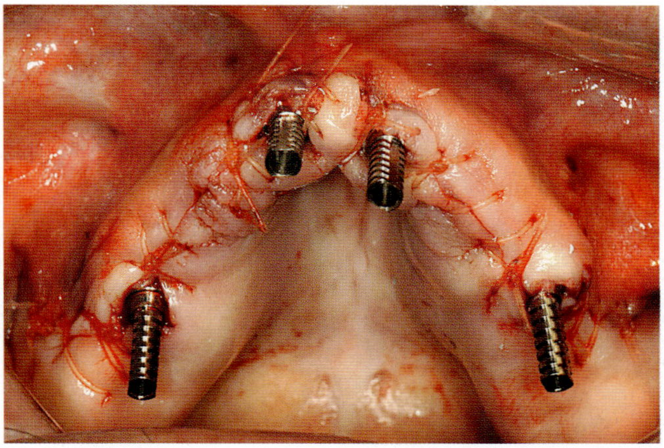

FIGURE 12-69 Temporary titanium cylinders are in place and ready for the conversion protocol.

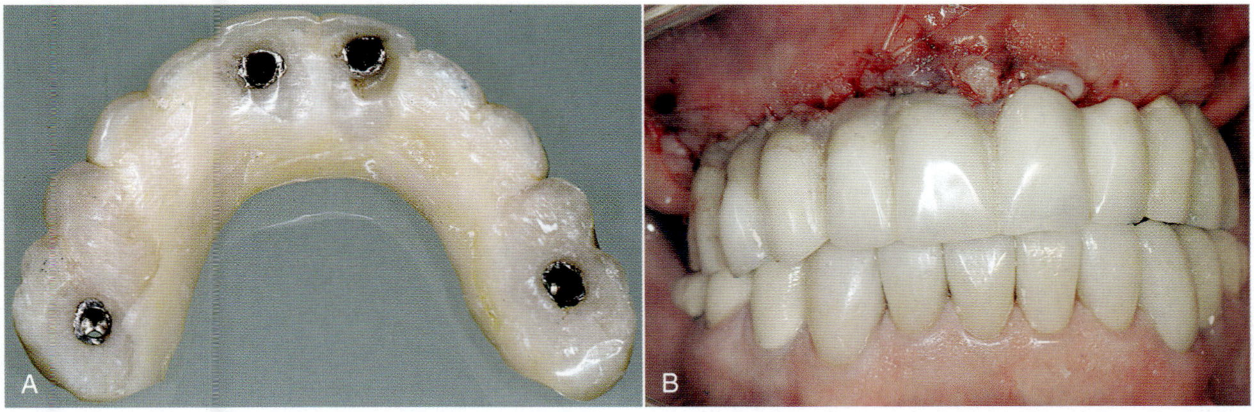

FIGURE 12-70 **A,** Converted provisional prosthesis. **B,** Attachment of the immediate-load prosthesis to the patient.

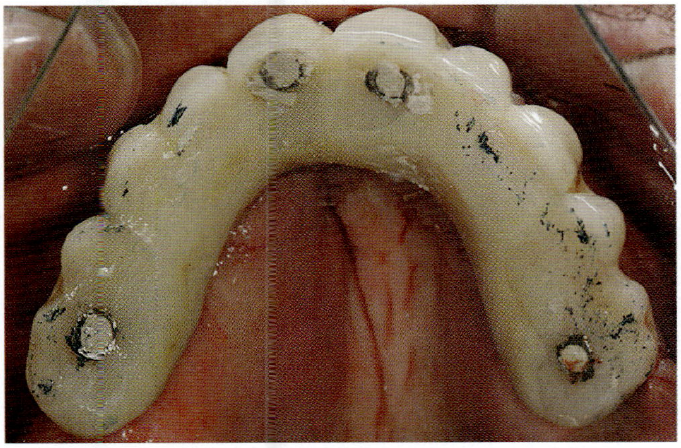

FIGURE 12-71 Bilateral group function.

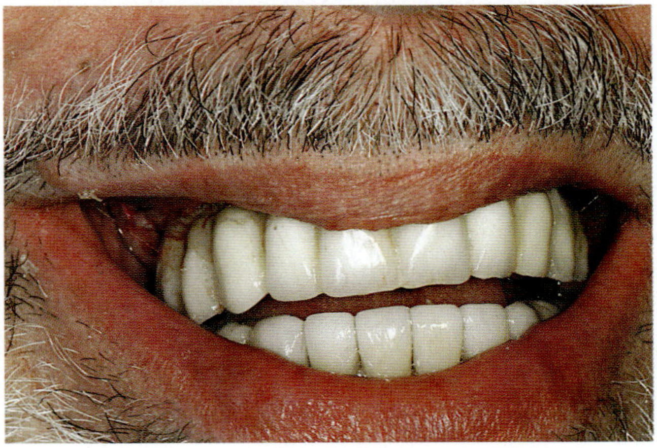

FIGURE 12-72 The hidden transition line allows for an aesthetically pleasing provisional prosthesis.

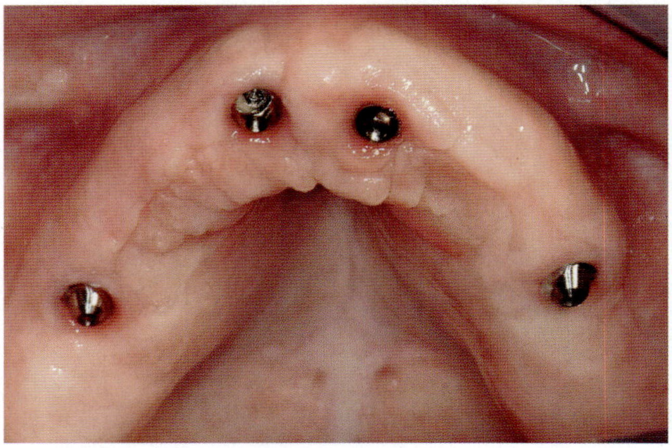

FIGURE 12-73 Evaluation of the implants 6 months after surgery.

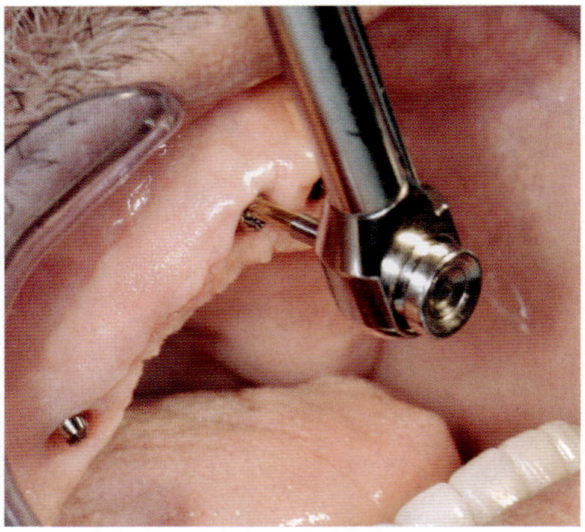

FIGURE 12-74 Touring the abutments prior to taking an impression.

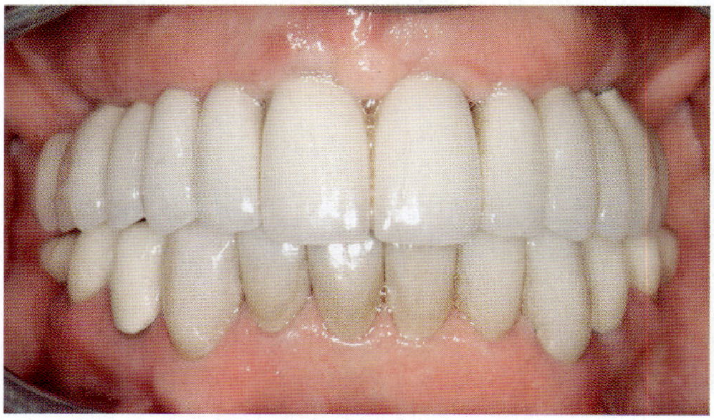

FIGURE 12-75 Completed fixed maxillary prosthesis.

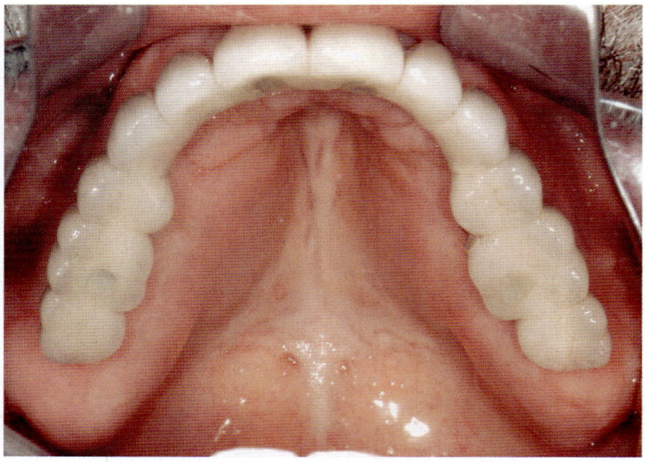

FIGURE 12-76 Occlusal view of the final fixed maxillary prosthesis.

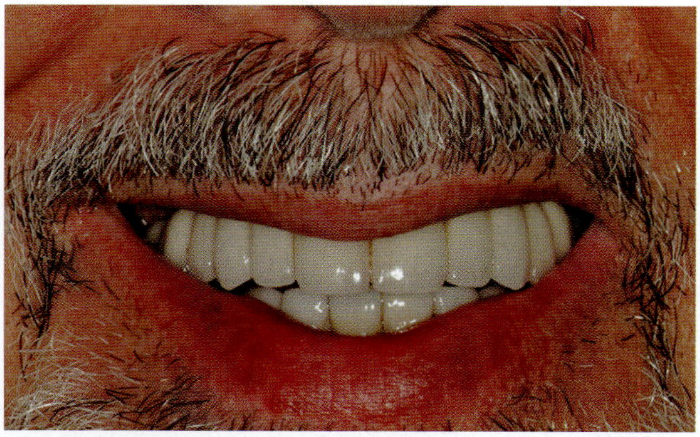

FIGURE 12-77 Aesthetic appearance of the final prosthesis during animation.

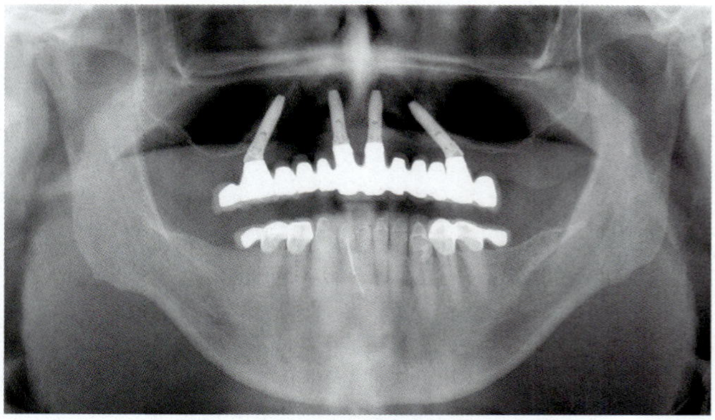

FIGURE 12-78 Final panoramic radiograph showing complete seating of the abutments and the final fixed maxillary prosthesis.

CHAPTER 13

CASE PRESENTATIONS: Immediate-Loading Zygoma Implant

IMMEDIATE-LOAD ZYGOMA PROTOCOL

The zygoma implant is unique because it has an angulated platform as well as two different length diameters. The zygoma concept is considered in patients who have zone I bone only in their edentulous maxilla (Figure 13-1).

Presence of Bone	Surgical Approach
Zones I, II, III	Traditional (axial)
Zones I, II	All-on-4
Zone I	Zygoma implants
Insufficient bone	Quad zygoma

FIGURE 13-1 The zygoma implant is considered when only zone I bone is available in the patient's residual maxillary alveolus.

Zygomatic implant specifications include:

Length: 30, 35, 40, 42.5, 45, 47.5, 50, and 52.5 mm
Platform: 45° angulated
Diameter: 5 mm crestal diameter and 4 mm apical diameter (Figures 13-2 and 13-3)

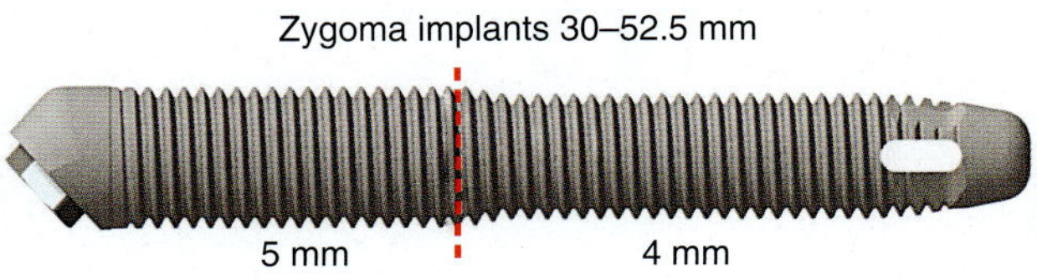

FIGURE 13-2 The zygomatic implant has two distinct diameters: 5 mm at the crest and 4 mm at the apical half. *(Courtesy Nobel Biocare, Yorba Linda, Calif.)*

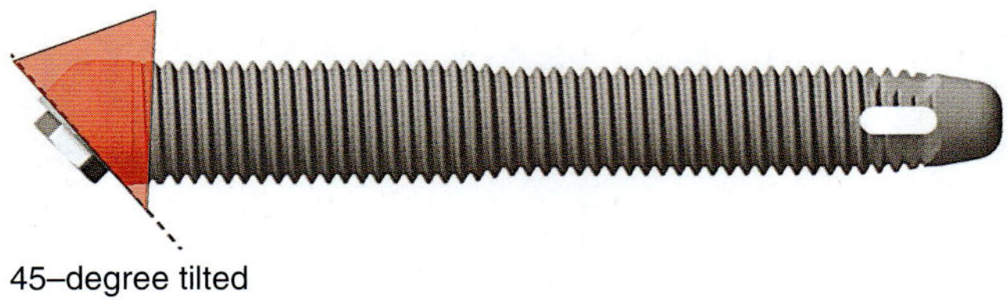

FIGURE 13-3 The implant platform is 45° and the soft tissue cuff is established around this portion of the platform and its corresponding abutment body. *(Courtesy Nobel Biocare, Yorba Linda, Calif.)*

The implant is generally placed between the first and second bicuspid position and is angled approximately 45° posteriorly as it traverses through the maxillary sinus and enters the body of the os zygomaticus. This is the only quad-cortically stabilized implant (Figures 13-4 to 13-6).

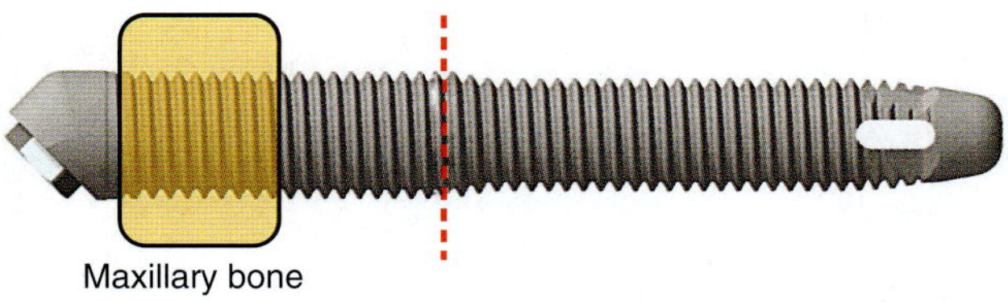

FIGURE 13-4 The crestal portion of the zygomatic implant is usually in 1 to 3 mm of alveolar bone because zones II and III bone is very limited or absent in this group of patients. *(Courtesy Nobel Biocare, Yorba Linda, Calif.)*

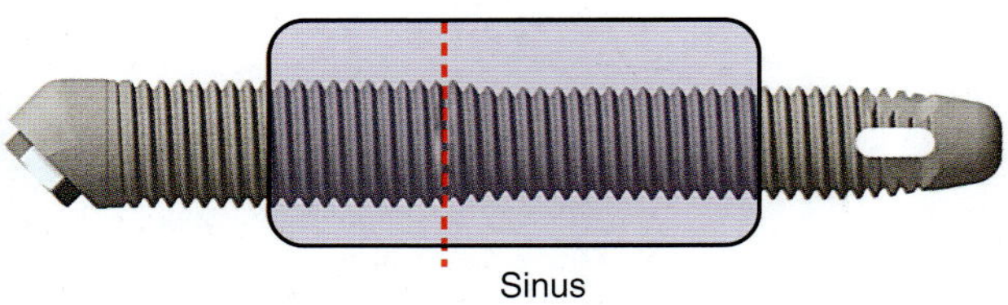

FIGURE 13-5 The majority of the mid-section of the zygomatic implant is traversing through the maxillary sinus without any bony contact. *(Courtesy Nobel Biocare, Yorba Linda, Calif.)*

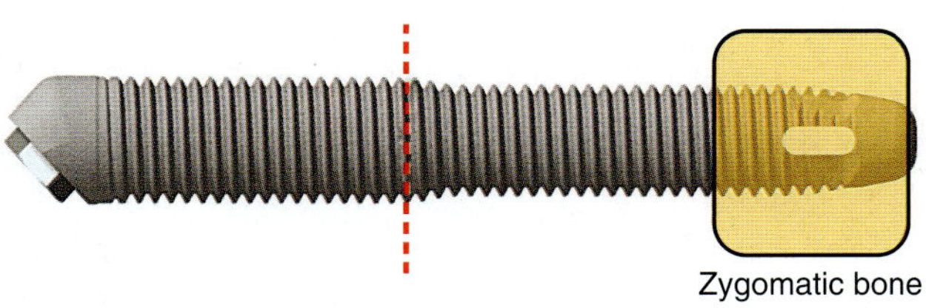

FIGURE 13-6 The apical portion of the implant is in approximately 4 to 10 mm of bone as it travels through the body of the os zygomaticus. *(Courtesy Nobel Biocare, Yorba Linda, Calif.)*

The four cortices include:

1. Maxillary lingual plate
2. Maxillary sinus floor
3. Maxillary sinus roof
4. lateral cortex of the os zygomaticus body (Figure 13-7)

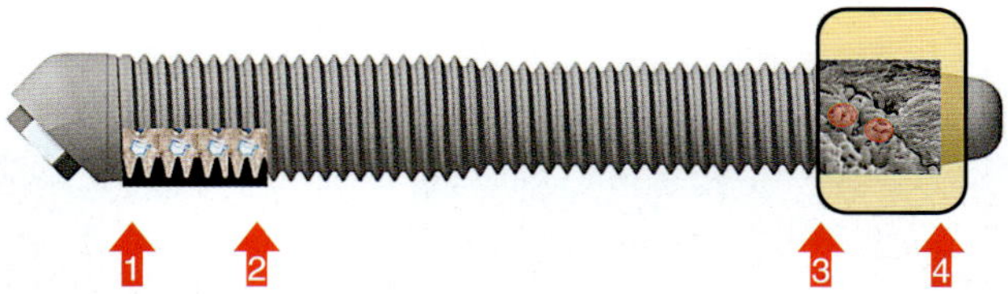

FIGURE 13-7 The quad-cortical stabilization of the zygomatic implants are at points 1, 2, 3, and 4. *(Courtesy Nobel Biocare, Yorba Linda, Calif.)*

Drill sizes include:

1. Round drill
2. 2.9 mm drill
3. 2.9- or 3.5-mm pilot drill
4. 3.5-mm drill
5. 4.2-mm drill (Figures 13-8 and 13-9)

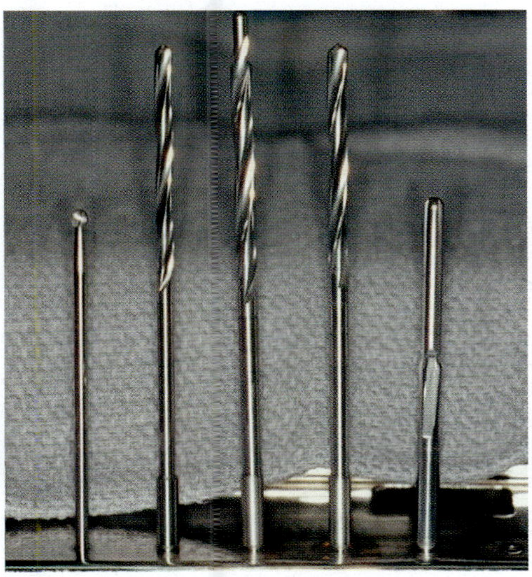

FIGURE 13-8 The drills have long shafts to allow access through the maxillary sinus and preparation of the osteotomy within the body of the os zygomaticus. Slightly shorter versions of the drills are also available.

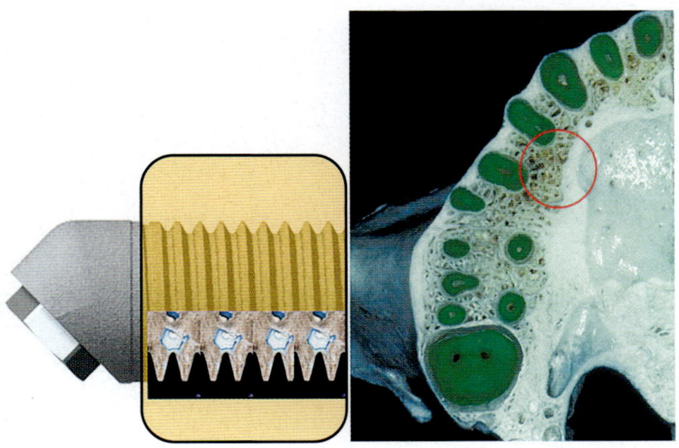

FIGURE 13-9 The crestal osteotomy is initiated between the first and second maxillary bicuspid region. *(Courtesy Nobel Biocare, Yorba Linda, Calif.)*

The three potential trajectories are:

1. Improper anterior position of the apical portion resulting in perforation into the orbit
2. Proper position of the apical portion of the implant within the body of the os zygomaticus
3. Improper posterior position of the apical position of the implant resulting in perforation of the posterior aspect of the os zygomaticus body into the infratemporal fossa (Figures 13-10 to 13-20)

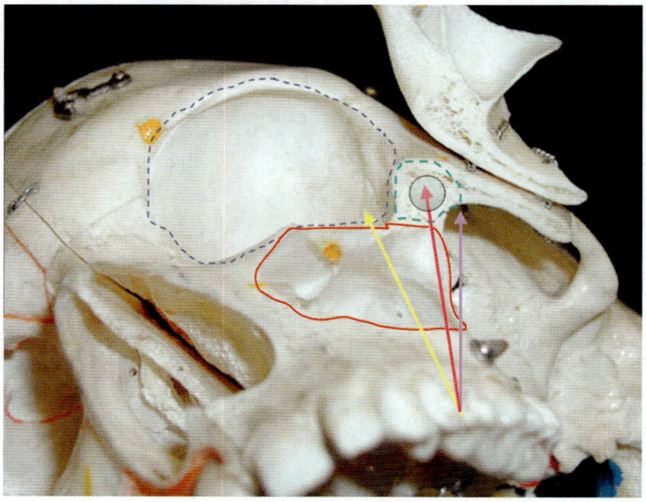

FIGURE 13-10 The *colored lines* represent the three trajectories of the zygomatic implant. The only proper trajectory is represented by the *red line*, placing the apex of the implant within the body of the os zygomaticus.

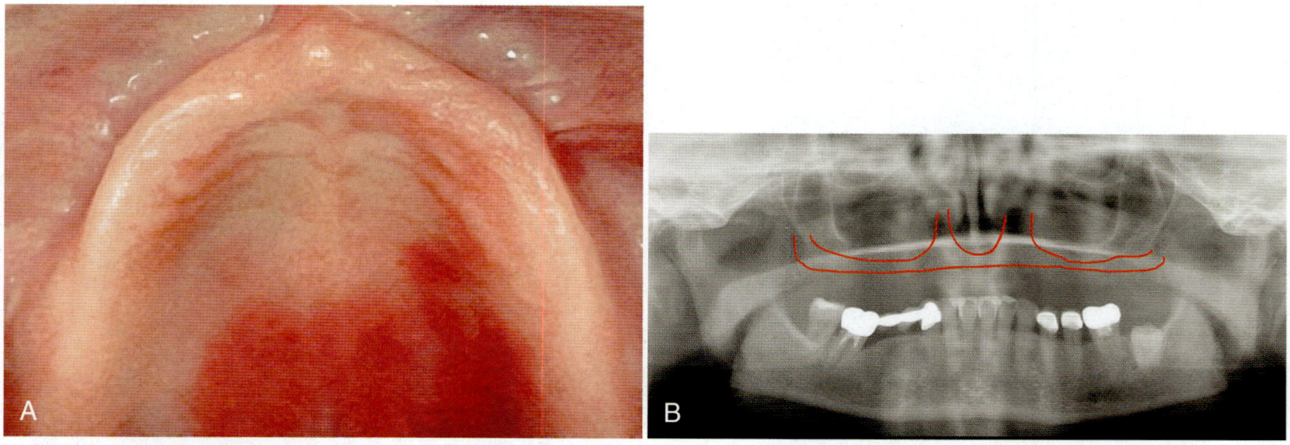

FIGURE 13-11 **A,** Shallow palatal vault and buccal vestibule are common in moderate to severely resorbed edentulous maxillae. **B,** Presence of zone I bone only is evident on the panoramic radiograph.

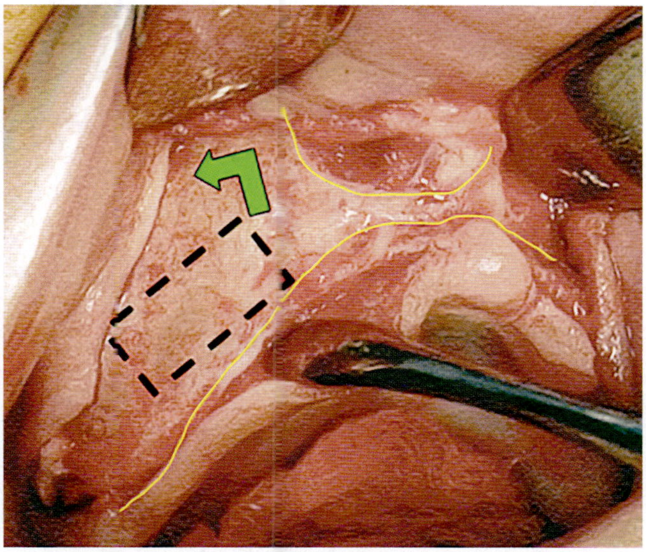

FIGURE 13-12 A full-thickness mucoperiosteal flap is raised, exposing the lateral maxillary wall. A modified sinus opening is made.

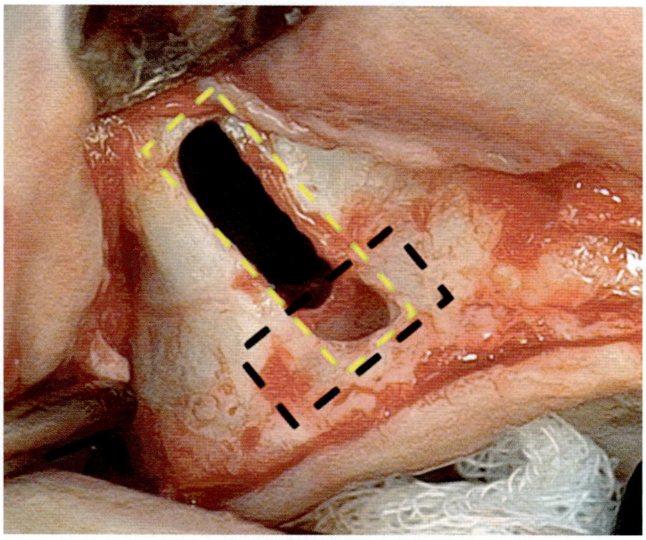

FIGURE 13-13 The sinus window made through the lateral wall of the maxillary sinus is established with a 90° counterclockwise rotation as compared with the outline made for a conventional sinus lift procedure.

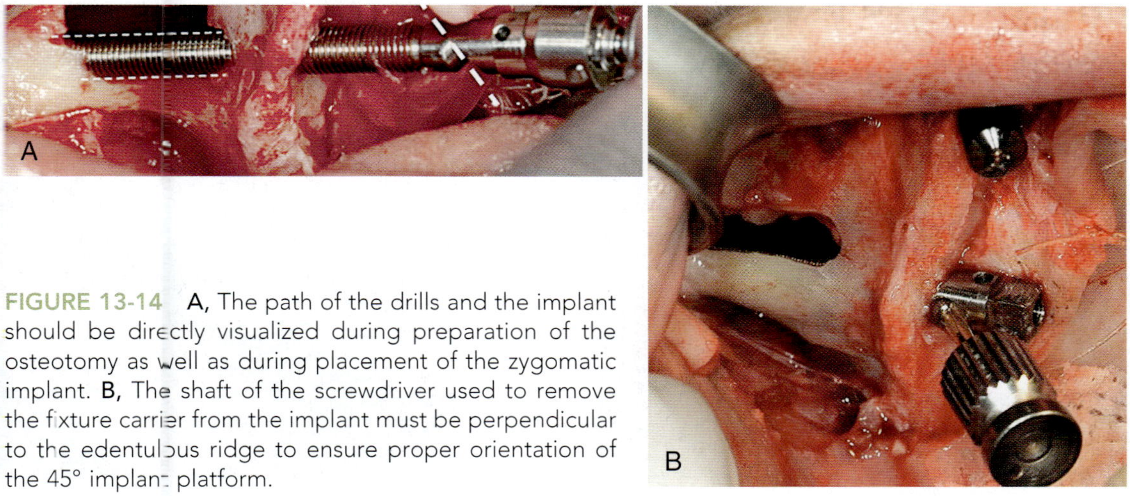

FIGURE 13-14 A, The path of the drills and the implant should be directly visualized during preparation of the osteotomy as well as during placement of the zygomatic implant. B, The shaft of the screwdriver used to remove the fixture carrier from the implant must be perpendicular to the edentulous ridge to ensure proper orientation of the 45° implant platform.

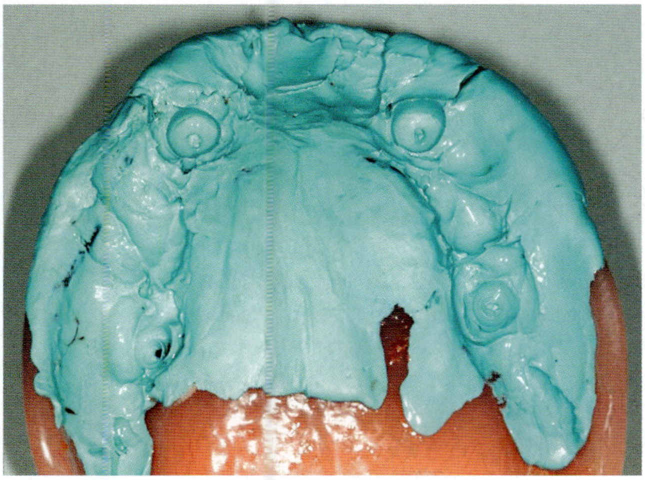

FIGURE 13-15 Indexing the denture with polyvinylsiloxane registration paste, allowing the transfer of the abutment positions onto the intaglio surface of the denture.

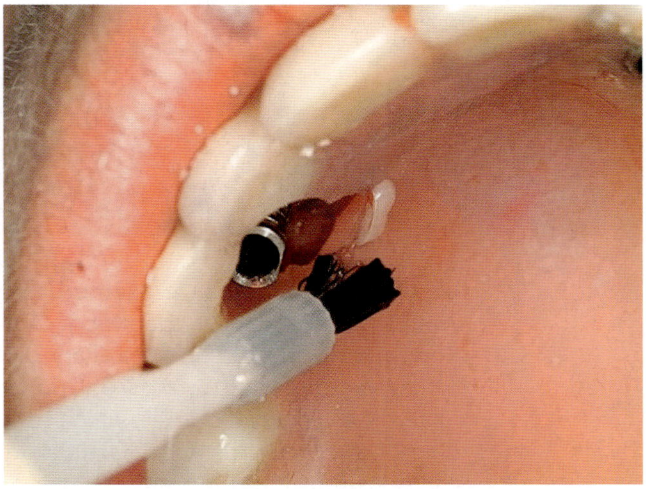

FIGURE 13-16 Luting the temporary titanium cylinders to the denture base using fast-setting acrylic.

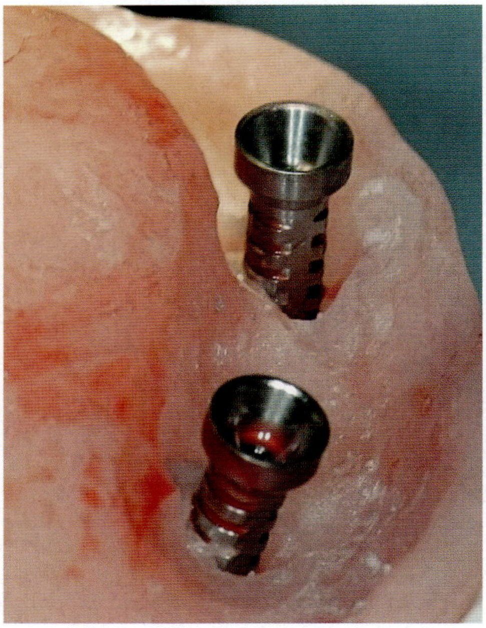

FIGURE 13-17 Luting the intaglio surface of the denture base to the titanium cylinders.

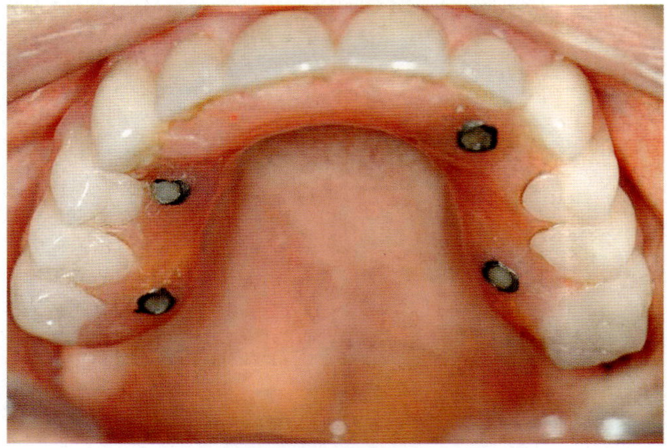

FIGURE 13-18 The immediate-load prosthesis 1 week after surgery.

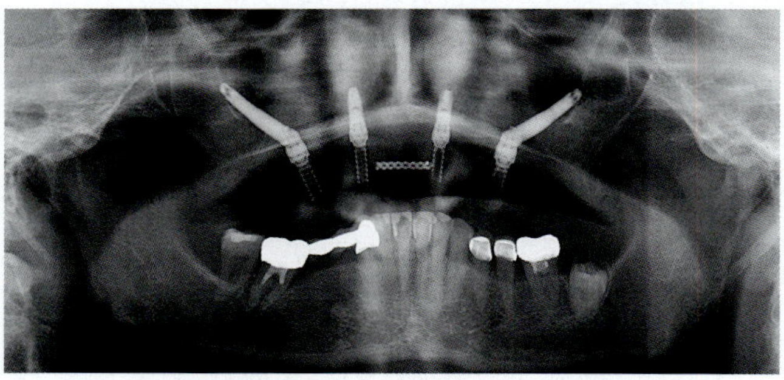

FIGURE 13-19 Postoperative panoramic radiograph of the immediate-load maxillary prosthesis supported by two premaxillary implants and two zygoma implants for posterior support.

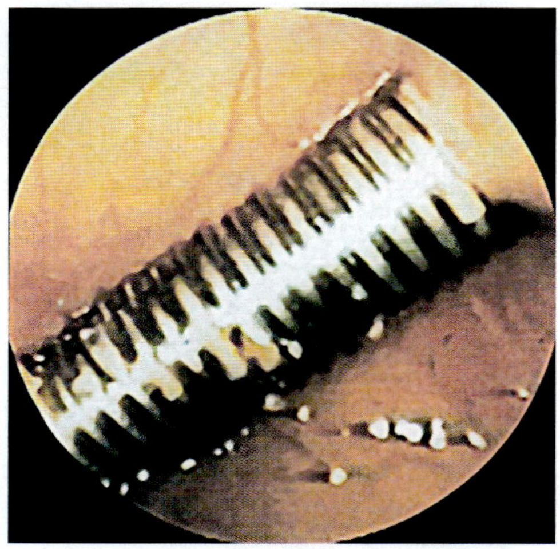

FIGURE 13-20 Endoscopic evaluation of the mid-portion of the zygomatic implant within the maxillary sinus demonstrates no adverse reaction of the Schneiderian membrane.

ZYGOMA CONCEPT: IMMEDIATE LOADING OF FAILING EXISTING TEETH AND IMPLANTS

A 47-year-old woman presented with failing implants at positions 6 and 10 as well as failing maxillary dentition. Clinical examination revealed asymmetric bone loss around the existing maxillary dentition and the presence of peri-implantitis of implant numbers 6 and 10. During animation, the patient displayed her maxillary-free gingival contour, which had to be considered in planning the transition line of the final prosthesis. Evaluation of the preoperative panoramic radiograph demonstrated zones I and II bone and limited zone III bone in the posterior maxilla (Figures 13-21 to 13-23).

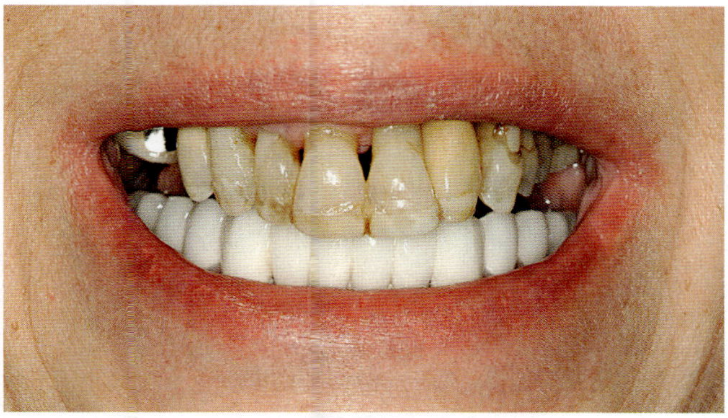

FIGURE 13-21 During animation the patient's maxillary free gingival margin is visible.

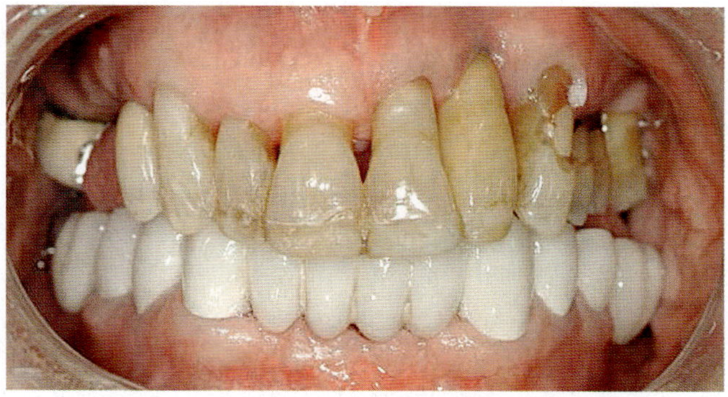

FIGURE 13-22 Uneven contour of the soft and hard tissues of the anterior maxilla indicates that an alveolectomy is appropriate to reposition the transition line after removal of the teeth and implants.

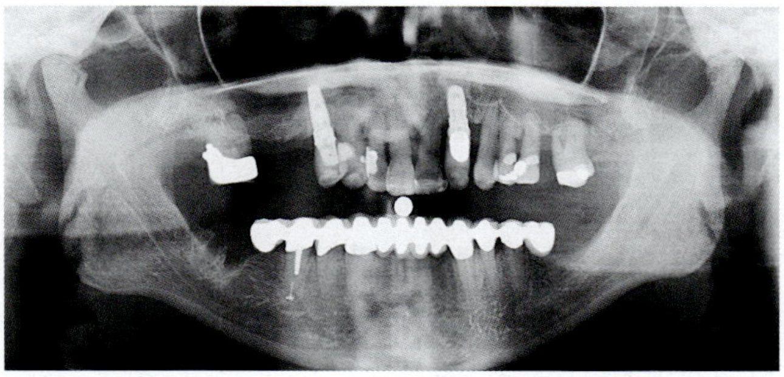

FIGURE 13-23 Preoperative panoramic radiograph demonstrates bone in zones I and II. Minimal zone III bone is available.

Treatment planning considerations include:

1. Removal of the existing maxillary teeth and failing implants
2. Maxillary alveolectomy to reposition the transition line apically
3. Immediate implant placement using the zygoma treatment concept
4. Conversion of a full maxillary denture into an immediate-load provisional prosthesis
5. Fabrication of a final metal-based profile prosthesis

After reflection of a full-thickness mucoperiosteal flap, the appropriate level of alveolectomy was evaluated before the existing teeth and implants were removed. Implant numbers 6 and 10 were trephined carefully. After removal of the maxillary teeth, an alveolectomy of the maxilla to create an even crestal topography was made. Two premaxillary implants and a single zygoma implant were placed. The full maxillary denture was converted to a provisional, immediate-load profile prosthesis. The immediate postoperative appearance of the smile line was aesthetically acceptable (Figures 13-24 to 13-29).

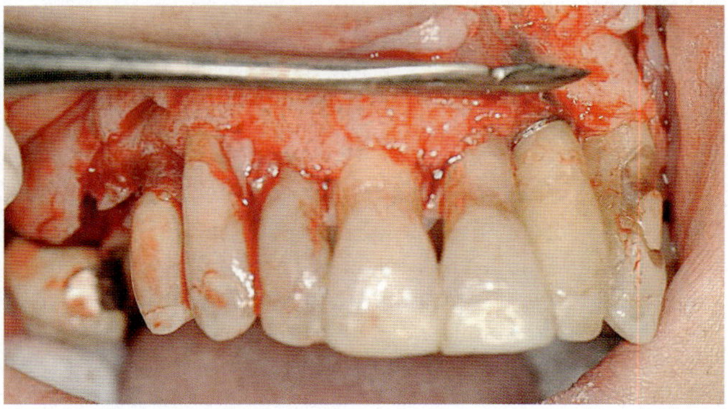

FIGURE 13-24 Prior to removal of the teeth, the appropriate level of alveolectomy is planned.

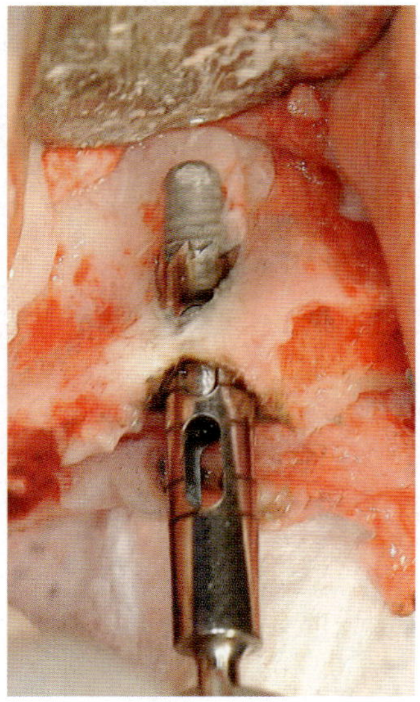

FIGURE 13-25 Trephining the failing implants is completed with minimal bone removal.

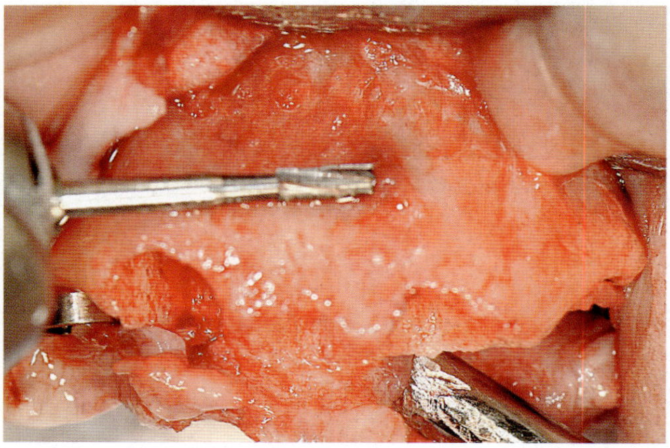

FIGURE 13-26 Alveolectomy of the premaxilla after removal of the teeth and failing implants is completed.

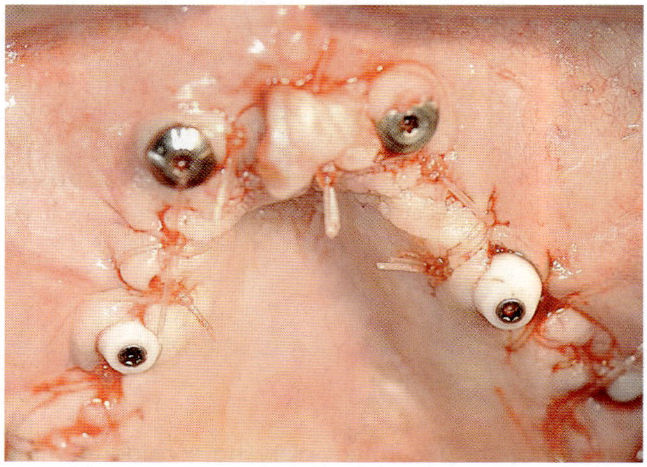

FIGURE 13-27 Soft tissue closure after placement of two premaxillary implants and two zygomatic implants.

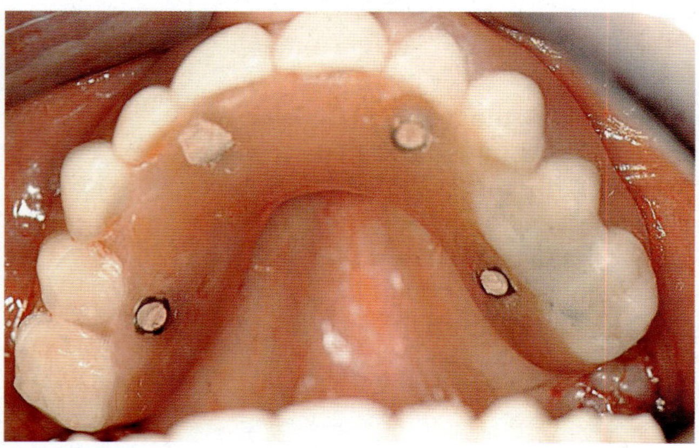

FIGURE 13-28 Conversion of the preoperative full upper denture into a provisional prosthesis is completed.

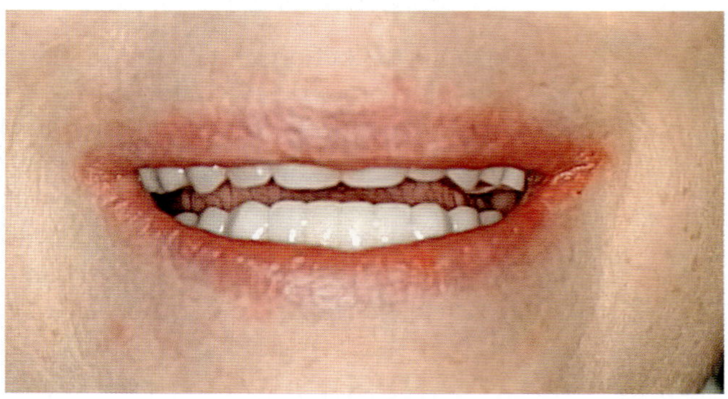

FIGURE 13-29 An aesthetically acceptable smile line is apparent immediately after surgery.

After the 6-month osseointegration period, the final profile prosthesis was fabricated. During animation, the patient was very satisfied with the aesthetic smile line and the filling of the buccal corridors. The final panoramic radiograph demonstrated complete seating of all components and will serve as the baseline radiograph to monitor the patient's progress in the future (Figures 13-30 to 13-32).

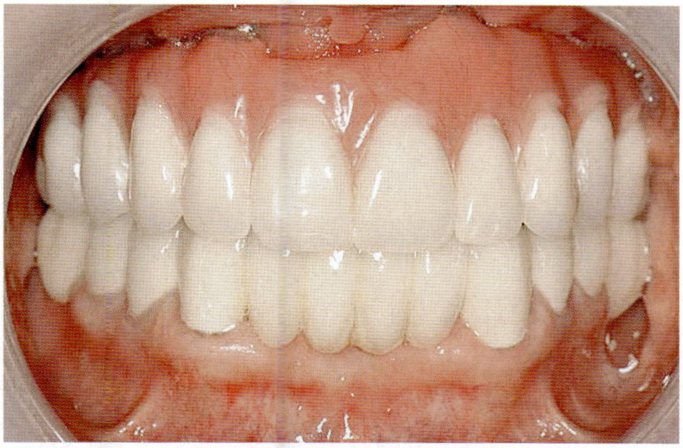

FIGURE 13-30 The completed final metal-based profile prosthesis.

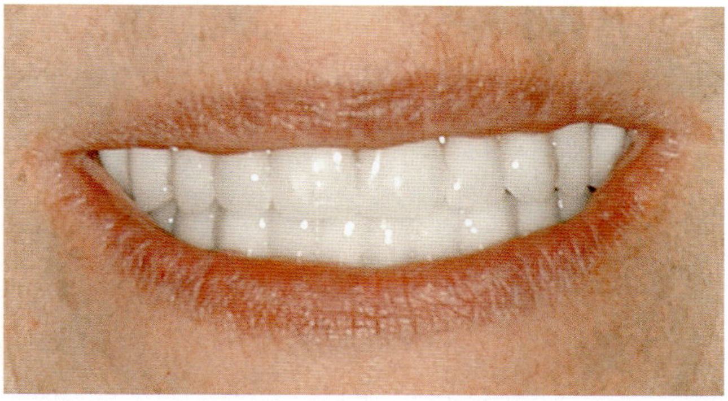

FIGURE 13-31 An aesthetically acceptable smile line with the hidden transition line.

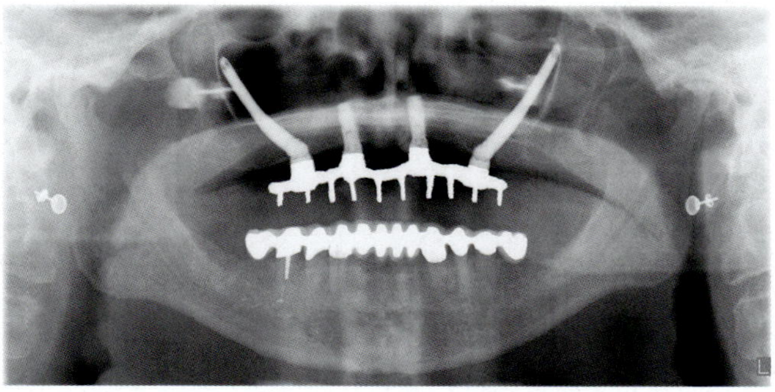

FIGURE 13-32 Final panoramic radiograph taken after delivery of the definitive profile prosthesis.

GUIDED ZYGOMA

A 34-year-old woman presented with a completely edentulous maxilla and a partially edentulous mandible. Her chief complaint was the inability to function with her newly fabricated full upper denture. After evaluation of the denture, it was determined that she would benefit from an implant-supported maxillary profile prosthesis. Her shallow maxillary vault and the presence of zone I bone only suggested that the Zygoma treatment concept was appropriate to support her final prosthesis (Figures 13-33 and 13-34).

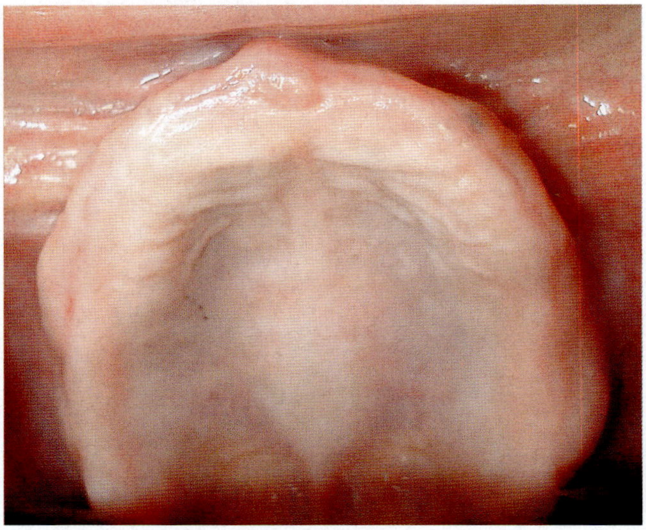

FIGURE 13-33 Preoperative, shallow maxillary vault and vestibule.

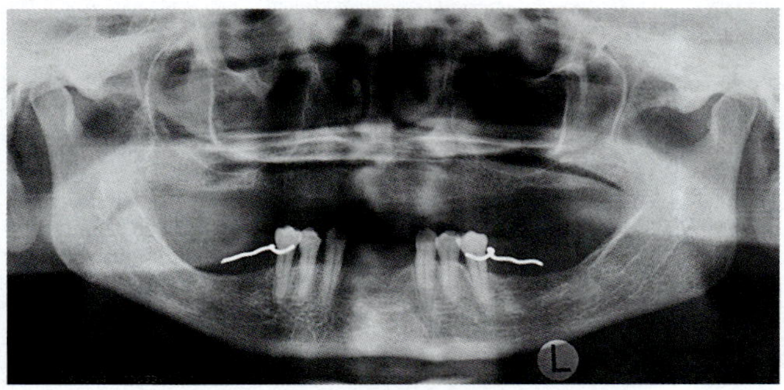

FIGURE 13-34 Preoperative pantomograph demonstrating zone I bone only in the maxilla.

After the dual-scan NobelGuide protocol was completed, two premaxillary implants in zone I and two zygoma implants in zone III were virtually placed (Figures 13-35 to 13-45).

Text continued on P. 212.

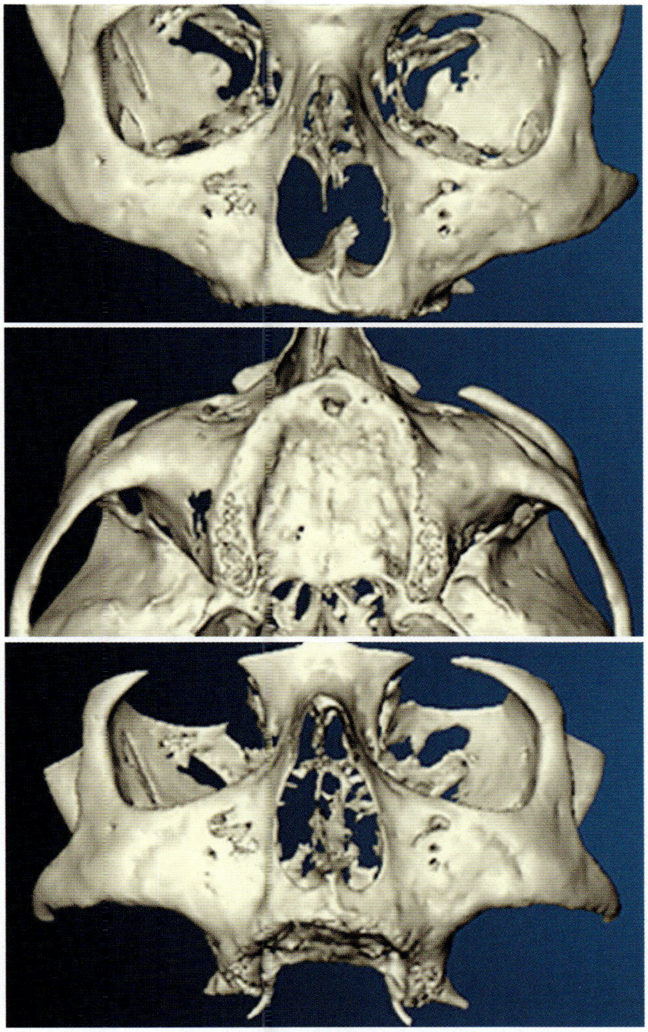

FIGURE 13-35 Three-dimensional imaging of the maxilla.

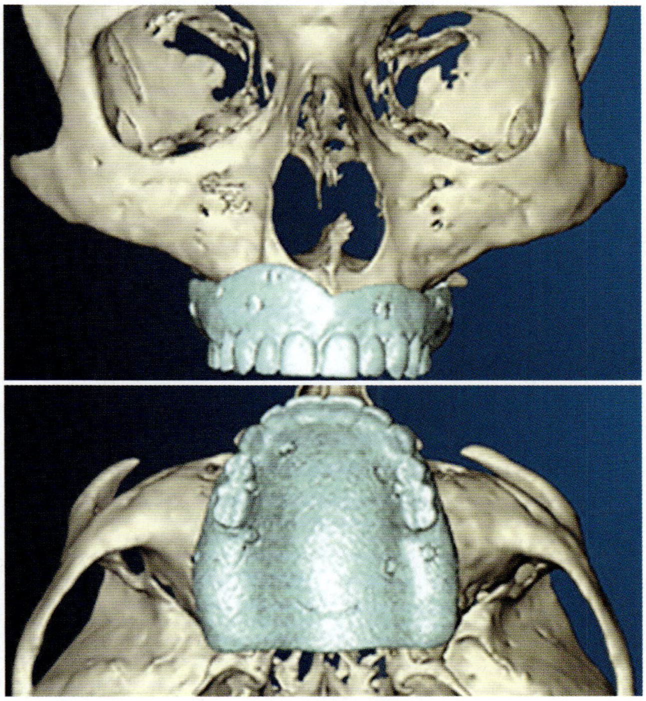

FIGURE 13-36 Three-dimensional imaging of the existing maxillary prosthesis.

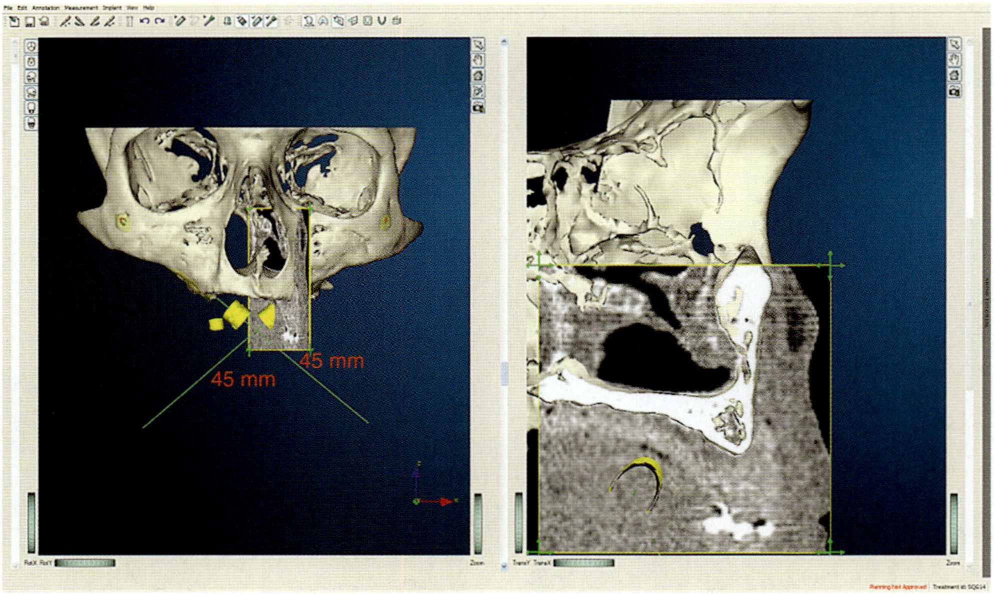

FIGURE 13-37 Evaluation of the width of zone I bone.

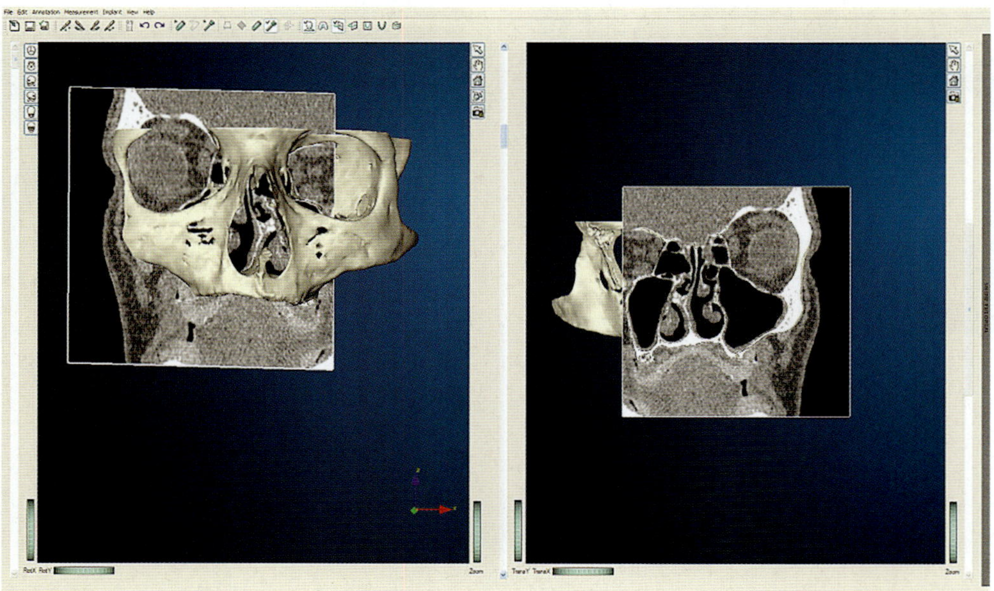

FIGURE 13-38 Evaluation of zone III bone, the maxillary sinus, and the body of the os zygomaticus.

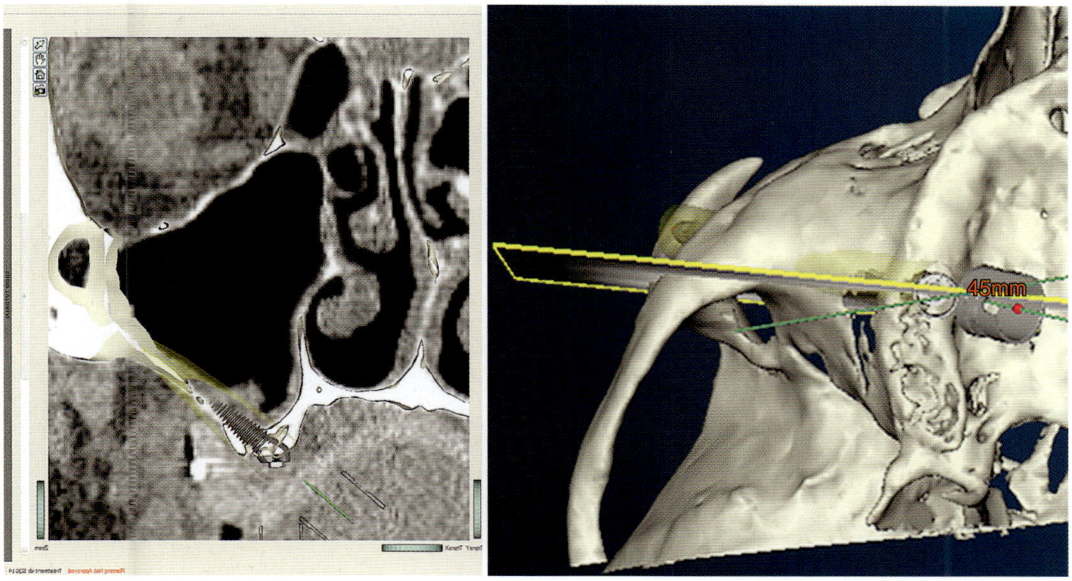

FIGURE 13-39 Virtual planning of the right zygomatic implant.

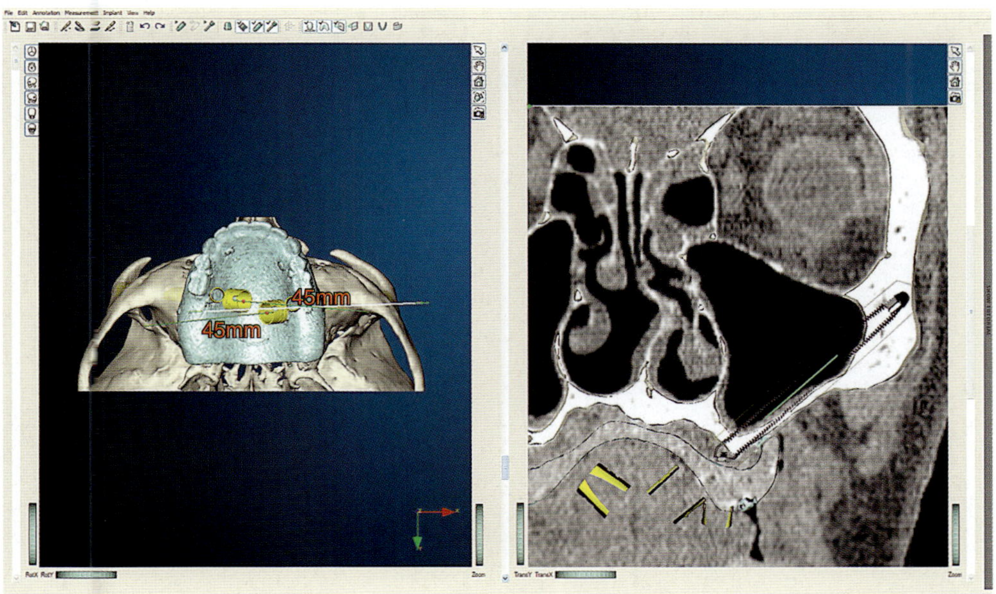

FIGURE 13-40 Virtual planning of the left zygomatic implant.

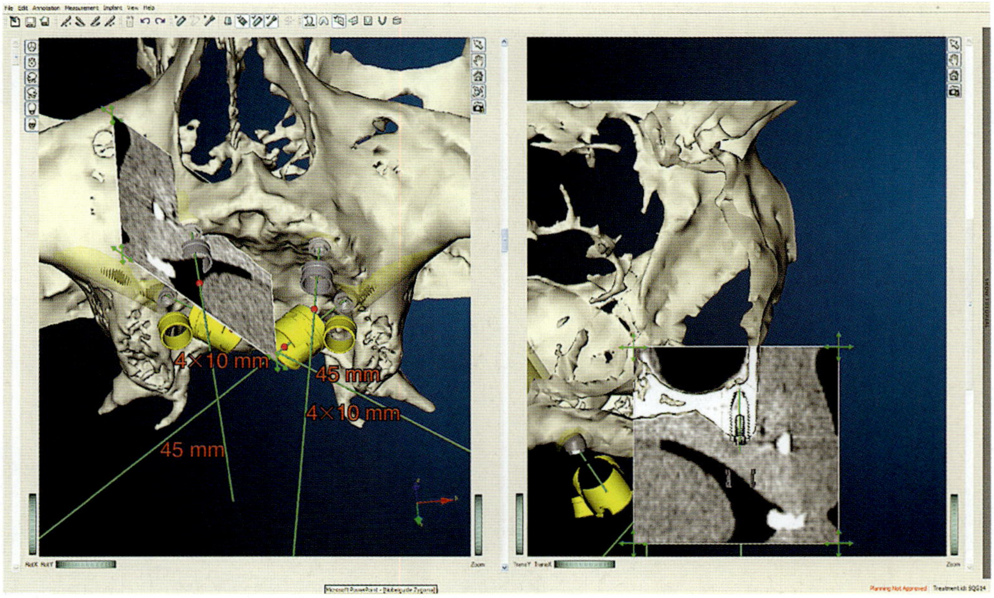

FIGURE 13-41 Virtual planning of the premaxillary implants.

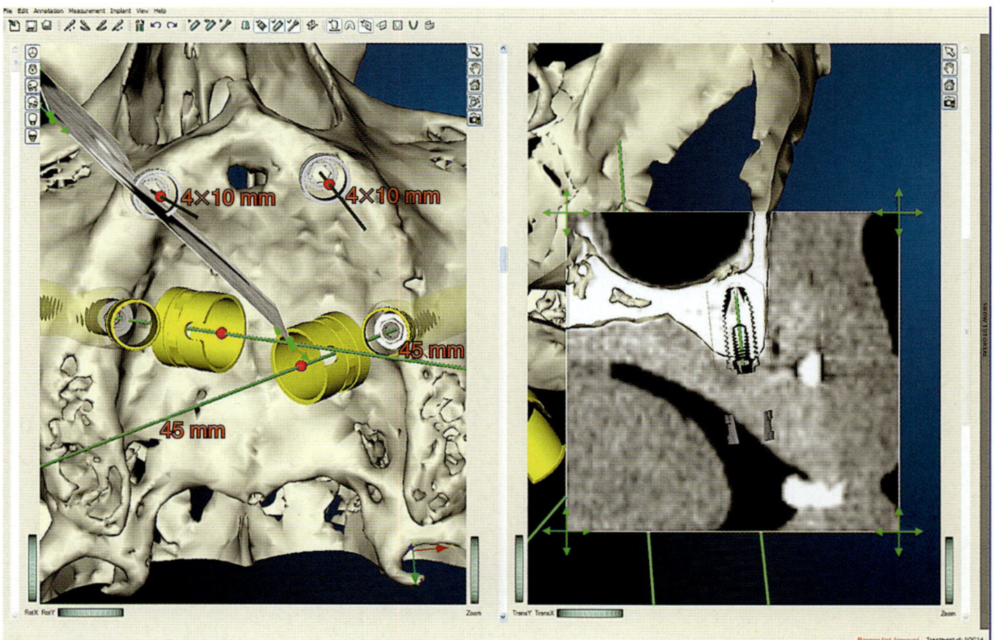

FIGURE 13-42 Confirmation of the properly positioned implant in zone I.

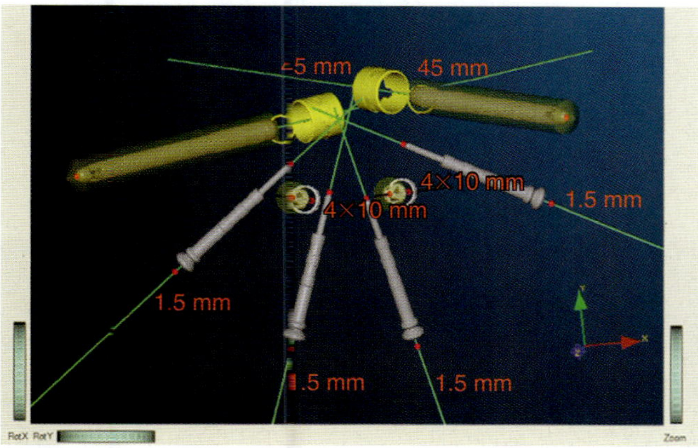

FIGURE 13-43 Confirmation of the lack of "collision" between the planned implants and the fixation pins.

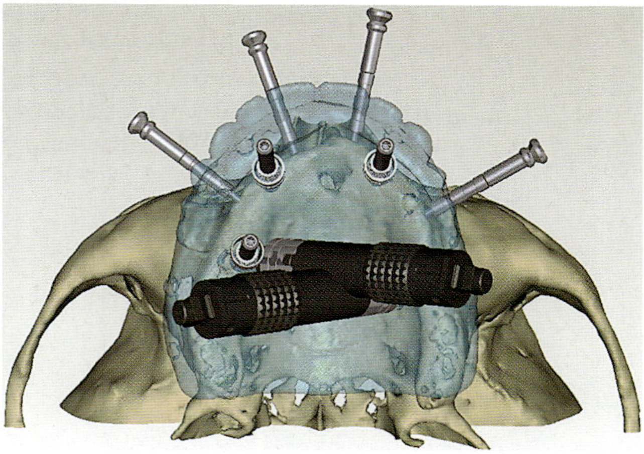

FIGURE 13-44 Virtual presentation of the completed computer-guided zygoma surgical template.

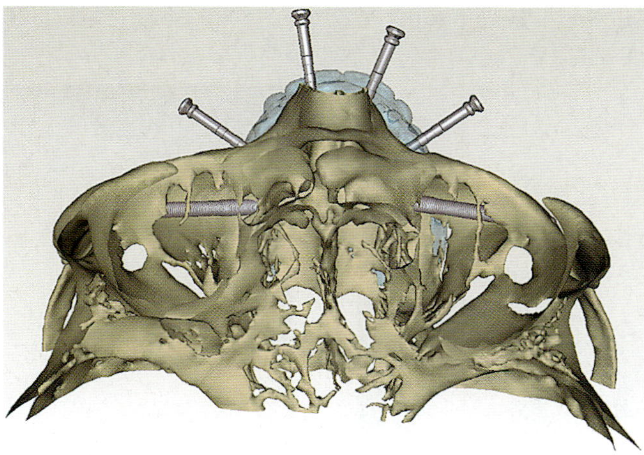

FIGURE 13-45 Virtual evaluation of the zygoma implant trajectory through the maxillary sinuses

After completion of the surgical template, the master cast was fabricated by attaching laboratory analogues to the template. After the master cast was poured, the duplicated denture was used to mount the master cast with the apposing dentition. The immediate-load provisional profile prosthesis was fabricated and, by replacing the profile prosthesis with the surgical template, the surgical bite registration was fabricated and was ready for surgery (Figures 13-46 to 13-50).

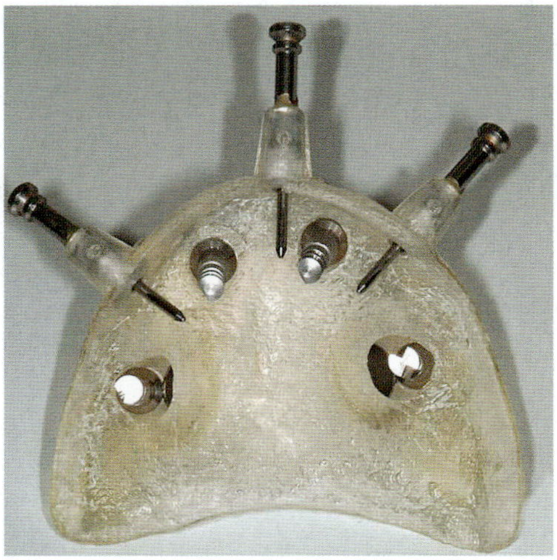

FIGURE 13-46 The completed surgical template with the laboratory fixture level analogues connected.

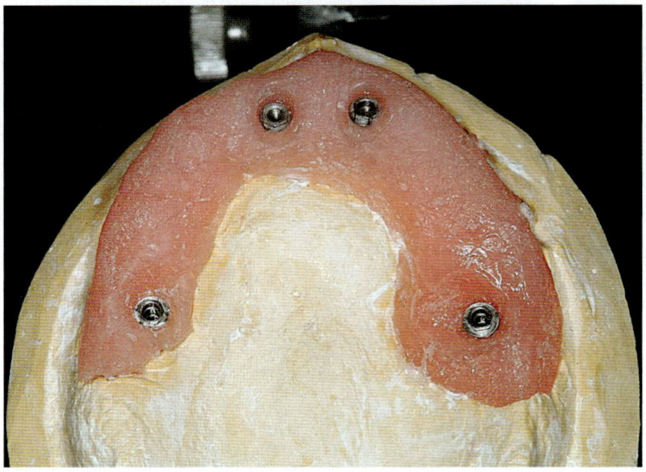

FIGURE 13-47 The completed master cast.

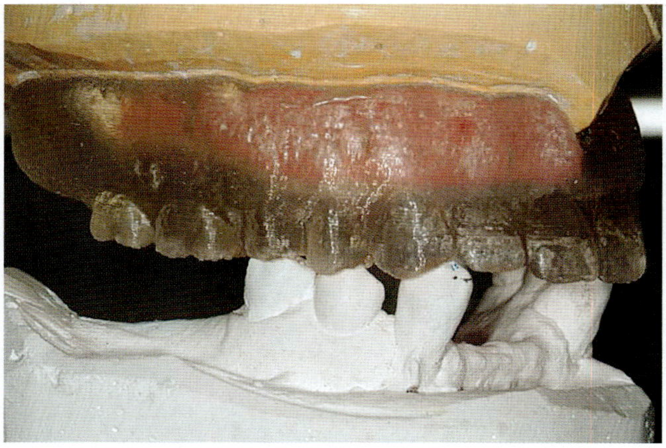

FIGURE 13-48 Mounting the master cast using the duplicated denture.

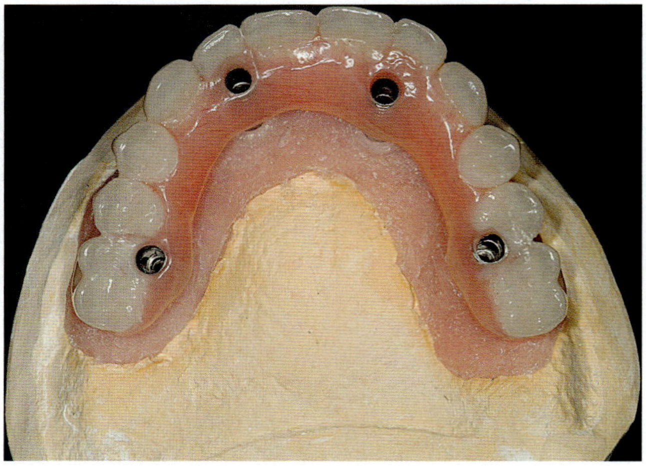

FIGURE 13-49 The completed immediate-load provisional profile prosthesis.

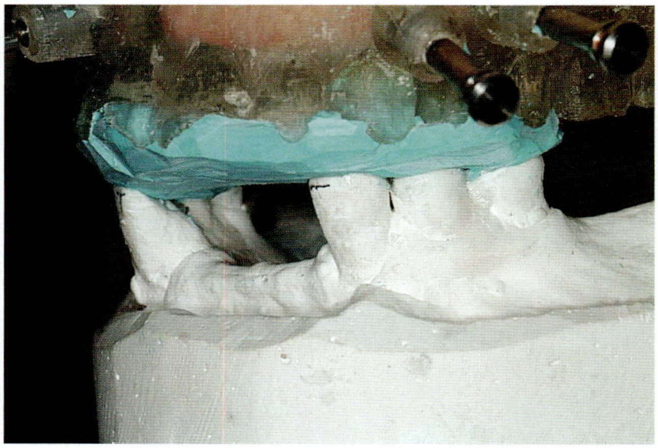

FIGURE 13-50 The surgical bite registration is fabricated.

The surgical bite registration was used to fix the surgical template to the patient's maxilla. After completion of the computer-guided zygoma sequential drilling protocol, the surgical template was removed and the computer-guided technique, which is minimally invasive, demonstrated soft tissue wounds at the implant and the fixation pin sites only. The provisional immediate-load profile prosthesis is connected to the implants using four computer-guided abutments (Figures 13-51 to 13-54).

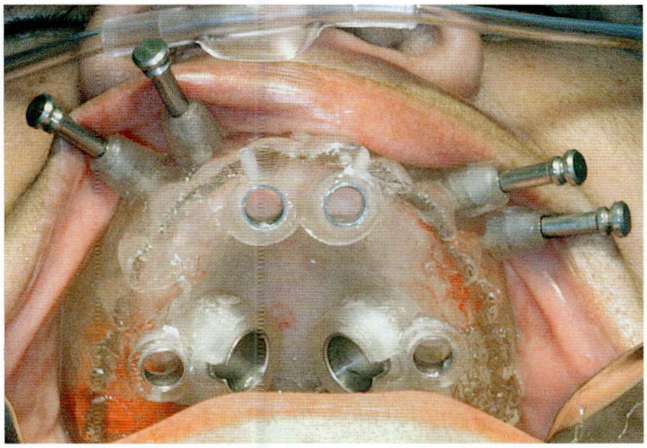

FIGURE 13-51 Seating the surgical template, which duplicates the virtual planning using the surgical bite registration index.

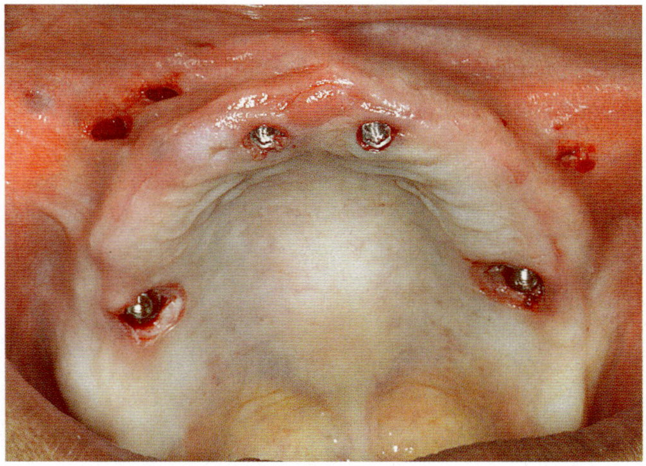

FIGURE 13-52 Completion of the computer-guided zygoma surgical protocol with minimal soft tissue trauma.

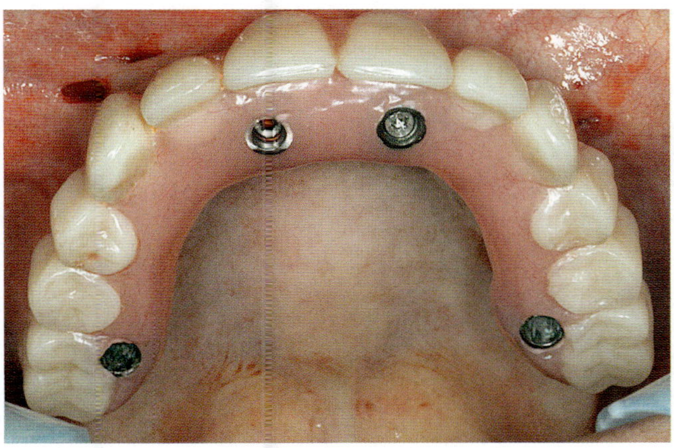

FIGURE 13-53 Connection of the provisional prosthesis using computer-guided abutments.

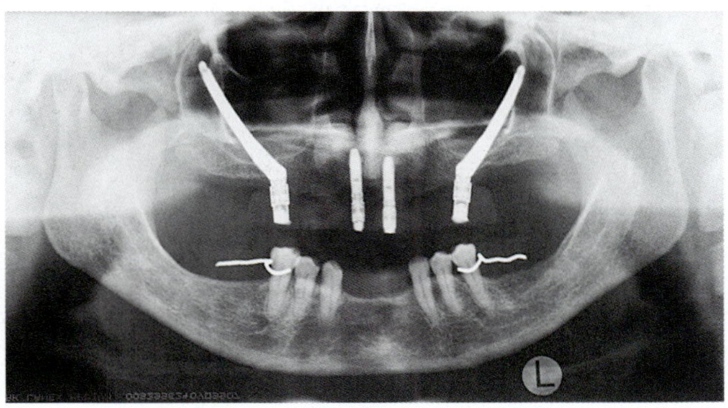

FIGURE 13-54 Postoperative panoramic radiograph confirming complete seating of all components.

After the 6-month osseointegration period, the provisional prosthesis was removed and osseointegration was confirmed using resonance frequency analysis and reverse-torquing the implants. To simplify fabrication of the final prosthesis, the guided abutments were replaced using standard multiunit abutments. After connecting the multiunit abutments to the anterior implants and torquing them to 35 Ncm, the two anterior temporary titanium cylinders were trephined from the provisional prosthesis and replaced with multiunit temporary cylinders. The same replacement protocol was followed for the posterior zygoma implants by first connecting and torquing two zygoma multiunit abutments and trephining and replacing the temporary cylinders (Figures 13-55 to 13-59).

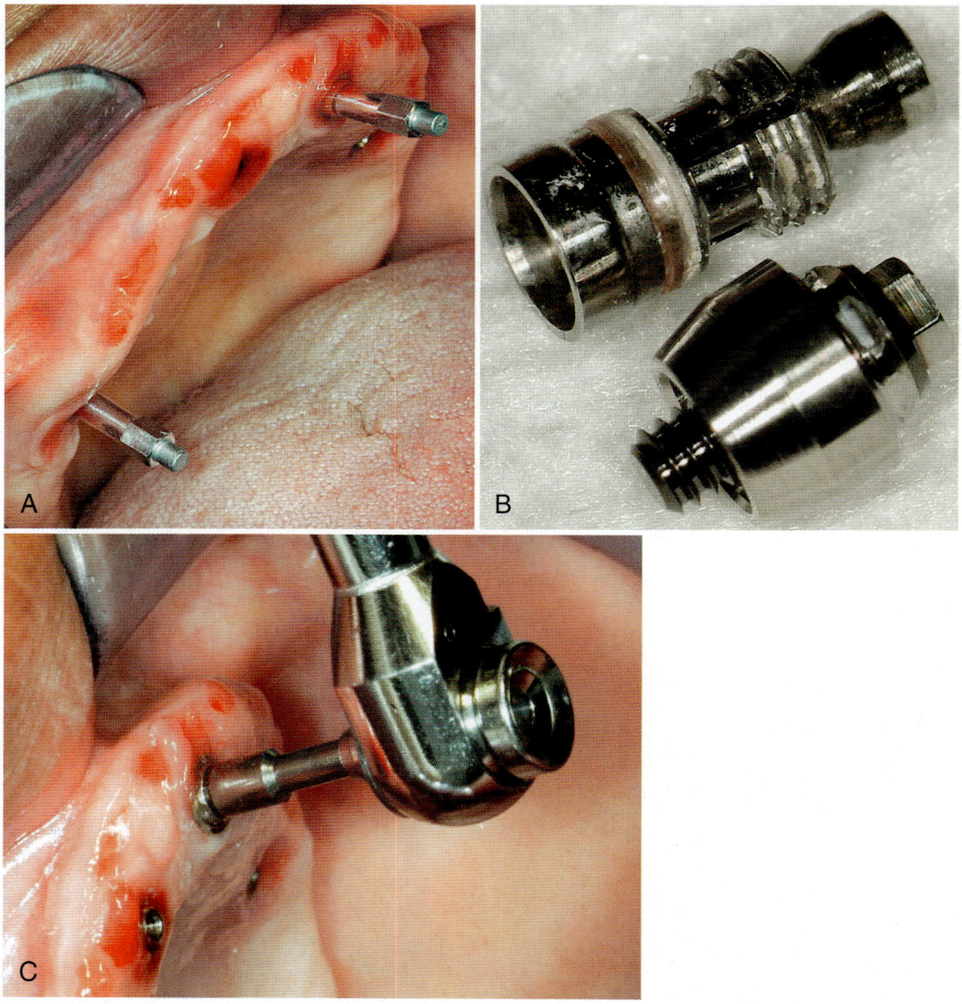

FIGURE 13-55 Recording the implant stability quotient values of the implants at the phase II appointment. The existing computer-guided abutments are replaced by multiunit abutments and torqued to 35 Ncm.

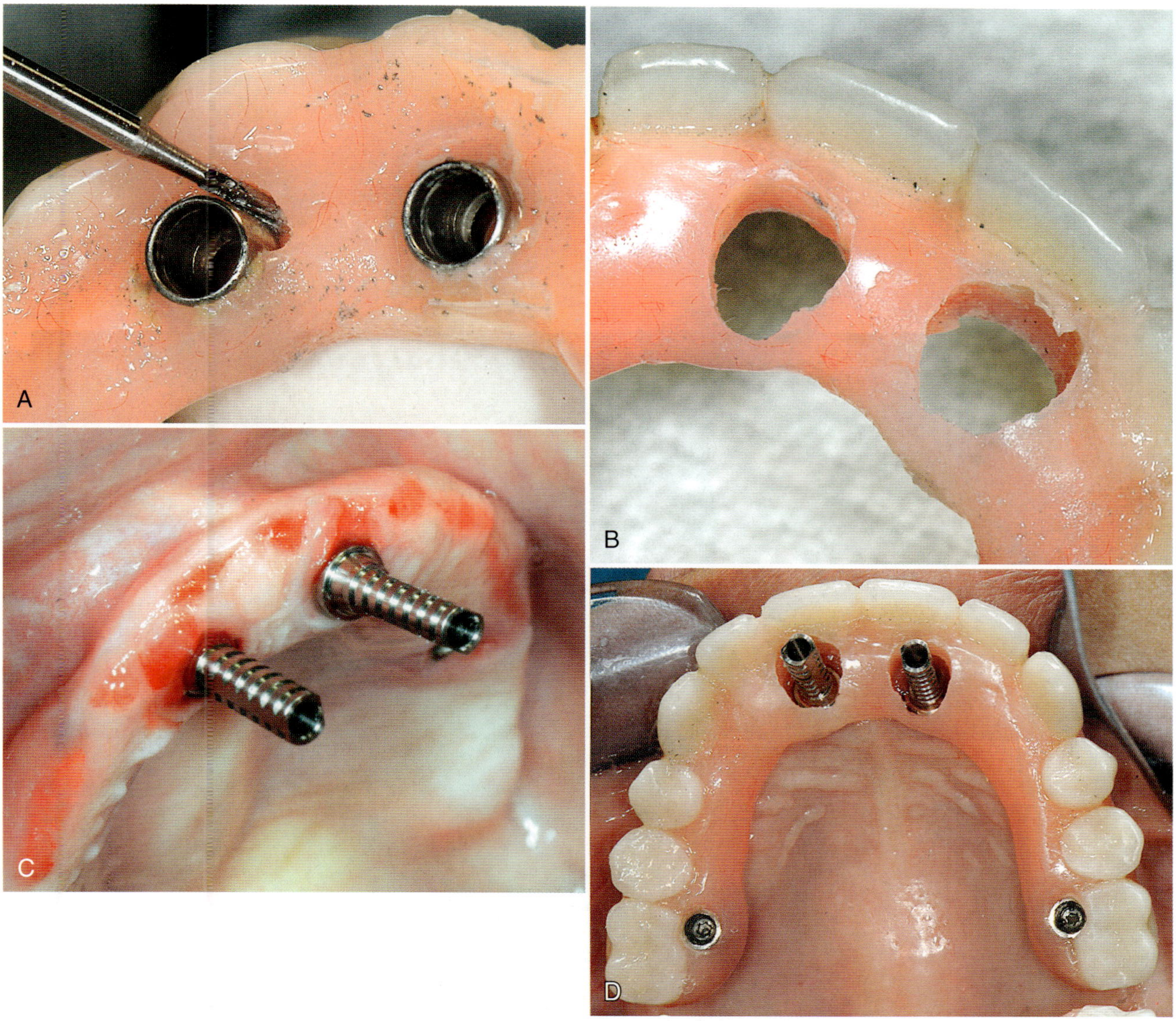

FIGURE 13-56 Trephining the existing computer-guided abutment cylinders from the two anterior implants. Connecting multiunit temporary cylinders to the anterior multiunit abutments with seating and stabilization of the provisional prosthesis on the existing computer-guided abutments on the zygomatic implants.

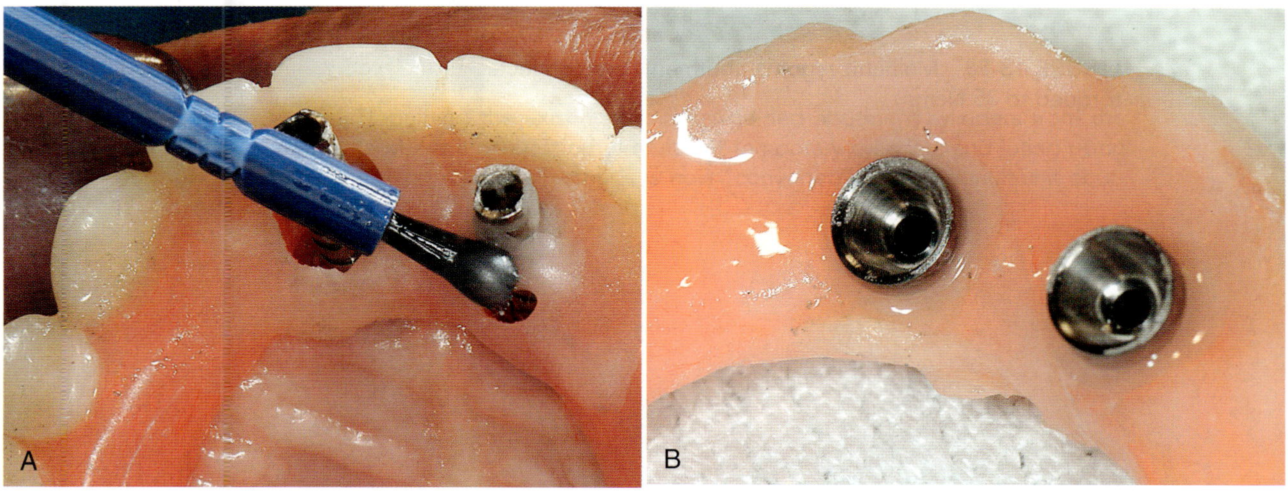

FIGURE 13-57 Quick-set acrylic is used to lute the temporary cylinders.

To initiate fabrication of the final prosthesis, a bite registration was made. The provisional prosthesis was removed, multiunit laboratory analogues were attached, and the prosthesis was mounted on the articulator. A putty index of the provisional prosthesis allowed for proper extensions for fabrication of the autopolymerized resin pattern. The pattern was indexed intraorally and used to pour the corrected cast. The pattern was scanned and the titanium framework milled. Confirmation of the passive fit of the titanium framework was made by connecting the framework to the implants using only one screw. The complete seating of all four abutment surfaces against the framework held in place by only one screw indicated a passive framework (Figures 13-60 to 13-66).

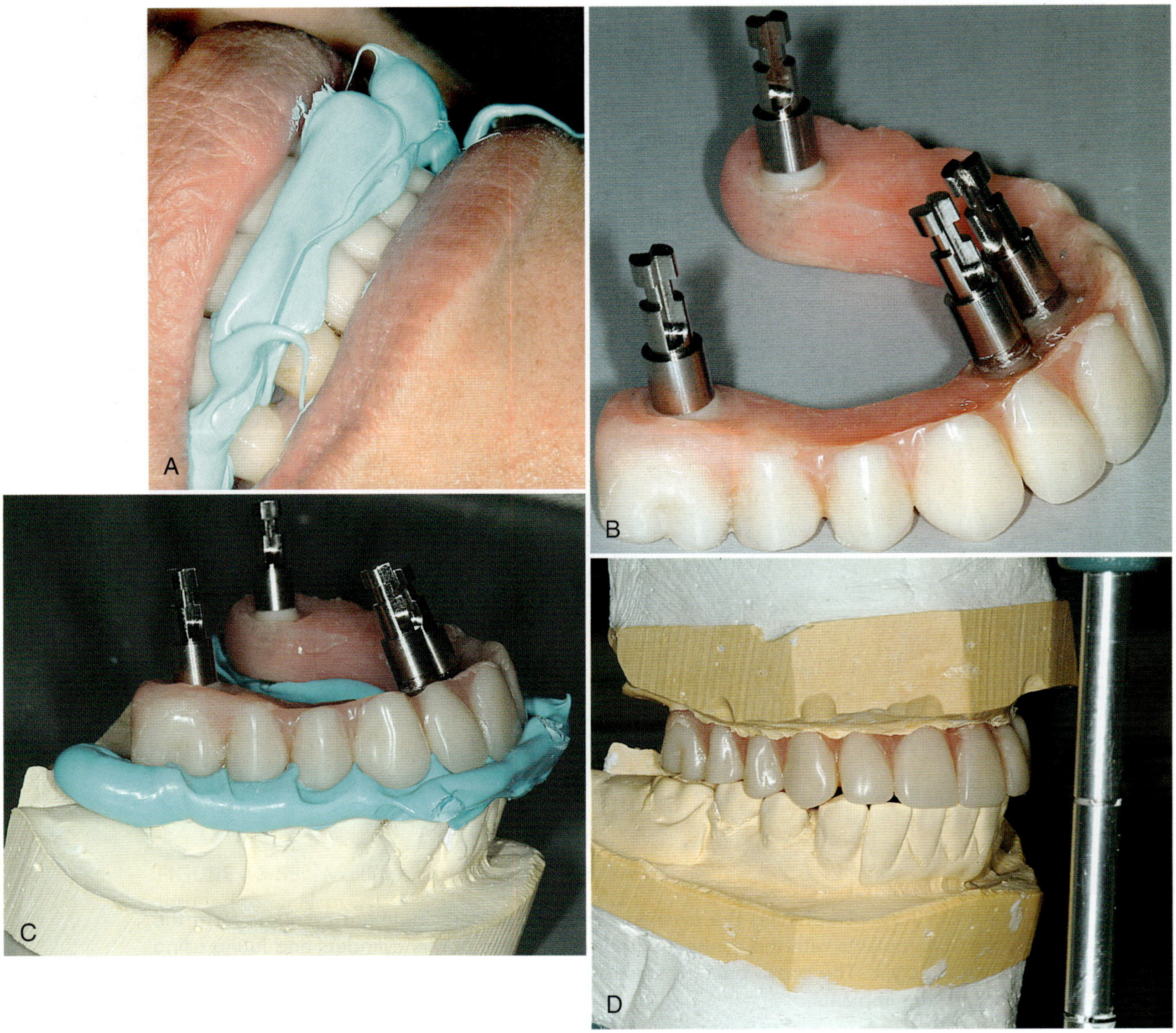

FIGURE 13-60 A new bite registration and connecting multiunit laboratory analogues to the provisional prosthesis allows articulation and mounting of the provisional prosthesis, which initiates fabrication of the final profile prosthesis.

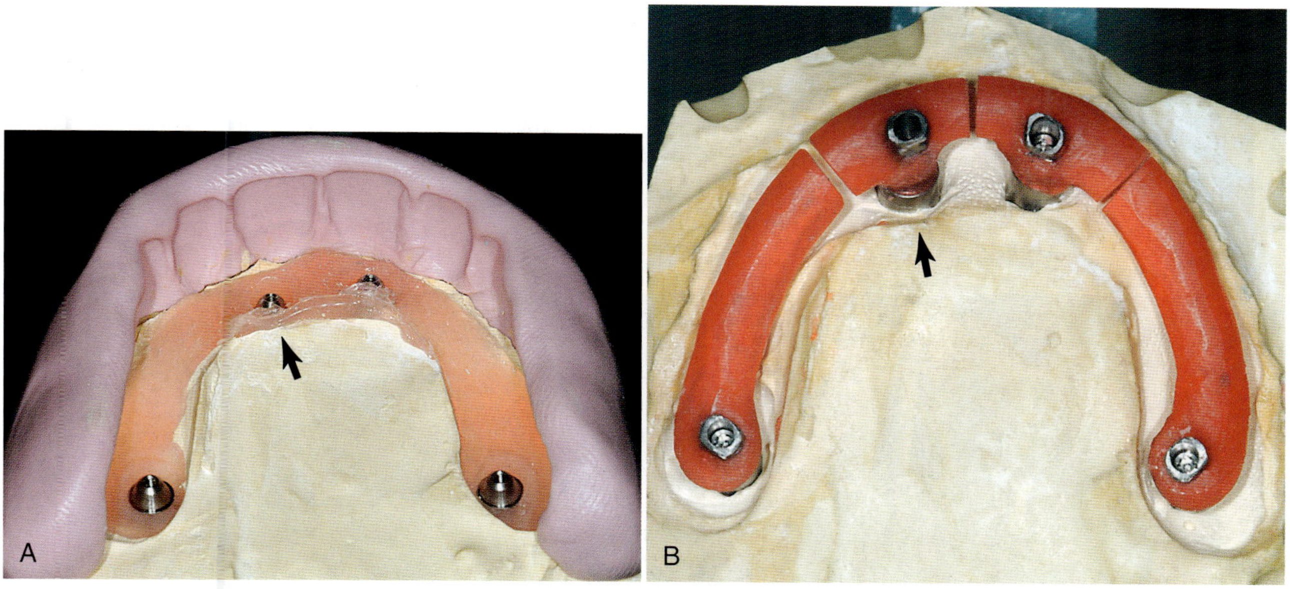

FIGURE 13-61 A putty index of the profile prosthesis guides the laboratory technician for the proper extensions of the autopolymerized resin pattern of the framework.

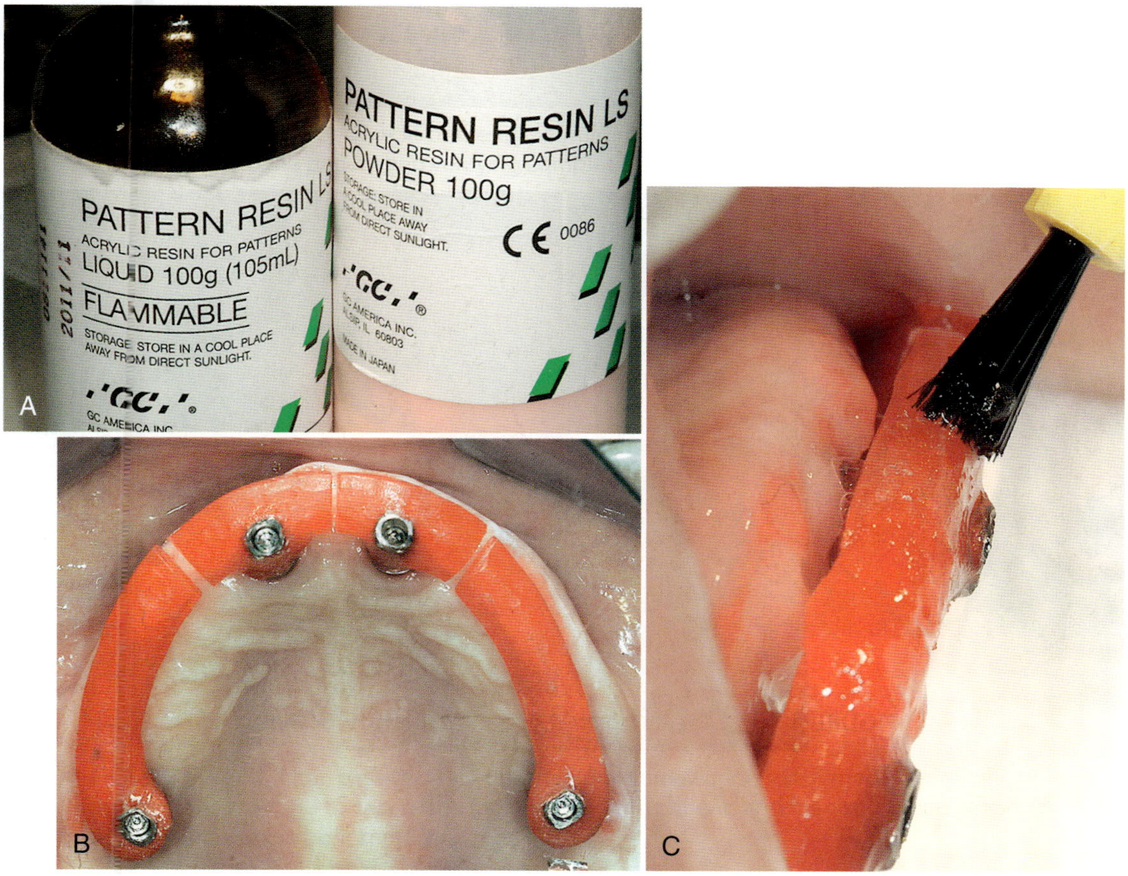

FIGURE 13-62 Pattern resin is used to connect the autopolymerized resin pattern intraorally.

Once the passive fit of the framework was confirmed, light body impression material was used to capture the relationship of the intaglio surface of the framework and the patient's soft tissues. A wax try-in of the final prosthesis allows evaluation of lingual contours, ensuring proper speech and proper anterior-posterior tooth positions for proper lip support and aesthetics during animation. After processing the prosthesis and establishing group function and proper maximum intercuspation, the screw access holes were sealed (Figures 13-67 to 13-71).

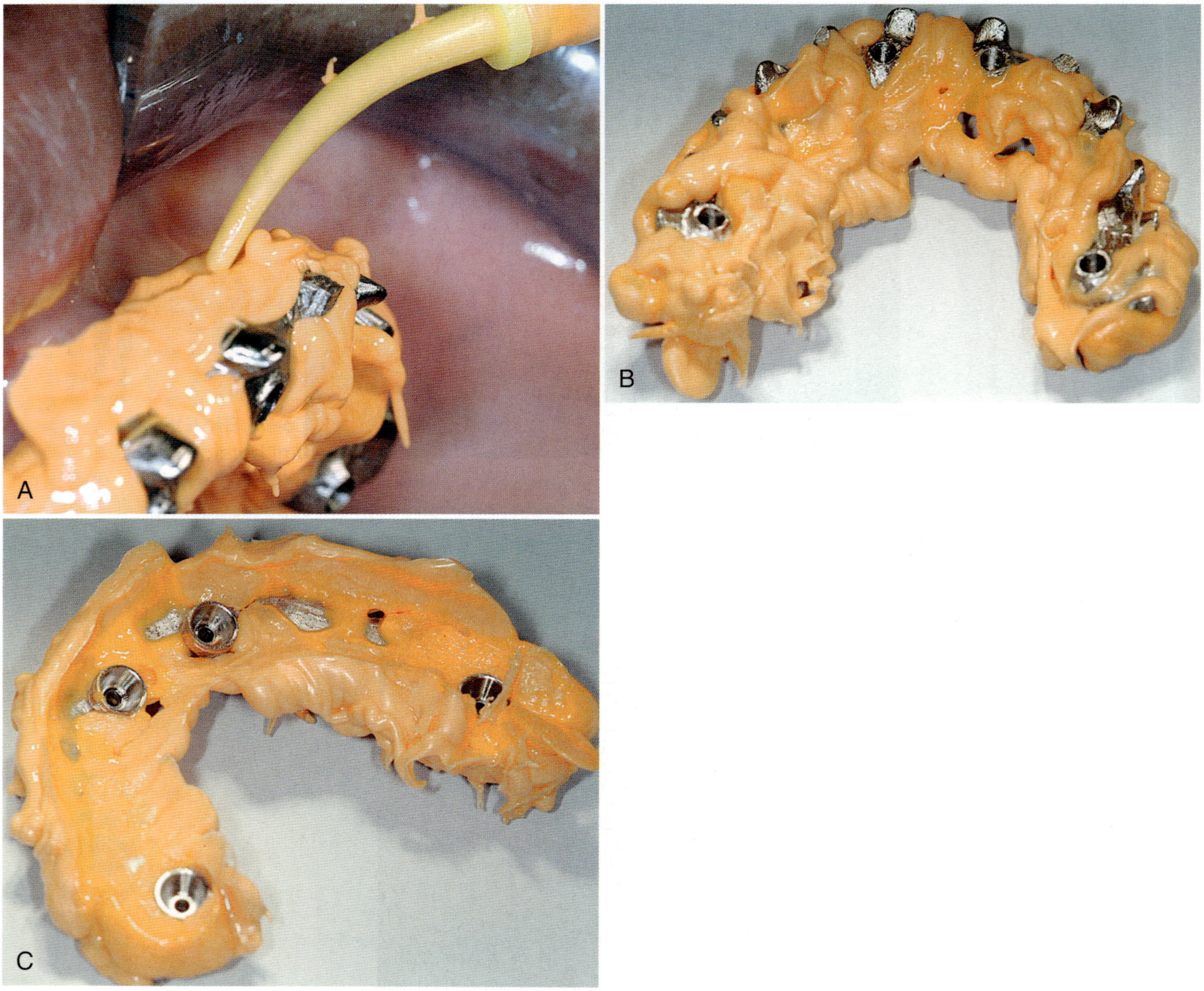

FIGURE 13-67 Soft tissue indexing: Light body impression material is used to capture the intaglio surface of the framework, allowing the proper contour of the profile prosthesis against the patient's soft tissues.

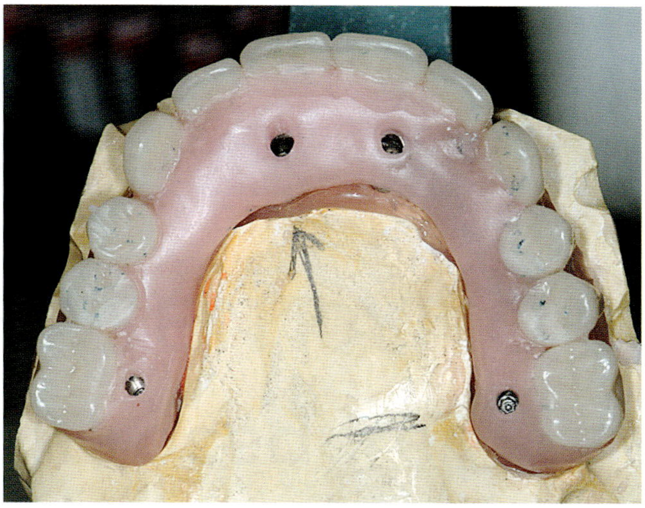

FIGURE 13-68 Wax try-in of the final prosthesis is completed prior to processing the final prosthesis.

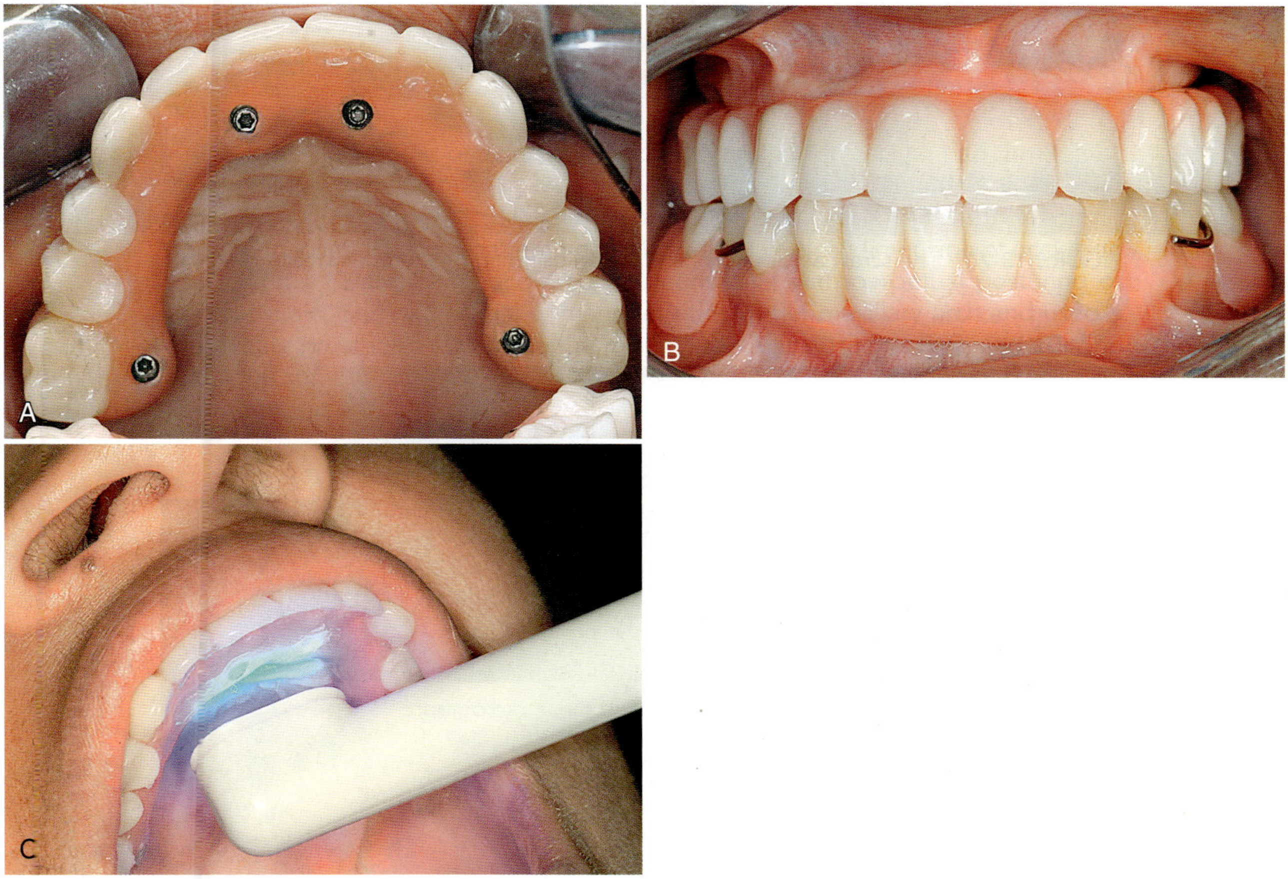

FIGURE 13-69 The completed final prosthesis.

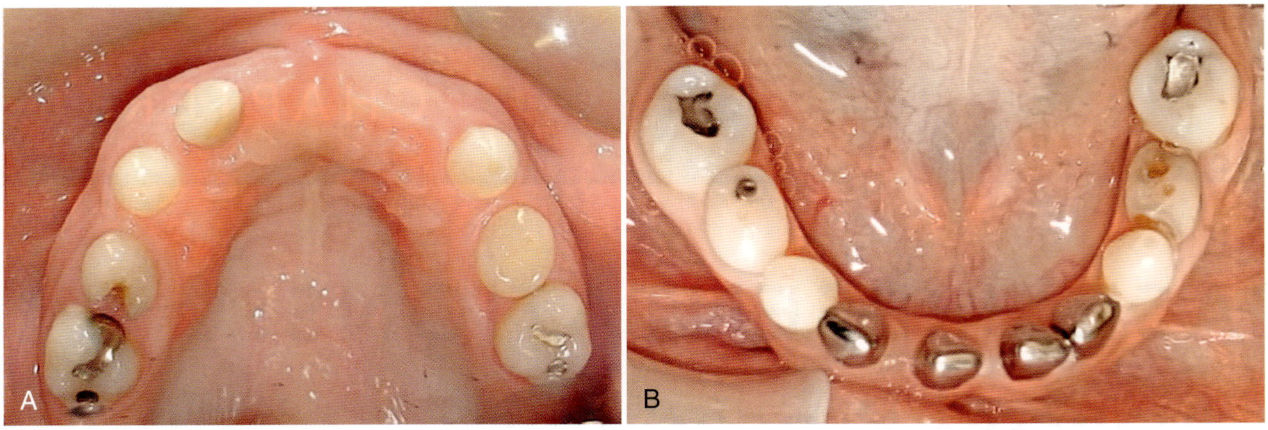

FIGURE 14-2 Maxillary and mandibular primary dentition with multiple restorations.

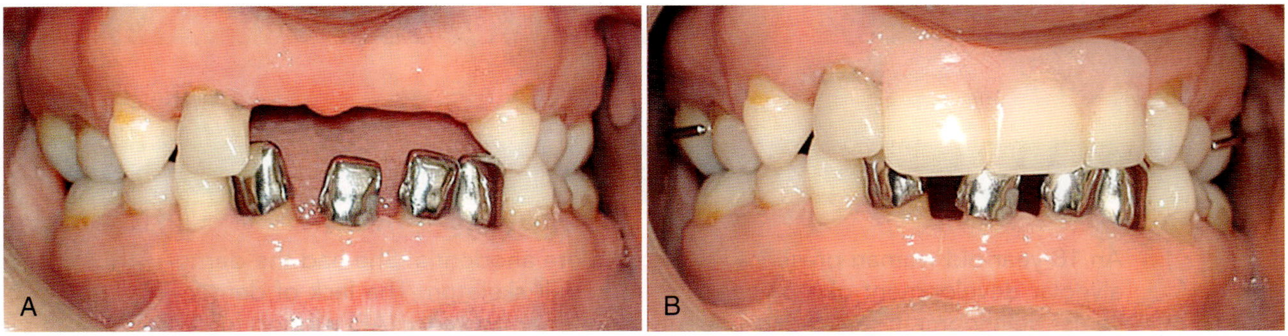

FIGURE 14-3 Replacement of the missing anterior maxillary teeth with an all-acrylic removable partial denture.

Her panoramic radiographic examination revealed the presence of zones I and II bone in the maxilla and adequate mandibular bony volume.

To plan treatment with an implant-supported prosthesis, it was paramount to establish the proper VDO, AP tooth position, and a stable and reproducible occlusion. To accomplish this goal, maxillary and mandibular overdentures were fabricated. Occlusal adjustments were made during the next 4 months to establish a reproducible occlusion (Figures 14-4 to 14-8).

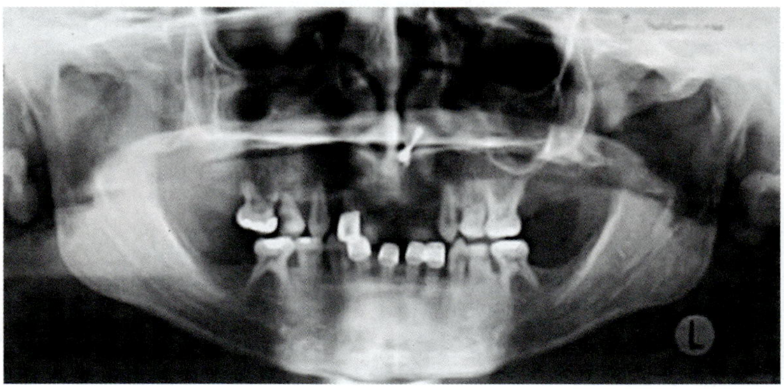

FIGURE 14-4 The patient's panoramic radiographic examination demonstrates a complete absence of adult dentition.

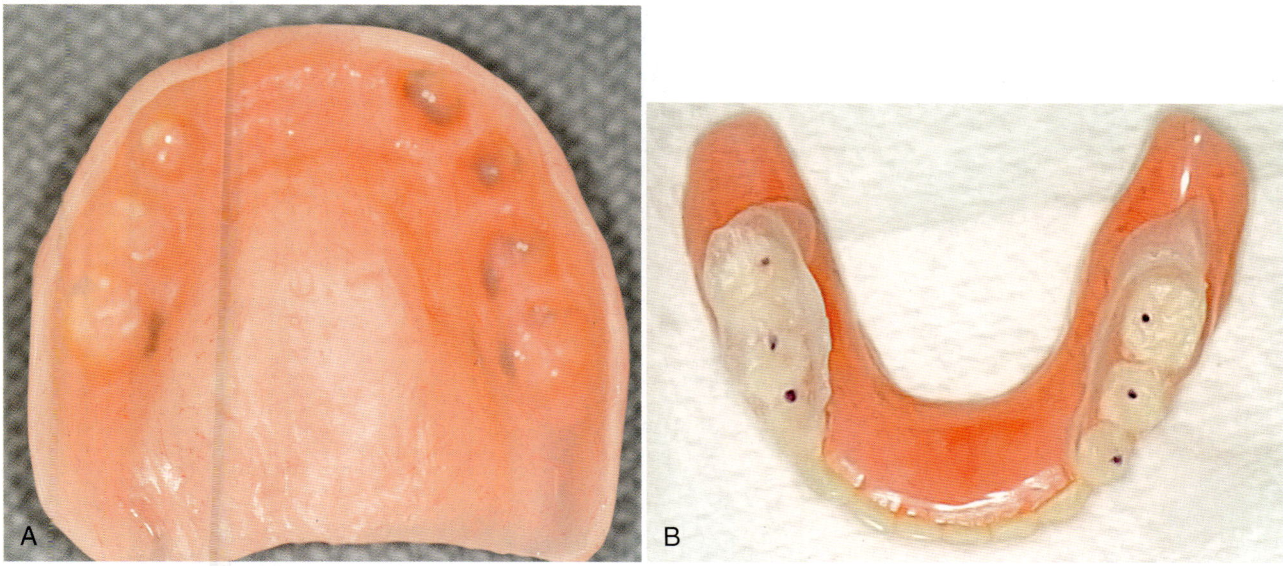

FIGURE 14-5 Maxillary and mandibular overdentures are used to re-establish the patient's vertical dimension of occlusion and anterior-posterior tooth position, and to establish a reproducible "adult" hinge axis.

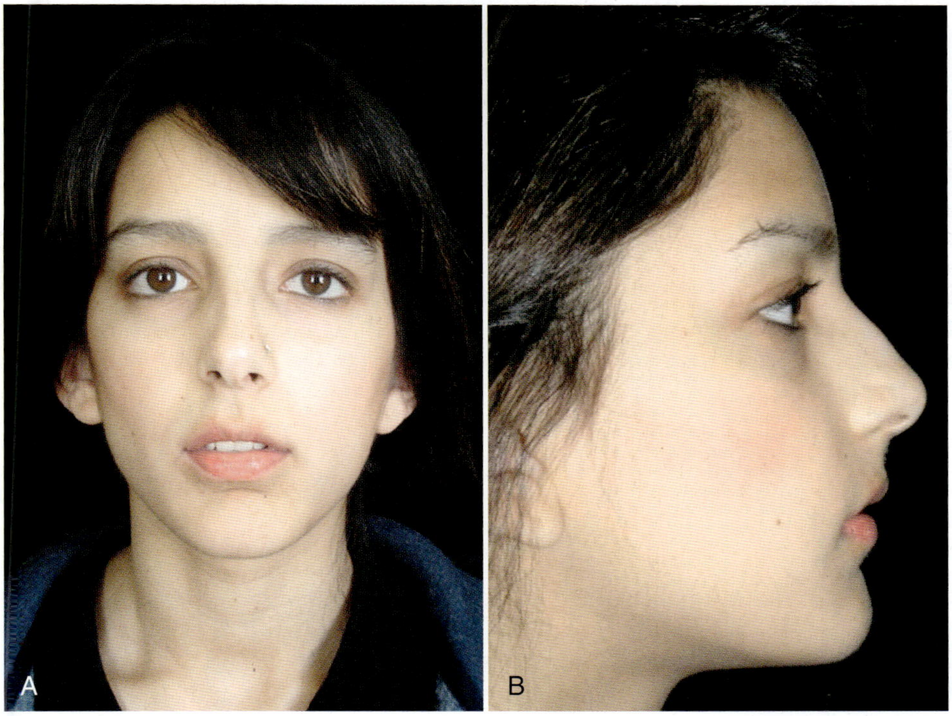

FIGURE 14-6 With the use of the overdentures, an increase in the height of the lower one-third of the face is observed, presenting a more balanced total facial height. Proper vertical dimension of occlusion and anterior-posterior tooth positioning allows for aesthetically acceptable nasolabial and labiomental profiles.

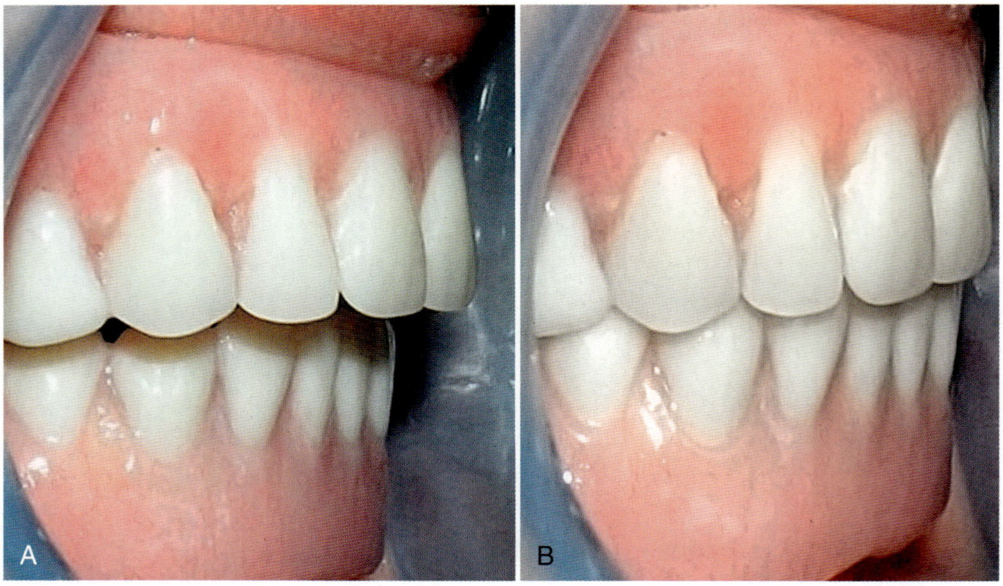

FIGURE 14-7 Anterior-posterior settling of the temporomandibular joints after 4 months of splint therapy and occlusal adjustment of the overdenture.

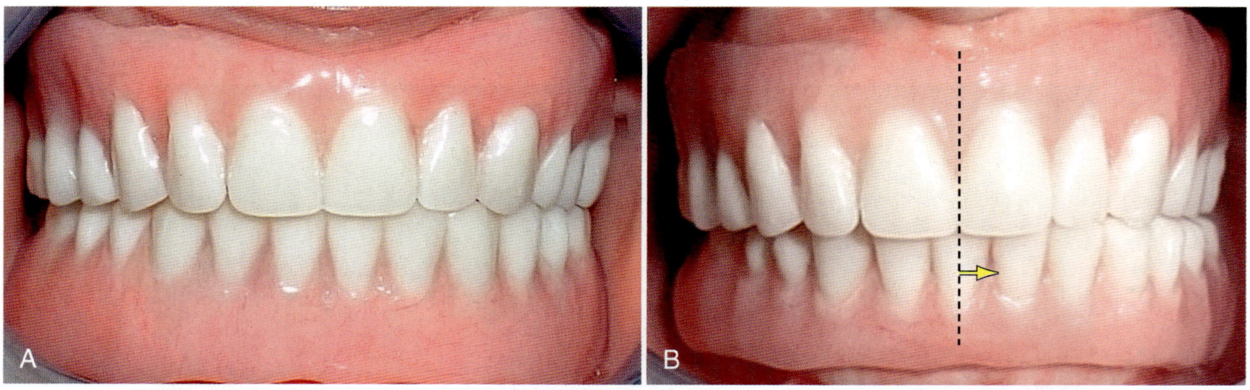

FIGURE 14-8 Lateral settling of the temporomandibular joints after 4 months of splint therapy and occlusal adjustment. Notice the deviation of the mandibular midline to the left.

Prior to planning treatment with implants, cone beam radiographic studies of the temporomandibular joints were completed. These studies demonstrated an absence of pathologic conditions in the joint and established a baseline study for comparison with future cone beam radiographic studies of the patient's joint (Figure 14-9).

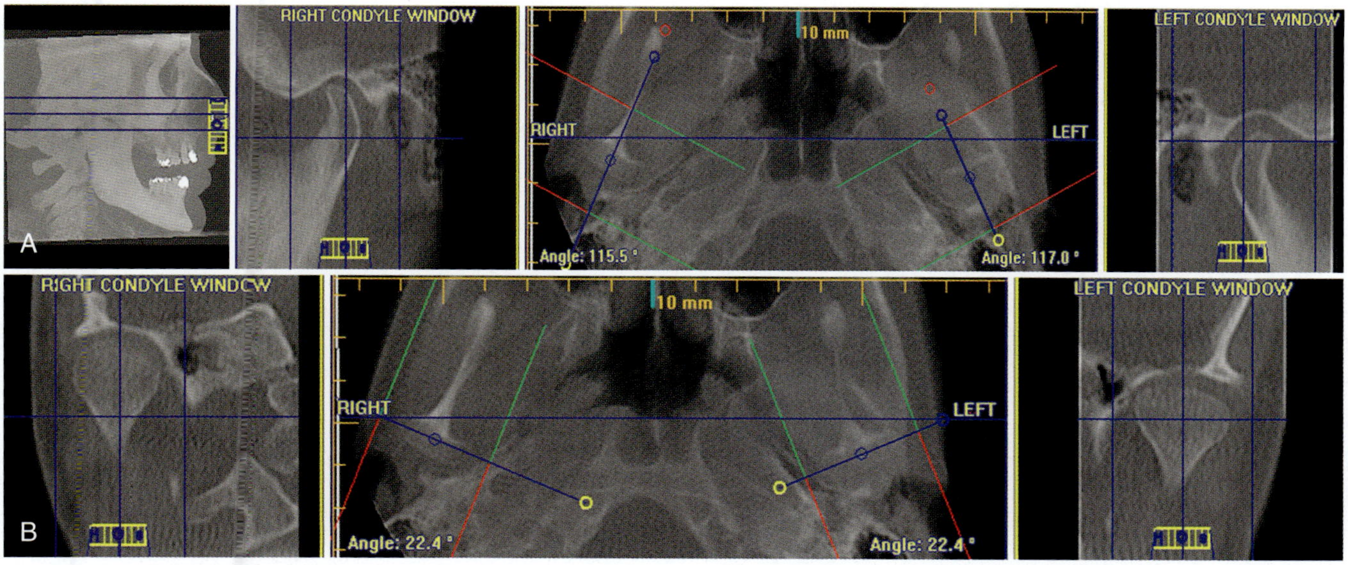

FIGURE 14-9 Sagittal and coronal cone beam radiographic studies establish a baseline for future reference.

Clear duplicated maxillary and mandibular dentures were made for systematic evaluation of an implant-supported prosthesis.

Systematic pretreatment evaluation of the patient:

1. Presence of both maxillary and mandibular composite defects
2. Favorable hidden maxillary transition line
3. Final prosthetic design consistent with maxillary and mandibular profile prosthesis
4. Presence of zones I and II bone in the maxilla, indicating that the tilted implant treatment concept is appropriate for the maxilla and the mandible

(Figures 14-10 to 14-12)

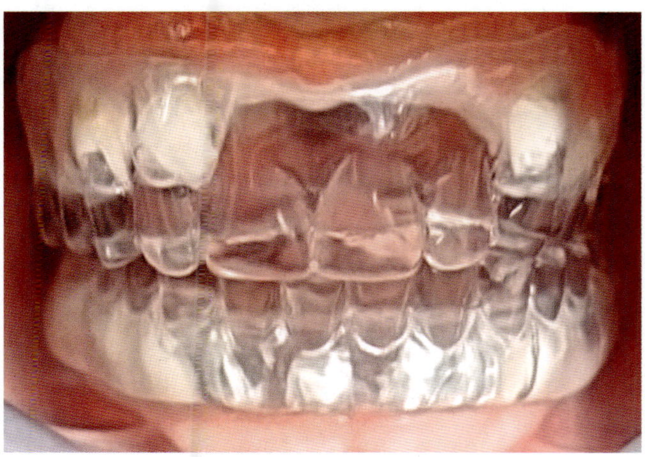

FIGURE 14-10 A composite defect is apparent when relating the cervical portion of the clear denture teeth to the patient's alveolar crest. This finding indicates that fabrication of a final profile prosthesis for both the maxilla and the mandible is appropriate.

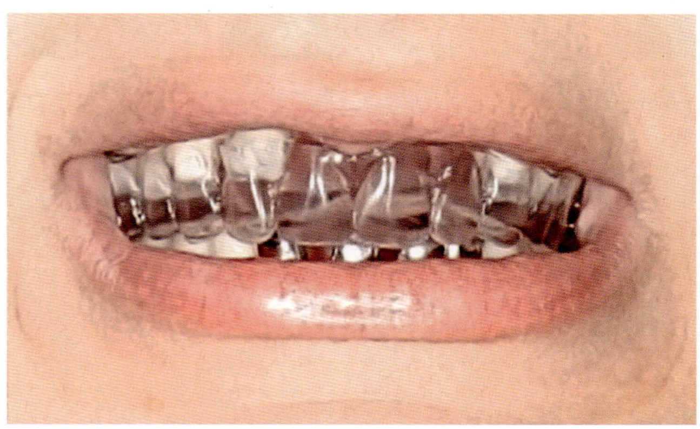

FIGURE 14-11 In animation, the soft tissue crest of the patient's alveolus is not visible, indicating a hidden, and therefore favorable, transition line of the proposed profile prosthesis.

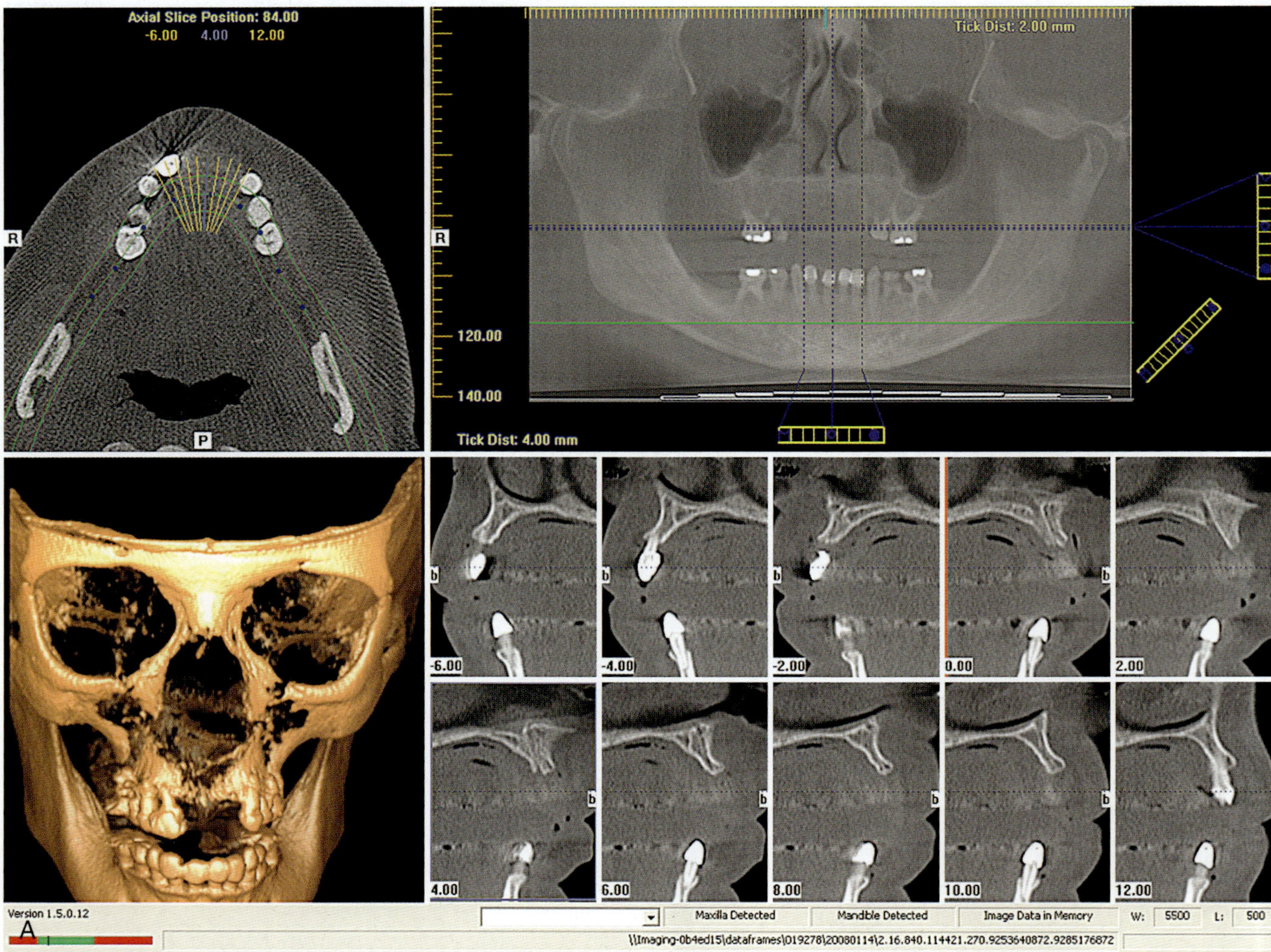

FIGURE 14-12 Maxillary and mandibular cone beam radiographic studies are consistent with narrow crestal alveolar width, which indicates the need for alveolectomies after removal of the maxillary and mandibular primary dentition.

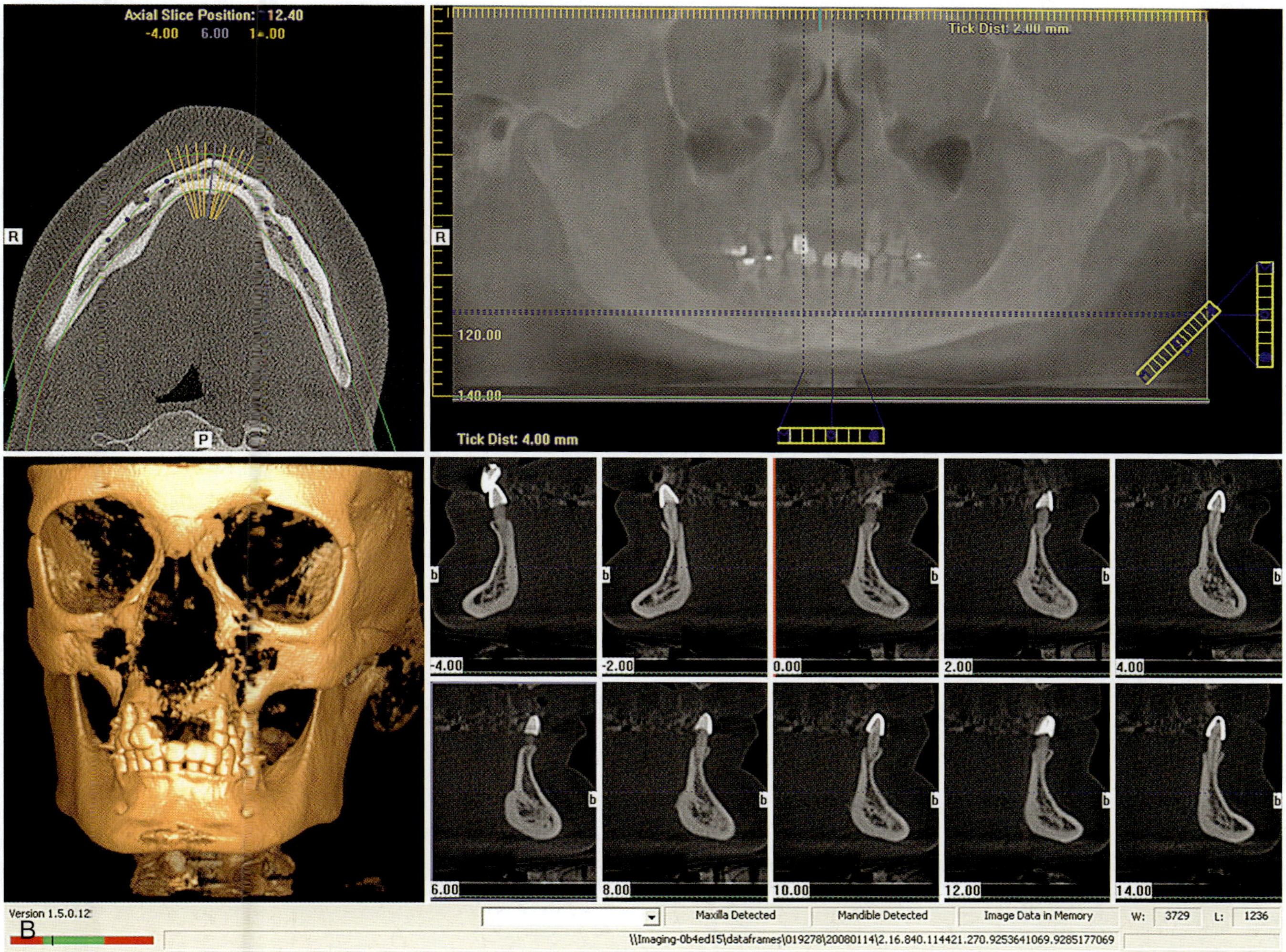

FIGURE 14-12, cont'd

Treatment plan:
Maxilla

1. Remove all existing maxillary primary dentition.
2. Perform alveolectomy to create a favorable width for implant placement.
3. Use the tilted implant treatment concept to establish adequate AP distribution.
4. Load immediately and convert the full maxillary denture to a provisional profile prosthesis.

(Figures 14-13 to 14-17)

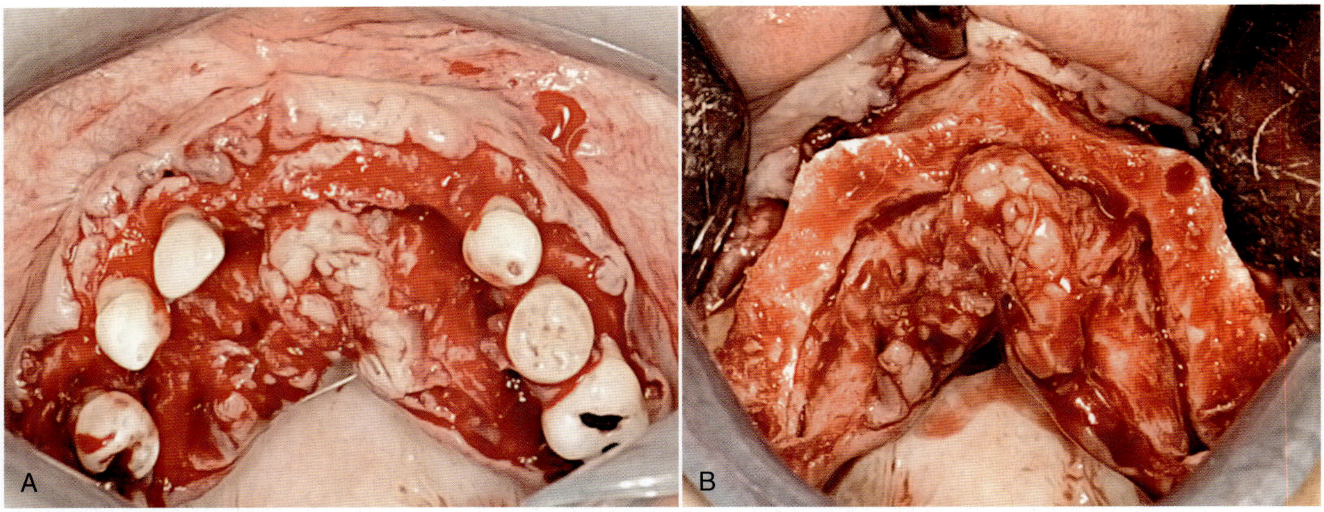

FIGURE 14-13 An envelope flap is placed, all maxillary primary teeth are removed, and alveolectomies are performed to establish adequate width for placement of regular platform NobelSpeedy implants.

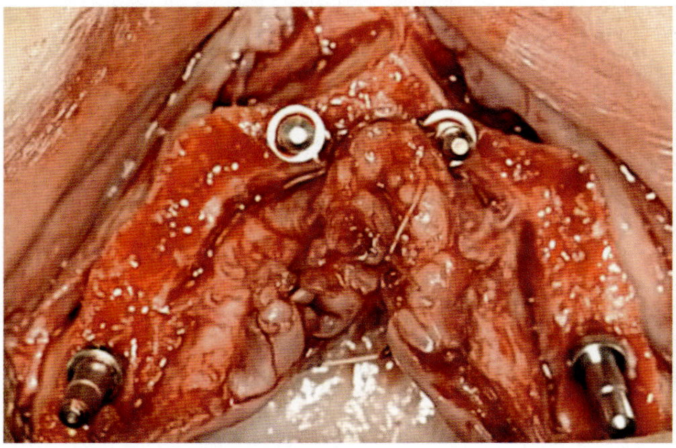

FIGURE 14-14 After establishing the desired implant length using the 2-mm start drill, paralleling pins are placed to allow better visualization of the proposed implant sites in the anterior-posterior dimension and in the buccal-palatal dimension (especially the posterior tilted implants).

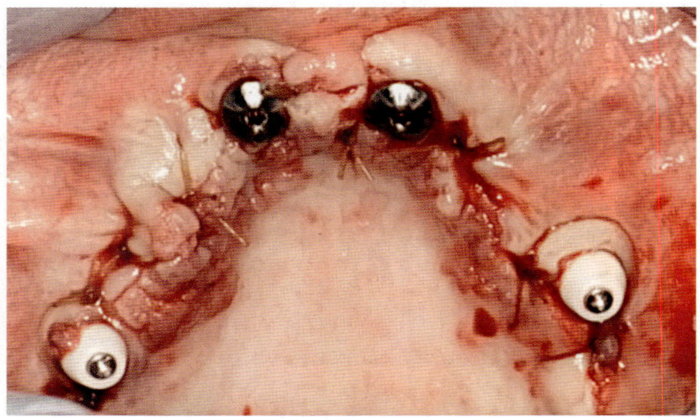

FIGURE 14-15 After implant placement with 40 Ncm insertion torque, 30° multiunit abutments are placed on the posterior tilted implants. For the anterior implants, temporary healing abutments are placed prior to indexing the positions of the implants with the intaglio surface of the denture.

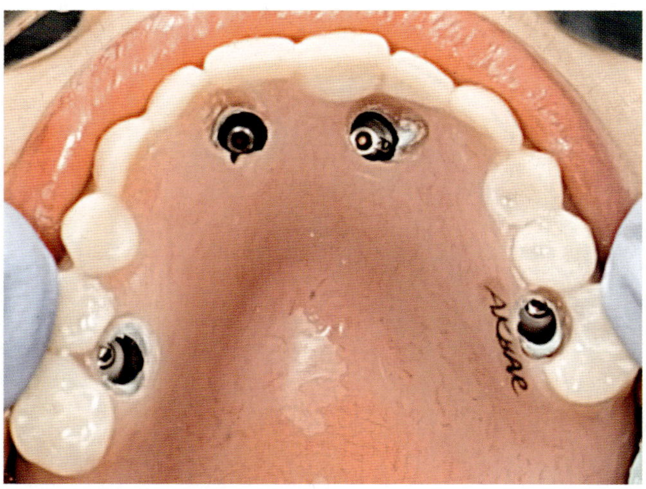

FIGURE 14-16 After indexing the position of the implants, the denture is placed passively over the abutments. At this point, the decision is made to either use straight multiunit abutments or 17° multiunit abutments for the anterior maxillary implants.

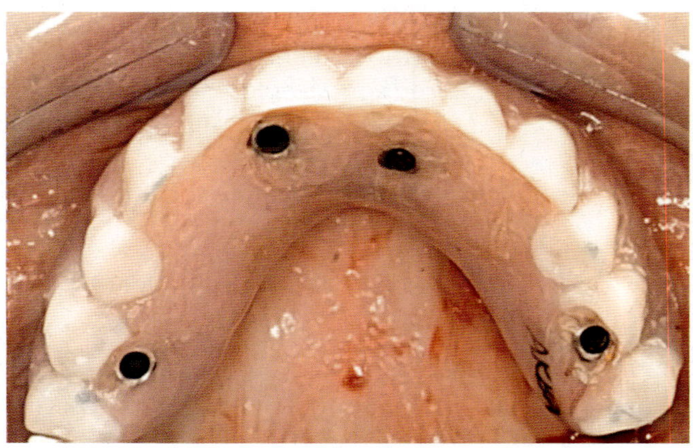

FIGURE 14-17 Completed maxillary provisional profile prosthesis.

Mandible

1. Remove all existing mandibular primary dentition.
2. Perform an alveolectomy to create a favorable width for implant placement.
3. Use the tilted implant treatment concept to establish adequate AP distribution.
4. Load immediately and convert the full mandibular denture to a provisional profile prosthesis.

(Figures 14-18 to 14-26)

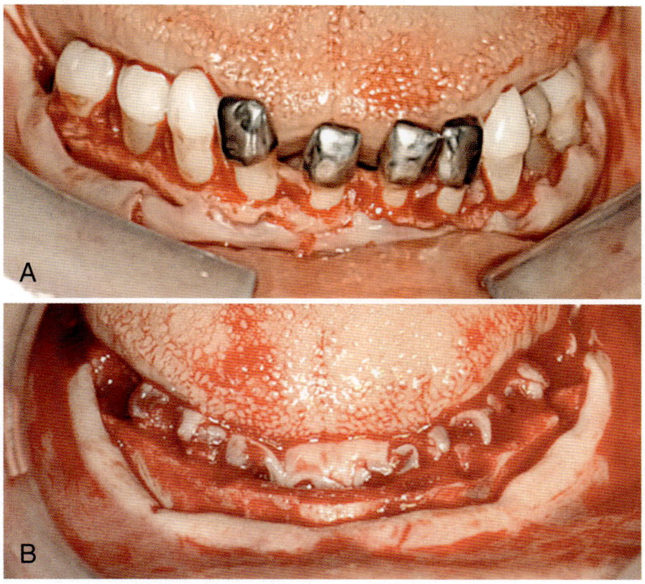

FIGURE 14-18 An envelope flap exposes the mandibular alveolus. The primary teeth are removed with a complete alveolectomy. The relationship of the mental foramina to the crest of the edentulous alveolus is observed bilaterally.

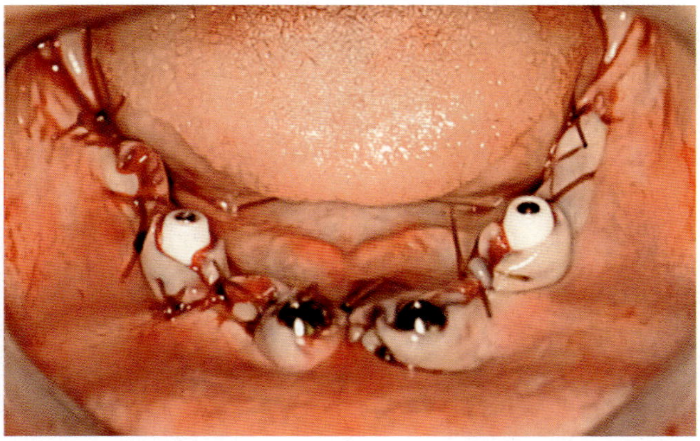

FIGURE 14-19 The implants are placed using the tilted treatment concept. If 40 Ncm insertion torque is maintained, 30° multiunit abutments are secured to the posterior implants, bringing the platform of the tilted implants in line with the platform of the anterior axial implants.

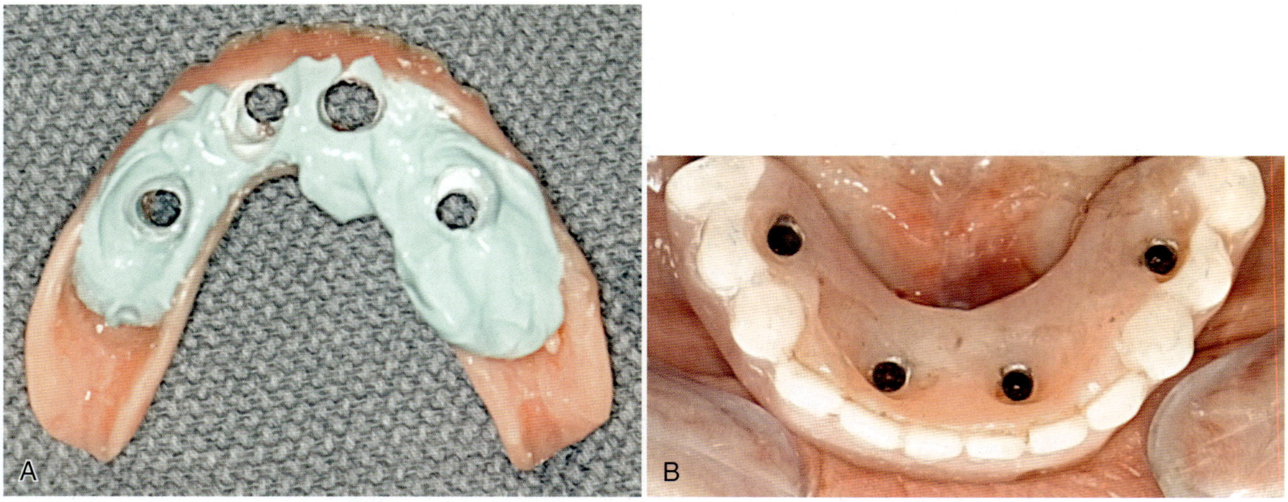

FIGURE 14-20 Indexing material is used to transfer the implant positions to the intaglio surface of the mandibular immediate denture. After choosing straight or 17° multiunit abutments for the anterior implants, the denture is converted to a provisional profile prosthesis and secured to the abutments with temporary titanium cylinders.

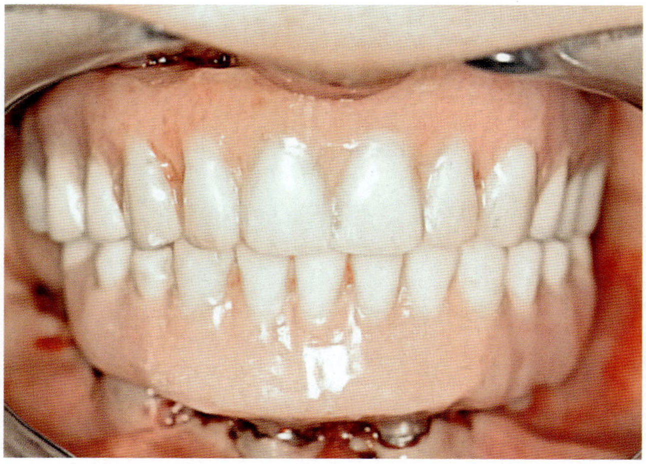

FIGURE 14-21 Completed maxillary and mandibular immediate-load prosthesis. The midline shift mimics the preoperative shift observed with the immediate overdentures.

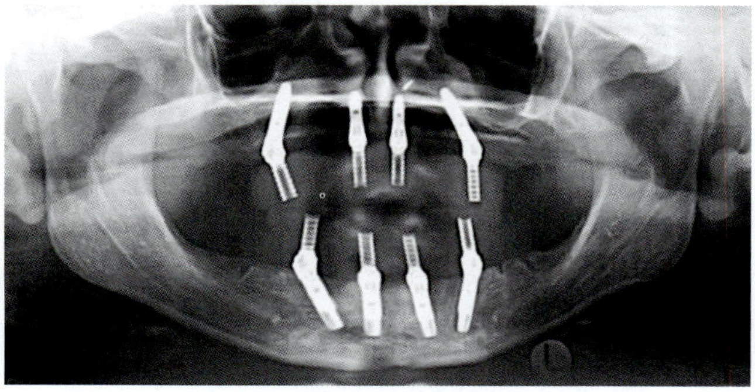

FIGURE 14-22 A panoramic radiograph taken immediately after surgery demonstrates a proper relationship between the tilted maxillary implants, the anterior maxillary wall, the tilted mandibular implants, the mental foramina, and the loop of the inferior alveolar nerve.

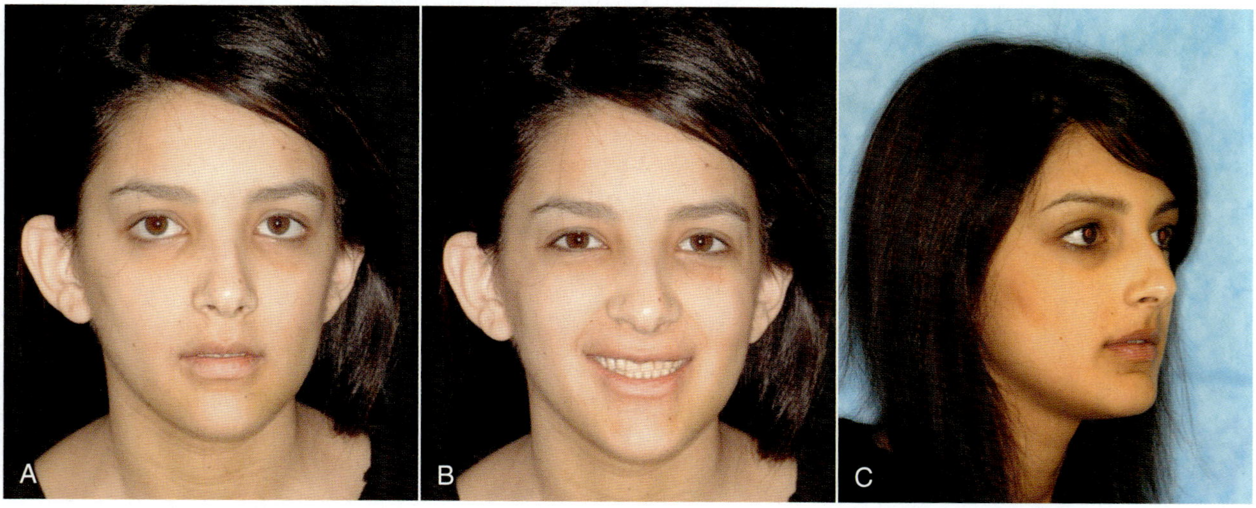

FIGURE 14-23 Photographs taken 1 week after surgery demonstrate proper vertical dimension of occlusion, balanced facial thirds, an aesthetically acceptable smile line, and a hidden maxillary transition lone.

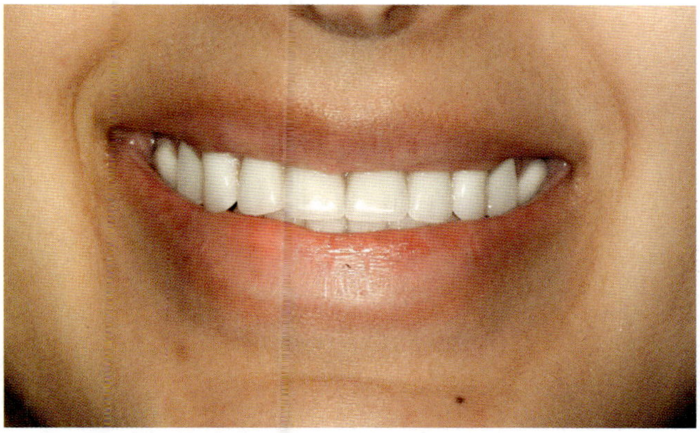

FIGURE 14-24 Six months after removal of the teeth, an alveolectomy, and immediate loading of the maxilla and the mandible, the final metal-based profile prosthesis is completed with a favorable hidden transition line.

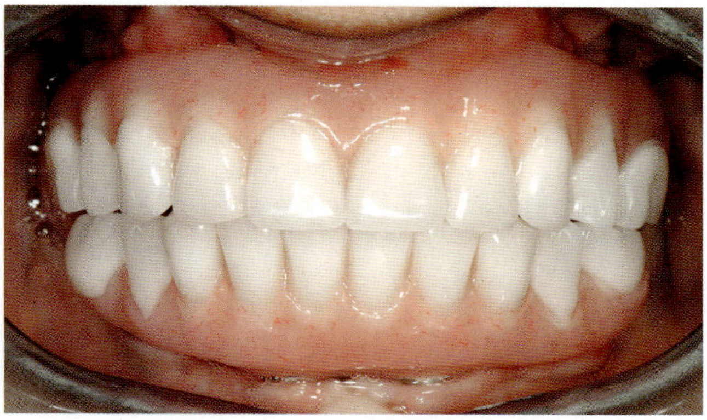

FIGURE 14-25 Correction of the vertical dimension of occlusion and the mandibular midline is observed in the final profile prosthesis.

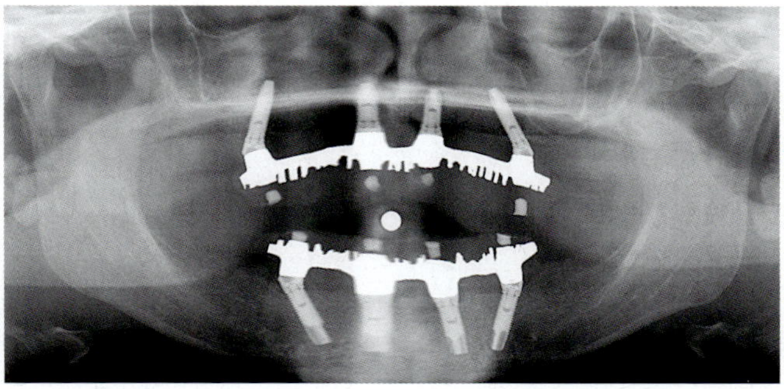

FIGURE 14-26 Final panoramic radiographic examination demonstrates complete seating of all abutments onto the implant platforms and seating of the maxillary and mandibular metal frameworks onto the abutments.

ECTODERMAL DYSPLASIA: THE ZYGOMA AND TILTED TREATMENT CONCEPTS

A 24-year-old healthy man presented with ectodermal dysplasia. The facial form indicated collapse of the nasolabial and labiomental angles. In the treatment planning phase, careful consideration must be given to the transition line of the final prosthesis. The intraoral presentation demonstrated partial maxillary and mandibular malformed teeth. A flat maxillary vault and advanced horizontal atrophy of the mandibular residual alveolus were also apparent. The patient maintained maxillary and mandibular removable partial dentures, which were not functional (Figures 14-27 to 14-31).

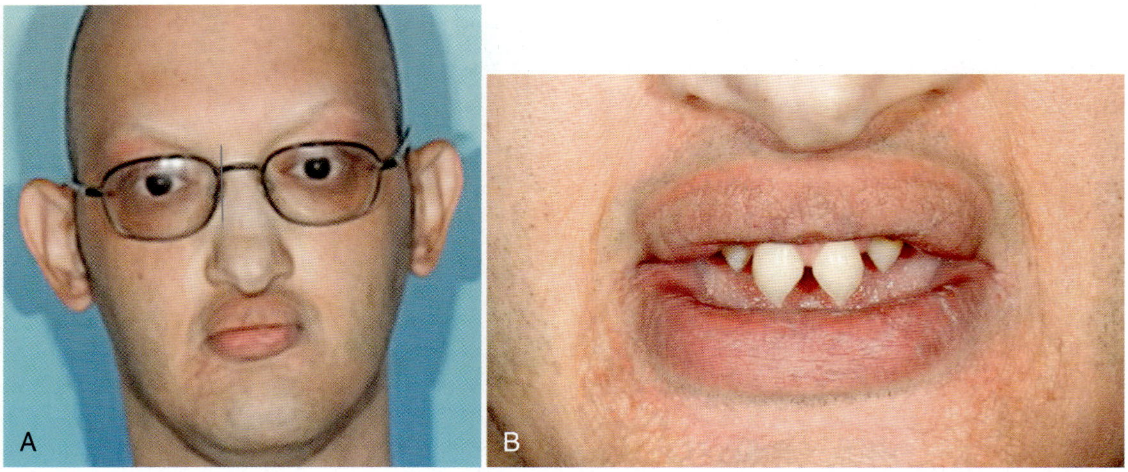

FIGURE 14-27 A, Improper vertical dimension of occlusion and anterior-posterior tooth support results in collapse of both the nasolabial and labiomental angles. B, The potential for a transition line visible during animation should be considered during treatment planning.

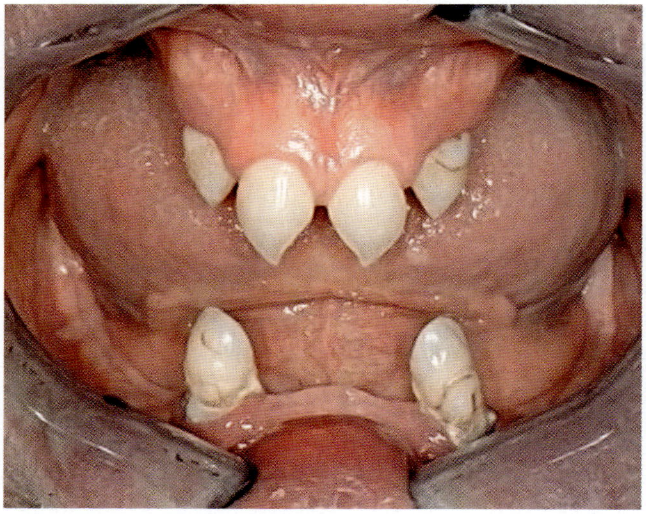

FIGURE 14-28 Only four anterior maxillary "peg" incisor teeth and two mandibular canines are present.

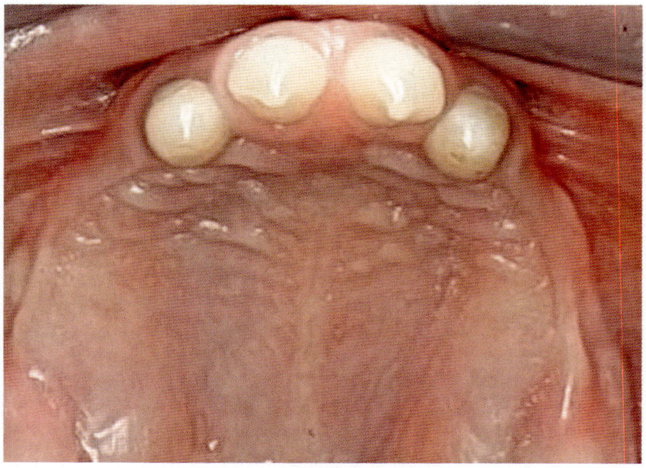

FIGURE 14-29 A flat maxillary vault and shallow maxillary vestibule are evident.

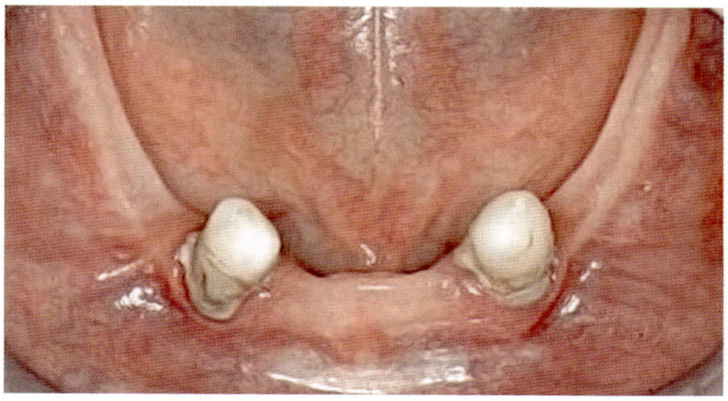

FIGURE 14-30 Advanced horizontal atrophy of the residual mandibular alveolar ridge is observed.

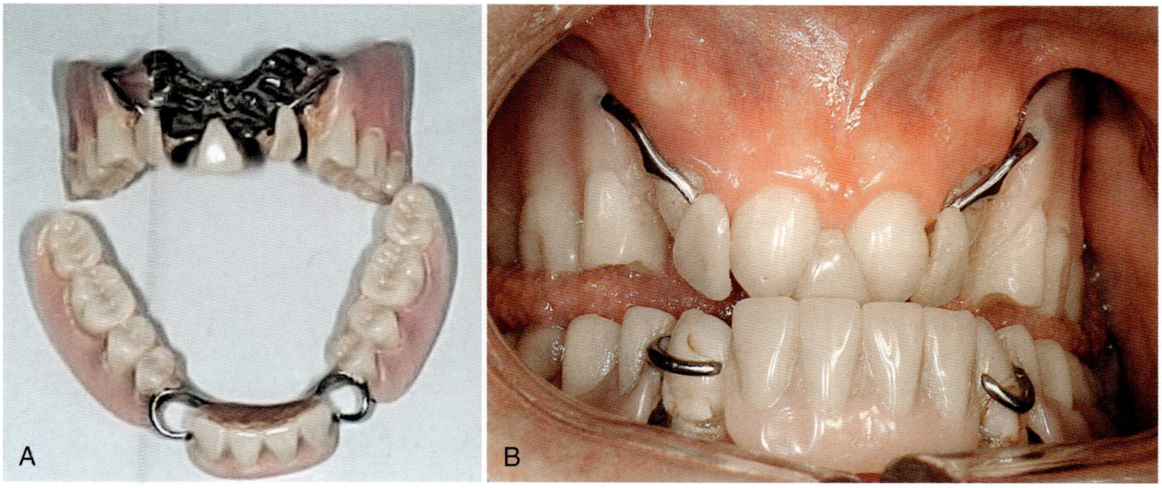

FIGURE 14-31 Nonfunctional maxillary and mandibular partial dentures with inadequate vertical dimension of occlusion are used by the patient.

The patient's panoramic radiographic examination demonstrated a prominent premaxilla and advanced resorption of the posterior maxillary alveolus. The mandible had moderate to advanced resorption in the vertical dimension with retained cuspids only. The presence of zone I bone only indicated that the zygoma treatment concept was appropriate for reconstruction of the maxillary dentition with a fixed profile prosthesis. The tilted implant concept may be considered for treatment of the mandible with a fixed, implant-supported prosthesis (Figure 14-32).

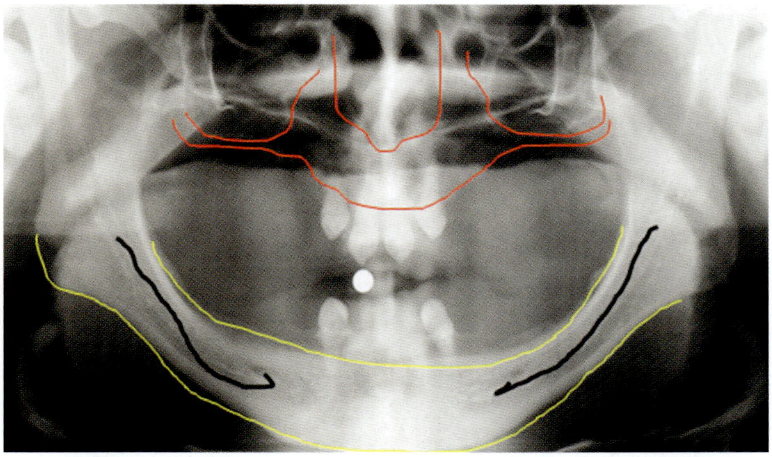

FIGURE 14-32 A prominent premaxilla with complete resorption of the posterior maxilla and advanced mandibular resorption is evident on the preoperative radiograph.

Treatment plan

1. Establish proper VDO and AP tooth position by using maxillary and mandibular overdentures.
2. Remove remaining maxillary teeth.
3. Perform a premaxillary alveolectomy.
4. Place two or four premaxillary implants in zone I.
5. Place a single zygoma implant in zone III.
6. Convert the preoperative full maxillary denture into a provisional fixed prosthesis.
7. Remove the remaining mandibular teeth.
8. Place four implants using the tilted treatment concept.
9. Convert the preoperative mandibular full denture into a provisional fixed prosthesis.
10. Fabricate the final maxillary and mandibular profile prosthesis.

To allow for an aesthetically acceptable final prosthesis, the transition line must be considered during treatment planning as well as intraoperatively. Removing the remaining maxillary teeth and performing an alveolectomy of the premaxilla resulted in a hidden transition line and an aesthetically acceptable final prosthesis. Placing two or four premaxillary implants in zone I and placing a single zygoma implants in zone III allowed adequate AP distribution and therefore proper support for an implant-supported, fixed profile prosthesis. For the mandible, removal of the remaining two cuspids and placement of four implants using the tilted treatment concept was considered. The patient's preoperative mounting with diagnostic overdentures demonstrated the increase in vertical dimension required for correction of the patient's collapsed maxillary-mandibular relationship (Figures 14-33 to 14-40)

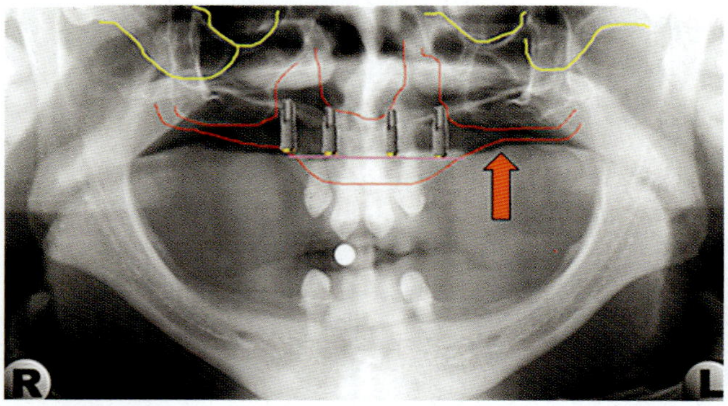

FIGURE 14-33 An alveolectomy is recommended after the remaining teeth are removed and before the premaxillary implants are placed.

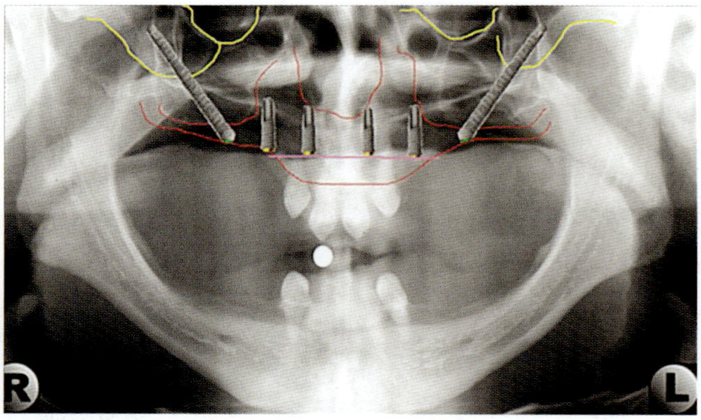

FIGURE 14-34 Placement of a single zygoma implant in zone III.

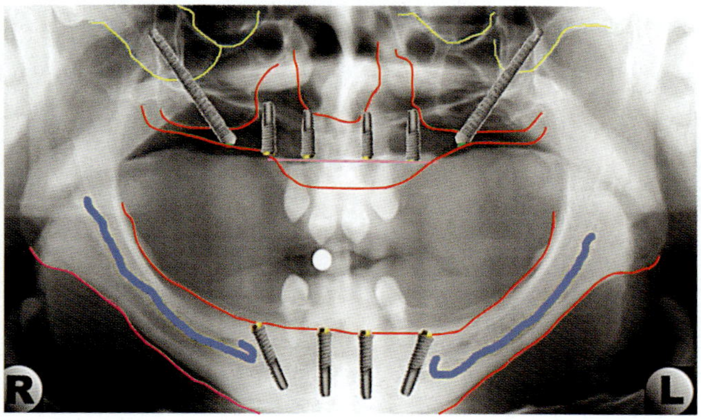

FIGURE 14-35 Placement of four mandibular implants using the tilted implant method.

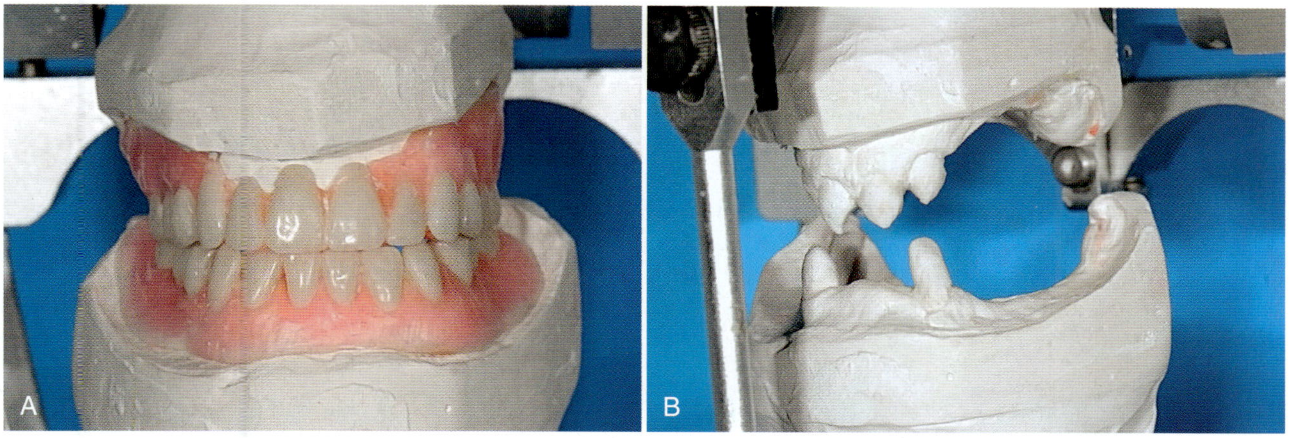

FIGURE 14-36 Diagnostic maxillary and mandibular overdenture permits establishment of proper vertical dimension of occlusion and anterior-posterior tooth position for proper lip support.

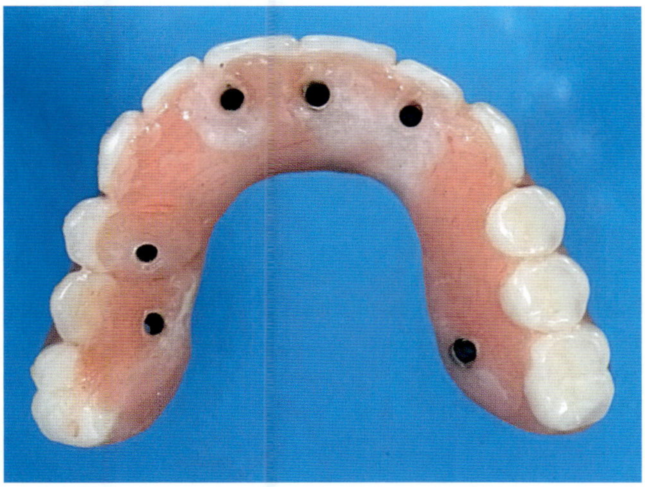

FIGURE 14-37 Completed provisional maxillary immediate-load prosthesis.

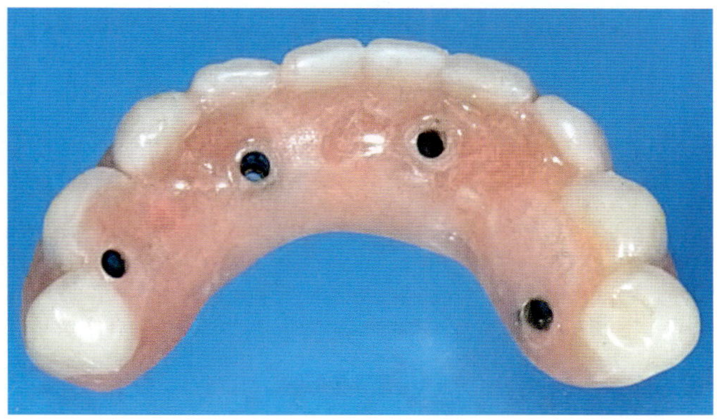

FIGURE 14-38 Completed provisional mandibular immediate-load prosthesis.

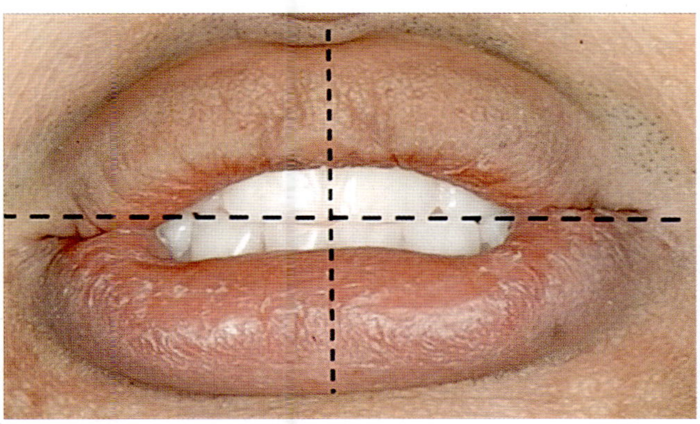

FIGURE 14-39 Clinical presentation of coinciding dental and facial midlines with proper maximum intercuspation.

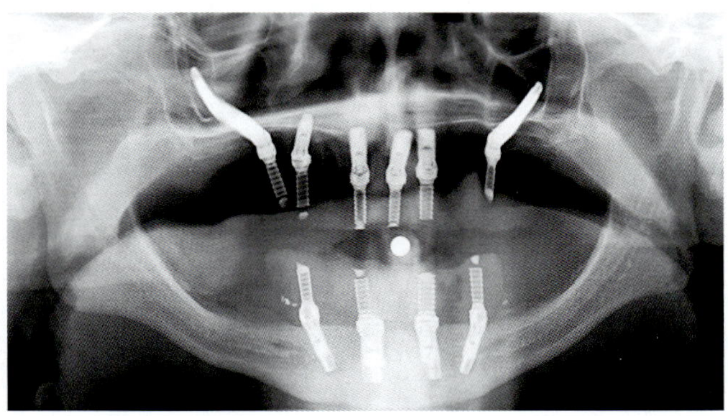

FIGURE 14-40 Immediate postoperative panoramic radiograph demonstrating complete seating of the abutments and temporary titanium cylinders onto the implants.

After allowing 6 months for osseointegration, the final metal-based, fixed maxillary and mandibular prosthesis is fabricated. Establishment of proper VDO and AP tooth position allowed for more aesthetically acceptable facial features. The transition line of the maxillary profile prosthesis was hidden and the patient demonstrated full and aesthetically acceptable buccal corridors and smile line during animation. The final panoramic radiograph demonstrated complete seating of the final maxillary and mandibular metal-based profile prosthesis. The premaxillary implant in position 6, although immediately loaded and incorporated in the provisional immediate load prosthesis, was not incorporated into the final prosthesis at the discretion of the restorative dentist (Figures 14-41 to 14-43).

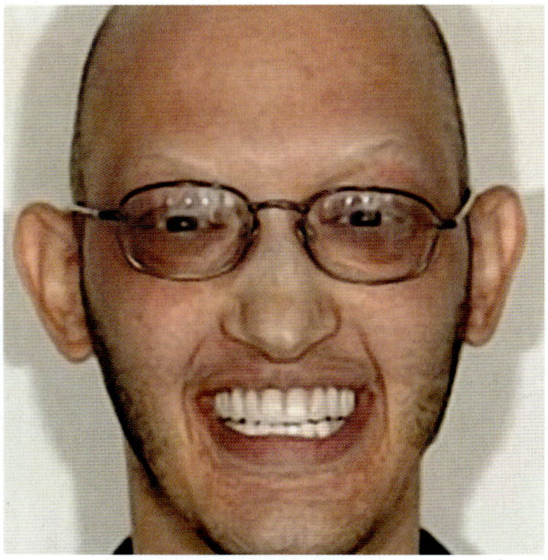

FIGURE 14-41 Dramatic improvement of the facial features resulting from proper vertical dimension of occlusion and anterior-posterior tooth position in the final prosthesis.

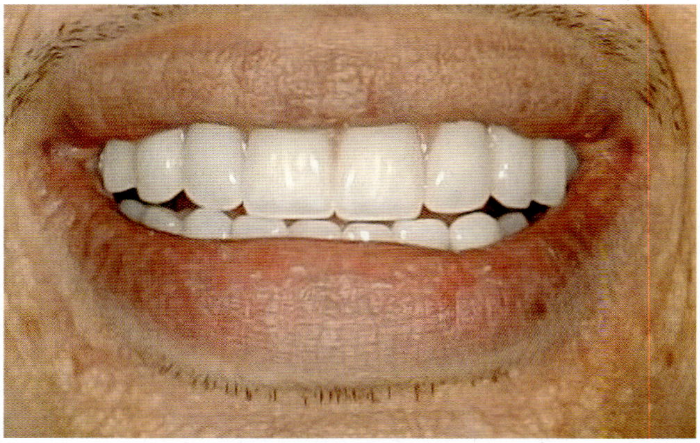

FIGURE 14-42 Aesthetically acceptable smile line is demonstrated during animation.

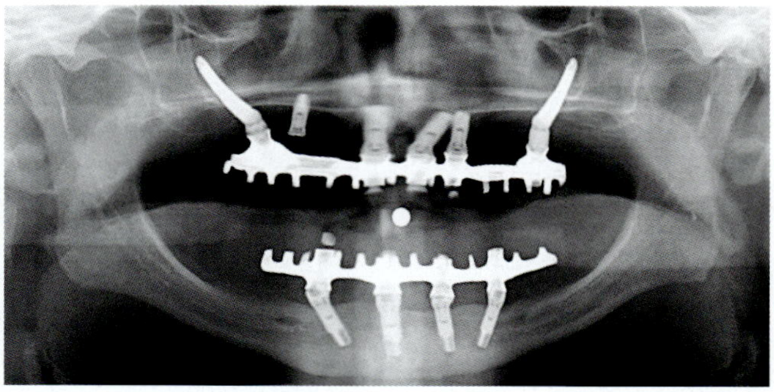

FIGURE 14-43 Final panoramic radiograph demonstrating complete seating of maxillary and mandibular components and frameworks. The decision was made by the restorative dentist not to incorporate the implant in the sixth position. (*Courtesy Dr. Lambert Stumpel, Restorative Dentist.*)

MANAGEMENT OF A PATIENT WITH A CLEFT PALATE

A 70-year-old patient with a left unilateral complete lip and alveolar cleft presented with a nonserviceable maxillary partial denture. The exiting abutment teeth retaining the maxillary partial denture were not restorable, and removal of the patient's maxillary teeth was planned. In anticipation of the patient's probable inability to retain and function with a full maxillary denture and function with it, extractions of the abutment teeth and immediate implant placement with immediate loading were planned.

The patient's panoramic radiographic examination demonstrated limited zone I bone volume available for implant placement. The complete alveolar cleft in the left maxilla further limited the bone available for implant placement.

The lateral reconstruction of the cone beam radiograph also demonstrated a lack of AP growth of the patient's maxilla.

The intraoral examination of the patient's maxilla was consistent with a shallow palatal vault and buccal vestibule. The two remaining nonrestorable abutment teeth had copings designed to allow retention of the existing maxillary partial denture clasps. The patient had a full complement of mandibular teeth and maintained a reproducible centric occlusion against the maxillary partial denture (Figures 14-44 to 14-51).

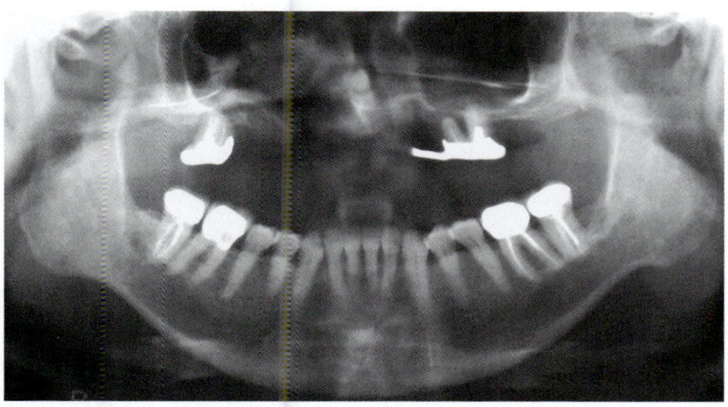

FIGURE 14-44 A panoramic radiograph demonstrates zone I bone and limited zones II and III alveolar bone.

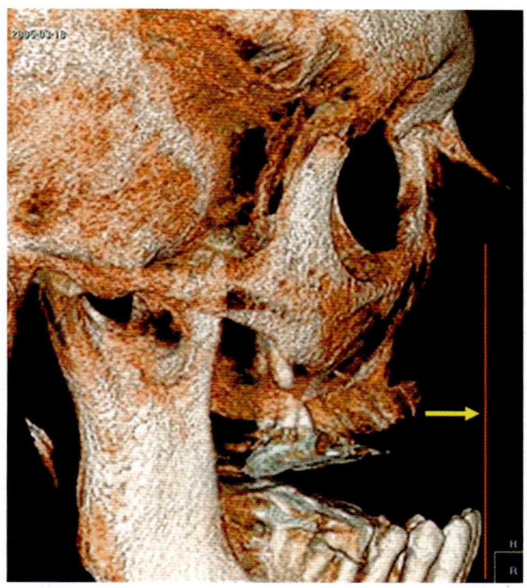

FIGURE 14-45 Three-dimensional, cone beam radiographic reconstruction of the lateral cephalometric view demonstrated a lack of anterior-posterior maxillary development, as is seen in patients with alveolar clefts. The patient's maxillary skeletal relationship was a "pseudo class III" as it related to his mandible.

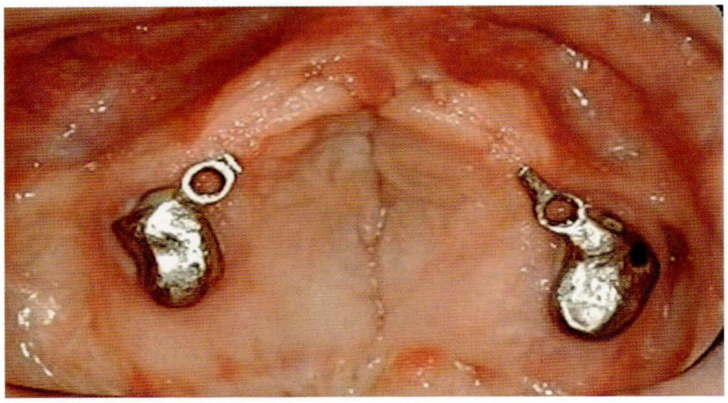

FIGURE 14-46 Flat maxillary vault and shallow buccal vestibule. Evidence of the alveolar cleft is seen at the junction of the left anterior-posterior maxilla.

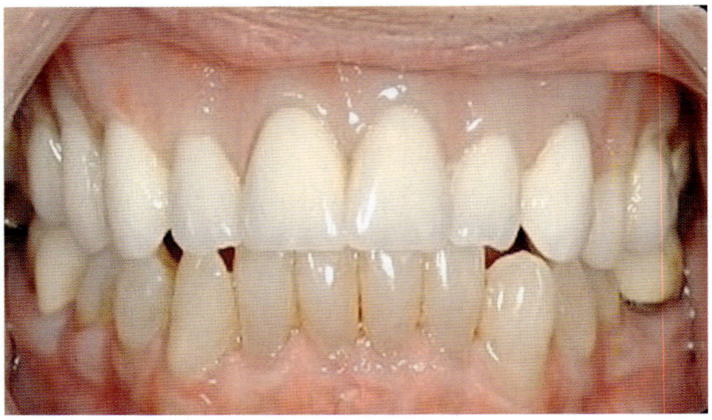

FIGURE 14-47 The patient's maxillary partial denture has a reproducible centric occlusion with apposing natural dentition.

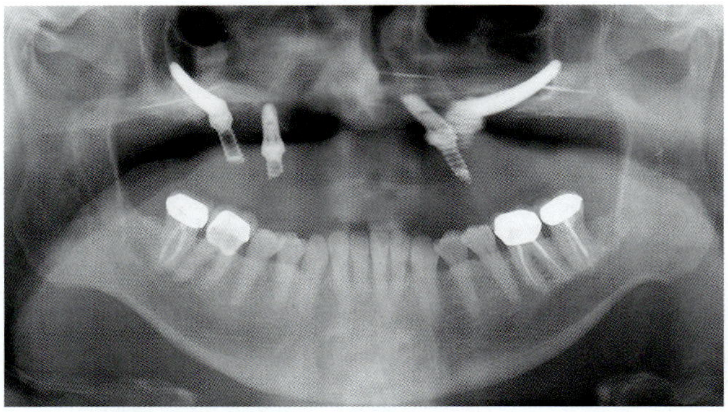

FIGURE 14-48 Immediate postoperative panoramic radiograph. Two zygomatic implants and two premaxillary implants were placed using the conventional protocol for placement of the zygoma implant. It was difficult to negotiate a stable alveolar bone in the area of the left premaxilla cleft.

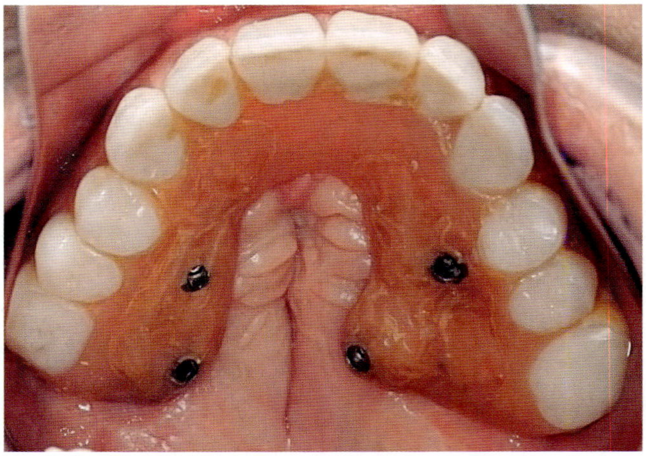

FIGURE 14-49 The patient's full maxillary denture was immediately converted into a provisional immediate-load prosthesis.

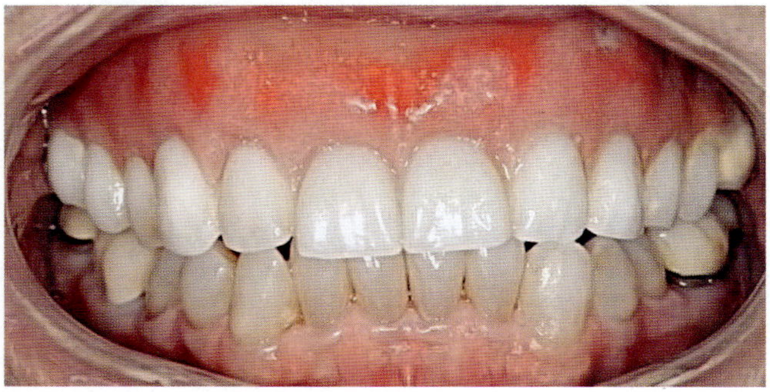

FIGURE 14-50 Stable occlusion with group function was established immediately after conversion of the prosthesis.

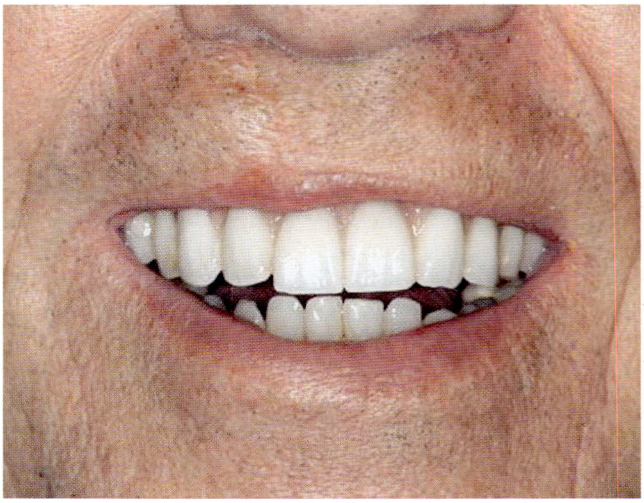

FIGURE 14-51 Appropriate aesthetics of the provisional prosthesis and the hidden transition line is evident in the photo taken 1 week after surgery.

Three months after placing and immediately loading four implants, the patient complained of a loose prosthesis. The prosthetic retaining screws (which were not loose) were removed, and the implant at position 11 was identified as mobile and removed. Anterior extension of the surgical field over the alveolar cleft site and into the limited bone mesial to the cleft site was investigated. A 10-mm Nobe Speedy implant was placed and the prosthesis was modified and delivered to the patient (Figures 14-52 to 14-56).

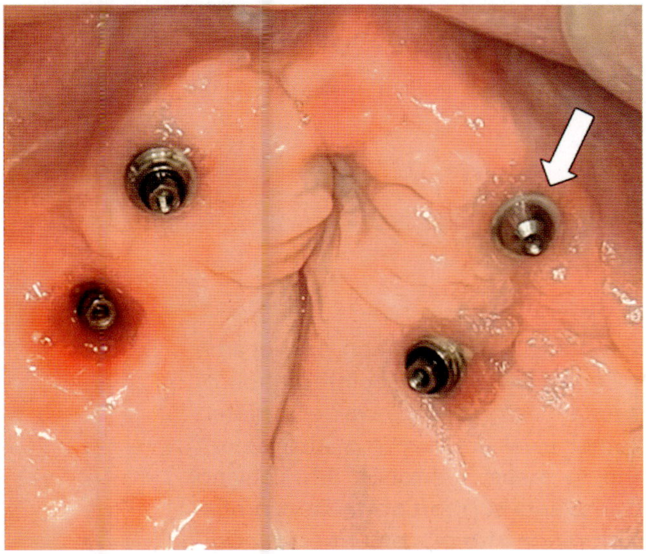

FIGURE 14-52 After removal of the provisional prosthesis at the 3-month postoperative appointment, the implant at position 11 is identified as mobile and removed.

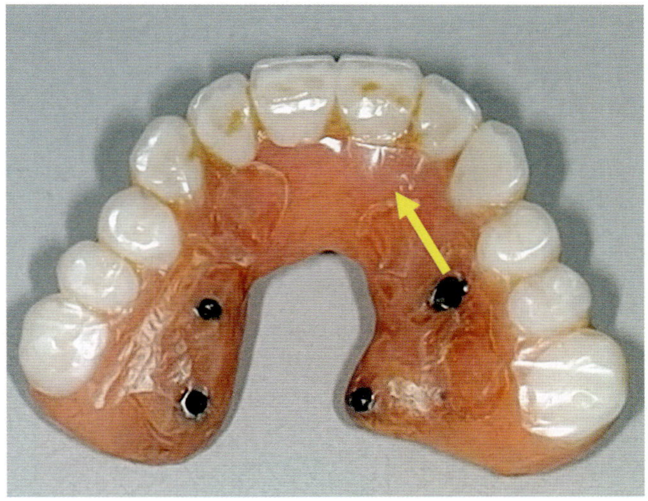

FIGURE 14-53 The temporary titanium cylinder in position 11 needs to be removed.

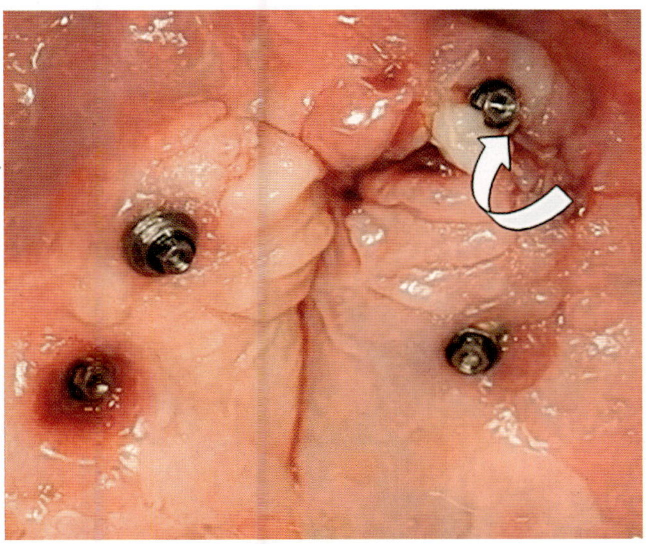

FIGURE 14-54 A new axial implant is placed on the mesial side of the alveolar cleft.

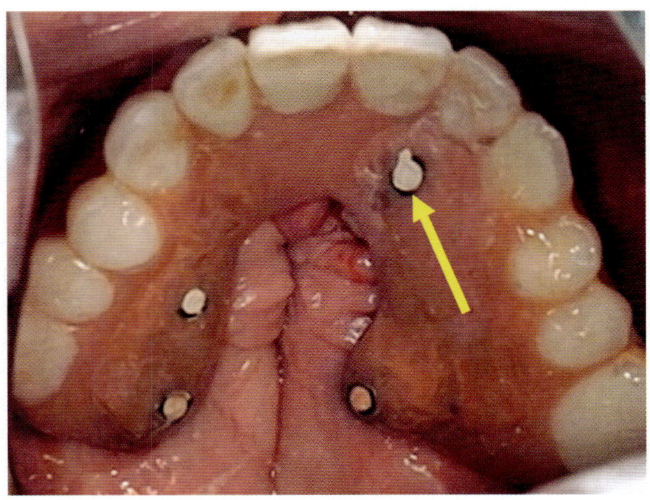

FIGURE 14-55 Incorporation of the temporary titanium cylinder of the newly placed implant into the provisional prosthesis.

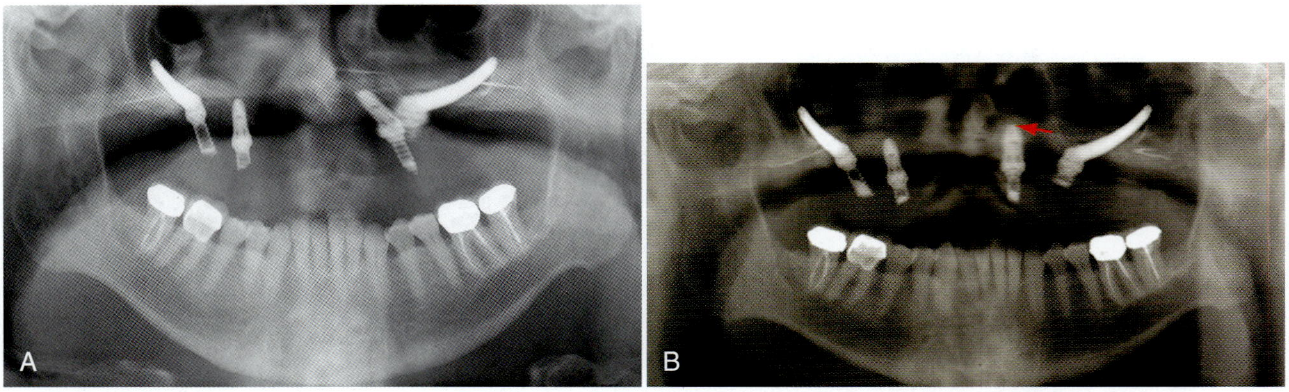

FIGURE 14-56 A panoramic radiograph demonstrates the failed implant at position 11, and the newly placed implant at position 10 (*red arrow*).

After 4 additional months, the newly placed implant at position 10 became loose and symptomatic, and was removed. Confirmation of osseointegration of the zygoma implants bilaterally and of the implant at position 8 was completed by reverse-torque testing. Placement of another axial anterior implant was not possible because of a lack of bony volume in areas 9 through 11. Leaving the patient with only three osseointegrated implants supporting a fixed profile prosthesis was not considered. Therefore, exploration into placement of an additional zygoma implant in the left body of the zygoma, which already housed a zygoma implant, was initiated (Figures 14-57 to 14-58).

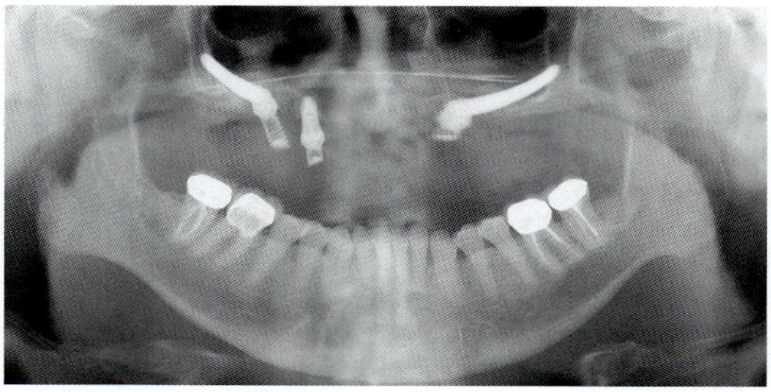

FIGURE 14-57 After removal of the failed implant at position 10, the three remaining implants supported the profile prosthesis.

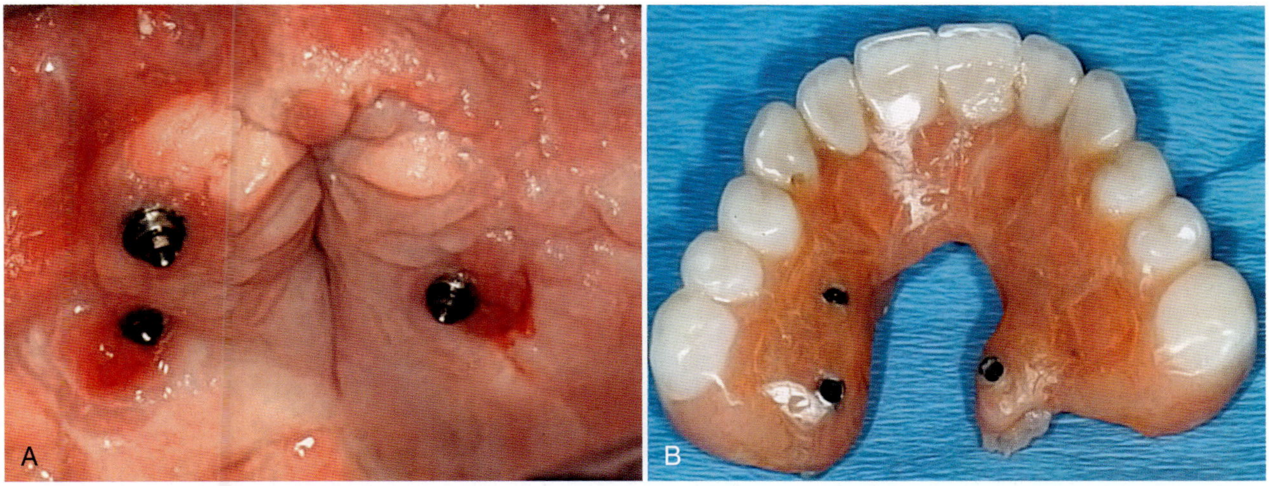

FIGURE 14-58 Removal of the profile prosthesis reveals healed soft tissues of the left premaxilla and the lack of anterior support of the left half of the provisional profile prosthesis.

A cone beam radiograph revealed adequate volume and contour of remaining bone in the body of the left zygoma to attempt placement of a second zygoma implant (Figures 14-59 to 14-60).

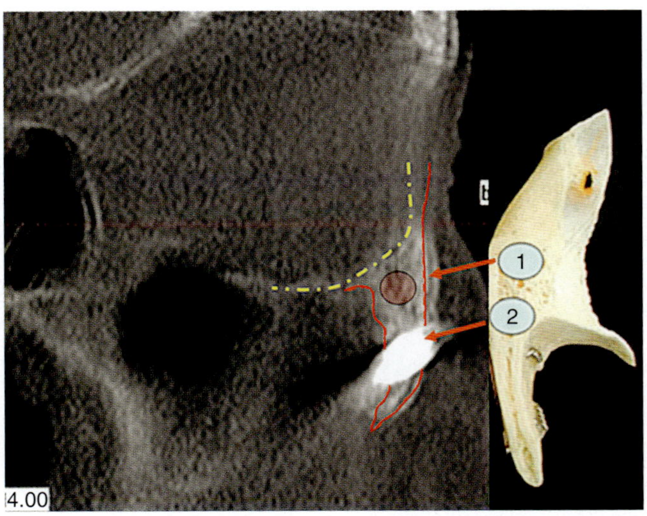

FIGURE 14-59 To plan placement of two zygomatic implants within the body of the os zygomaticus, a dry skull is used to demonstrate the "stacked" relationship of the apical portion of the zygomatic implants. Position 1 corresponds with the anterior zygoma implant in the cuspid area and position 2 corresponds with the posterior zygoma implant in the bicuspid area.

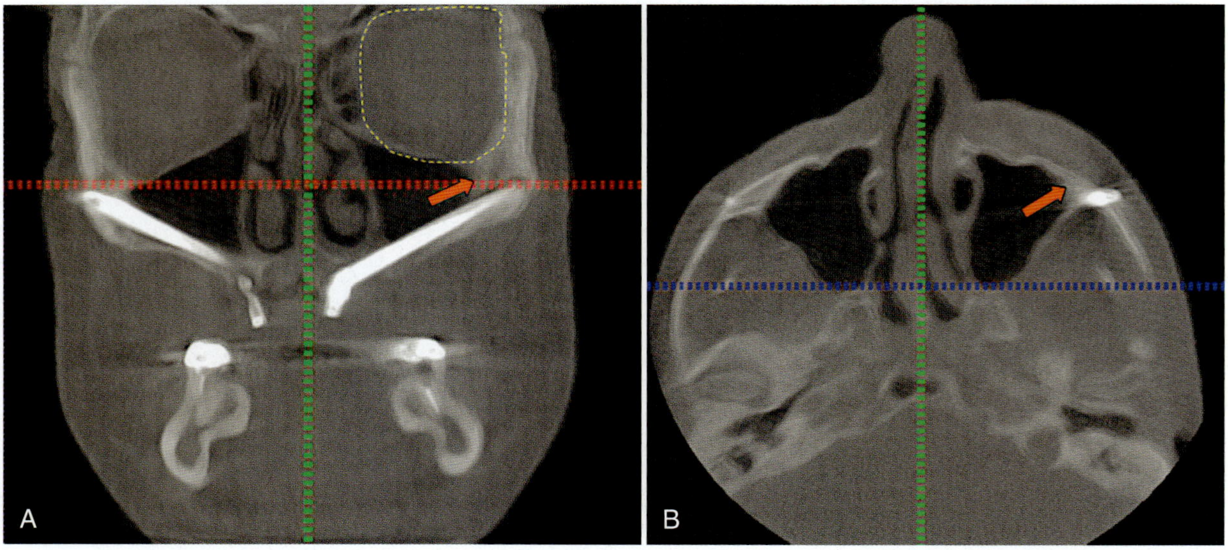

FIGURE 14-60 Cone beam radiographic views show the availability of bone for placement of a zygoma implant in position 1.

A local flap was established to expose the previous bony window, which was developed for placement of the initial zygoma implant. Osseointegration of the initial implant was confirmed by reverse-torque testing at 35 Ncm. Careful negotiation of the superior-medial aspect of the zygomatic bone was made with the placement of the zygomatic implant platform in positions 11 and 12. After a multiunit abutment was placed and torqued to 35 Ncm, the immediate-load prosthesis was modified to incorporate the temporary titanium cylinder of the newly placed zygomatic implant (Figures 14-61 to 14-64).

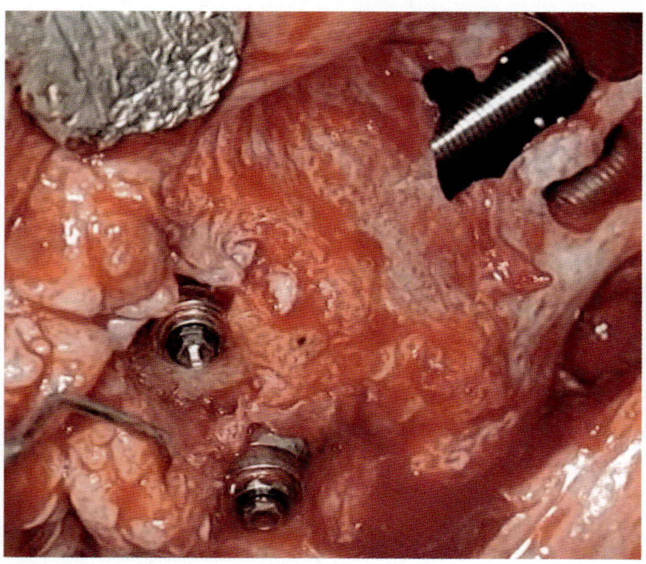

FIGURE 14-61 Direct visualization of the insertion path of the newly placed second zygoma implant.Isquissi musdae.

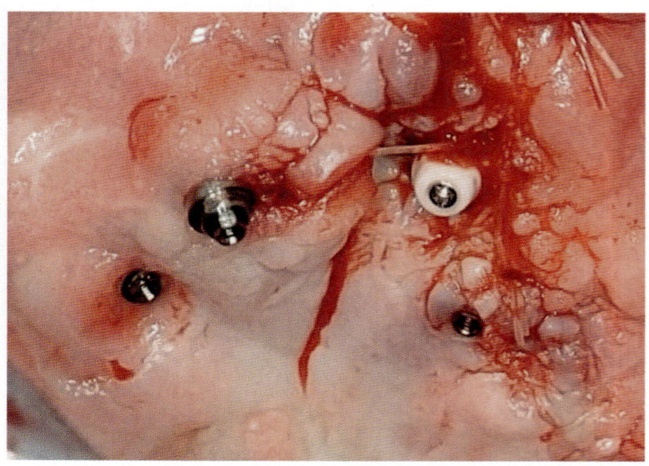

FIGURE 14-62 Placement of the multiunit abutment.

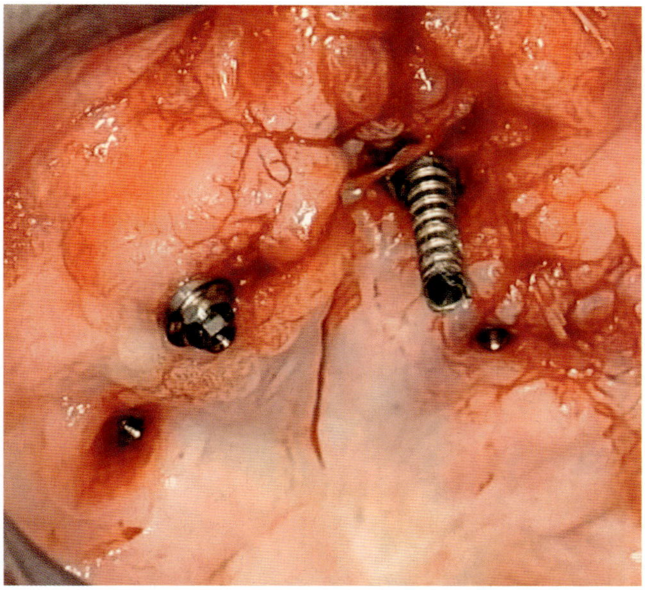

FIGURE 14-63 Connection of a temporary titanium cylinder.

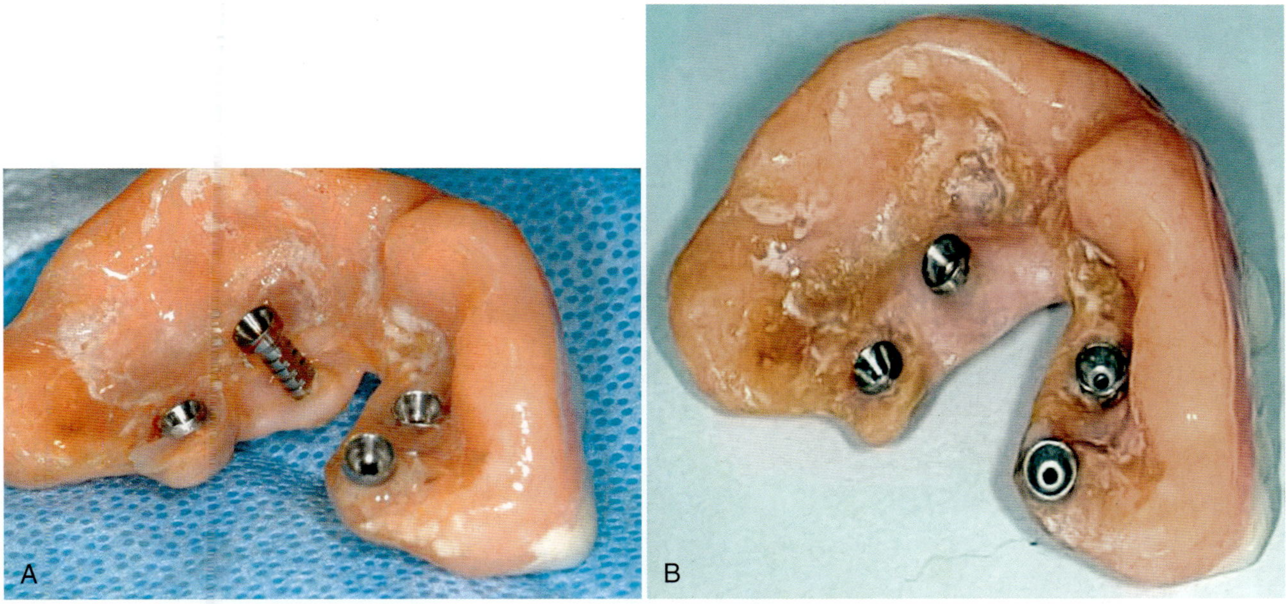

FIGURE 14-64 Incorporation of the newly placed zygomatic implant into the existing provisional prosthesis.

Six months of further osseointeqration is allowed for the newly placed zygoma implant. At the 6-month appointment, cone-beam evaluation of the position of the implants was studied (Figures 14-65 to 14-69).

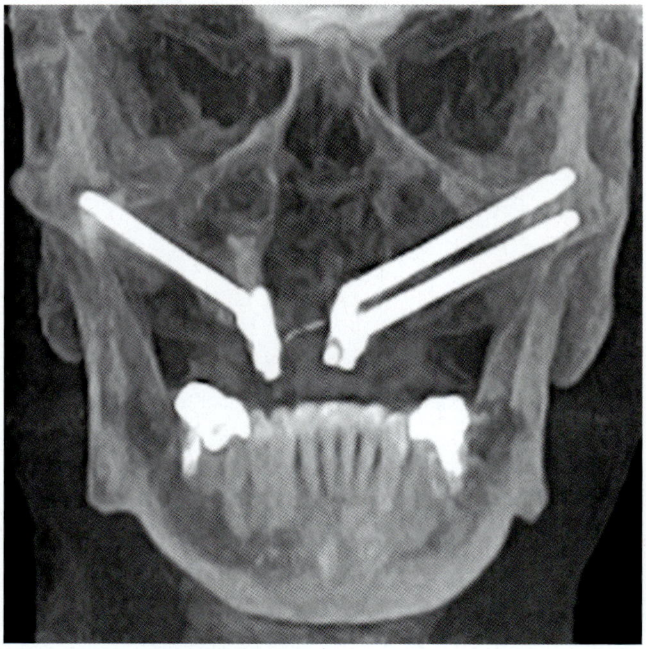

FIGURE 14-65 A cone beam radiograph demonstrates the relationship of the two zygoma implants within the sinus.

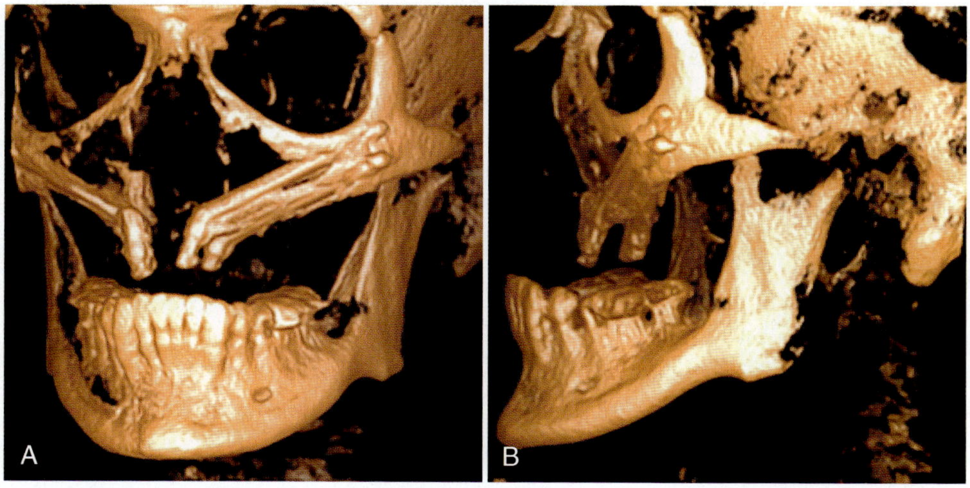

FIGURE 14-66 Three-dimensional reformatting of the cone beam radiograph demonstrates the relationship at the apical portion of the two zygomatic implants.

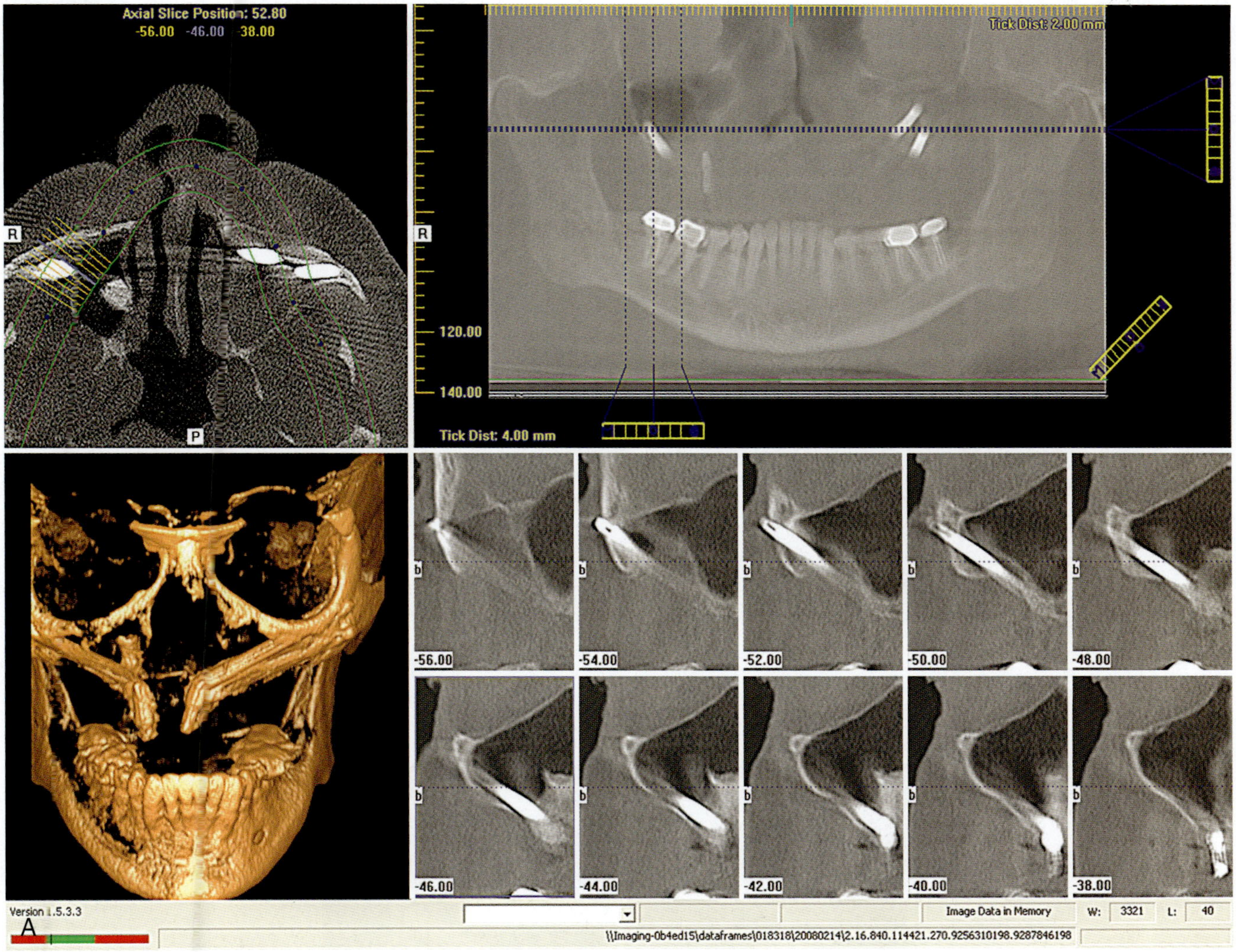

FIGURE 14-67 The path of the zygomatic implants from the crest of the maxilla through the maxillary sinus and their termination in the body of the zygoma is clearly demonstrated in the cone beam radiograph.

continued

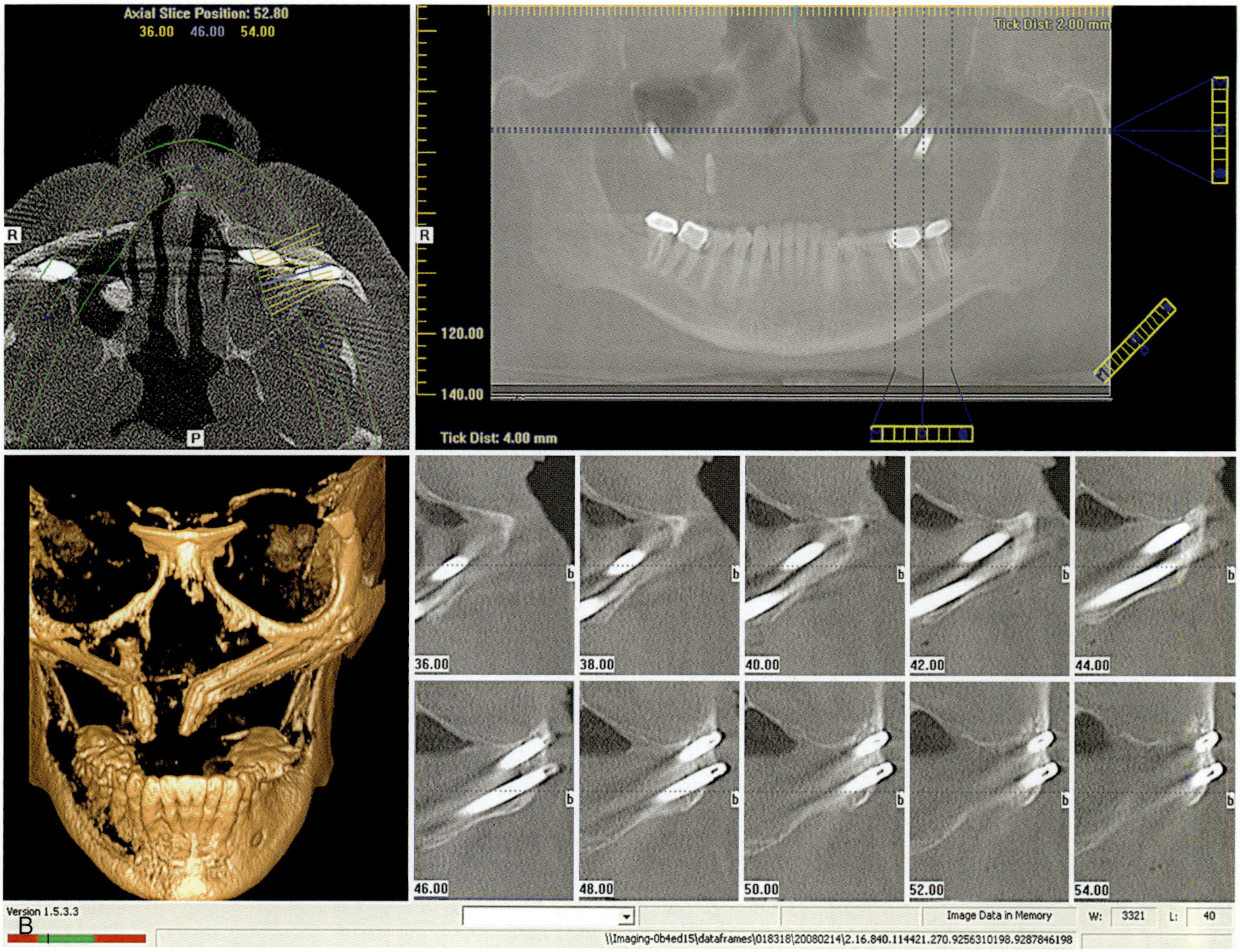

FIGURE 14-67, cont'd

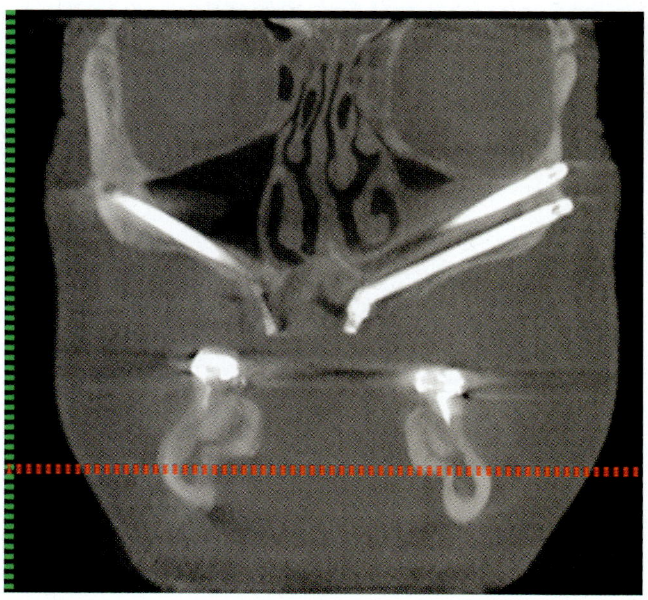

FIGURE 14-68 Immediate postoperative anterior-posterior cephalometric reformatted view using a cone beam radiograph to illustrate the apical "stacking" of two zygoma implants.

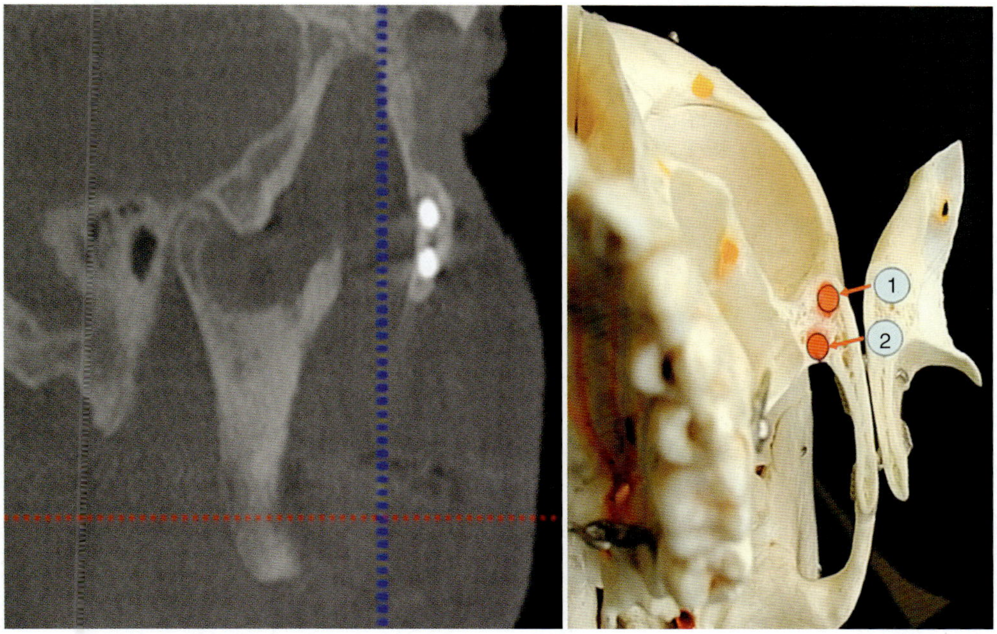

FIGURE 14-69 The apical positioning of the two zygomatic implants mimics the intended positioning as demonstrated on the dry skull model.

Reverse torque text confirms osseointegration of the new zygomatic implant in position number 11 (Figures 14-70).

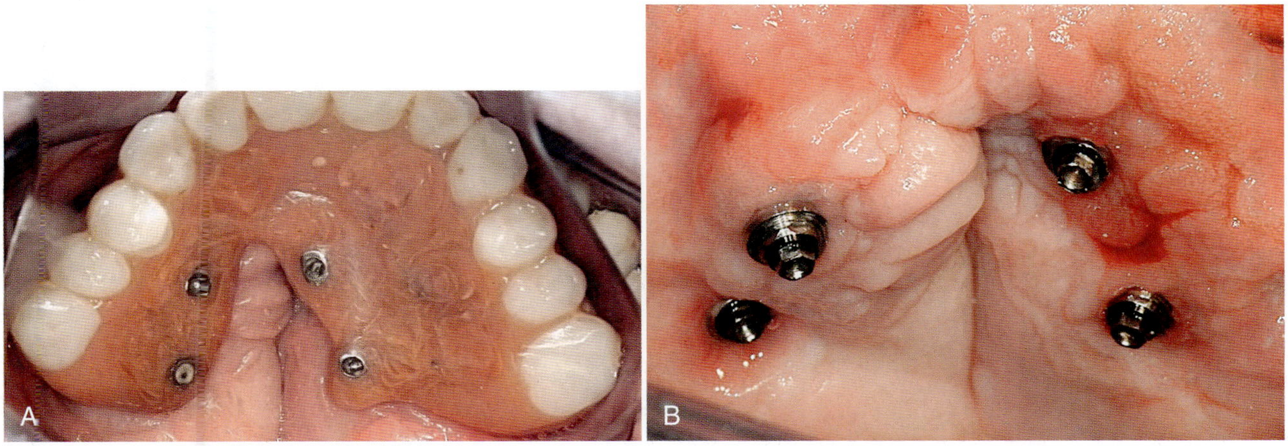

FIGURE 14-70 Six months after placement of the new zygoma implant, osseointegration of all implants were confirmed by reverse-torque testing.

After confirmation of osseointegration of all implants, fabrication of the final metal-based profile prosthesis was made (Figures 14-71 to 14-75).

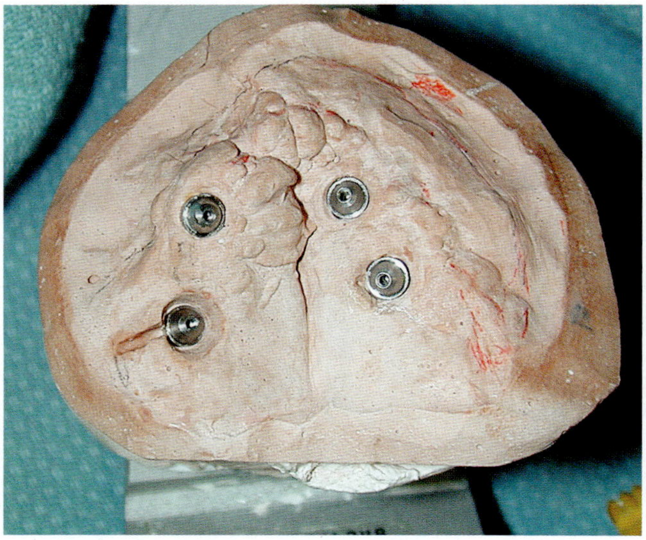

FIGURE 14-71 Master cast in preparation for fabrication of the final prosthesis.

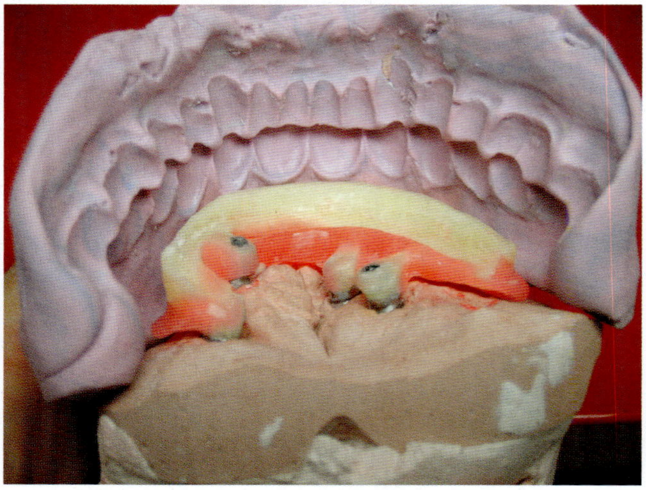

FIGURE 14-72 A putty index of the desired teeth positions guides the metal framework design.

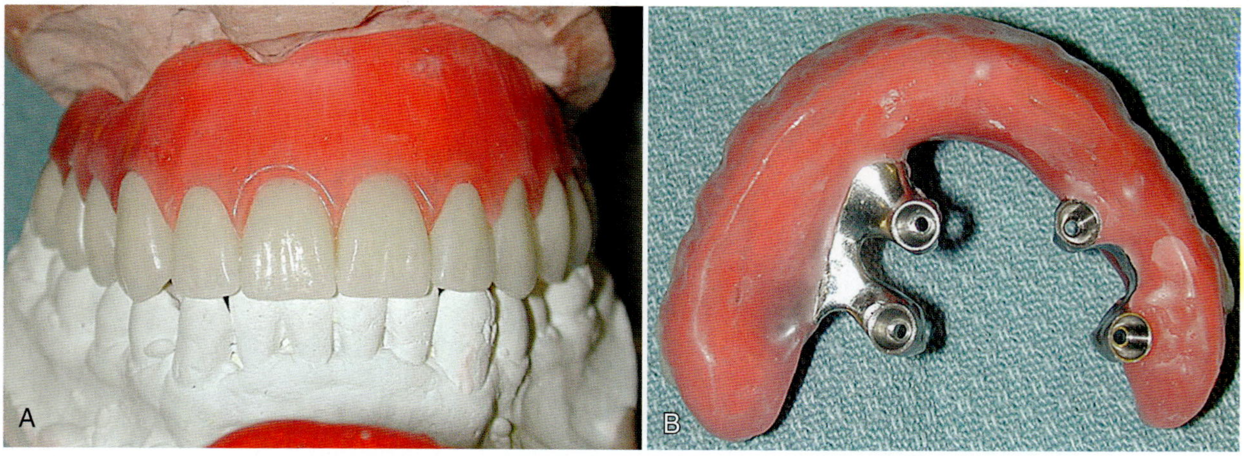

FIGURE 14-73 Completed maxillary profile prosthesis.

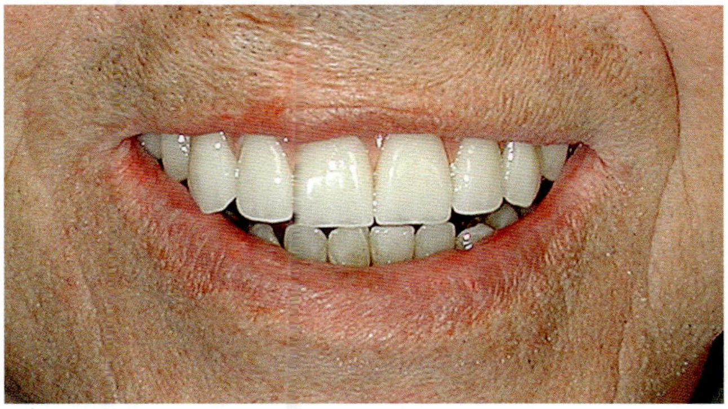

FIGURE 14-74 Hidden transition line and an aesthetically acceptable smile during animation of the final profile prosthesis.

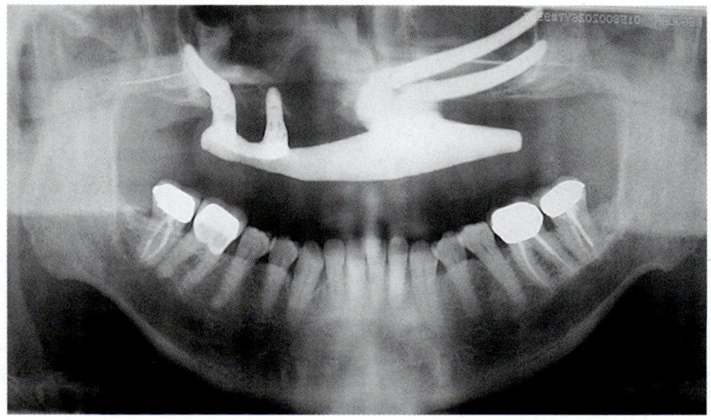

FIGURE 14-75 Final panoramic radiograph. (*Courtesy Dr. Paul Binor Prosthodontist.*)

FAILING IMPLANTS

A 62-year-old woman presented with a history of having "press fit" implants placed 15 years earlier for support of a fixed maxillary and mandibular prosthesis. 7 years after implant placement, mandibular swelling and infection developed, which was managed with antibiotics and local debridement as needed. Eventual loss of several implants in the lower left quadrant occurred, however. At the time of examination, the patient presented with an inability to function with her mandibular partial denture, periodontally involved anterior mandibular teeth, and peri-implantitis associated with the implants in the mandibular right quadrant. The remaining maxillary fixed prosthesis was stable; moderate to advanced bone loss was associated with each implant, however, resulting in intermittent pain and swelling associated with peri-implantitis around each of the abutments. The patient's initial priority was treatment of the mandibular arch (Figure 14-76).

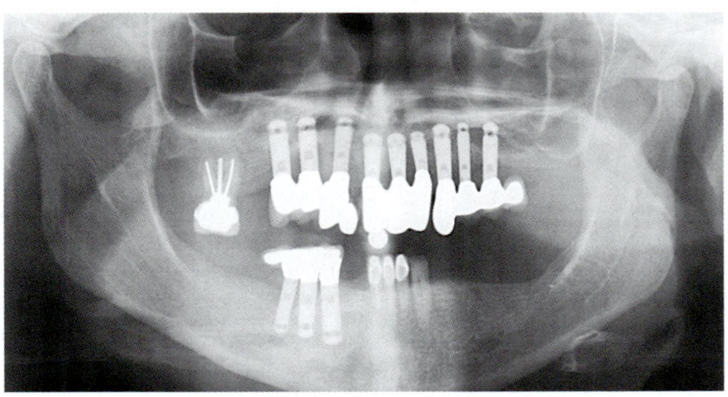

FIGURE 14-76 Preoperative radiograph with failing implants and anterior mandibular dentition.

Overall treatment plan

1. Remove the mandibular implants and teeth with immediate loading of the mandibular arch.
2. Remove the failing maxillary implants, place new implants, and load immediately.

The initial phase of the patient's treatment included removal of the failing teeth and implants in the lower right quadrant with simultaneous placement of new implants and immediate loading (Figure 14-77).

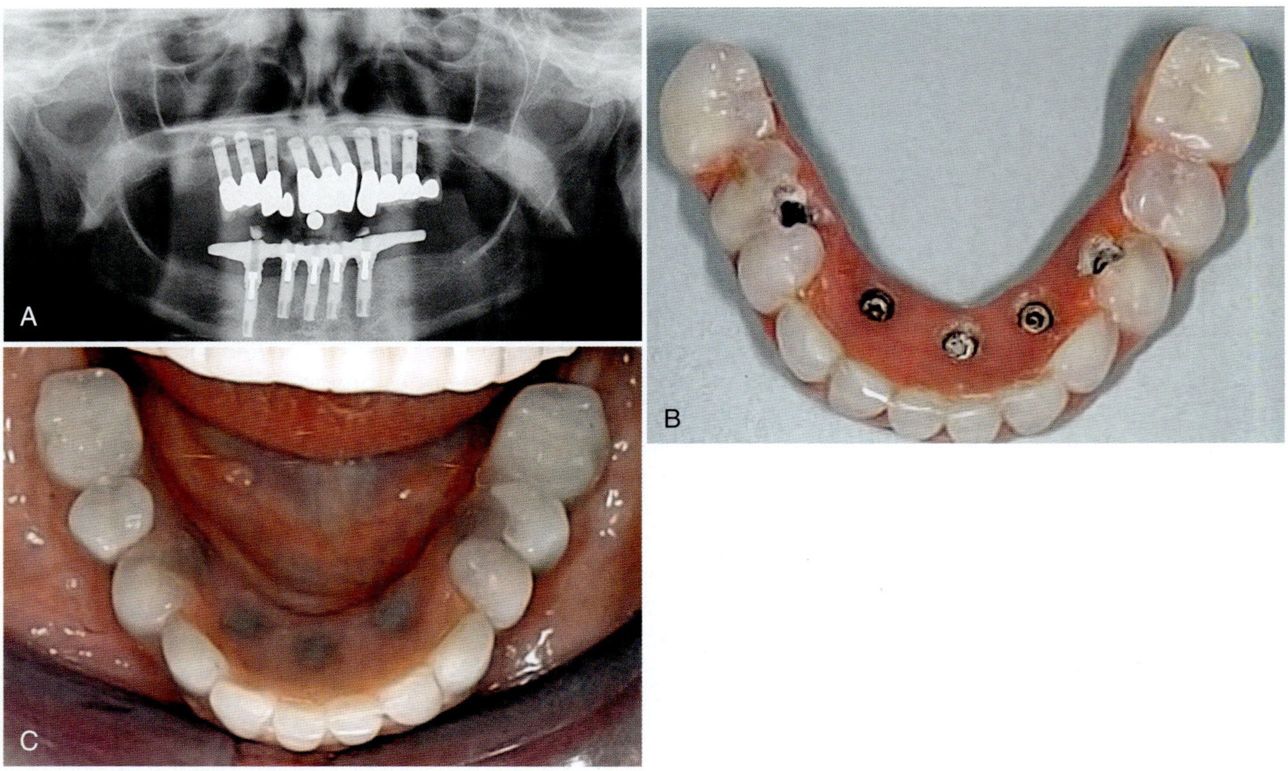

FIGURE 14-77 Completed mandibular treatment with removal of the anterior teeth and the posterior implants with simultaneous immediate loading of the new implants paced in the mandibular arch.

Two years after treatment of the mandibular arch, the patient presented with continuous maxillary gingival pain with inflammation and drainage from the soft tissues around the abutments (Figure 14-78).

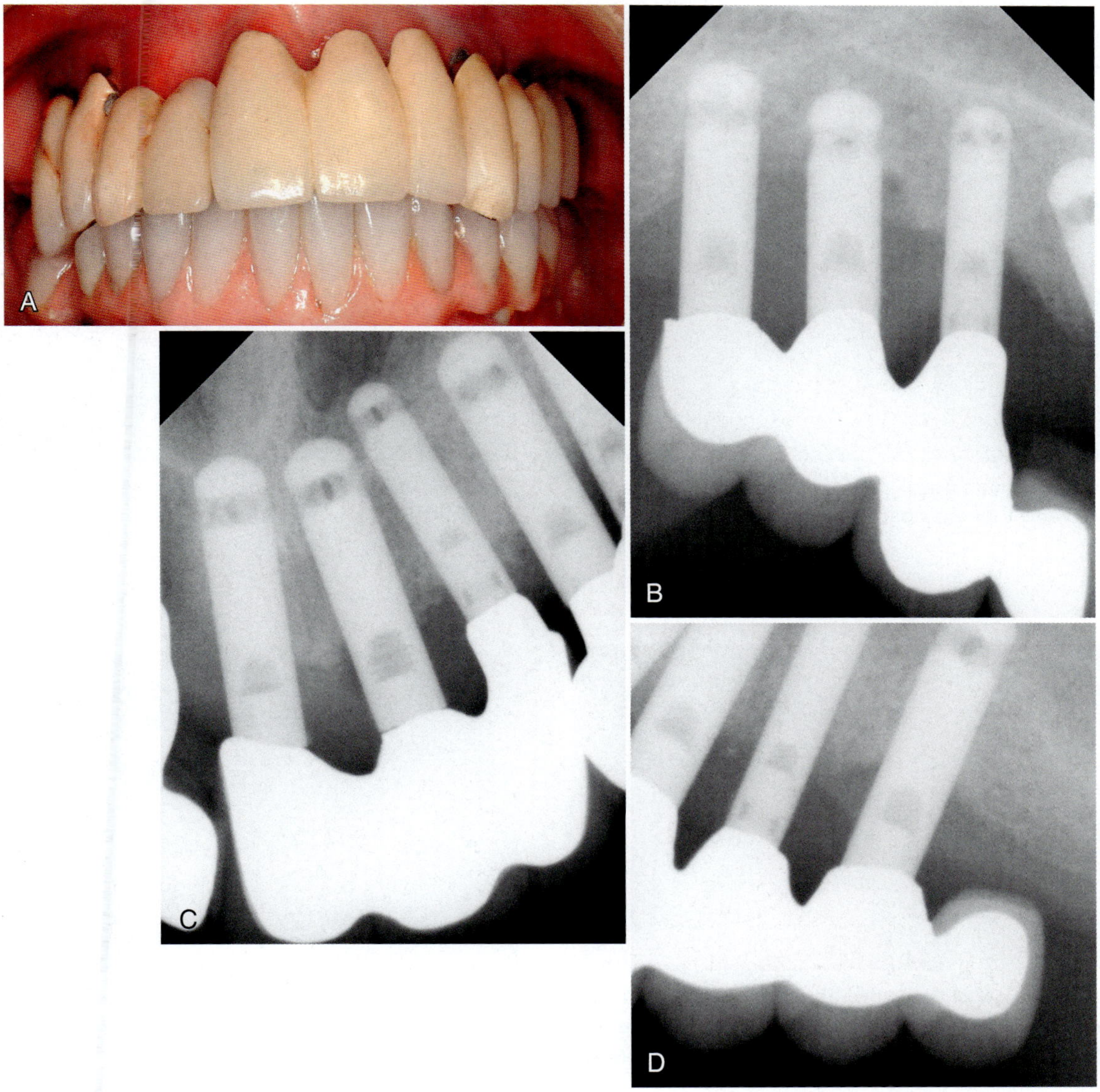

FIGURE 14-78 A, Maxillary prosthesis with evidence of peri-implantitis. B, Periapical radiographs of the maxillary right quadrant showing more than 75% vertical bone loss. C, Periapical radiographs of the anterior maxillary implants. D, Periapical radiographs of the maxillary right quadrant showing cupping defect of the implants.

Maxillary treatment plan

1. Trephine the existing failing implants.
2. Place immediate-load implants using the zygoma protocol.
3. Load the implants immediately with a profile prosthesis.
4. Fabricate a final metal-based profile prosthesis.

(Figures 14-79 to 14-83)

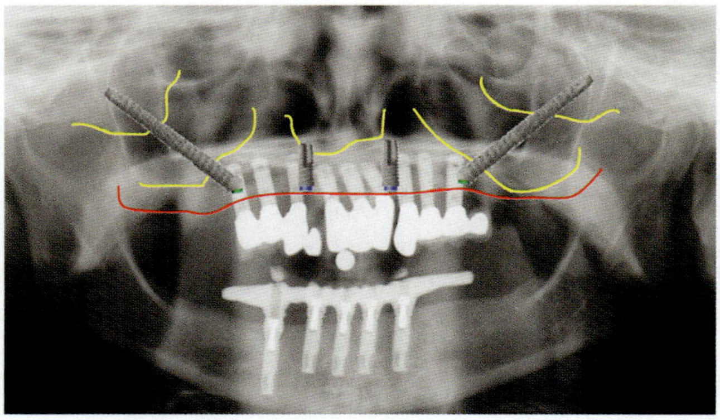

FIGURE 14-79 Planning of the positions of the premaxillary implants and the two posterior zygoma implants.

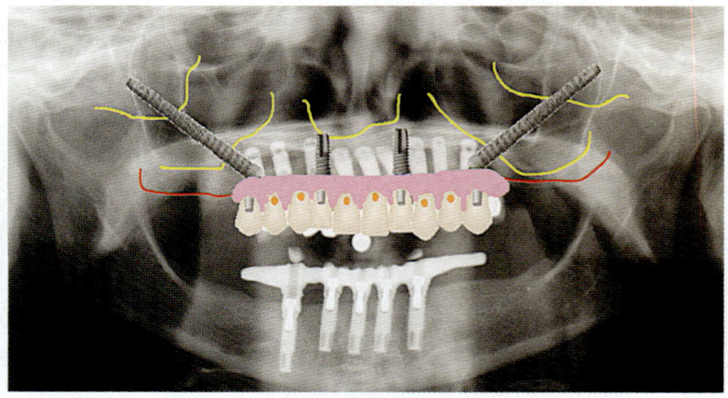

FIGURE 14-80 Planning of the provisional prosthesis supported by the four implants.

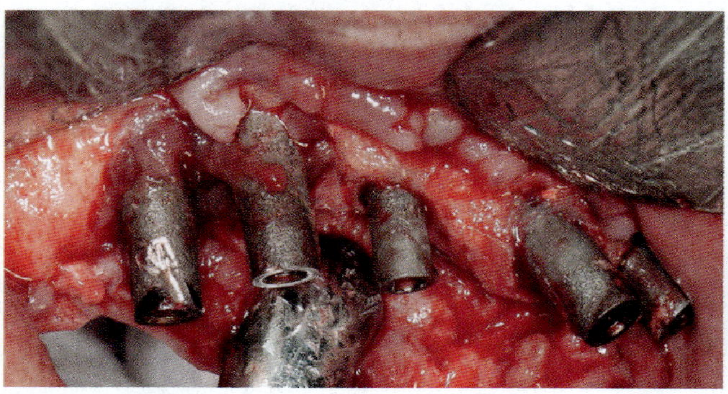

FIGURE 14-81 Exposure of the implants in the maxillary right quadrant. Direct visualization of the bony defect consistent with the radiographic findings and the clinical symptoms.

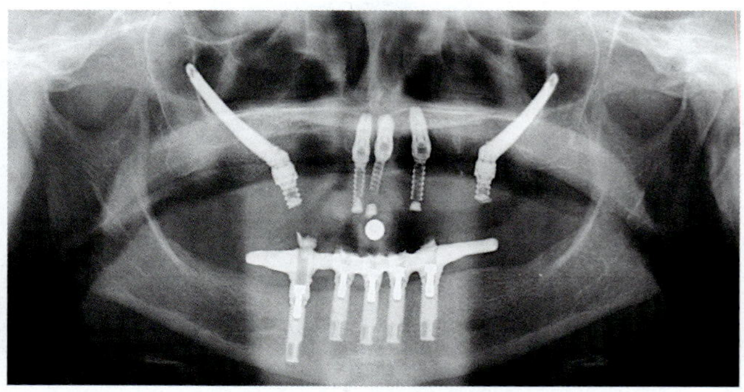

FIGURE 14-82 Immediate postoperative panoramic radiograph. The third premaxillary implant was placed because the implant in position 9 was seated with only 20 Ncm insertion torque, which is inadequate for immediate loading. Therefore, implant 10 was placed with an insertion torque of 40 Ncm.

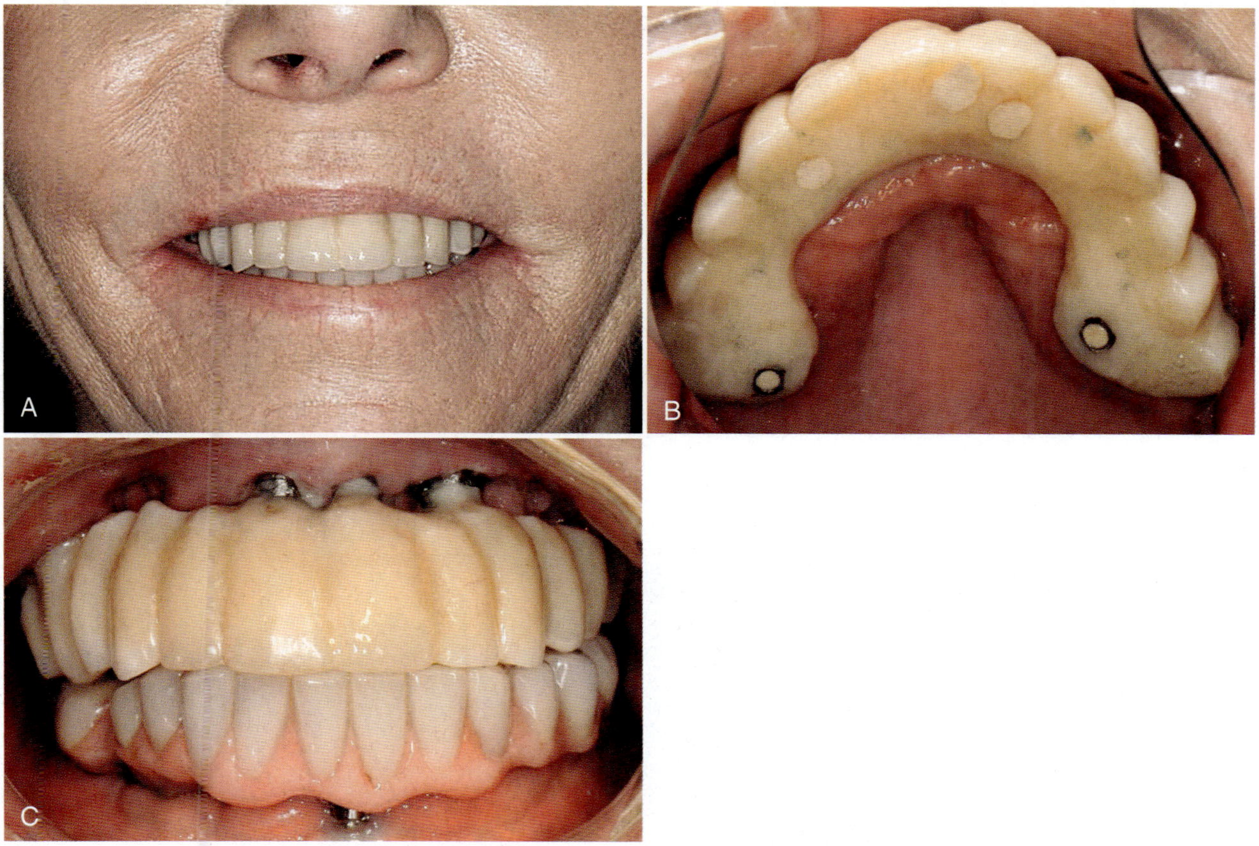

FIGURE 14-83 An aesthetically acceptable and functional provisional prosthesis. **A,** One week after trephining the implants. **B,** Immediate placement of the new implants. **C,** The immediate chairside conversion of the maxillary prosthesis to a fixed provisional prosthesis. Stable occlusion with bilateral group function is essential.

The implants were allowed to osseointegrate for 6 months, at which time the provisional prosthesis was removed and the stability of the abutment screws and implants were confirmed by retorquing the abutment screws. The final prosthesis was then fabricated.

The provisional prosthesis can be used until it is no longer functional, at which point one of the following treatment options may be chosen:

1. Fabricate an all-acrylic, laboratory-processed maxillary profile prosthesis.
2. Fabricate a metal framework final profile prosthesis.
3. Fabricate a titanium framework, Procera profile prosthesis.

For this patient, a metal framework profile prosthesis was fabricated.

(Figures 14-84 to 14-87)

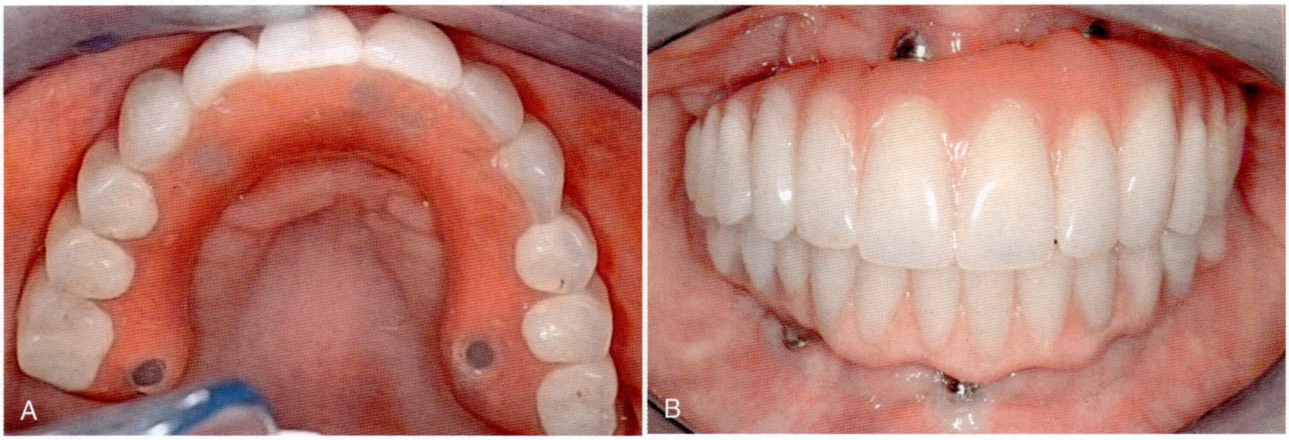

FIGURE 14-84 Final metal-based profile prosthesis.

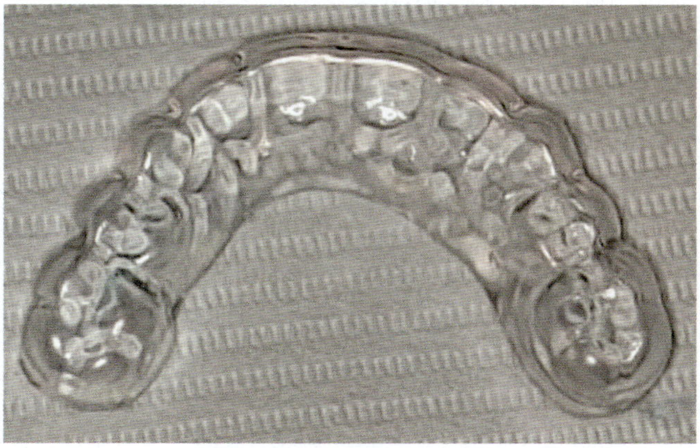

FIGURE 14-85 An occlusal splint may be fabricated as indicated after completion of the final prosthesis.

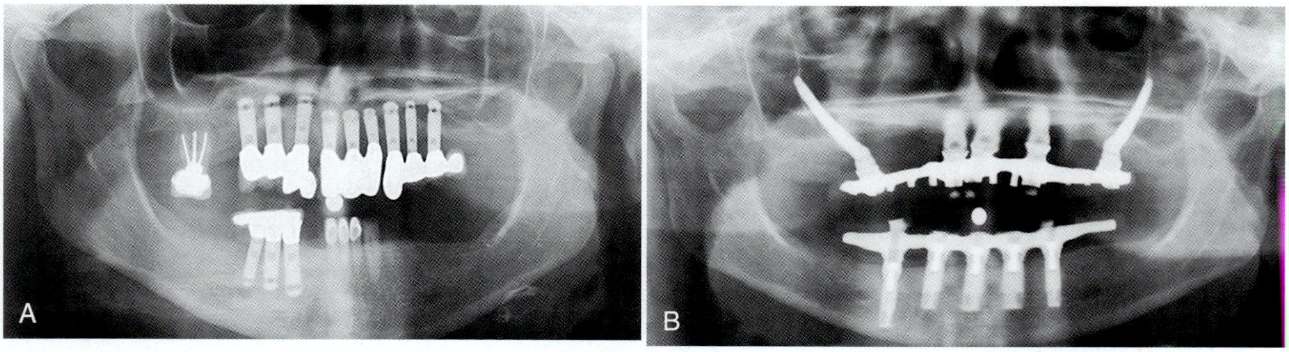

FIGURE 14-86 Preoperative (A) and postoperative (B) radiographs.

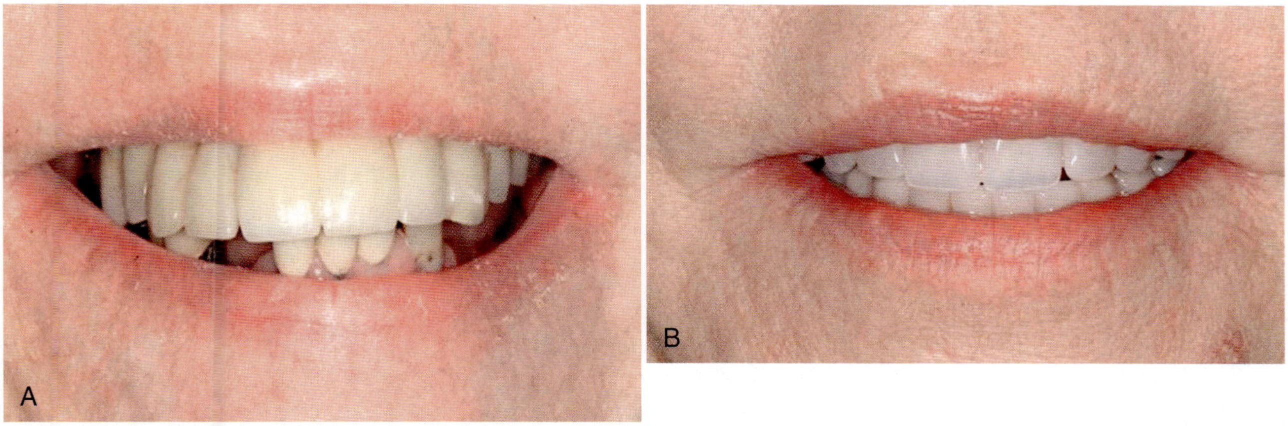

FIGURE 14-87 Preoperative and postoperative clinical presentation of the patient's smile.

FAILING IMPLANT-SUPPORTED MAXILLARY OVERDENTURE

A 47-year-old female presents with a 10-year history of utilizing an implant-supported maxillary overdenture. The existing implants have had an intermittent history of gingival irritation and purulent exudates, which have failed to respond to oral hygiene treatment as well as multiple regimens of antibiotic therapy. The intraoral examination is consistent with the presence of an implant-supported overdenture bar. Upon its detachment from the existing implants, drainage of purulence was evident around each implant platform (Figures 14-88 to 14-91).

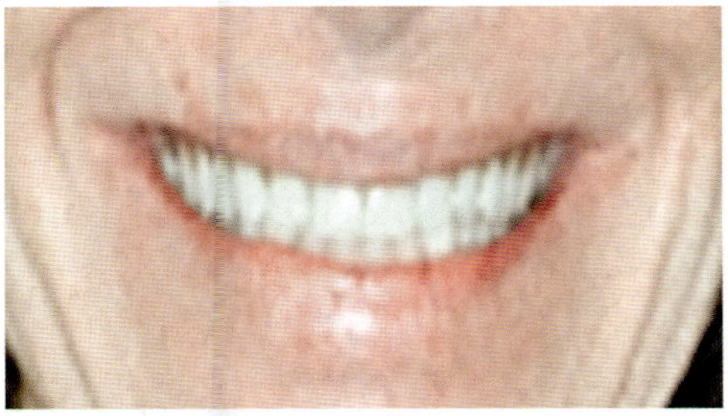

FIGURE 14-88 Aesthetic smile line of an existing maxillary implant-supported overdenture.

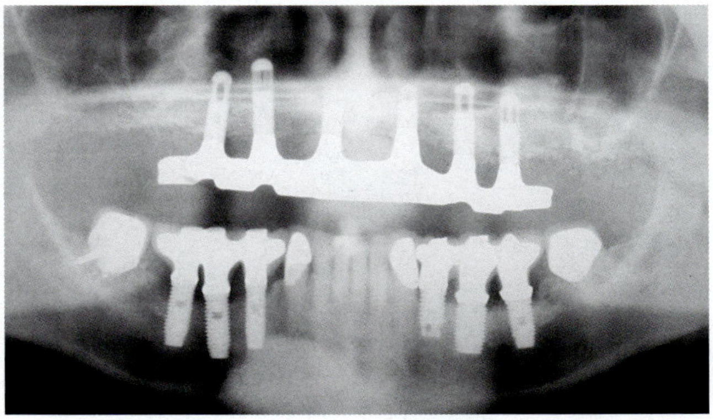

FIGURE 14-89 Preoperative panoramic radiograph.

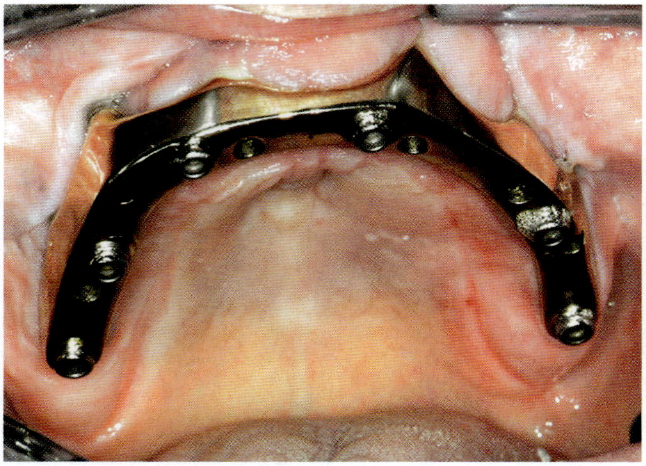

FIGURE 14-90 Existing overdenture framework.

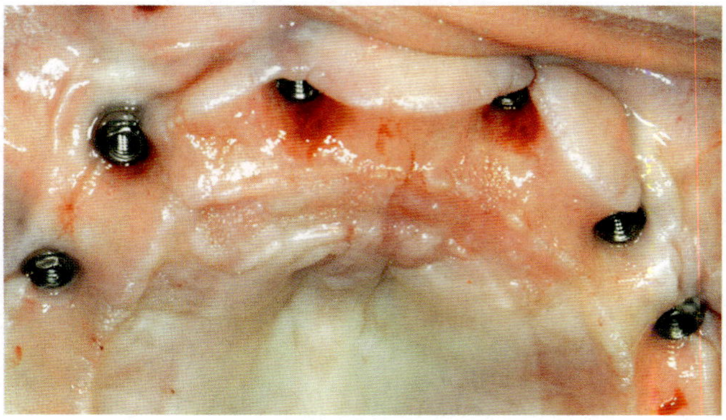

FIGURE 14-91 Evidence of peri-implantitis after removal of the metal overdenture bar.

Treatment planning:

1. Fabrication of a new full maxillary denture.
2. Removal of all existing failing implants.
3. Immediate placement of two premaxillary and two zygomatic implants.
4. Immediate conversion of a full maxillary denture into a provisional profile prosthesis.
5. Final fabrication of a fixed, implant-supported profile prosthesis.

(Figures 14-92 to 14-103)

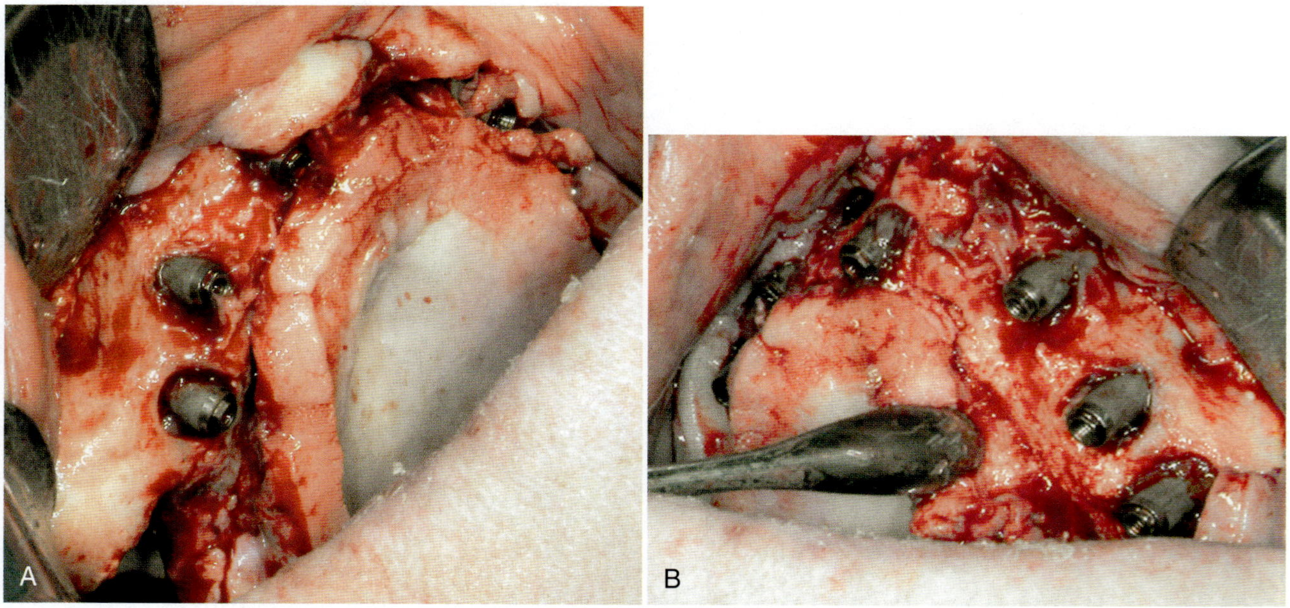

FIGURE 14-92 Evidence of the peri-implant bone loss on all existing implants.

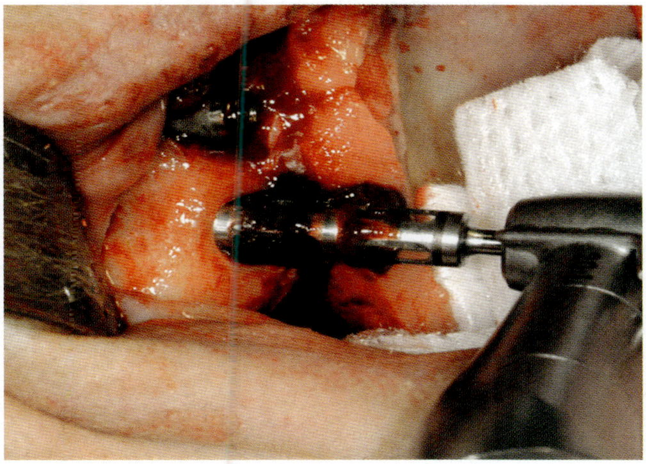

FIGURE 14-93 Trephining of the existing failing implants.

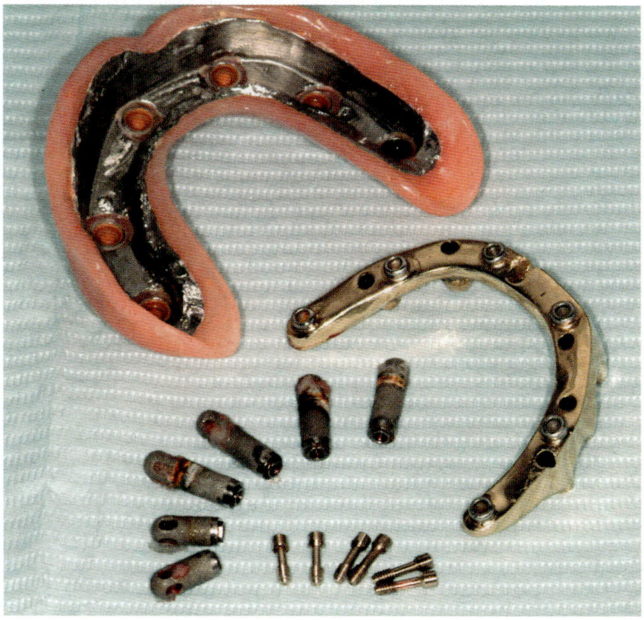

FIGURE 14-94 Existing overdenture, overdenture bar, and the trephined implants.

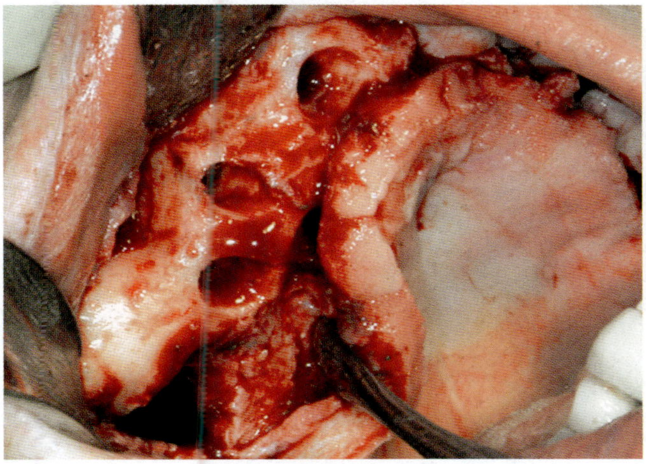

FIGURE 14-95 Residual defects after trephining of the implants.

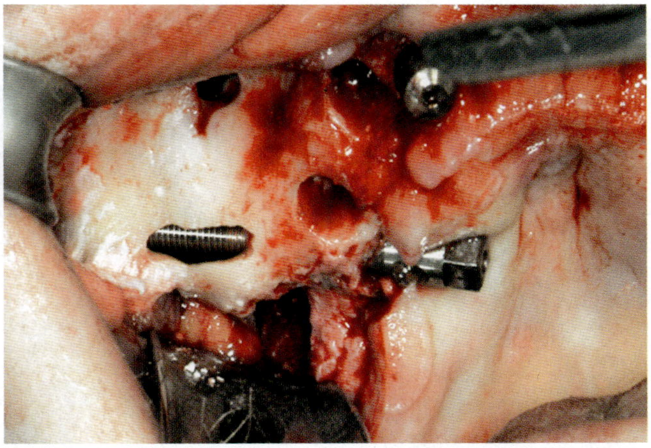

FIGURE 14-96 Immediate placement of the zygomatic implants.

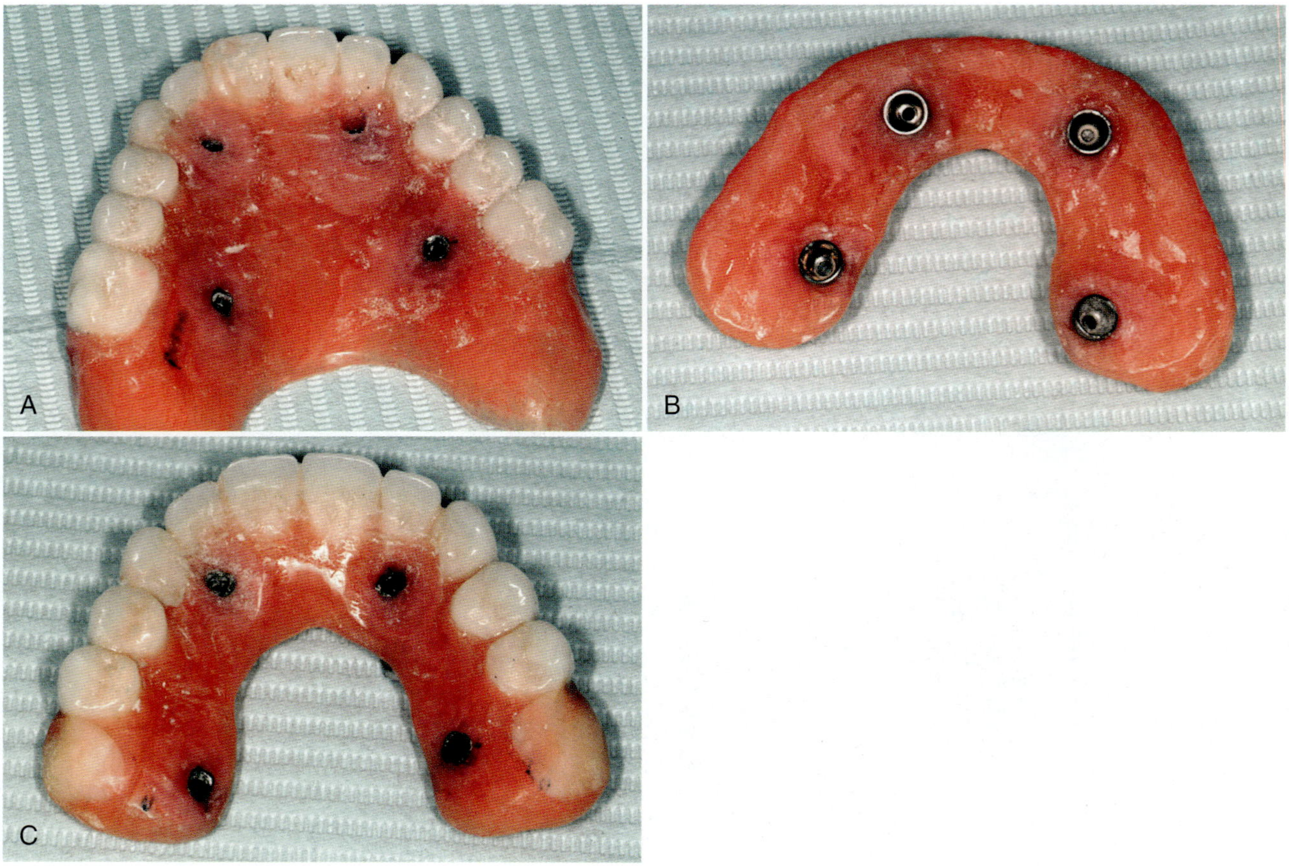

FIGURE 14-97 Completed conversion of the full maxillary denture into a provisional profile prosthesis.

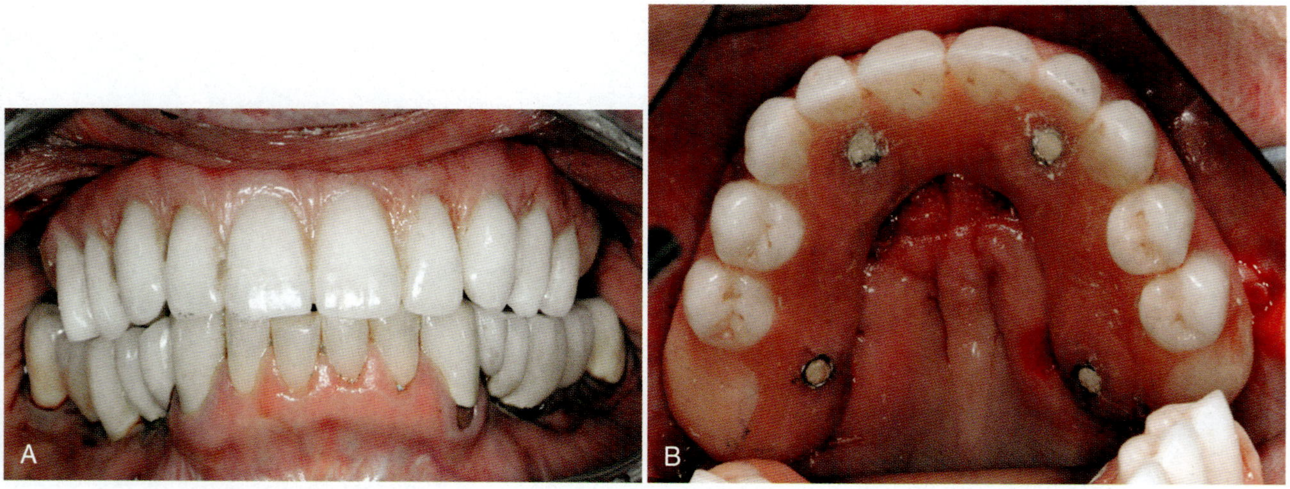

FIGURE 14-98 Stable maximum intercuspation of the completed provisional prosthesis.

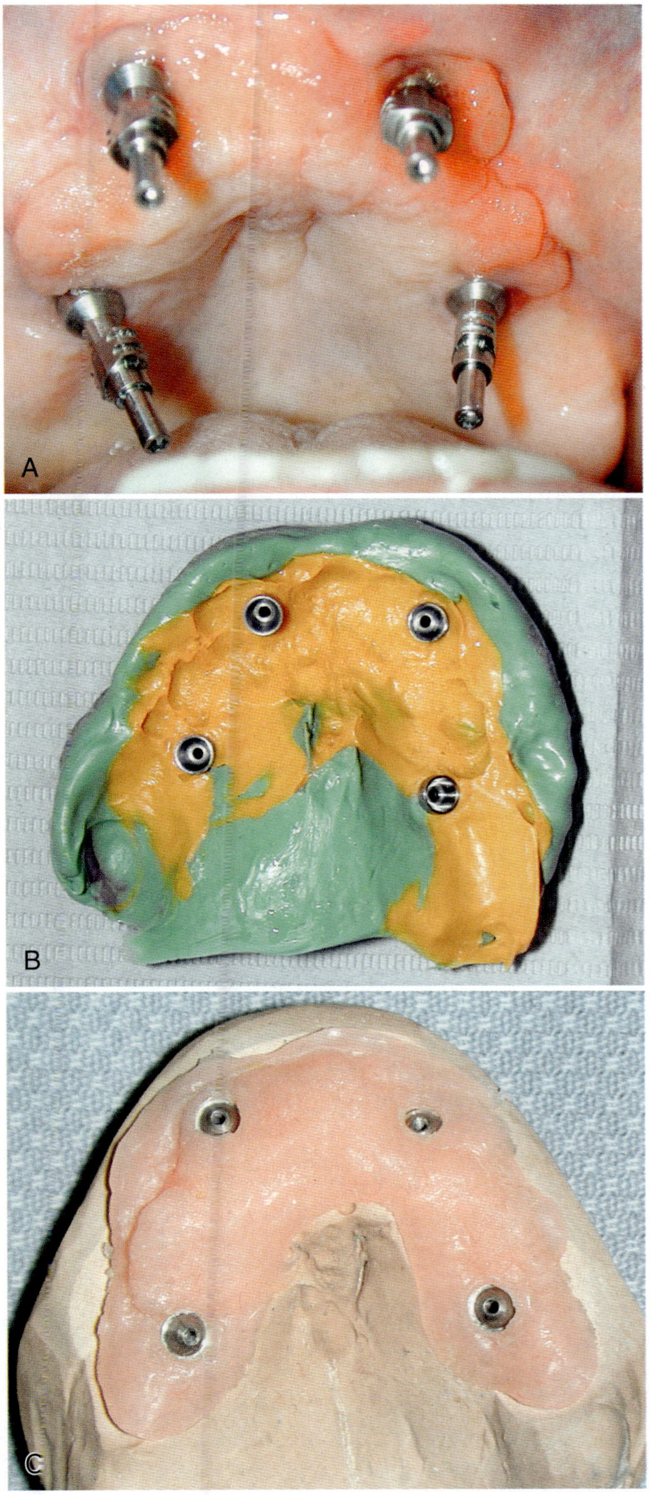

FIGURE 14-99 Six months after implant placement, abutment level impression and the pouring of the maxillary soft tissue model is done.

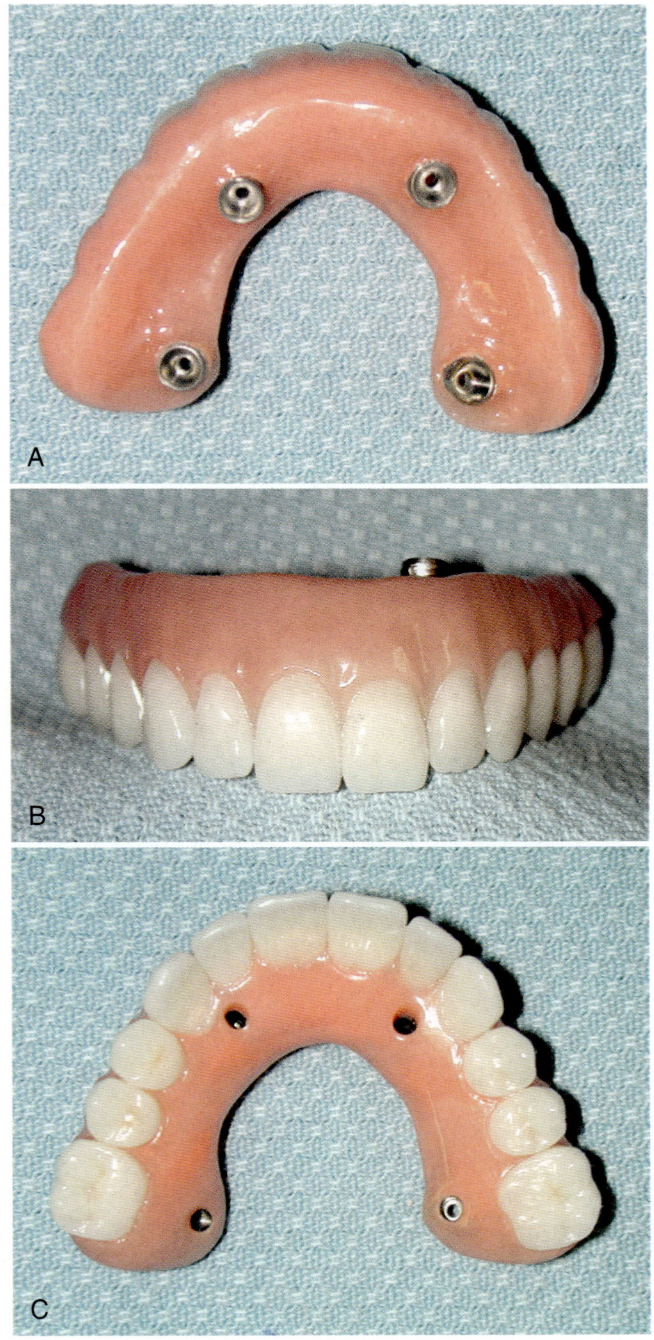

FIGURE 14-100 Final metal-based profile prosthesis.

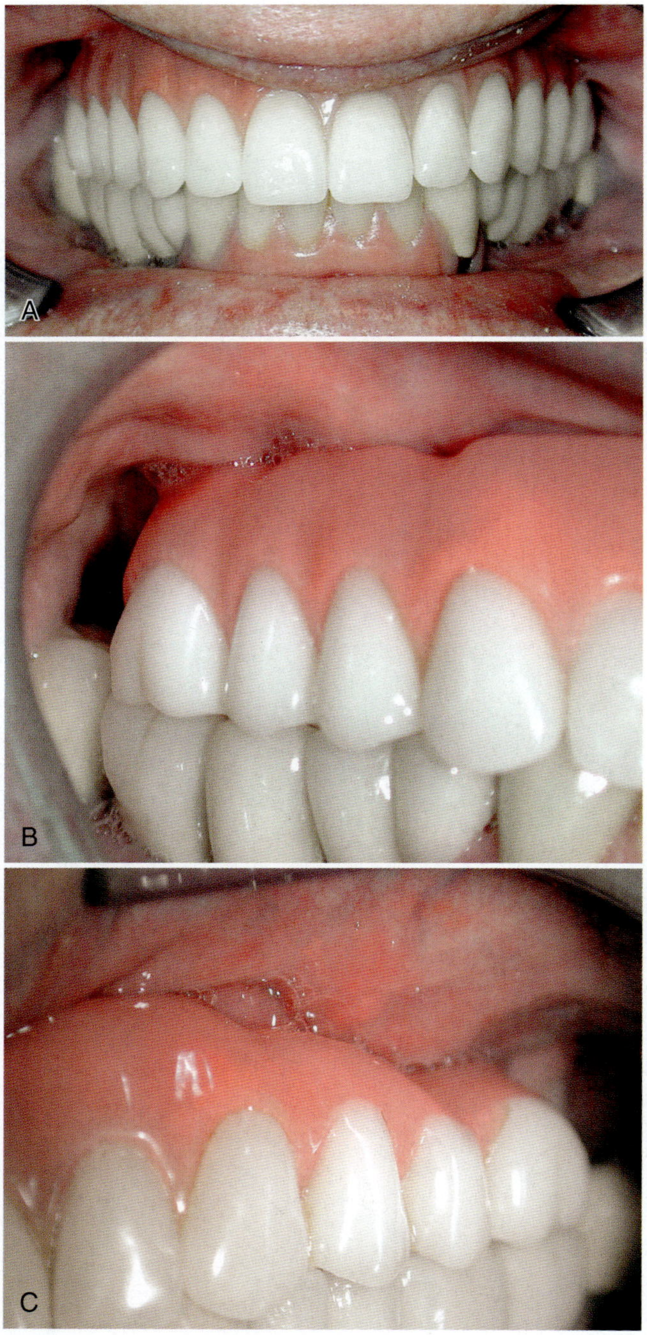

FIGURE 14-101 Bilateral group function of the final profile prosthesis.

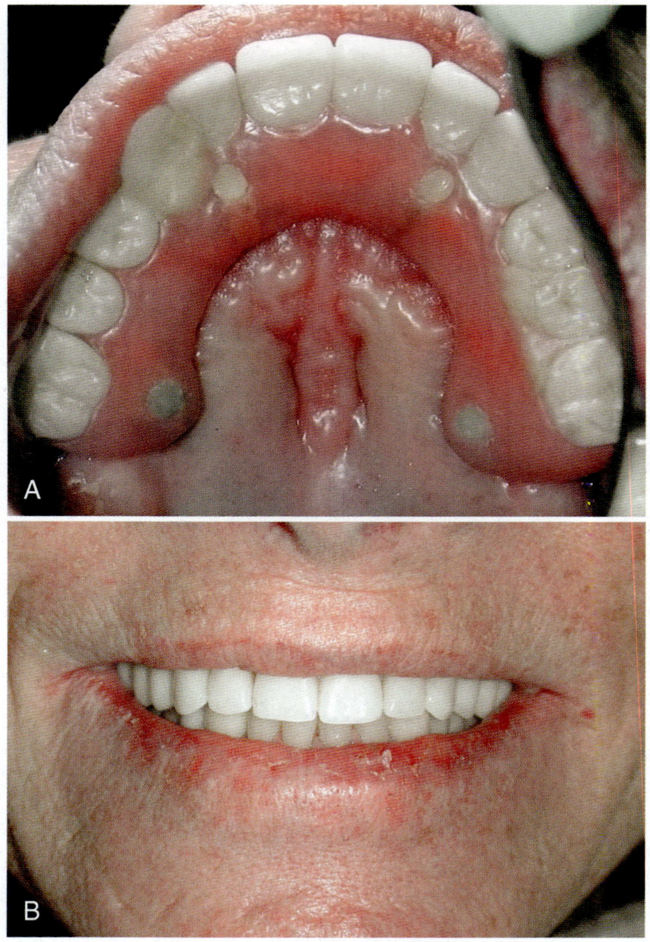

FIGURE 14-102 Palatal seal allowing for proper enunciation as well as a hidden transition line and an aesthetic smile.

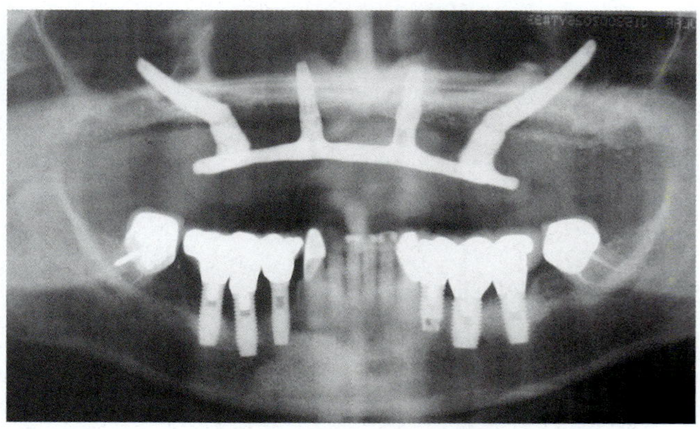

FIGURE 14-103 Final panoramic radiograph. (*Courtesy Dr. Paul Binon, Prosthodontist.*)

CHAPTER 15

CASE PRESENTATIONS: Management of Complications

MANAGEMENT OF FAILED IMMEDIATELY-LOADED ZYGOMATIC IMPLANTS

A 64-year-old woman presented with no restorable mandibular dentition and an ill-fitting maxillary full denture. The clinical and radiographic studies demonstrated multiple periodontally involved and nonrestorable teeth. The panoramic study demonstrated advanced resorption of the maxillary alveolar bone and residual alveolar bone in zone I only. The patient's priority was treatment of the mandibular arch. After fabrication of a full mandibular denture, the mandibular teeth were removed; mandibular implants were placed immediately and the mandibular denture was converted into an immediate-load mandibular provisional, implant-supported bridge. After 3 months of osseointegration, the mandibular implants were checked for the presence of osseointegration and the final profile prosthesis was fabricated and delivered (Figures 15-1 to 15-3).

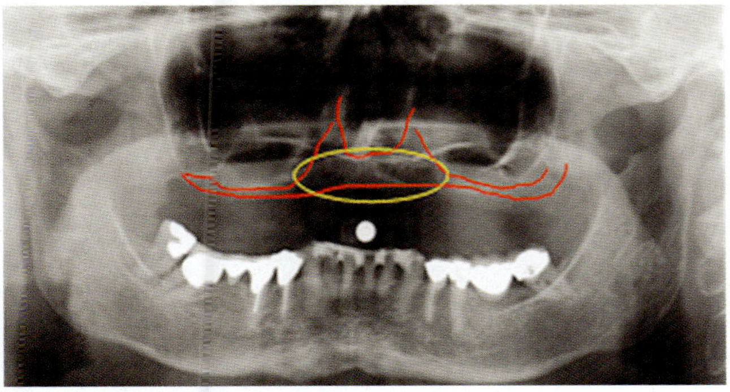

FIGURE 15-1 Preoperative panoramic radiograph with evidence of nonrestorable mandibular teeth and presence of zone I alveolar bone only in the edentulous maxilla.

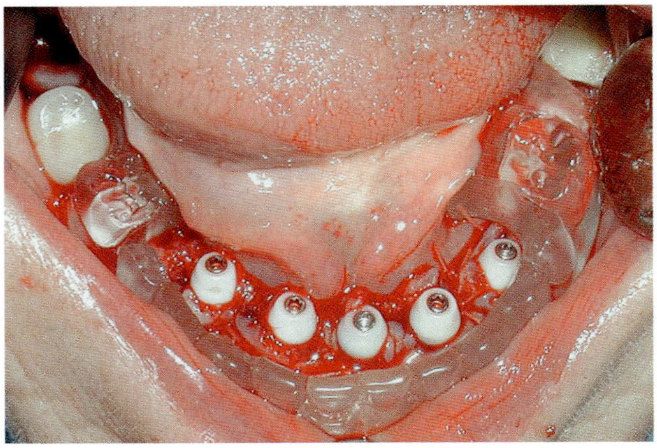

FIGURE 15-2 Removal of the mandibular teeth and simultaneous placement of mandibular implants.

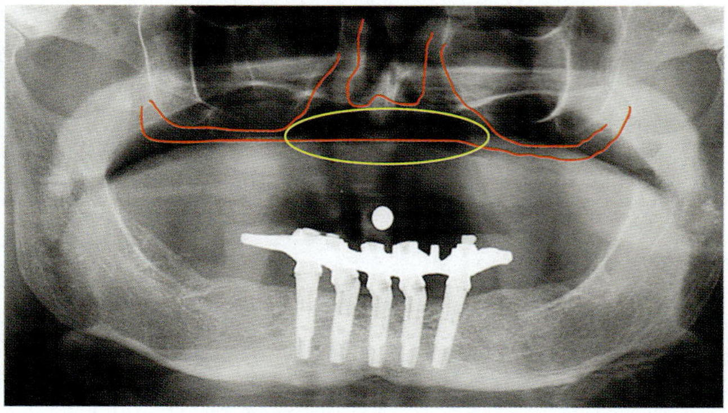

FIGURE 15-3 Radiograph taken 5 years after surgery with the completed mandibular profile prosthesis and the existing edentulous maxilla.

Five years after treatment of the mandible, the patient requested treatment of her maxillary arch with an implant-supported fixed bridge. Because of the presence of zone I bone and an inadequate volume of zones II and III bone, the zygomatic treatment method was used. Using the protocol for the zygomatic method, two premaxillary implants and two zygomatic implants were placed and the patient's full maxillary denture was converted to a provisional, immediate-load prosthesis (Figures 15-4 to 15-7).

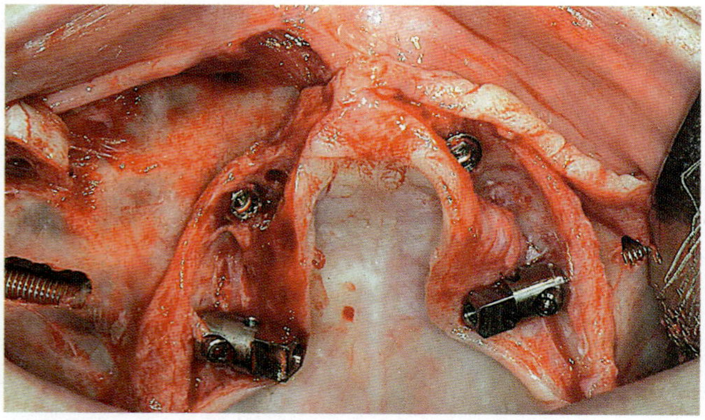

FIGURE 15-4 Placement of the maxillary implants using the zygoma concept for the posterior maxilla and placement of two premaxillary implants.

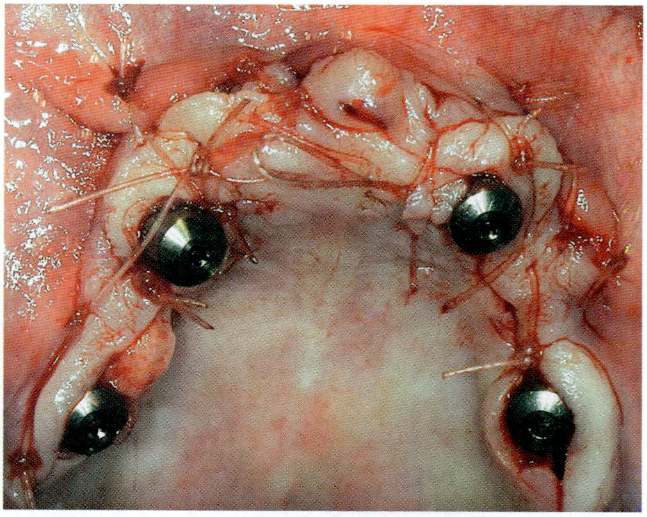

FIGURE 15-5 Placement of abutments and completed soft tissue closure.

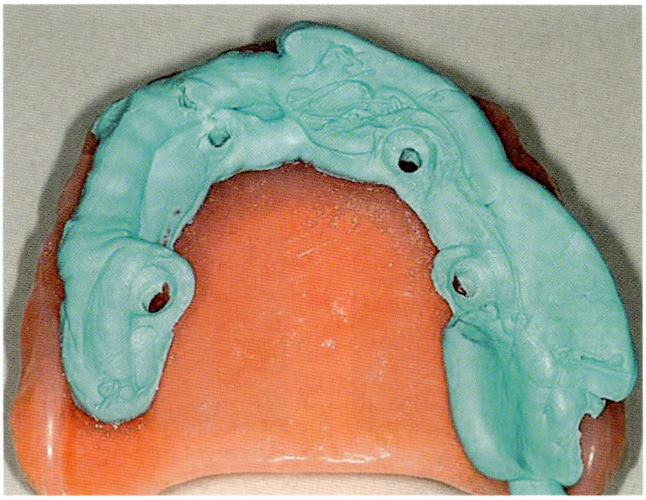

FIGURE 15-6 Indexing the implant positions on the intaglio surface of the full maxillary denture.

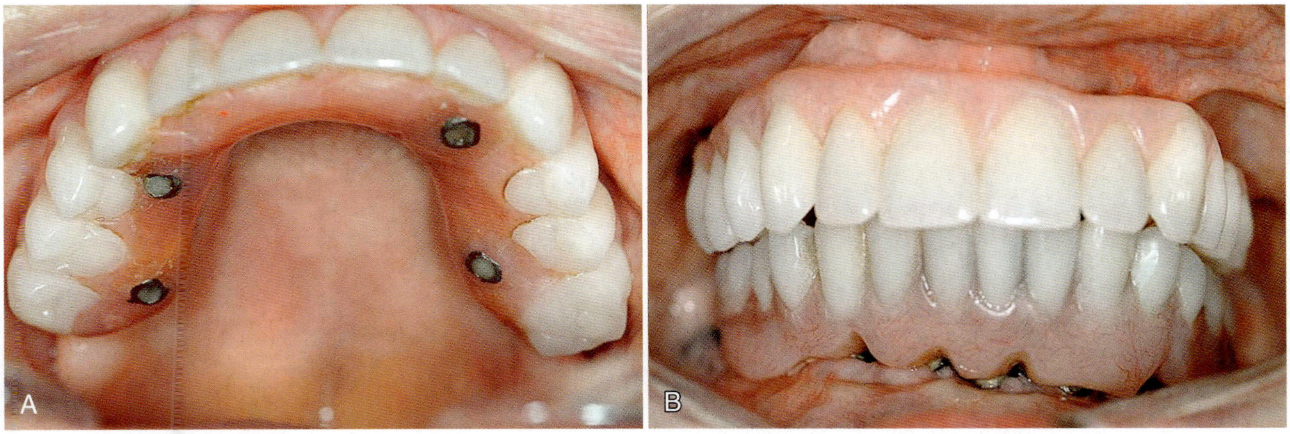

FIGURE 15-7 Completed conversion of the full maxillary denture into an immediate-load maxillary provisional prosthesis.

Six months after the maxillary procedure, the patient presented for phase II with stable occlusion and without any complaints. Osseointegration was confirmed and fabrication of the final profile prosthesis was planned. After removal of the provisional prosthesis, osseointegration was checked by applying the torque driver to each implant. The right zygomatic implant rotated on its axis, demonstrating a lack of osseointegration. The remaining premaxillary and left zygomatic implants were stable without any rotation or symptoms during torquing of their abutment screws. The decision to replace the right zygomatic implant was made.

In preparation for replacement of the failed zygoma implant, reformatted views of the patient's cone beam radiographic study demonstrate the availability of bone above the existing implant. The intention of the procedure was to remove the failed implant, with immediate placement of a new zygoma implant with the apex in the os zygomaticus and above the failed implant apex (Figures 15-8 to 15-16).

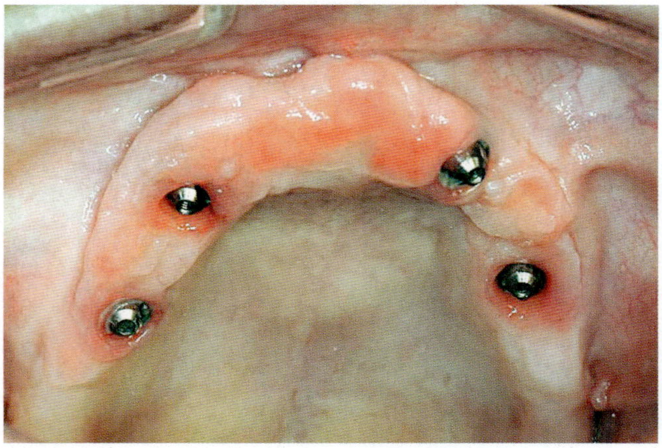

FIGURE 15-8 When 20 Ncm of torque is applied to confirm osseointegration, the right zygomatic implant demonstrates rotation.

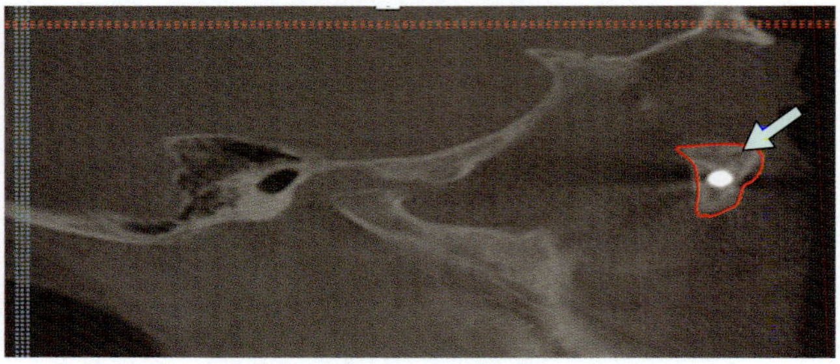

FIGURE 15-9 Cone beam radiographic study demonstrates availability of bone in the body of the zygoma immediately above the existing failed implant.

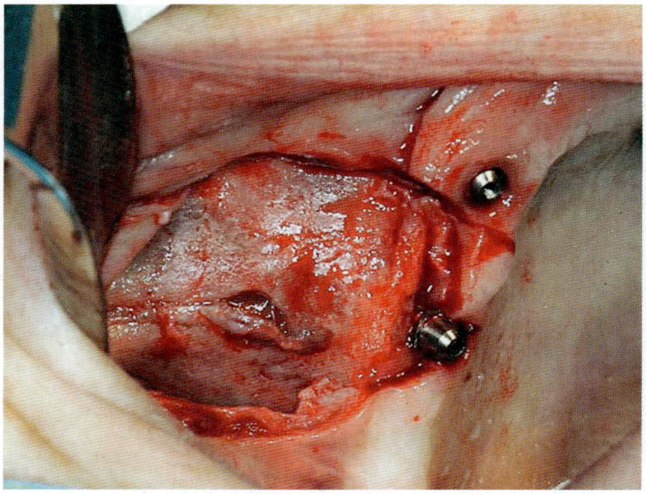

FIGURE 15-10 A full-thickness mucoperiosteal implant demonstrates coverage of the previous osteotomy into the maxillary sinus by the re-established Schneiderian membrane.

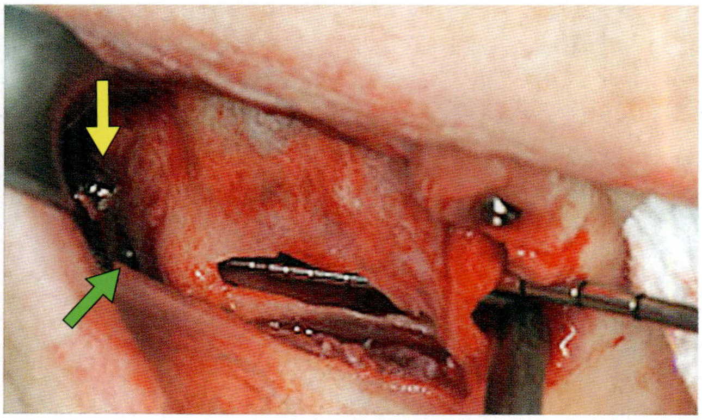

FIGURE 15-11 The *yellow arrow* points to the depth gauge instrument placed in the new osteotomy. The *green arrow* demonstrates the inferior position of the removed failed implant.

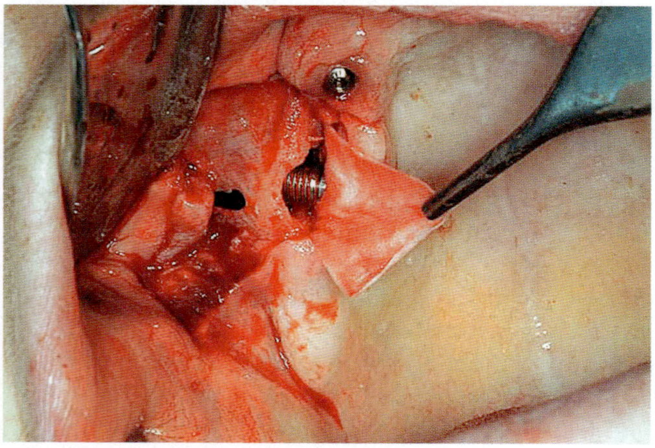

FIGURE 15-12 Placement of the new zygomatic implant at 40 Ncm or more.

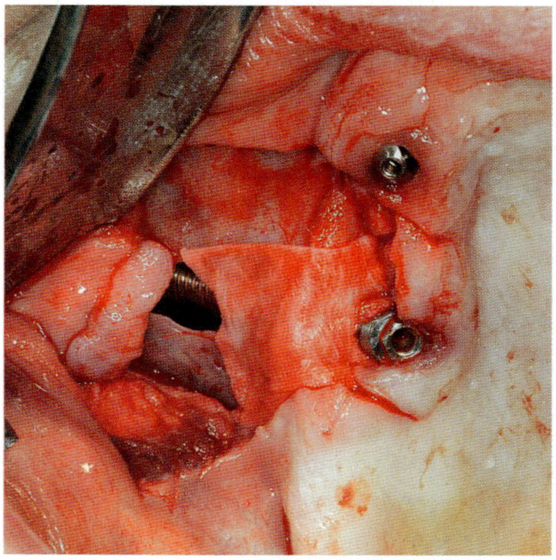

FIGURE 15-13 To prevent soft tissue breakdown over the crestal bony defect, a resorbable membrane is placed over the implant platform.

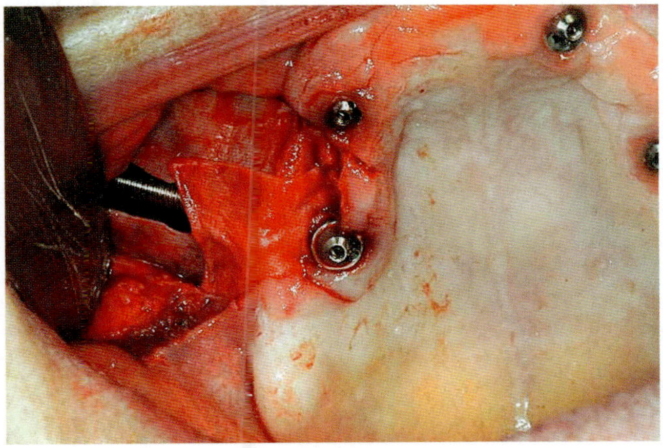

FIGURE 15-14 The membrane is tailored over the defect and stabilized using 1.5-mm fixation screws.

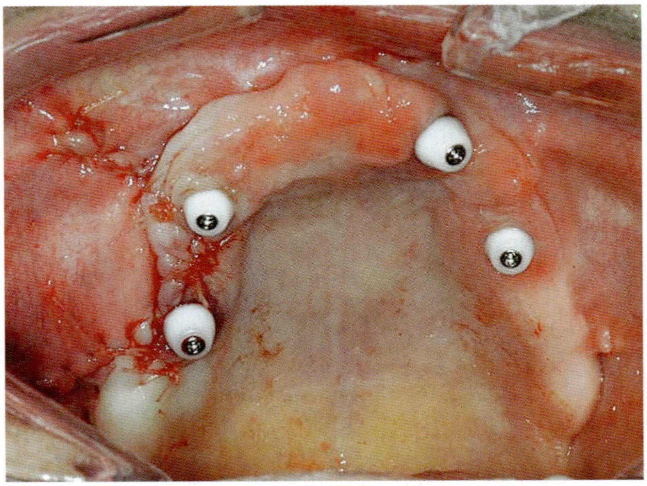

FIGURE 15-15 Closure of the soft tissues after connection and torquing of a new multiunit abutment at 35 Ncm.

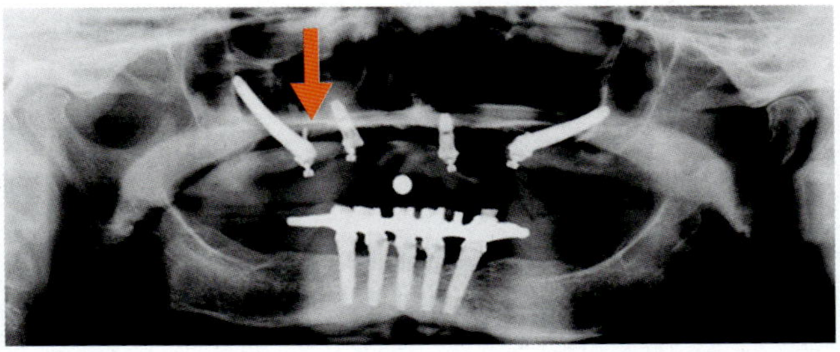

FIGURE 15-16 Immediate postoperative radiograph demonstrating the new right zygoma implant and the fixation screws of the membrane.

To reconnect the immediate-load provisional prosthesis to the new implant, the existing right posterior maxillary titanium cylinder was removed. The provisional prosthesis was connected to the existing three implants by their retention screws and the new implant was "salt and peppered" to the new titanium cylinder. The patient was discharged with the corrected prosthesis. An additional 6 months of osseointegration was allowed prior to checking the right maxillary implant for osseointegration. After osseointegration of all four implants was confirmed, the final metal-based profile prosthesis was fabricated (Figures 15-17 to 15-22).

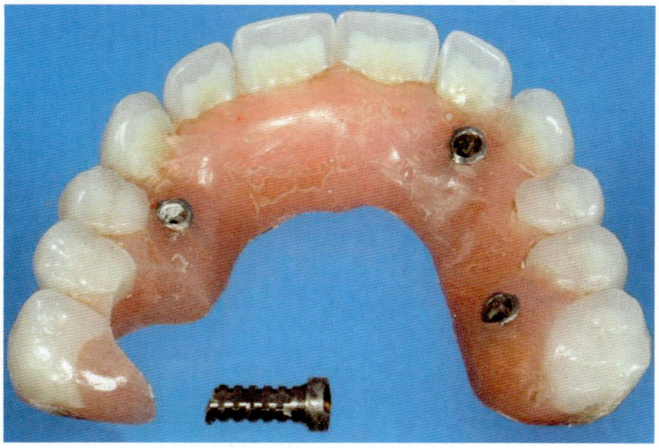

FIGURE 15-17 The existing temporary titanium cylinder is removed from the provisional bridge.

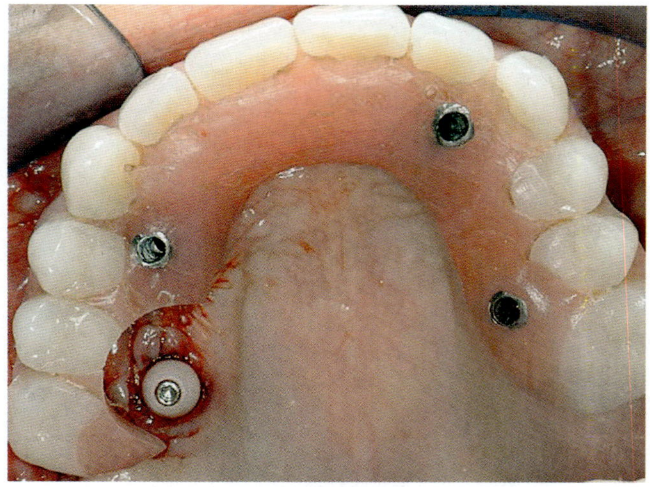

FIGURE 15-18 The provisional prosthesis is reconnected to the existing osseointegrated implants.

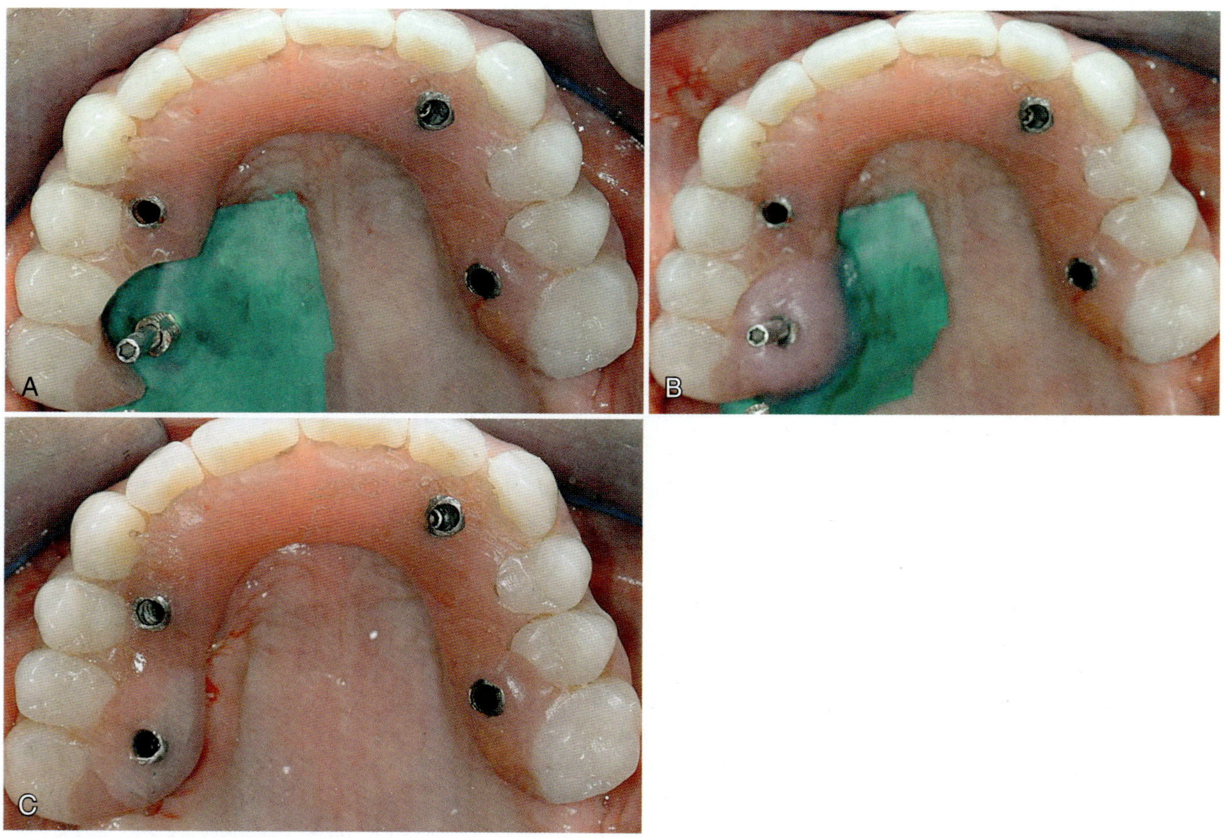

FIGURE 15-19 After the new implant is connected to the prosthesis, an additional 6-month osseointegration period is allowed for the right zygoma implant.

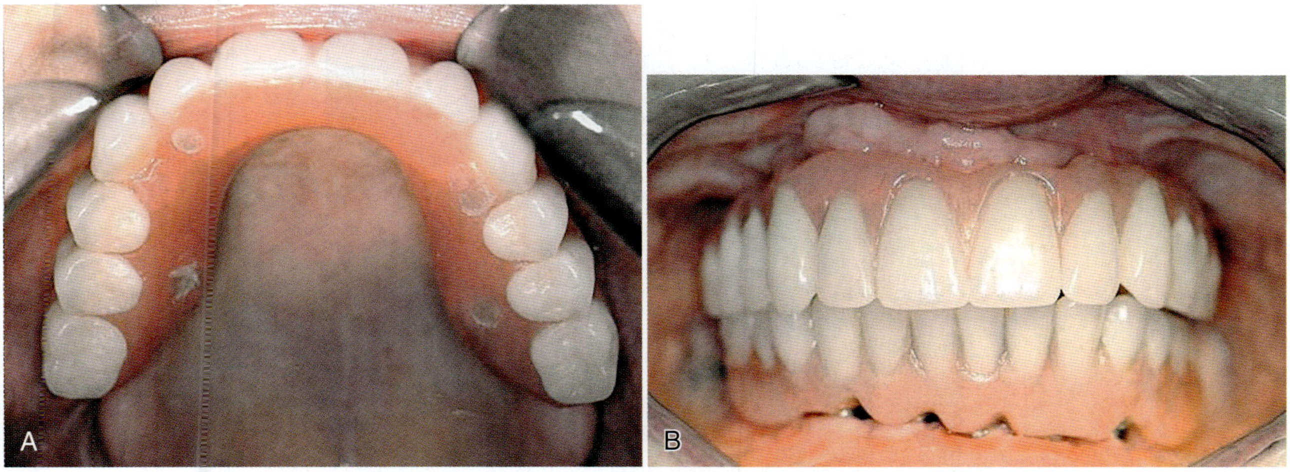

FIGURE 15-20 Completed metal-based final provisional prostheses.

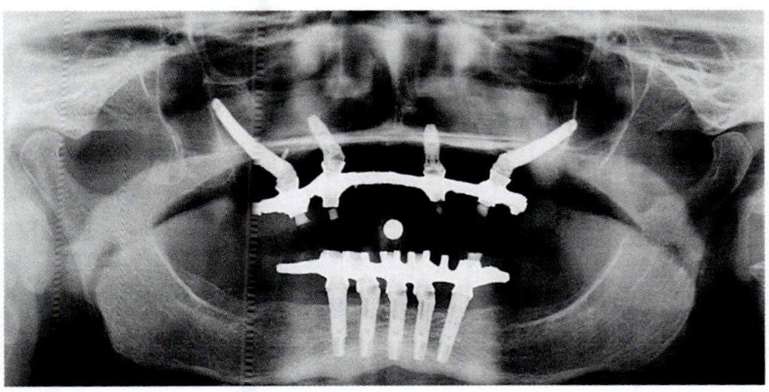

FIGURE 15-21 Final panoramic radiograph with complete seating of all components.

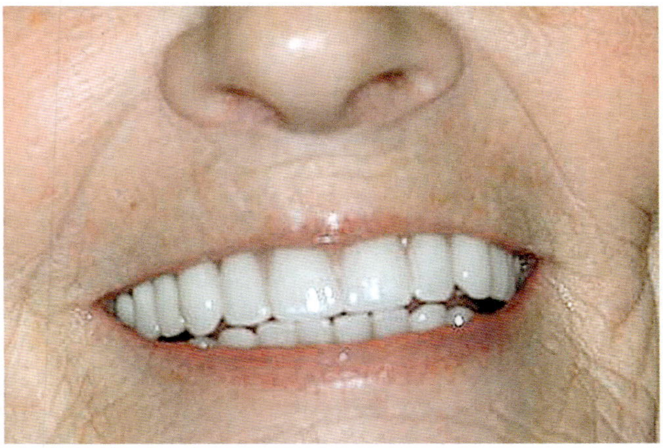

FIGURE 15-22 An aesthetically acceptable smile line with hidden transition line and full buccal corridor.

SINUS INFECTIONS AFTER PLACEMENT OF ZYGOMATIC IMPLANTS

At times, delayed unilateral infection of the maxillary sinus is apparent after placement and immediate loading of zygomatic implants (Figure 15-23). The initial concern is that, because the implant is a foreign body, it is responsible in part for the persistence of the infection and its removal may be indicated. The *unilateral* infection in the presence of *bilateral* zygomatic implants, however, suggests another cause.

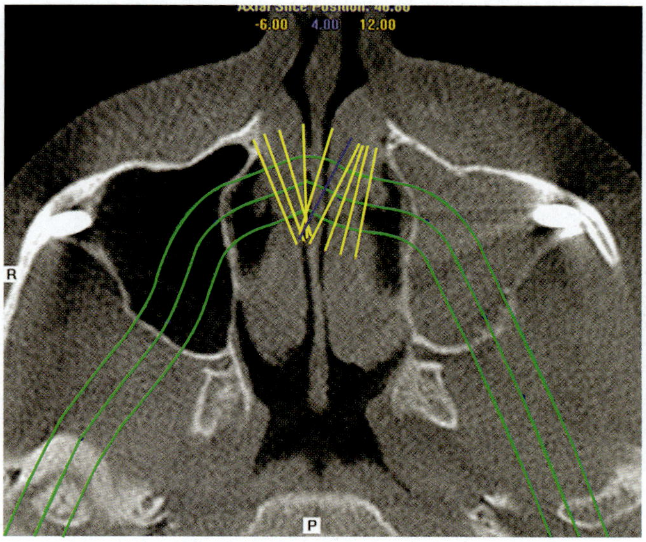

FIGURE 15-23 Unilateral maxillary sinus infection after placement of bilateral zygoma implants and immediate loading 36 months earlier.

For the maxillary sinus to drain, a patent osteomeatal complex is necessary (Figure 15-24). If congenital or traumatic deformities of the osteomeatal complex constrict this passageway, then slight swelling of the overlying soft tissues may completely block the drainage of not only the maxillary sinus, but the ethmoid and frontal sinuses, as well (Figure 15-25). Physical blockage of the maxillary ostium with postsurgical debris left inside the sinus may also contribute to postsurgical maxillary sinus infection without involvement of the ethmoid or frontal sinuses (Figure 15-26).

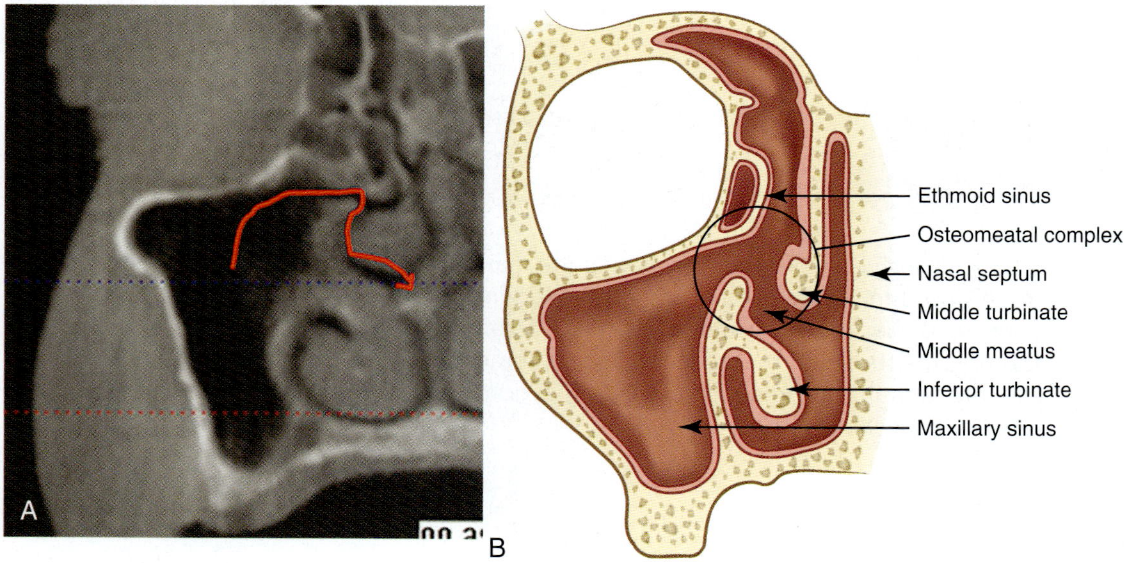

FIGURE 15-24 A patent osteomeatal complex is needed for the normal passive drainage of the maxillary, ethmoid, and sphenoid sinuses.

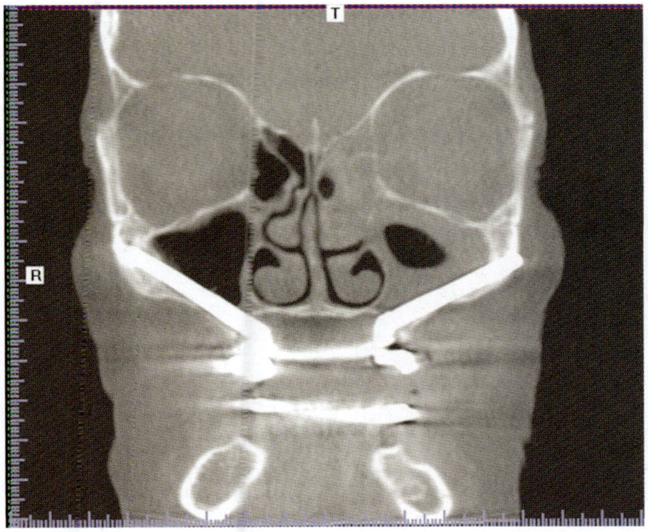

FIGURE 15-25 Unilateral left maxillary, ethmoid, and sphenoid pansinusitis secondary to soft tissue edema and blockage of the left osteomeatal complex.

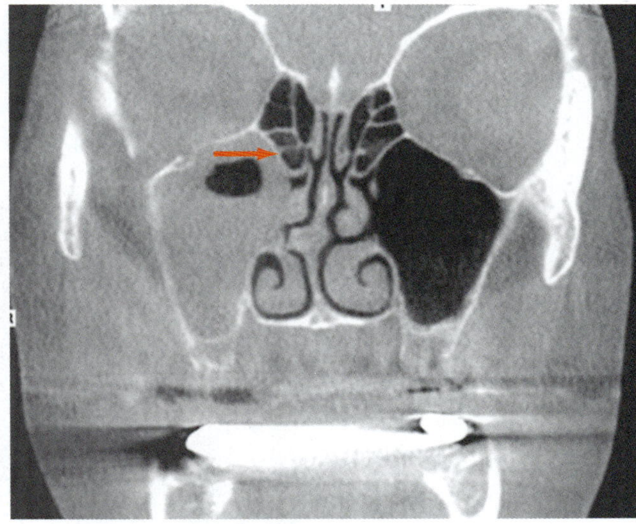

FIGURE 15-26 Unilateral right maxillary sinus infection secondary to blockage of the maxillary ostium only. Note the patent ethmoid sinuses.

Bjorn Peterson reported on foreign bodies in the maxillary sinus (Figure 15-27) by reviewing 14 patients 1 year after placement of zygomatic implants using an endoscope for rhinoscopy and sinoscopy. He found no signs of infection or inflammation in the mucosa around the fixtures.[1] Delayed, acute sinusitis was reported by Aparicio,[2] however, at 14, 23, and 27 months after surgical procedures. The maxillary infections were resolved at onset using an oral antibiotic regimen. There were no further complications. In cases in which the infections persist, however, the inflamed soft tissues of the maxillary ostium create a "domino effect" in which the inflammation of the soft tissues of the osteomeatal complex causes blockage of the natural drainage path of the ethmoid and frontal sinuses.

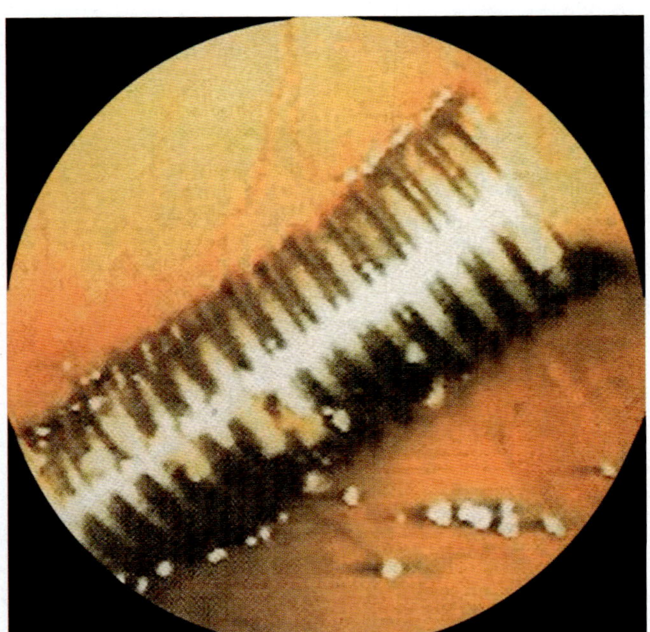

FIGURE 15-27 Transnasal endoscopic view of a zygoma implant.

Failure to resolve the infection with antibiotics warrants functional endoscopic sinus surgery (FESS) to establish a patent osteomeatal complex and allow drainage of the maxillary, ethmoid, and frontal sinuses. FESS involves removal of the middle turbinate, the bulla, and the uncinate processes. The ethmoid air cells are opened (Figure 15-28), allowing passive drainage.

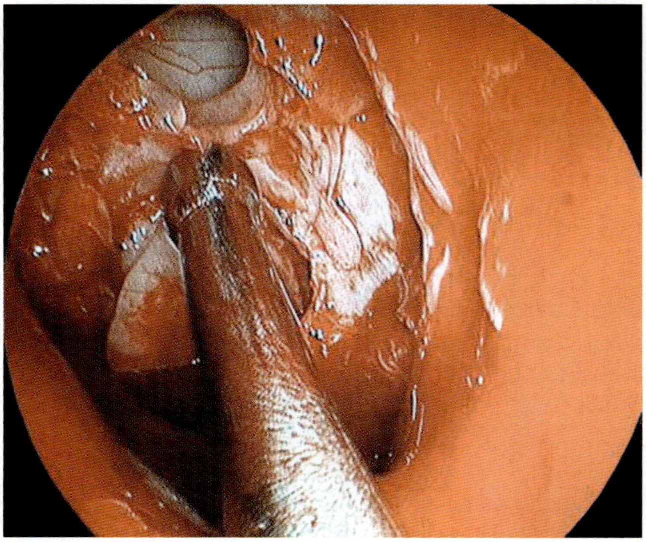

FIGURE 15-28 "Unroofing" of the ethmoid air cells via a functional endoscopic sinus surgery to establish passive drainage.

After FESS is complete, a patent osteomeatal complex is created, which allows passive drainage (Figure 15-29). Postoperative oral antibiotic treatment helps resolve the infection completely.

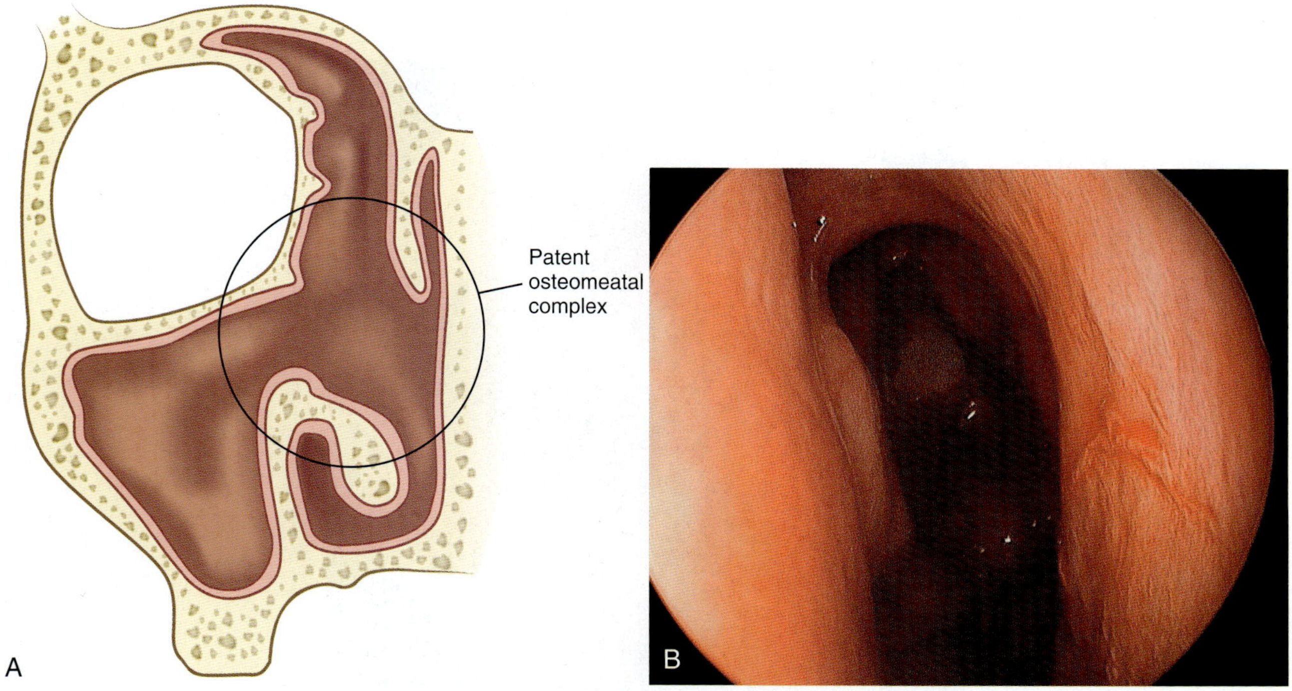

FIGURE 15-29 After functional endoscopic sinus surgery with patent osteomeatal complex.

A comprehensive discussion with an otolaryngologist to consider FESS is strongly recommended if oral antibiotic treatments do not resolve the maxillary sinus infection.

FAILED TILTED IMPLANT: IMMEDIATE TREATMENT

A 62-year-old man presented with recurrent caries in his remaining maxillary teeth. Examination revealed no soft or hard tissue defect. Therefore, a tooth-only defect was present and restoration with a porcelain-fused-to-metal prosthesis was planned.

In animation, the patient's transition line was present. The radiographic evaluation demonstrated zones I and II bone. The plan for the removal of the patient's maxillary dentition and placement of four implants using the tilted treatment concept and immediate loading with a "white denture" has been described in earlier chapters (Figures 15-30 to 15-32).

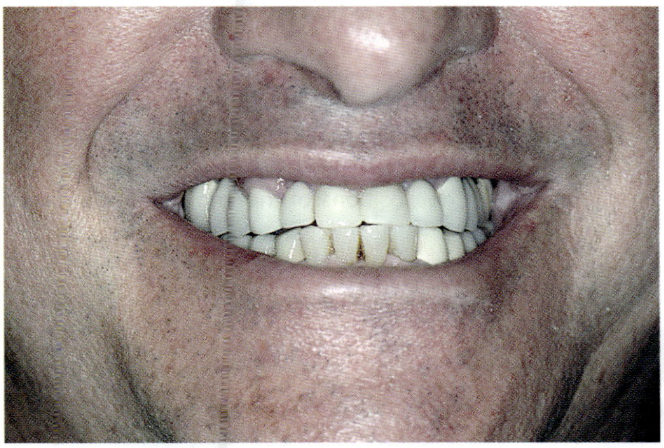

FIGURE 15-30 Preoperative smile line demonstrates a visible transition line.

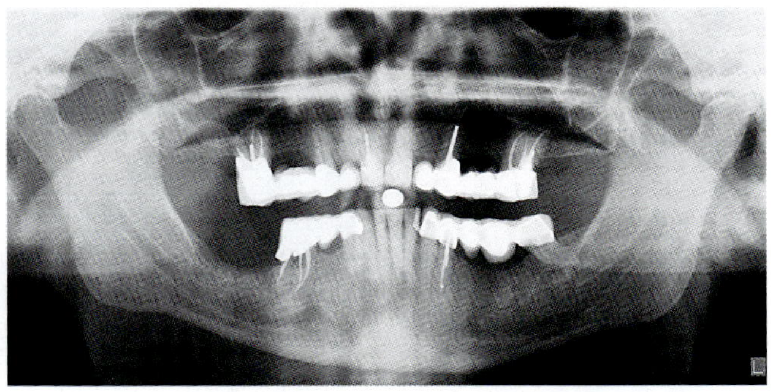

FIGURE 15-31 Preoperative radiograph demonstrates zones I and II bone.

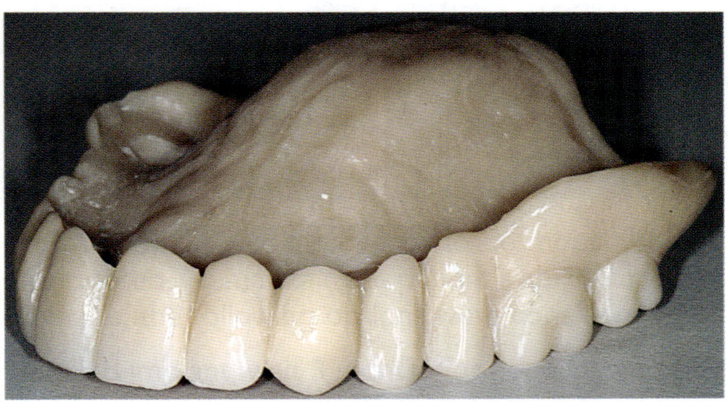

FIGURE 15-32 A "white denture" is a provisional prosthesis that can be converted into a provisional fixed prosthesis.

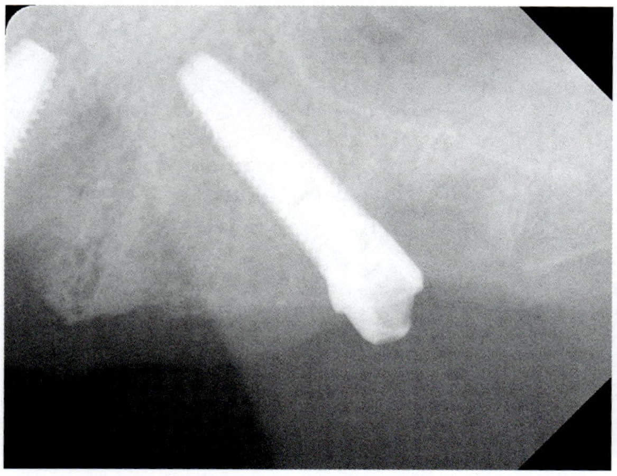

FIGURE 15-38 Periapical radiograph of the mobile implant at position 14.

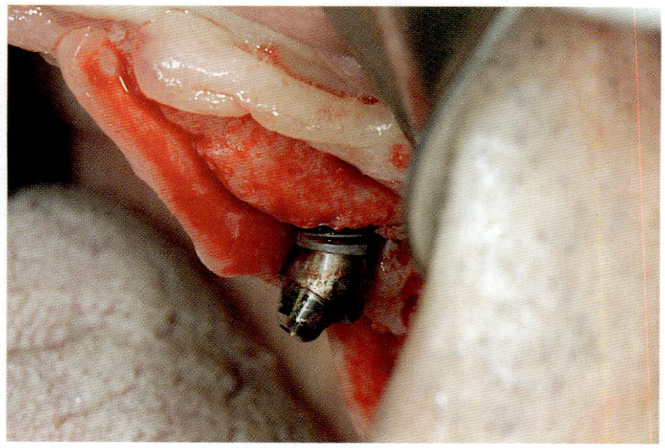

FIGURE 15-39 Exposure of the mobile implant; the existing 30° abutment and implant were removed by counterclockwise rotation.

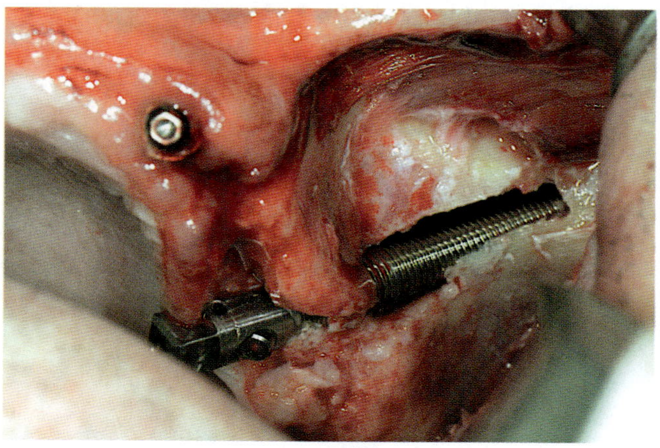

FIGURE 15-40 Placement of a zygomatic implant. The platform of the zygomatic implant is in the same position as the tilted implant platform.

After the zygomatic implant was placed, a straight multiunit abutment was connected and torqued to 35 Ncm. The existing temporary titanium cylinder was trephined out of the provisional prosthesis and a new cylinder was connected to the zygoma implant and reconnected to the provisional prosthesis. The "rescued" provisional was reconnected to the abutments and the implants were allowed to osseointegrate for 6 months (Figures 15-41 to 15-43).

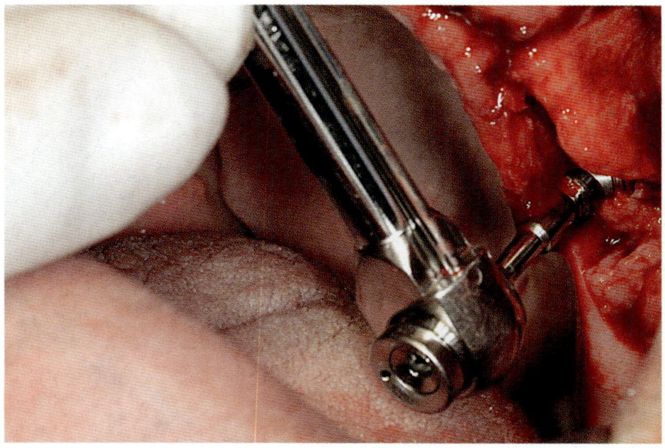

FIGURE 15-41 Connection and torquing of a straight multiunit abutment to the new zygoma implant to 35 Ncm.

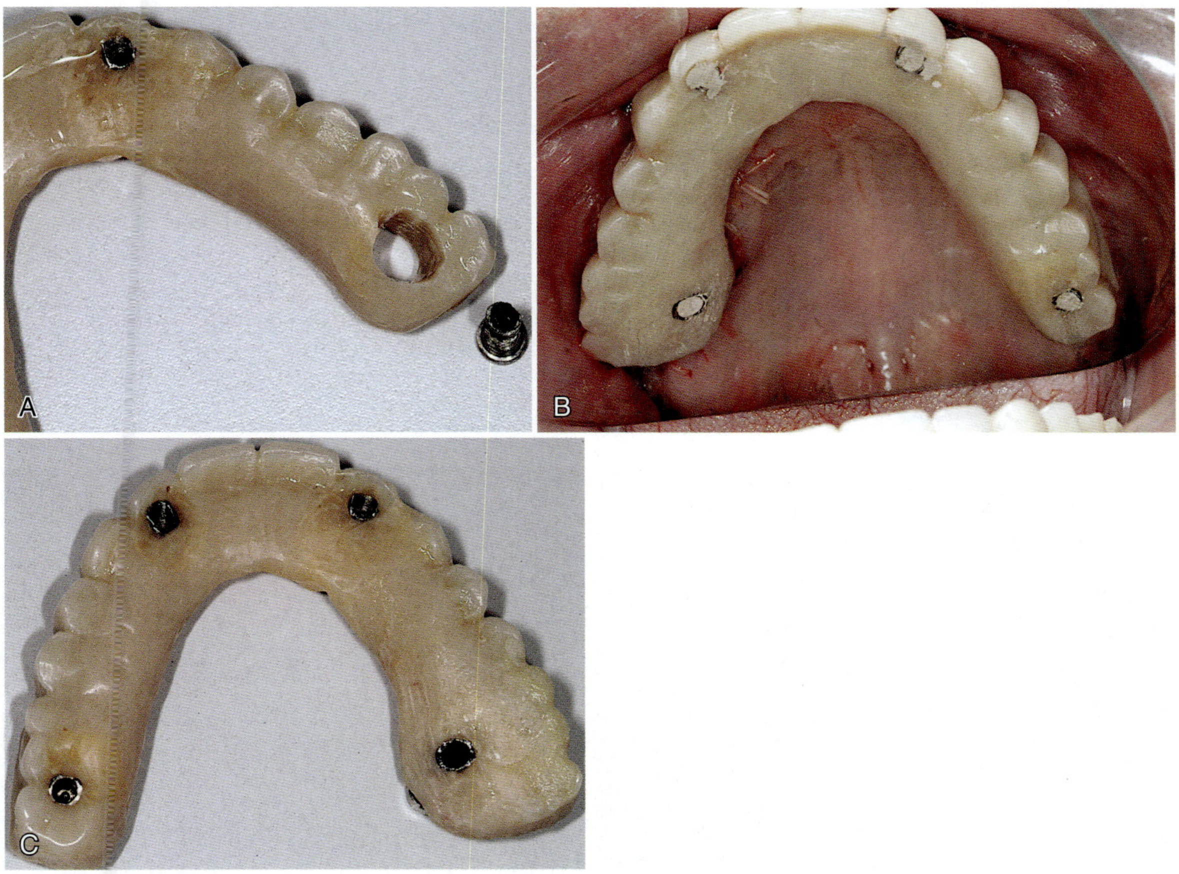

FIGURE 15-42 Removal of the existing temporary cylinder and reconnection of the temporary cylinder to the newly placed zygoma implant.

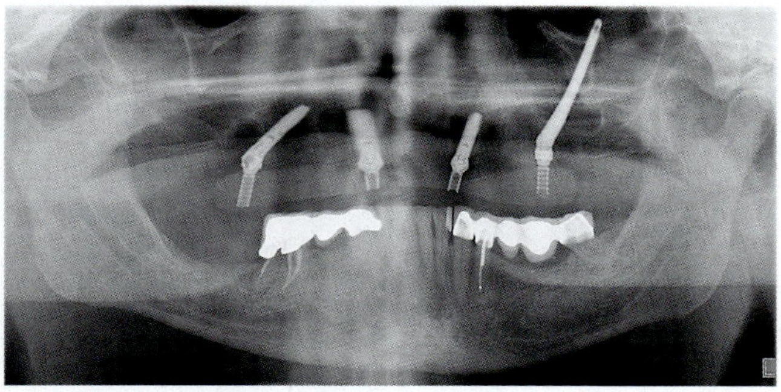

FIGURE 15-43 Immediate postoperative panoramic radiograph with the newly positioned "rescue" zygoma implant.

An additional 6-month osseointegration period was allowed for the newly placed zygomatic implant. After the osseointegration period, the provisional prosthesis was removed and each implant was evaluated for sensitivity and motion. During the final prosthetic fabrication, the decision was made to use the profile prosthesis method because the patient preferred shorter teeth. Therefore, confirmation of proper phonetics and aesthetics was made during the wax try-in appointment prior to processing the final profile prosthesis. The final profile prosthesis was supported by the four implants and allowed for an aesthetically acceptable smile line during animation (Figures 15-44 to 15-47).

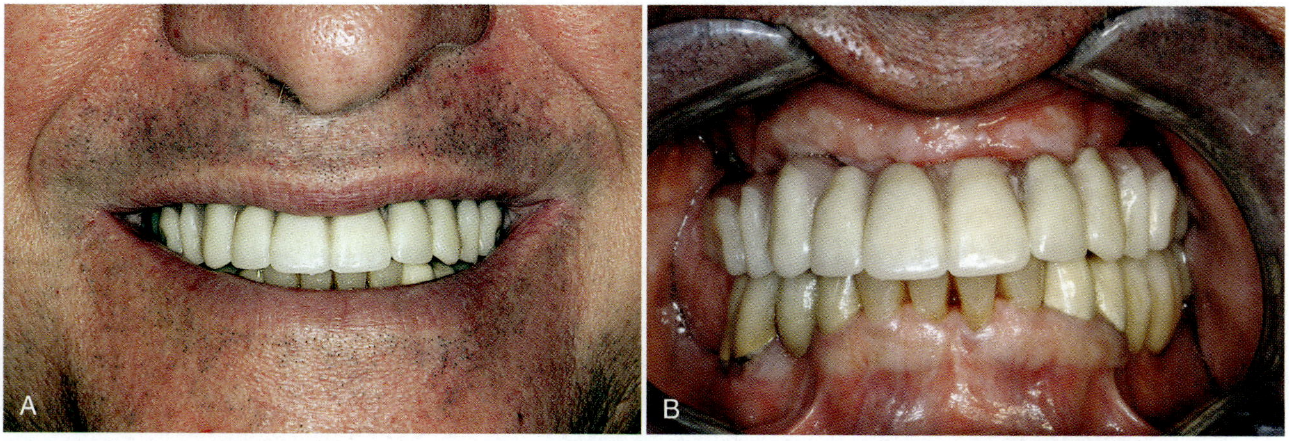

FIGURE 15-44 The decision to convert the porcelain-fused-to-metal final prosthesis to a profile prosthesis is made at the wax try-in appointment. The hidden transition line allows an aesthetically acceptable smile line.

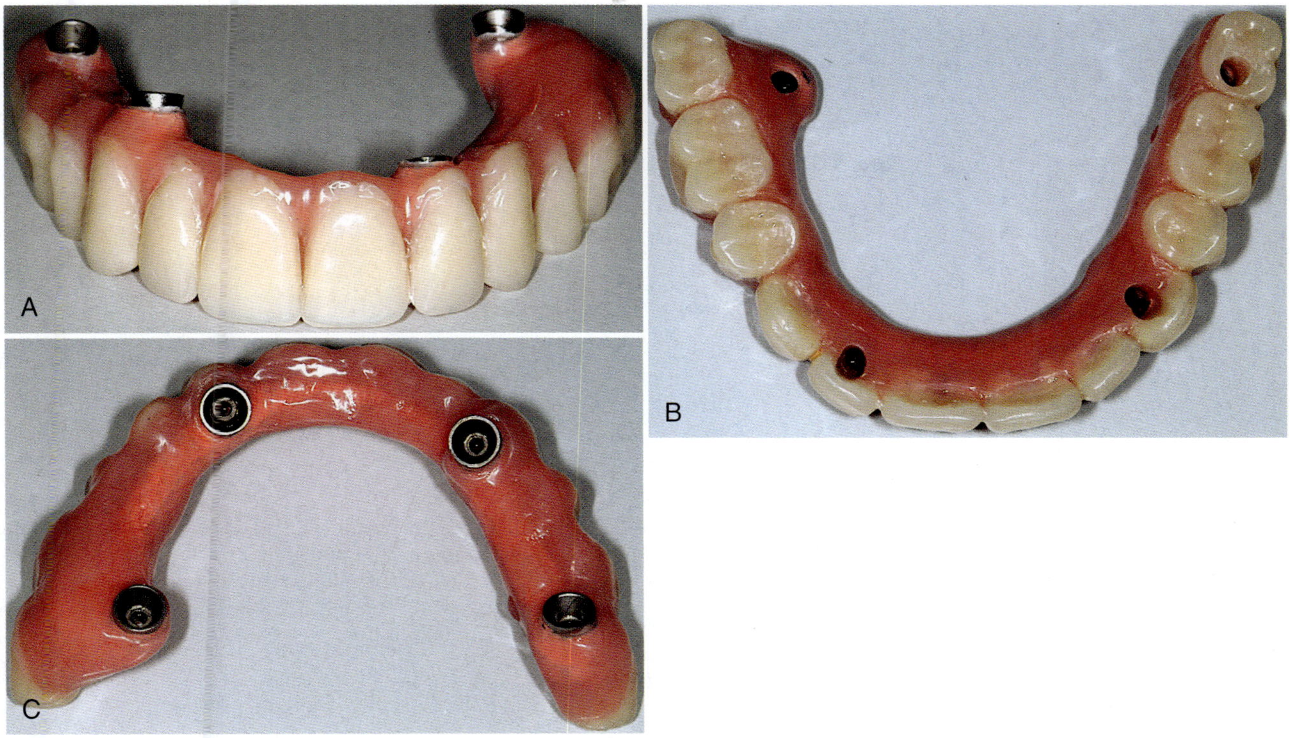

FIGURE 15-45 Final processed profile prosthesis.

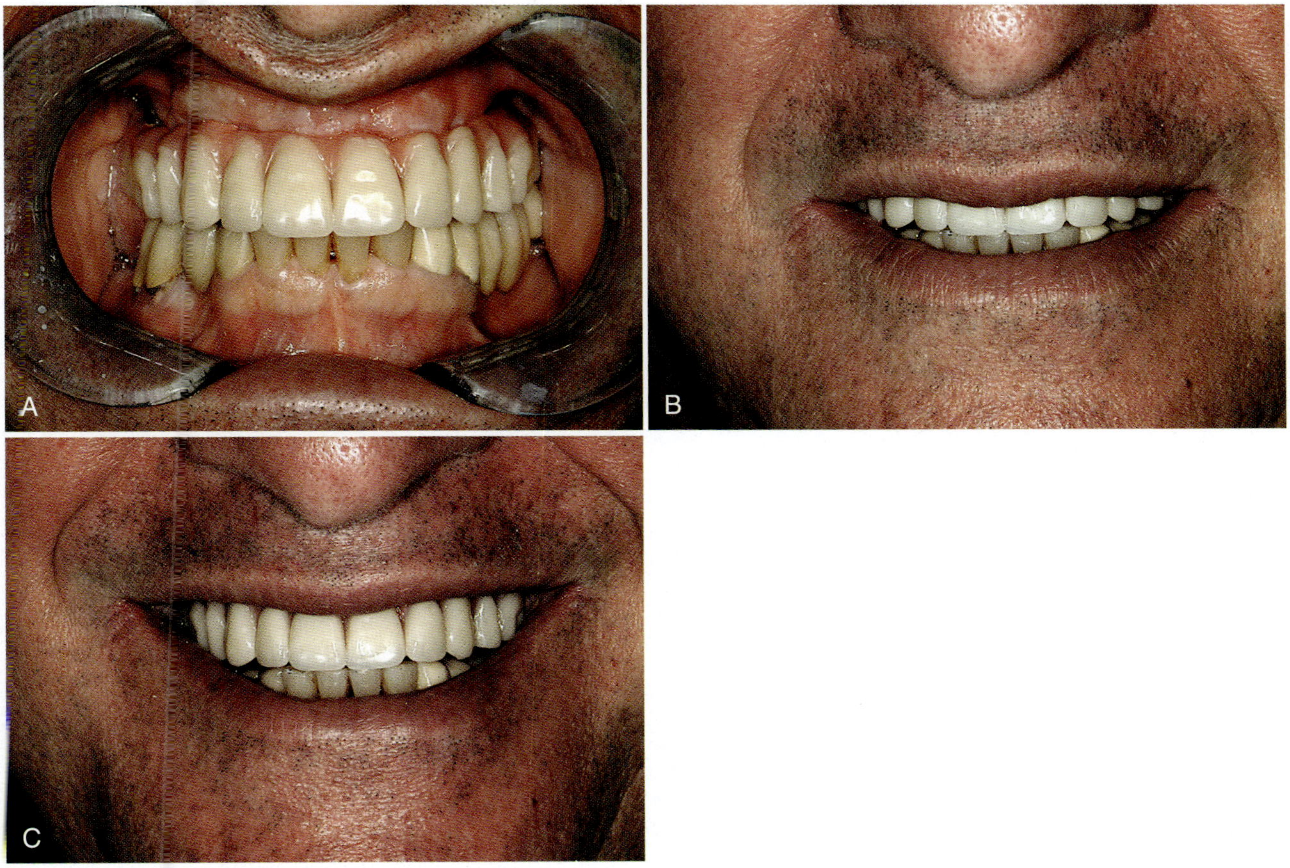

FIGURE 15-46 Final prosthesis delivered. Bilateral group function exists. The hidden transition line allows for an aesthetically acceptable smile line during animation as well as extreme animation.

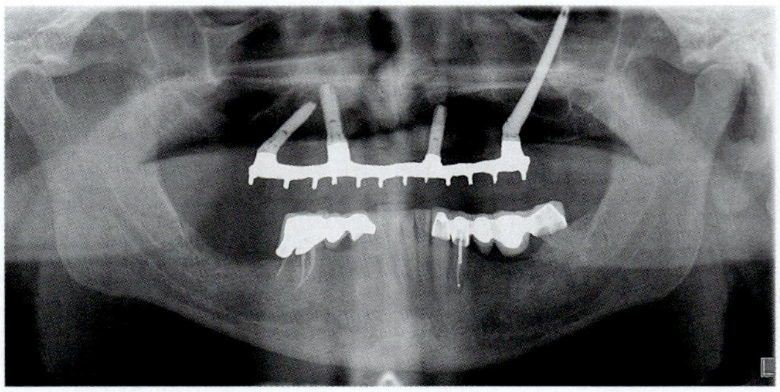

FIGURE 15-47 Final panoramic radiograph demonstrating complete seating of all components.

REFERENCES

1. Petruson B: Sinoscopy in patients with titanium implants in the nose and sinuses. *Scand J Plast Reconstr Surg Hand Surg* 38:86-93, 2004.

2. Aparicio C, Ouazzani W, Garcia R, et al: A prospective clinical study on titanium implants in the zygomatic arch for prosthetic rehabilitation of the atrophic maxilla: A follow-up of 6 months to 5 years. *Clin Implant Dent Res* 8:114-122, 2006.

CHAPTER 16

CASE PRESENTATIONS: Quad Zygoma

PRELIMINARY PRESENTATION

Complete maxillary alveolar resorption results in lack of bony volume in zones I, II, and III. Retention of a removable prosthesis is not possible with the remaining maxillary basal bone. When the maxillary alveolus is completely resorbed, clinical examination reveals a flat palatal vault and absence of a maxillary vestibule. Patients are unable to function with their conventional complete dentures. Such patients present with a significantly thick denture base and a thick circumferential flange, confirming the presence of horizontal and vertical composite defects. Physiologic reconstruction of this group of debilitated patients requires adequate implant support to stabilize an implant-supported prosthesis. To enable prosthetic rehabilitation of such patients, Brånemark introduced the idea of using extensive onlay bone grafts in conjunction with bilateral sinus inlay grafts for placement of six implants. The Brånemark "horseshoe" graft requires hospitalization and harvesting of autogenous iliac bone from the patient. During the 6-month osseointegration period, the patient is unable to wear his or her denture, which is generally not well-received by patients. An alternative graftless approach uses four zygomatic implants. The placement of two zygomatic implants in each zygoma allows for fabrication of an implant-supported fixed maxillary prosthesis without bone grafting and can be accomplished in an office setting.

The implants are placed in a "stacked" manner, with the superior implant emerging at the cuspid position and the inferior implant emerging in the bicuspid position (Figures 16-1 and 16-2).

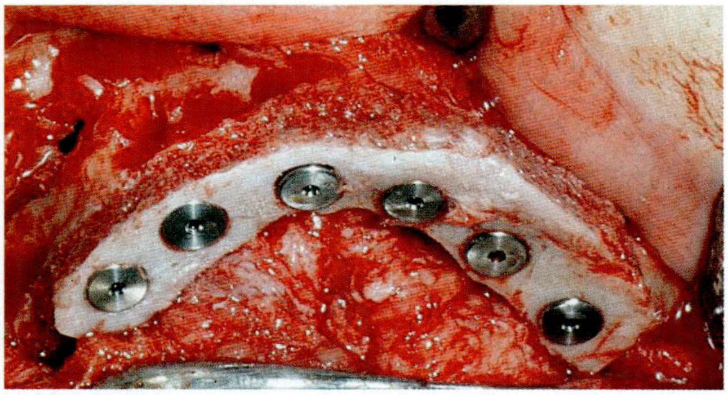

FIGURE 16-1 The Brånemark "horseshoe" graft with two-stage protocol and fabrication of an implant-supported, fixed maxillary prosthesis.

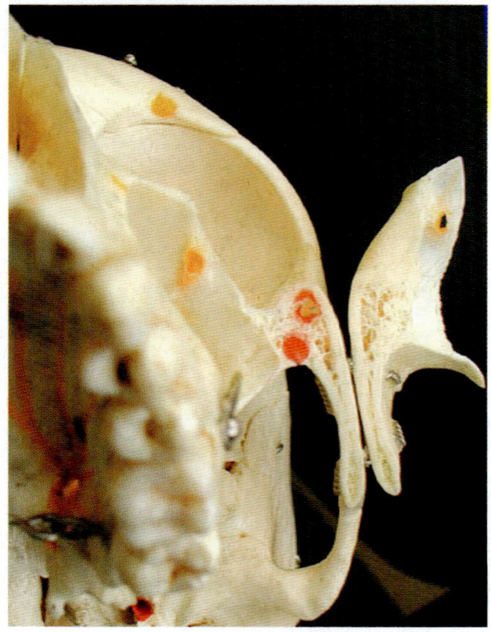

FIGURE 16-2 Placement of two zygoma implants within the body of the zygoma in a "stacked" configuration.

The preoperative panoramic radiograph demonstrates a lack of maxillary alveolar bone in all three zones. The surgical protocol for implant placement is very similar to the single zygoma implant protocol, with the exception that care must be taken to identify the most inferior lateral corner of the infraorbital rim. This reference is used while preparing the superior osteotomy to avoid penetration into the bony orbit. The implants are stabilized at 40 Ncm or greater. The two-stage protocol is followed by securing cover screws and submerging the implants for the 6-month osseointegration period (Figures 16-3 to 16-6).

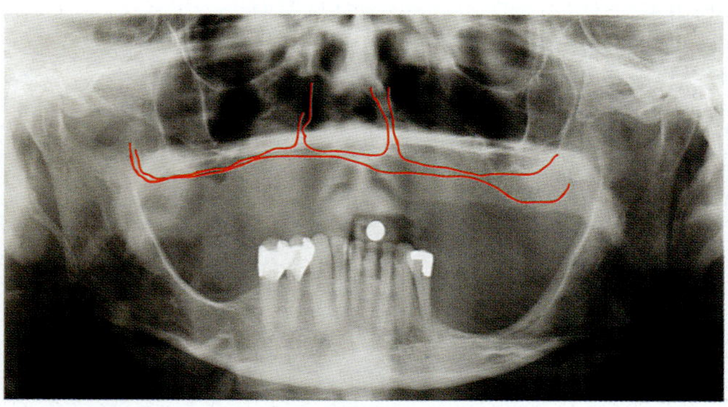

FIGURE 16-3 Preoperative radiograph demonstrating complete absence of zones I, II, and III bone.

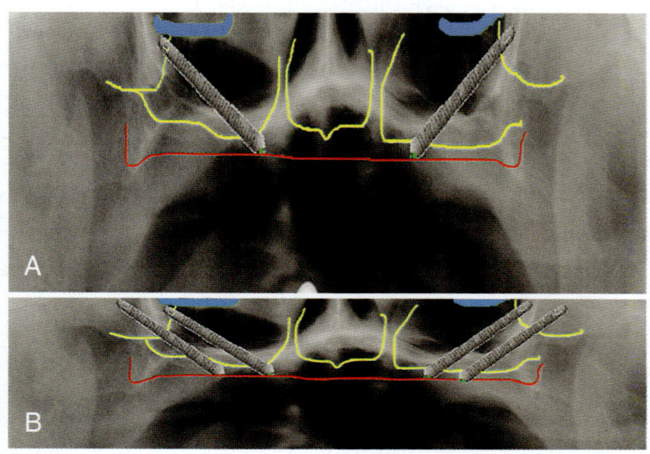

FIGURE 16-4 The superior implant is planned with its platform in the cuspid position. The inferior implant is planned with its platform in the bicuspid position.

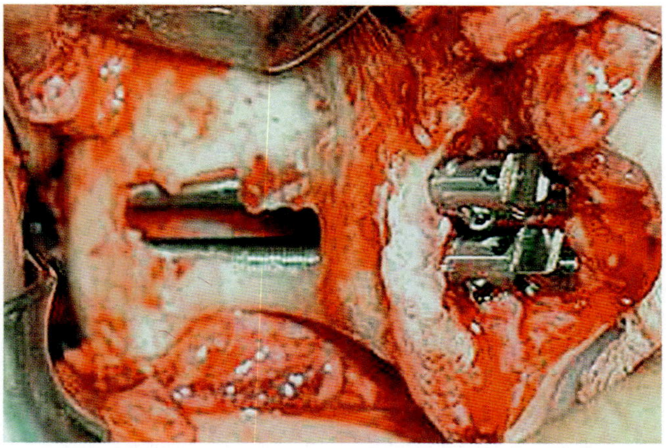

FIGURE 16-5 Opening the lateral maxillary wall for direct visualization of the drills during preparation of the osteotomy, as well as visualization of the implants during placement into the prepared osteotomy.

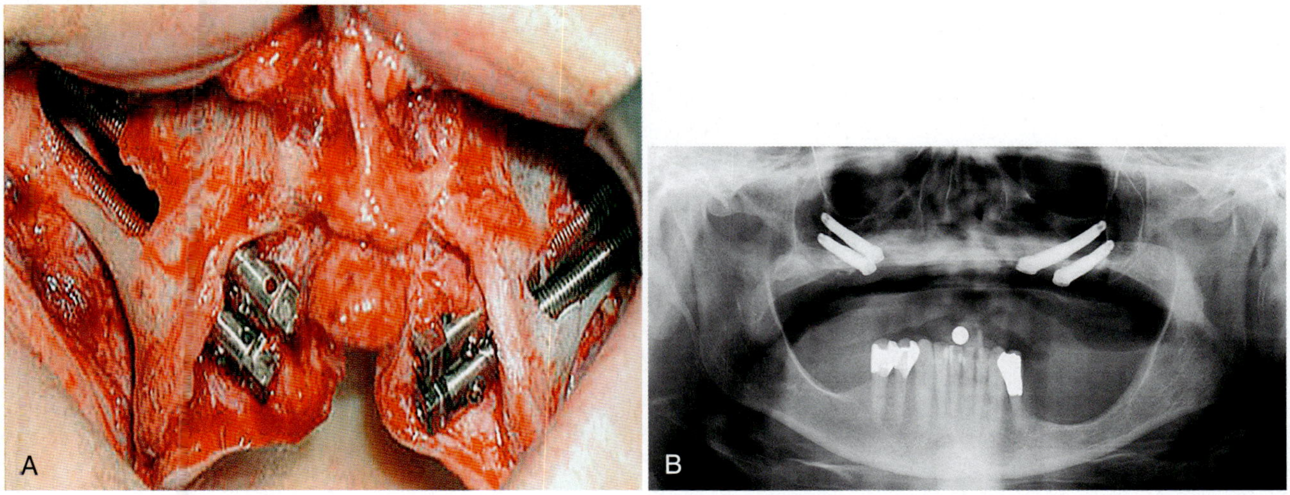

FIGURE 16-6 A, Completed surgical procedure. B, Postoperative radiograph with cover screws in place.

During stage II surgery, 6 months after implant placement, osseointegration is confirmed and multiunit abutments are placed. The full denture is converted into a provisional fixed bridge using the same immediate-loading conversion protocol.

The completed fixed provisional is secured to the multiunit abutments and the patient's occlusion is checked for bilateral group function. Radiographs taken after stage II surgery confirm complete seating of all components (Figures 16-7 to 16-9).

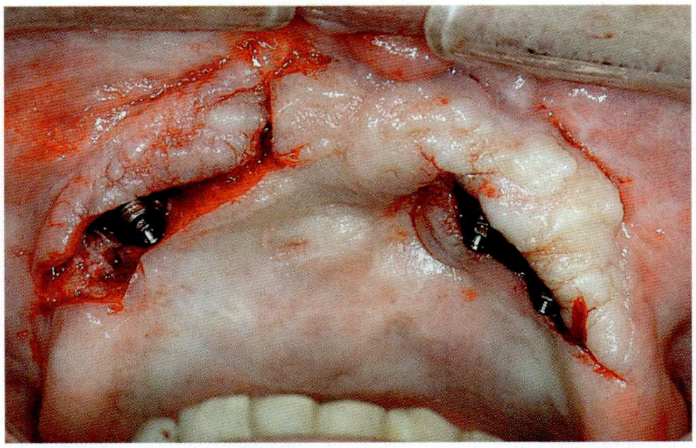

FIGURE 16-7 After 6 months of osseointegration, stage II surgery is performed.

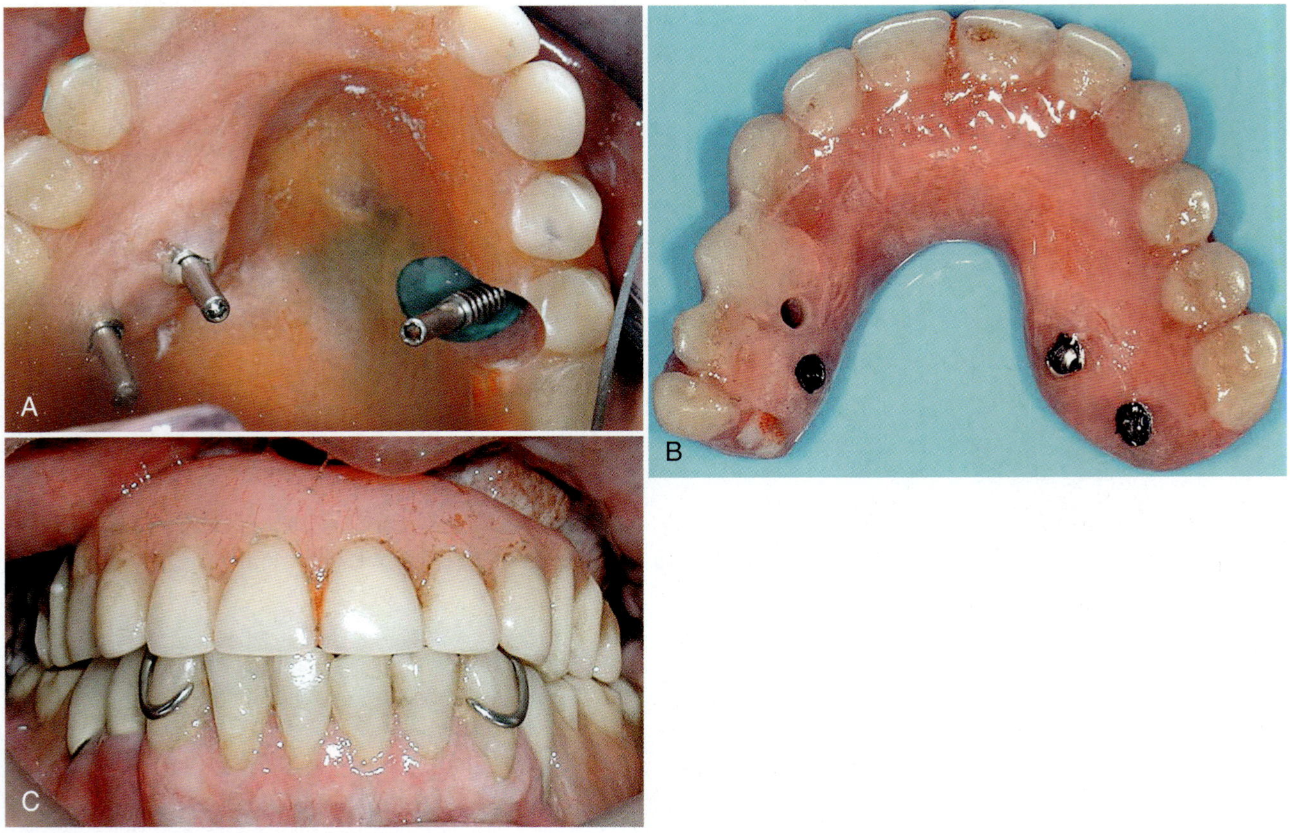

FIGURE 16-8 Placement of multiunit abutments and conversion of the full denture into a provisional fixed prosthesis.

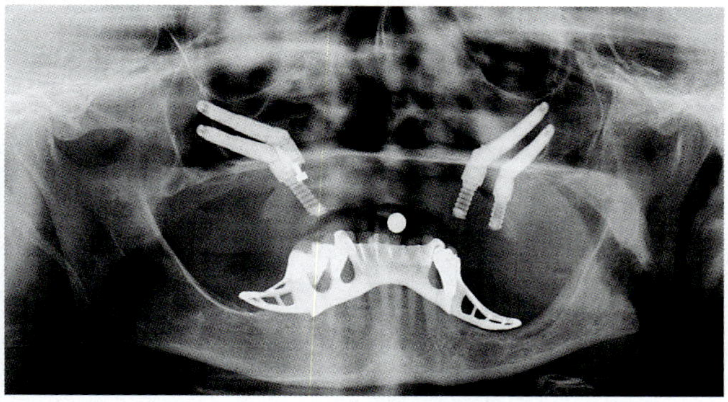

FIGURE 16-9 Radiograph taken immediately after stage II surgery.

The soft tissues are allowed to heal for a period of 6 to 8 weeks prior to initiation of the fabrication steps for the final profile prosthesis (Figures 16-10 to 16-12).

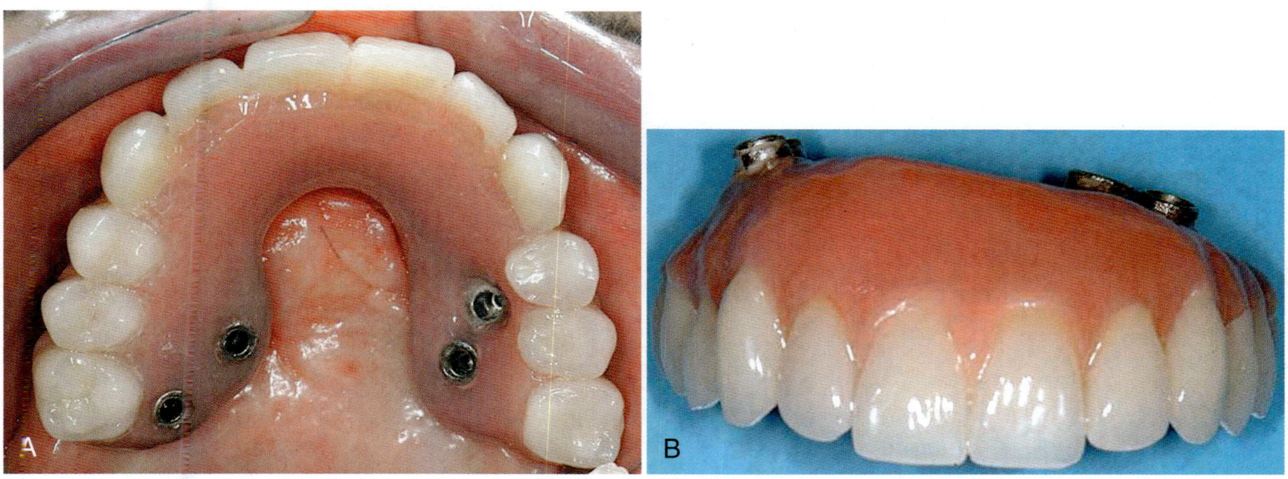

FIGURE 16-10 Completed final fixed maxillary implant-supported profile prosthesis.

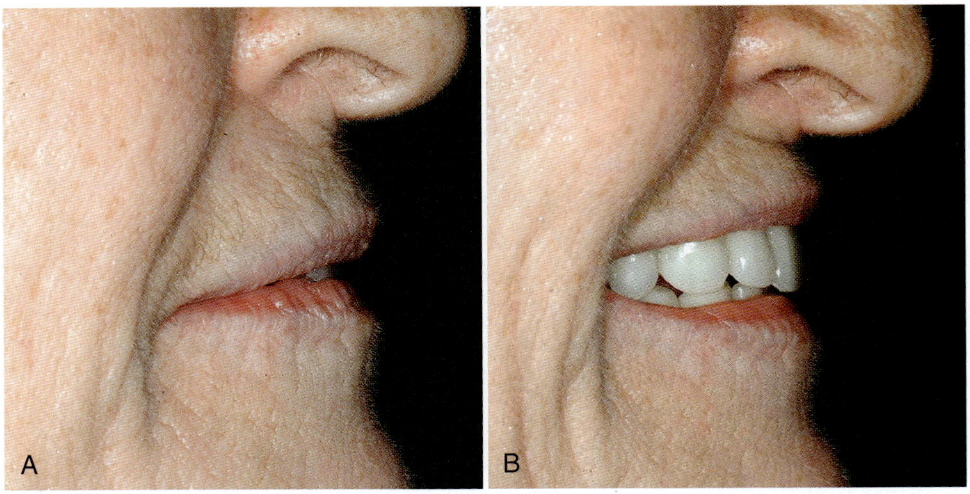

FIGURE 16-11 Aesthetically acceptable profile in repose and in animation with the fixed profile prosthesis.

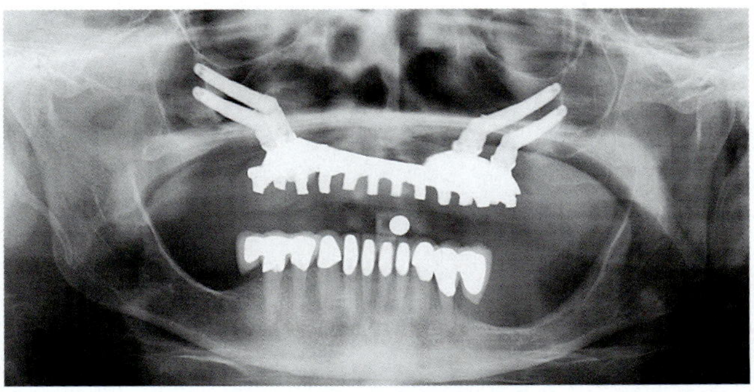

FIGURE 16-12 Panoramic radiograph taken 5 years after surgery demonstrating complete seating of all components. (*Courtesy Lambert Stumpel, Restorative Dentist.*)

FAILED MAXILLARY OVERDENTURE

A 57-year-old patient presented with a 14-year-old maxillary overdenture. The overdenture bar was mobile, but the patient did not complain of any painful symptoms. During clinical examination, the overdenture bar was removed easily without anesthesia and with digital pressure only, as were the four implants (Figures 16-13 to 16-15).

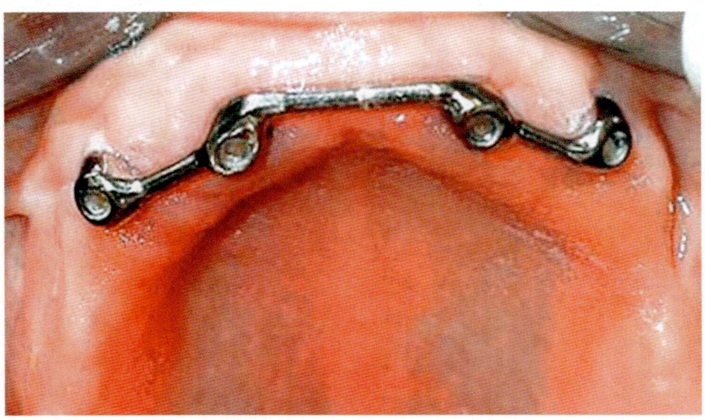

FIGURE 16-13 Maxillary overdenture bar stabilized by four implants in zone I.

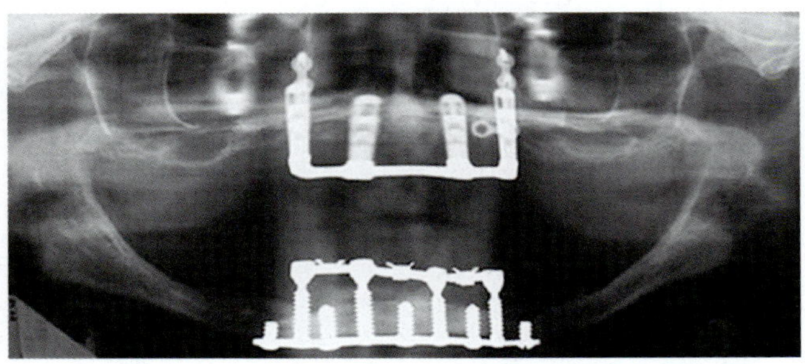

FIGURE 16-14 Panoramic radiograph demonstrates a transmandibular implant system in the mandible and four premaxillary implants in the maxilla.

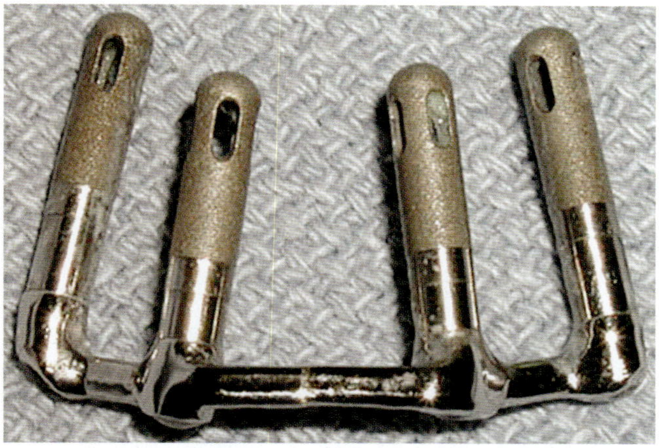

FIGURE 16-15 All four implants attached to the overdenture bar were easily removed by a coronal pull on the bar.

The residual soft tissue defect and the underlying bony defect were clinically consistent with lack of maxillary alveolar bone in zones I, II, and III. The treatment of this patient with a fixed, implant-supported prosthesis included the quad zygoma treatment method. The four zygoma implants were placed using the two-stage protocol (Figures 16-16 and 16-17).

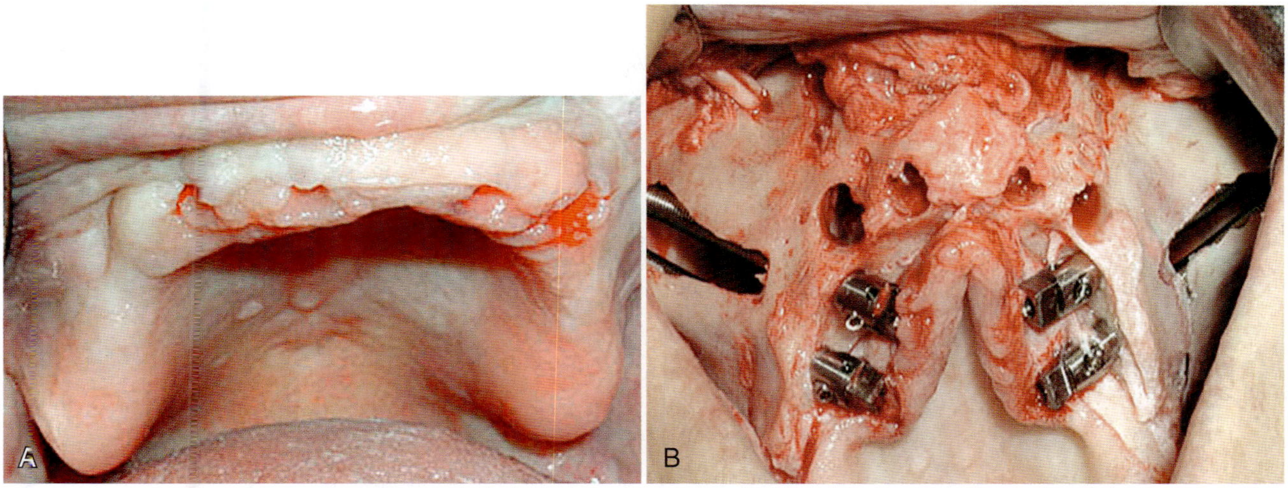

FIGURE 16-16 The residual defects are consistent with a lack of all three zones of the maxillary alveolus.

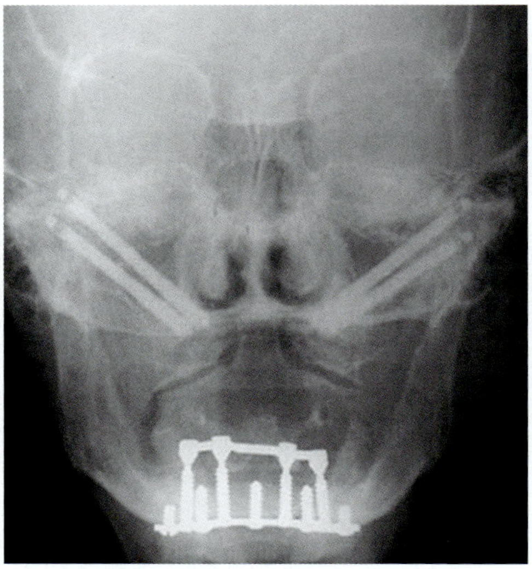

FIGURE 16-17 Immediate postoperative radiograph with the four zygoma implants in place and cover screws attached.

After 6 months of osseointegration, the implants were uncovered and cross-arch linked by conversion of the full maxillary denture into a provisional fixed prosthesis. The soft tissue was given 6 to 8 weeks to heal, and then the final profile prosthesis was fabricated. The final prosthesis demonstrated good lip support, excellent speech, and an aesthetically acceptable facial profile and smile line (Figures 16-18 to 16-20).

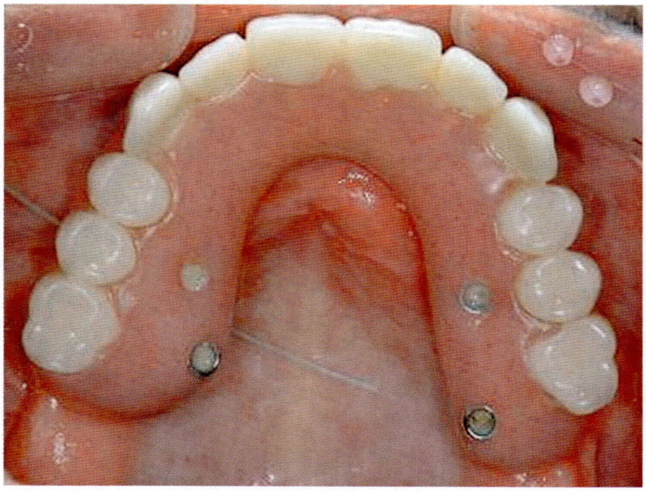

FIGURE 16-18 Final maxillary implant-supported profile prosthesis.

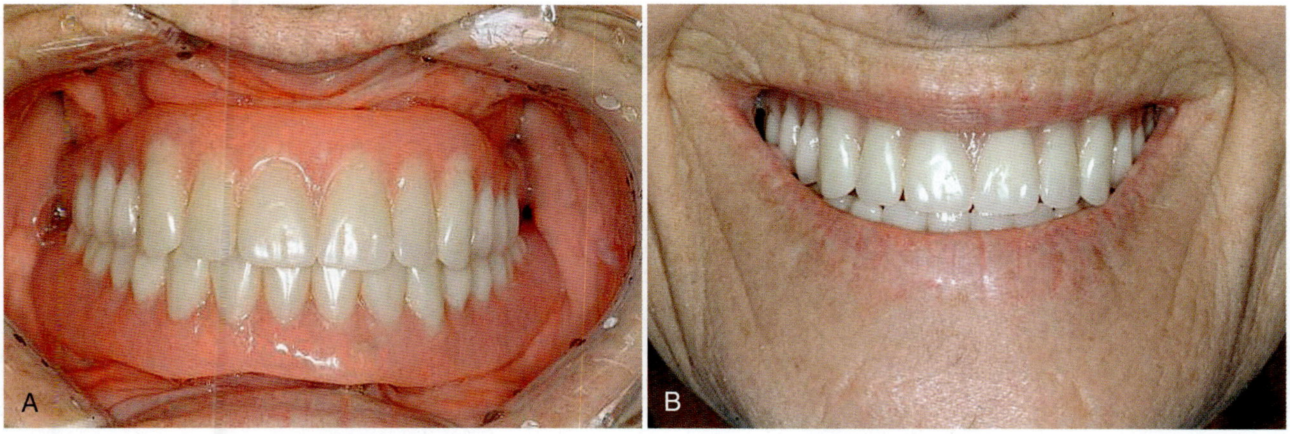

FIGURE 16-19 The final profile prosthesis with stable occlusion and good facial form and smile line.

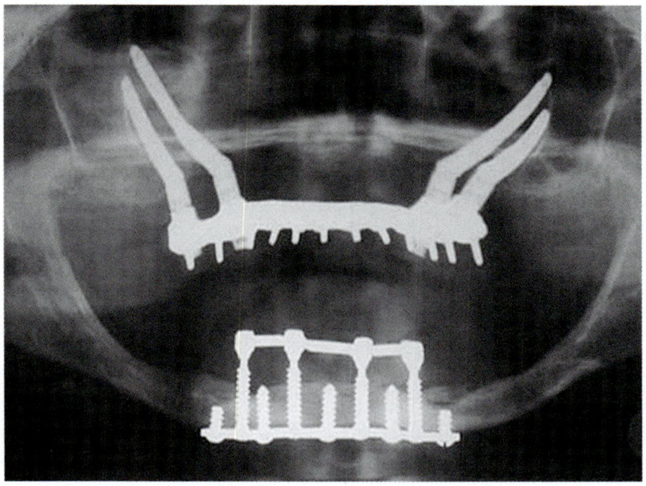

FIGURE 16-20 Radiograph taken 7 years after surgery demonstrating complete seating of all components.

"ACCESSORY" NASAL FLOOR IMPLANT

A 67-year-old patient presented with complete alveolar resorption. Two-dimensional and three-dimensional radiographic studies demonstrated complete maxillary alveolar resorption and therefore a lack of bony volume in zones I, II, and III. Final treatment planning involved placement of four zygomatic implants to support a fixed maxillary profile prosthesis (Figures 16-21 to 16-23).

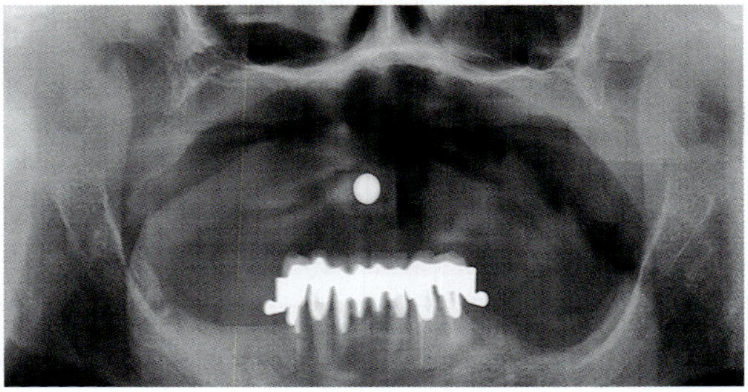

FIGURE 16-21 Preoperative panoramic radiograph demonstrating an absence of zones I, II, and III.

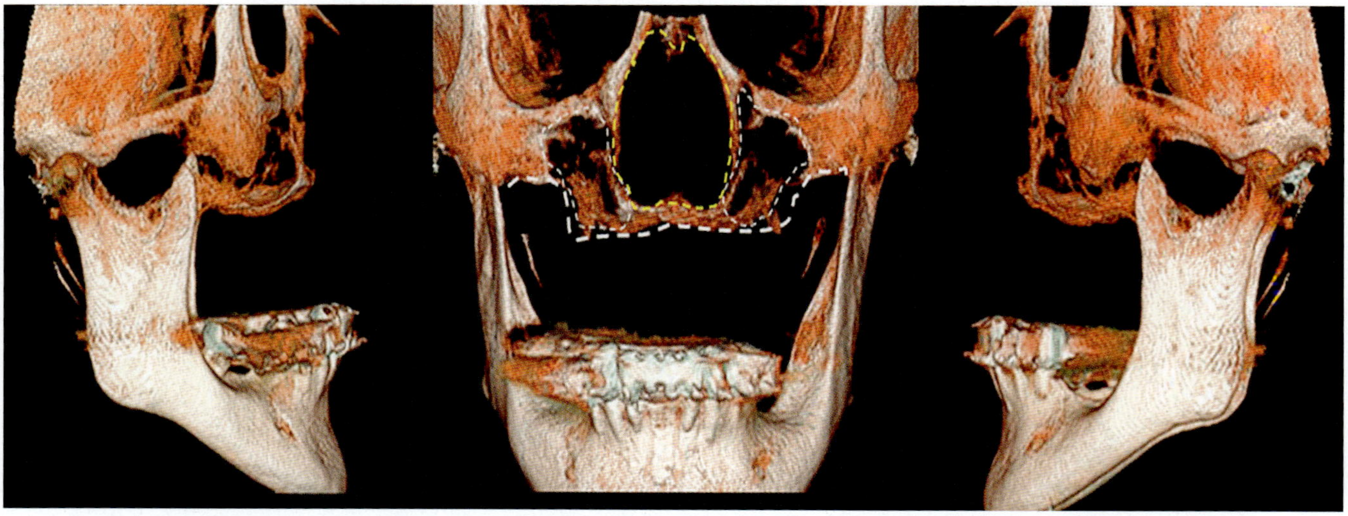

FIGURE 16-22 Three-dimensional radiograph demonstrating the complete absence of the maxillary alveolus and the pseudo class III skeletal relationship between the maxilla and the mandible.

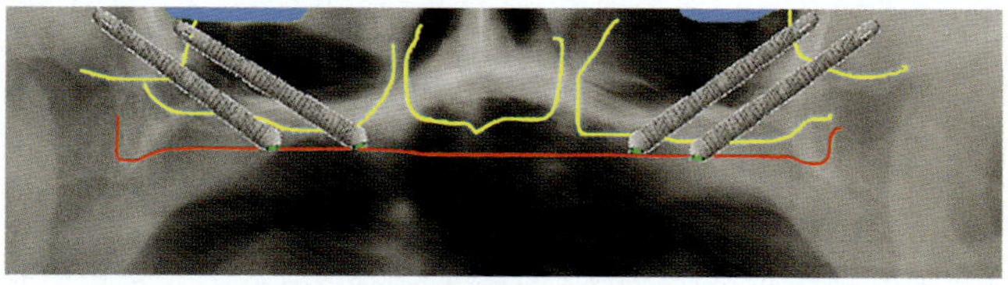

FIGURE 16-23 Four zygomatic implants are placed in a "stacked" manner.

After placement of the zygoma implants, the floor of the right nasal aperture was elevated and bovine-derived bone substitute grafting material was placed between the periosteum of the nasal cavity and the floor of the right nose, very similar to a maxillary sinus lift procedure. A 7-mm NobelSpeedy implant was placed in this position with 20 Ncm of insertion torque. After securing the cover screws, the soft tissues were primarily closed over the five implants (Figures 16-24 to 16-26).

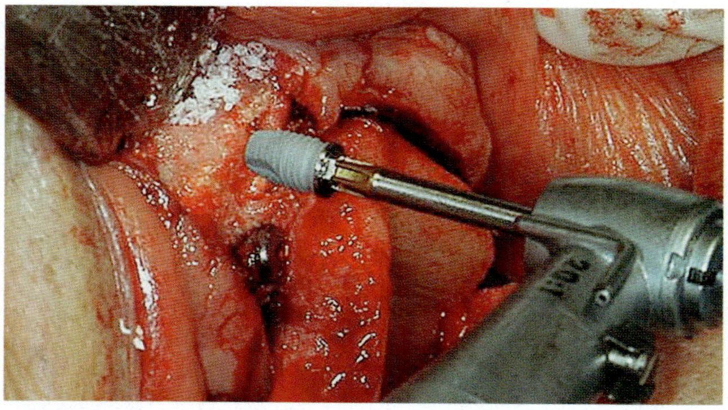

FIGURE 16-24 Grafting of the right nasal floor with placement of a 7-mm implant in position 8.

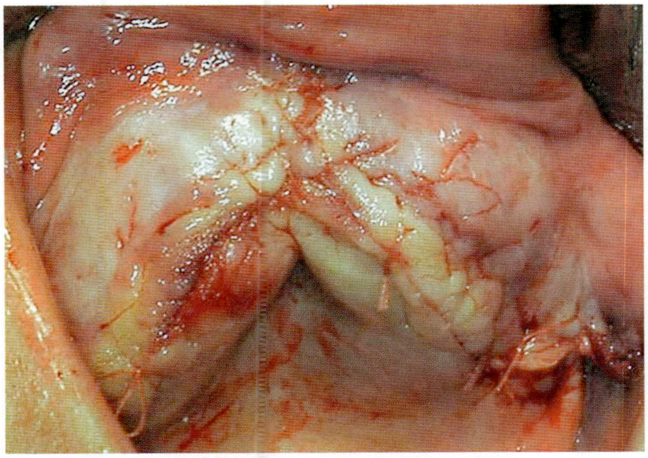

FIGURE 16-25 Primary closure of the soft tissues after connection of the cover screws.

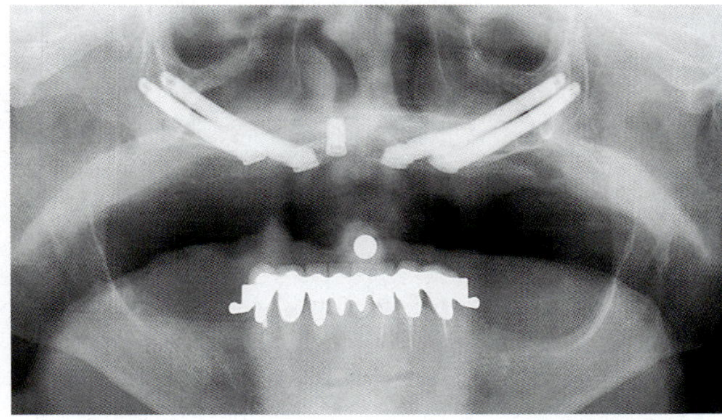

FIGURE 16-26 Postoperative radiograph demonstrating the five implants with cover screws attached.

After the 6-month osseointegration period, the cover screws were removed, osseointegration was confirmed, and multiunit abutments were placed for stage II conversion of the patent's full maxillary denture into a provisional, fixed bridge.

A 17° multiunit abutment was connected to the nasal floor implant, bringing the access the prosthetic screw into a more favorable lingual position. The conversion process began by indexing the implant positions onto the intaglio surface of the existing denture. The provisional prosthesis was screw-retained and in bilateral equal group function. The panoramic radiograph taken immediately after stage II surgery demonstrated full seating of all five implant components. The lip support and phonetics were aesthetically acceptable and functional (Figures 16-27 to 16-31).

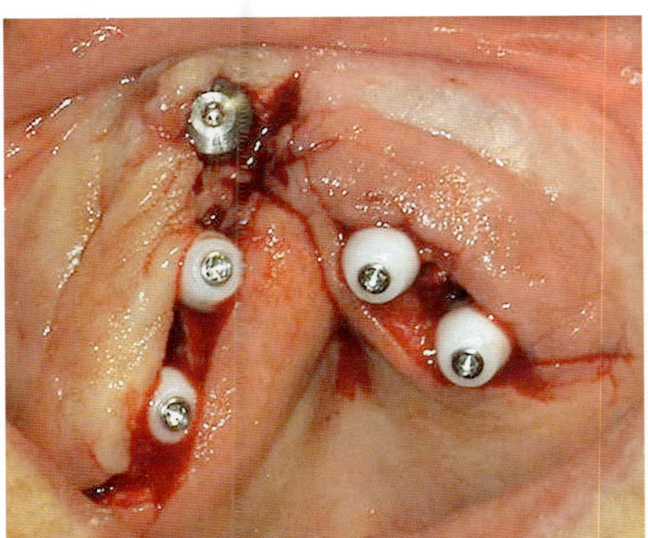

FIGURE 16-27 Placement of multiunit abutments at stage II surgery.

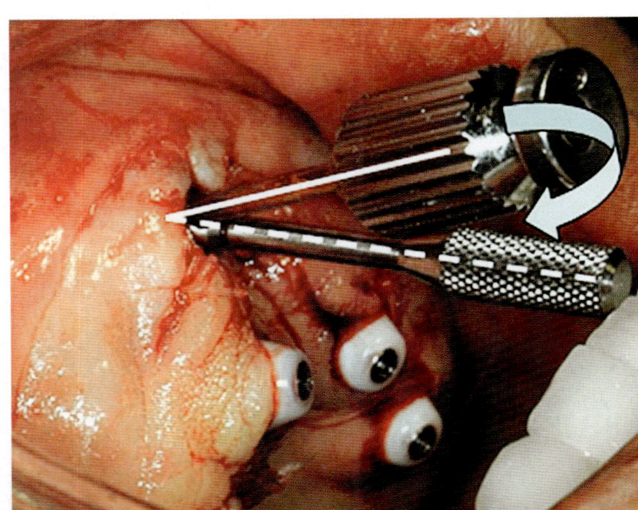

FIGURE 16-28 Multiunit, 17° abutment is connected to the premaxillary implant.

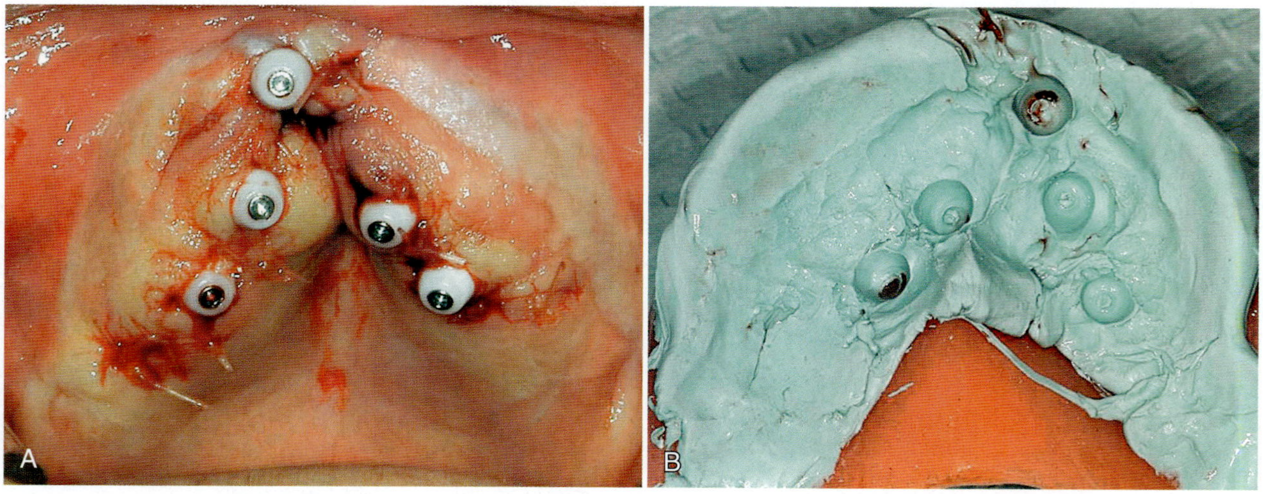

FIGURE 16-29 Indexing of the implant positions onto the intaglio surface of the maxillary denture.

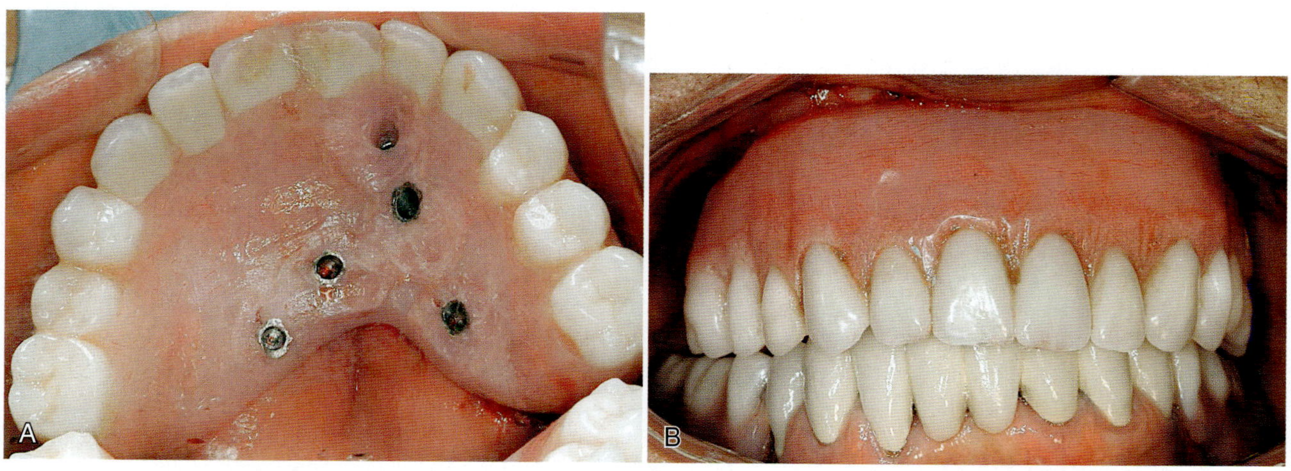

FIGURE 16-30 Completed provisional prosthesis with bilateral group function.

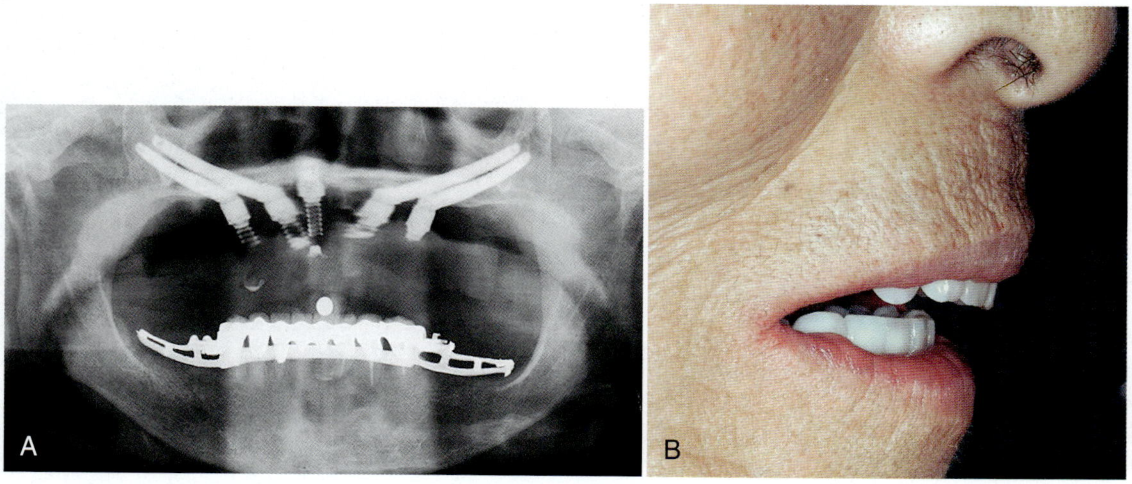

FIGURE 16-31 The completed provisional prosthesis with complete seating of all components and an aesthetically acceptable nasolabial angle.

After 6 to 8 weeks of soft tissue healing, the final prosthetic fabrication with a metal-based final profile prosthesis began. The final screw-retained prosthesis was delivered with good aesthetics and phonetics (Figures 16-32 to 16-37).

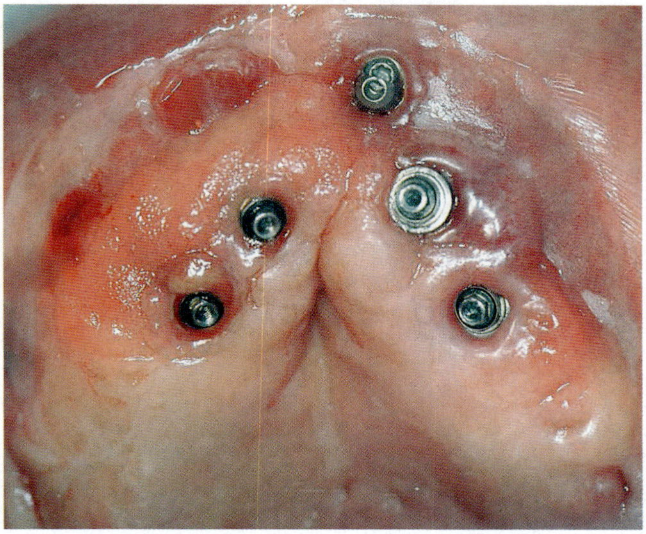

FIGURE 16-32 Presentation of the soft tissues 7 weeks after stage II surgery and provisional loading.

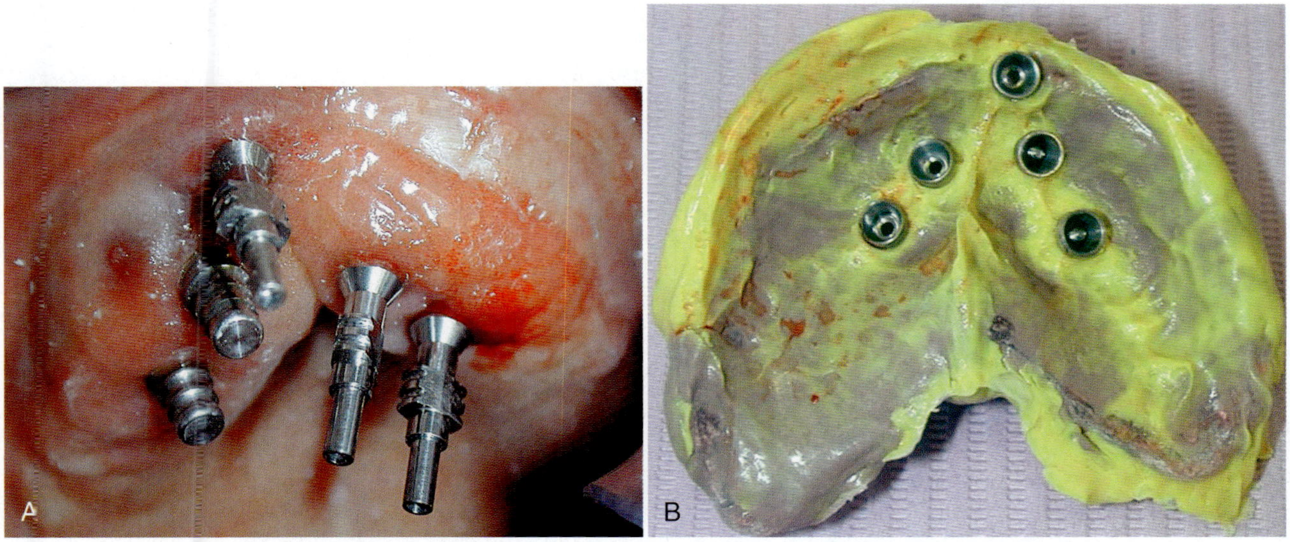

FIGURE 16-33 Open-tray impression technique is used to initiate fabrication of the final profile prosthesis.

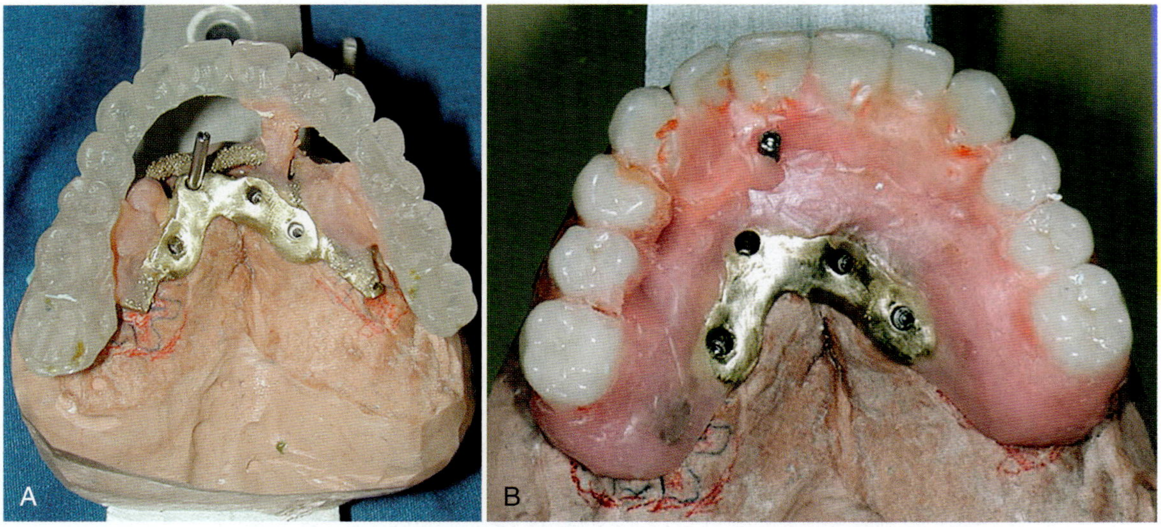

FIGURE 16-34 A, Fabrication of the metal framework and (B) the initial wax try-in of the final profile prosthesis.

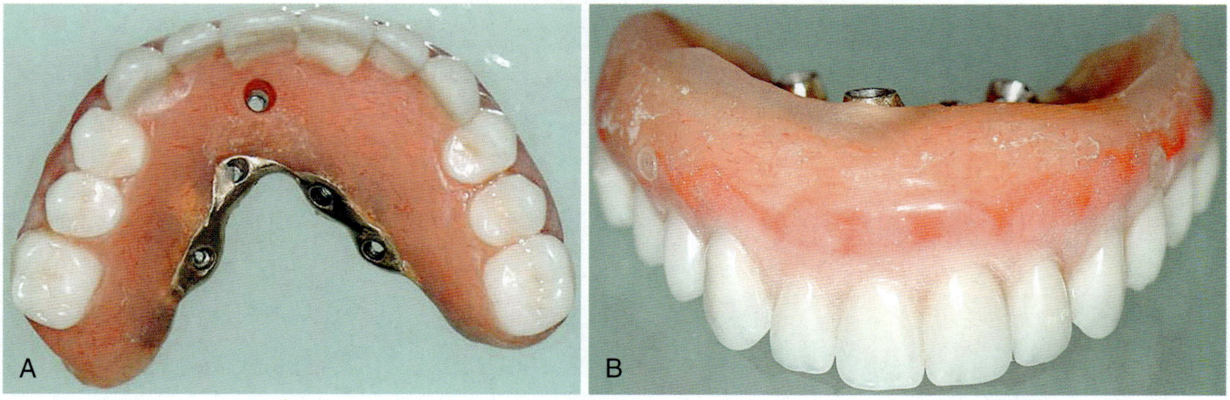

FIGURE 16-35 Completed final profile prosthesis.

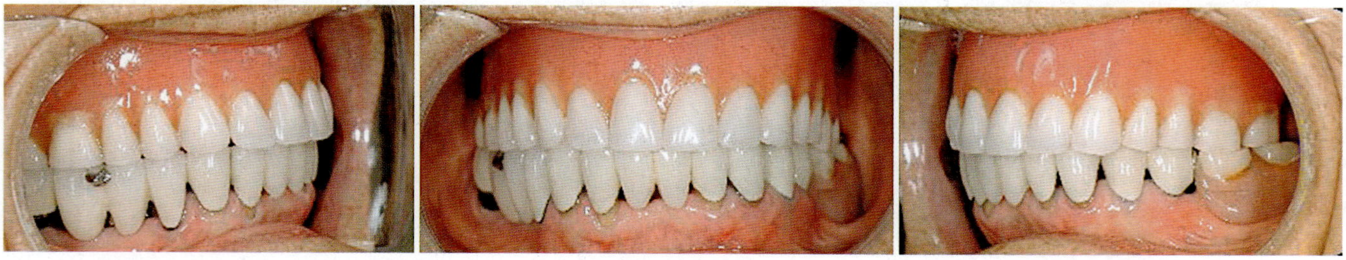

FIGURE 16-36 Completed final provisional prosthesis.

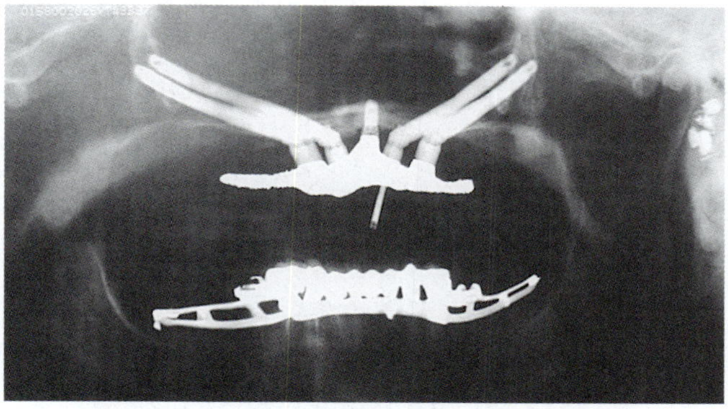

FIGURE 16-37 Panoramic radiograph taken 3 years after surgery.

THROUGH-AND-THROUGH PALATAL DEFECT

A 54-year-old woman presented with a 30-year history of maxillary edentulism. The clinical examination demonstrated a flat maxillary vault and shallow vestibule. A preoperative panoramic radiograph demonstrated complete resorption of the maxillary alveolus. The absence of zones I, II, and III bone indicated that an adaptation of the quad zygoma concept would be beneficial for support of a fixed maxillary profile prosthesis.

After reflection of a full-thickness mucoperiosteal flap, a through-and-through defect of the right alveolar crest was identified. To directly visualize the path of the drills and the implants, the traditional sinus opening into the maxillary sinus was made (Figures 16-38 to 16-40).

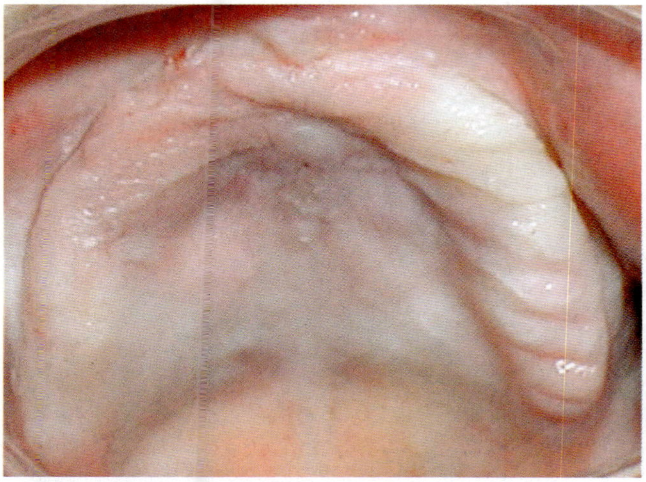

FIGURE 16-38 Intraoral presentation of a flat maxillary vault and shallow vestibule.

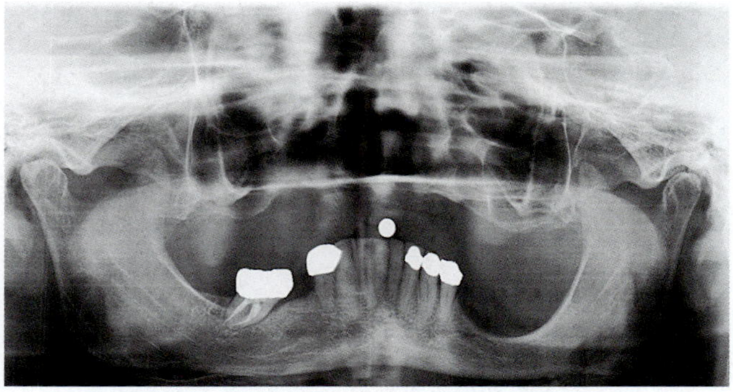

FIGURE 16-39 Preoperative panoramic radiograph demonstrates the absence of zones I, II, and III.

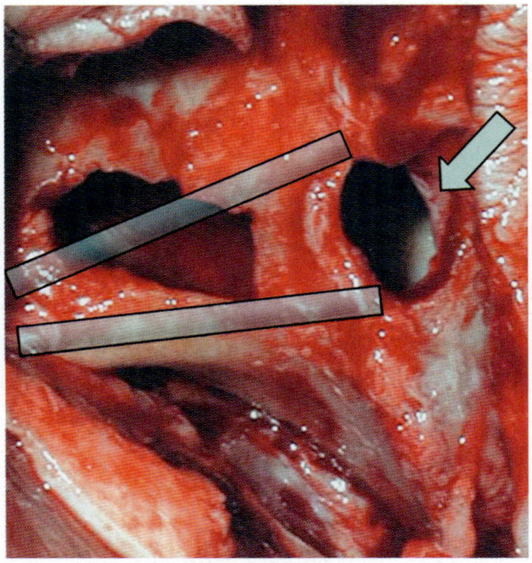

FIGURE 16-40 Existing through-and-through defect from the maxillary crest to the right maxillary sinus.

After placement of the two right maxillary zygoma implants, a resorbable collagen membrane was secured to the implant platforms with a cover screw. Mini-screws with a diameter of 1.5 mm were used to drape the membrane across the defect, stabilizing the superior aspect of the membrane. The left maxillary implants were placed using the quad zygoma protocol.

After the cover screws were connected to the soft tissue closure, the immediate postoperative panoramic radiograph was taken (Figures 16-41 to 16-43).

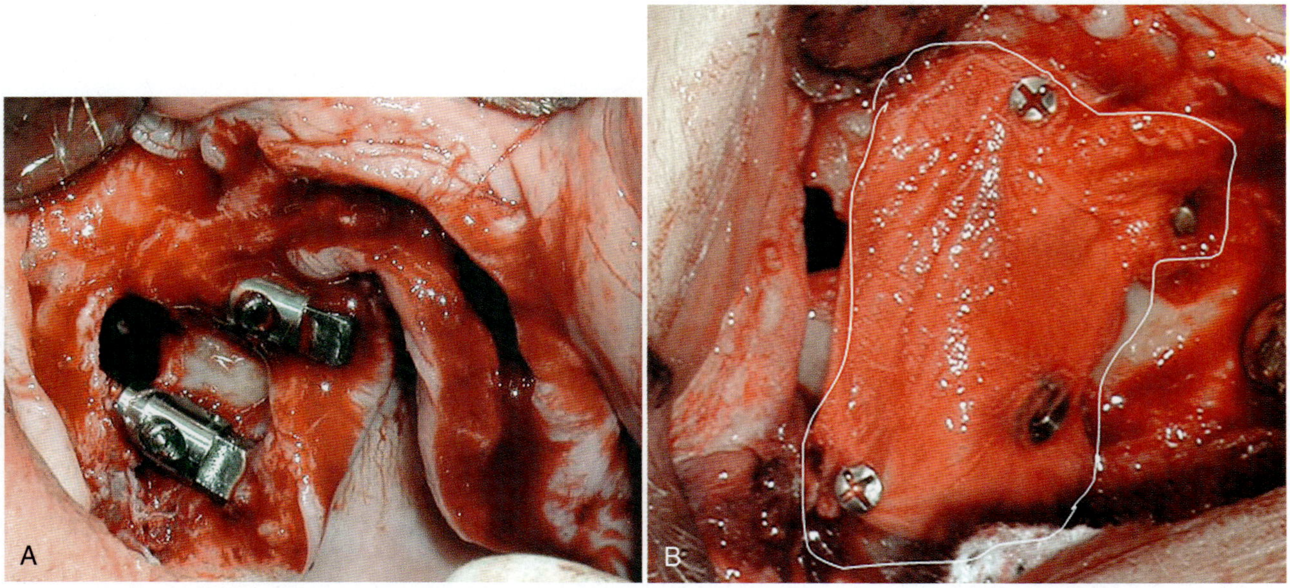

FIGURE 16-41 **A,** Placement of the two zygoma implants in front and behind the existing defect. **B,** Stabilization of the collagen membrane with cover screws and 1.5-mm mini-screws.

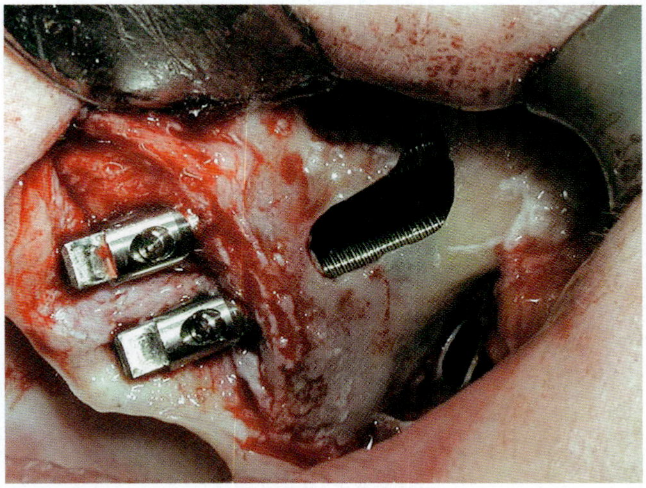

FIGURE 16-42 Placement of the two left zygomatic implants.

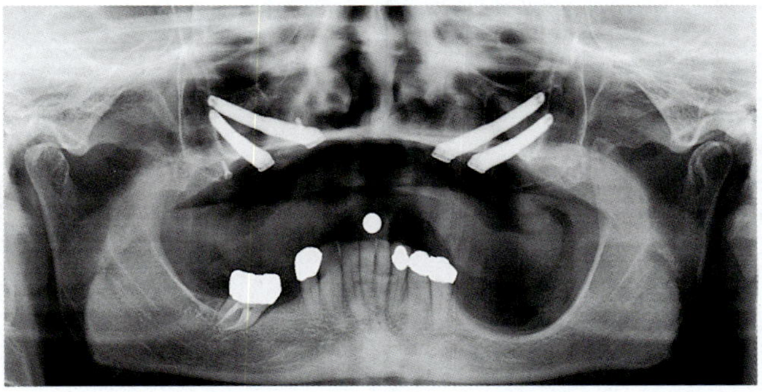

FIGURE 16-43 Immediate postoperative radiograph demonstrates complete seating of the cover screws and the 1.5-mm mini-screws.

After 6 months of osseointegration and conversion of the full maxillary denture into a provisional fixed bridge, an abutment level impression was taken to begin fabrication of the final profile prosthesis (Figures 16-44 to 16-46).

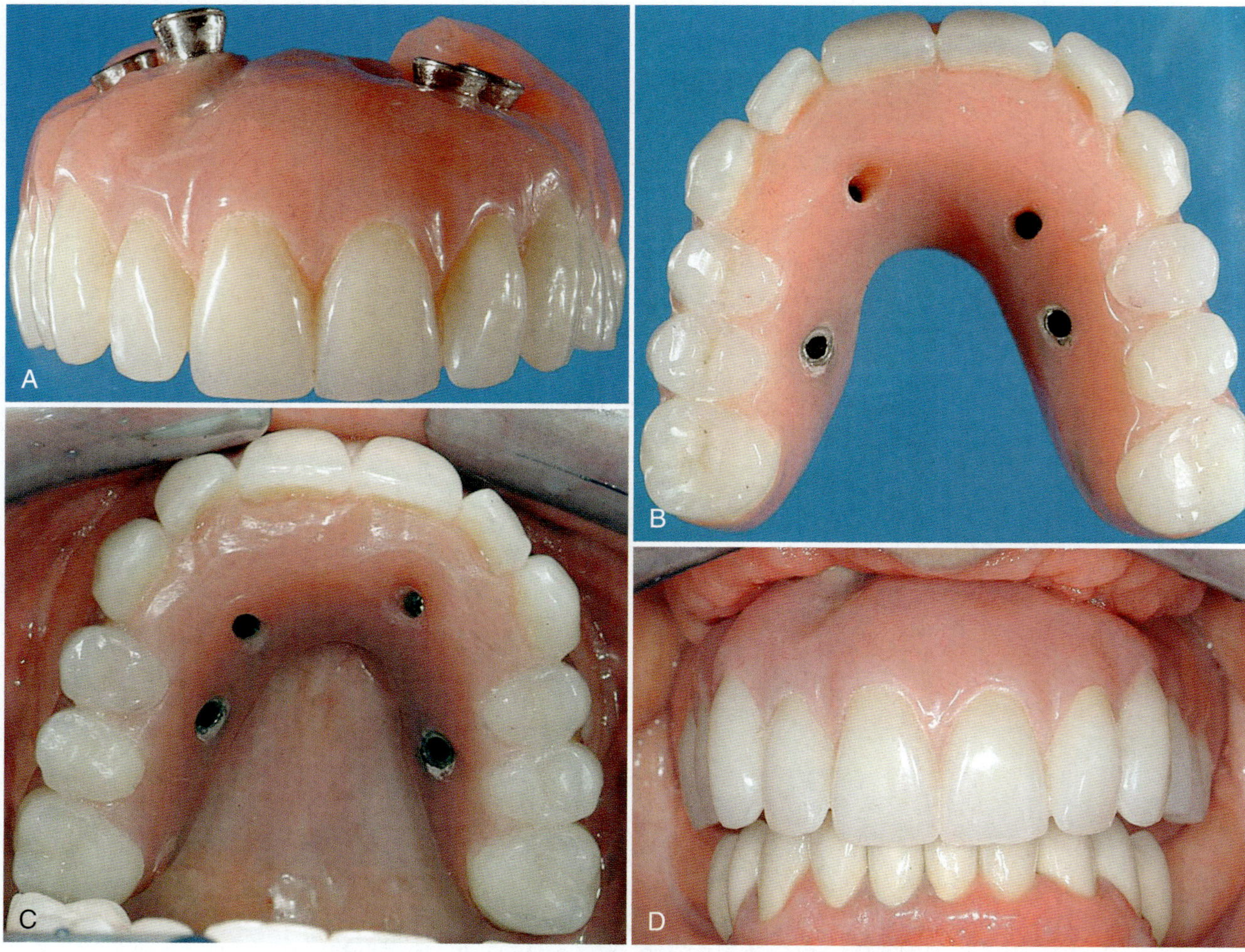

FIGURE 16-44 Final metal-based profile prosthesis.

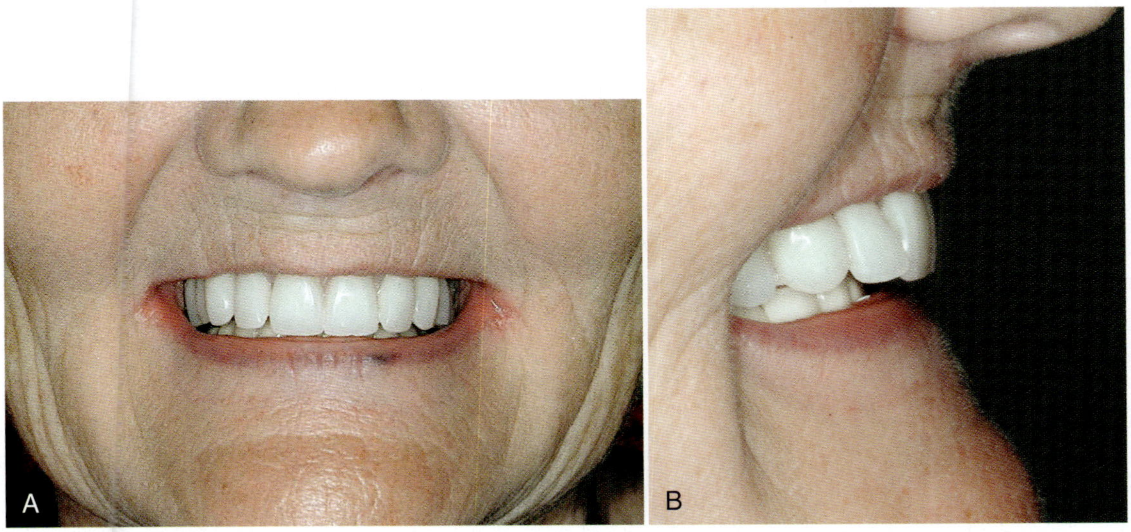

FIGURE 16-45 Aesthetically acceptable final smile line and nasolabial angle.

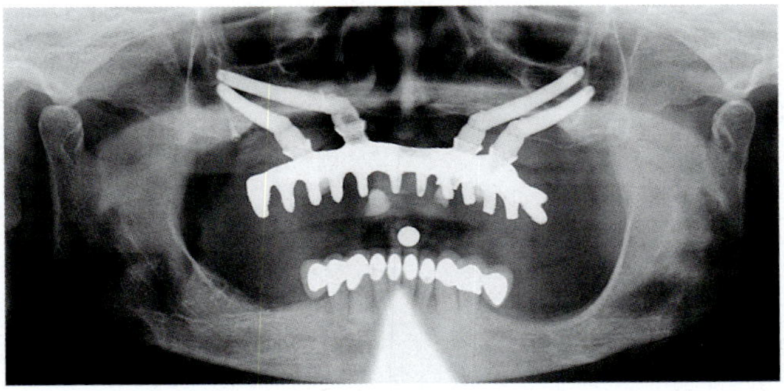

FIGURE 16-46 Panoramic radiograph taken 5 years after surgery demonstrates complete seating of all components. (*Courtesy Dr. Lambert Stumpel, Restorative Dentist.*)

f indicates figure; b, box; t, table.